The Duration and Safety of Osteoporosis Treatment

The Duration and Safety of Osteoporosis Treatment

Anabolic and Antiresorptive Therapy

Stuart L. Silverman • Bo Abrahamsen

Editors

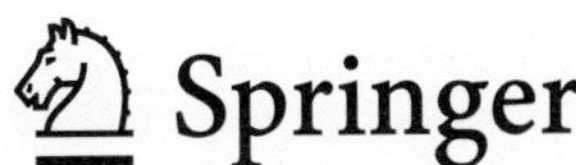

Springer

Editors
Stuart L. Silverman, MD, FACP, FACR
Cedars-Sinai Medical Center
Division of Rheumatology
Department of Medicine
Los Angeles, CA, USA

University of California Los Angeles
David Geffen School of Medicine
Los Angeles, CA, USA

Bo Abrahamsen, MD, PhD
University of Southern Denmark
Odense Patient Data Explorative
  Network
Institute of Clinical Research
Odense, Denmark

Holbæk Hospital
Department of Medicine
Holbæk, Denmark

ISBN 978-3-319-23638-4   ISBN 978-3-319-23639-1   (eBook)
DOI 10.1007/978-3-319-23639-1

Library of Congress Control Number: 2015957990

Springer Cham Heidelberg New York Dordrecht London

Printed on acid-free paper

Springer International Publishing AG Switzerland is part of Springer Science+Business Media (www.springer.com)

Foreword

Advances in the management of osteoporosis in the last two to three decades have exceeded that of most other chronic diseases of aging, yet suboptimal rates of treatment are widely reported. These arise partly from underrecognition of osteoporosis as a disease but also from concerns about the safety of treatment and the related issue of for how long treatment should be given. Rare but serious side effects such as atypical femoral fractures and osteonecrosis of the jaw have received much attention in the media and have made many patients and their doctors reluctant to embark on or continue therapy. In addition, the evidence base on which to develop advice about duration of therapy is incomplete. Despite these difficulties, however, there is consensus in the field that when appropriately targeted, the benefits of treatment outweigh the risks. In addition, there is increasing agreement that after 3–5 years treatment with the most commonly used intervention, bisphosphonate therapy, it may be possible to stop treatment for a limited period of time in some people, although in those at high risk of fracture, long-term continuous therapy is often required.

In their book "The Safety and Duration of Osteoporosis Treatment," Stuart Silverman and Bo Abrahamsen address these difficult and critical issues against a background of the epidemiology and pathophysiology of osteoporosis, approaches to the assessment of fracture risk, and the efficacy and safety of pharmacological interventions to reduce fracture risk. Detailed coverage is given to the epidemiology, diagnosis, clinical presentation, and management of atypical femoral fractures and osteonecrosis of the jaw. The controversial topic of treatment failure is discussed, and approaches to improving adherence to therapy are considered. Potential nonskeletal benefits of treatments and effects of therapy on fracture healing are included and regulatory perspectives are covered. The closing chapter of the book presents an integrated approach to the long-term management of osteoporosis in the light of what is known about efficacy and safety of existing interventions.

This book, edited and written by leading experts in the field, provides a welcome update on some of the most topical but challenging issues in the management of osteoporosis. While many gaps in knowledge remain, there have also been advances that allow more accurate assessment of the balance of risk and benefit in individual patients. For healthcare professionals involved in the care of osteoporosis, this book offers a balanced perspective that will aid decision making about when to start treatment, how long to continue it, and how to ensure that patients understand the safety issues involved. It also provides a glimpse of the future, with treatment individualized according to the specific disease characteristics and preferences of the patient to achieve optimal efficacy, safety, and adherence.

Cambridge Biomedical Campus   Juliet Compston, MBBS, MD,
Addenbrooke's Hospital   FRCP, FRCPath, FMedSci
Cambridge, UK

Preface

In the past three decades, clinicians treating osteoporosis have seen the disease change from being a debilitating chronic disease with few treatment options and little chance of real improvement. However, with the introduction of the bisphosphonates and later the SERMs, parathyroid hormone-based anabolics, and more recently the biologicals, our viewpoint has changed enormously. Unlike other chronic diseases such as hypertension or asthma where we try to stabilize the condition, in osteoporosis we have the promise of improving skeletal health, increasing bone mineral density, and reducing risk of fracture. However, how much do we really know about the long-term management of osteoporosis in the current era of potent antiresorptive and anabolic medications? The mainstay of osteoporosis treatment remains the affordable bisphosphonates. However, from the initial introduction of bisphosphonates, the first antiresorptive drugs, there was the nagging doubt that they were almost too good to be true. Surely we will have developed bone remodeling for a reason. For how long can we safely put a dampener on bone resorption without some cost in the form of accumulation of old bone tissue of potentially poorer strength and increased brittleness?

Patients, clinicians, specialty societies, and health authorities are legitimately concerned about side effects of osteoporosis medications, both short and long term. Though still rare, atypical femur fractures and osteonecrosis of the jaw are legitimate concerns and the time has certainly come to collect the scientific information on the safety and duration of osteoporosis therapies that is currently available and to digest and interpret it.

As Editors we asked top scientists and clinicians in the bone field to review and update the reader on the pathophysiology of osteoporosis and the principles behind our present and future drugs for osteoporosis, both antiresorptive and anabolic. This book contains a comprehensive compendium of short- and long-term adverse events that have been suspected or demonstrated for osteoporosis drugs. We asked for chapters covering prediction of fracture risk, monitoring of response to treatment, and identification of treatment failure. The practical management of drug holidays and tools for improving adherence are comprehensively dealt with in the subsequent chapters.

We hope this book will give clinicians a practical compendium of evidence that will allow them to continue to make the best informed decisions together with their patients about important decisions including when to modify, stop, or reinitiate osteoporosis treatment. The book is also intended to facilitate the work of health planners and regulatory authorities and help researchers and funding bodies set the future research agenda for management of osteoporosis.

Los Angeles, CA, USA   Stuart L. Silverman, MD, FACP, FACR
Odense, Denmark   Bo Abrahamsen, MD, PhD

Acknowledgment

The coeditors (Stuart L. Silverman and Bo Abrahamsen) both wish to acknowledge the importance of mentorship by colleagues during their journey in Bone disease.

Stuart L. Silverman would like to acknowledge the late Louis Avioli who encouraged him to study clinical bone disease and the late Moise Azria with whom he spent years together traveling and debating the safety of osteoporosis therapies.

Bo Abrahamsen would like to acknowledge his mentor, the late Sandy Marks, Jr., from UMASS Medical Centre, Erik Eriksen his PhD supervisor, and Richard Eastell who introduced him to atypical femur fractures and to how to set up an integrated osteoporosis service.

Contents

Contributors

Bo Abrahamsen, MD, PhD Institute of Clinical Research, OPEN, University of Southern Denmark, Odense, Denmark

Arnav Agarwal, BHSc Faculty of Medicine, University of Toronto, Toronto, ON, Canada

Yelena Bogdan, MD Department of Orthopaedic Surgery, Boston University Medical Center, Boston, MA, USA

Adele L. Boskey, PhD Mineralized Tissue Research, Musculoskeletal Integrity Program, Hospital for Special Surgery, New York, NY, USA

Mary L. Bouxsein, PhD Department of Orthopedic Surgery, Beth Israel Deaconess Medical Center, Boston, MA, USA

Karine Briot, MD, PhD Service de Rhumatologie, Hôpital Cochin, Paris, France
INSERM U1153, Paris-Descartes University, Paris, France

Susan V. Bukata, MD Department of Orthopaedics, UCLA, Santa Monica, CA, USA

Abigail L. Campbell, MD, MSc, BSE Orthopaedic Surgery, NYU Hospital for Joint Diseases, New York, NY, USA

Andrew D. Chantry, MD, PhD Department of Oncology and Human Metabolism, The Mellanby Centre for Bone Research, The University of Sheffield Medical School, Sheffield, UK

Juliet Compston, MBBS, MD, FRCP, FRCPath, FMedSci Bone Medicine, Cambridge Biomedical Campus, Addenbrooke's Hospital, Cambridge, UK

Cyrus Cooper, OBE, FMedSci MRC Lifecourse Epidemiology Unit, Southampton General Hospital, University of Southampton, Southampton, UK

Elisa Torres del Pliego, MD Department of Internal Medicine, Hospital del Mar-IMIM, Autonomous University of Barcelona and RETICEF, Instituto Carlos III, Barcelona, Spain

Adolfo Díez-Perez, MD, PhD Department of Internal Medicine, Hospital del Mar-IMIM, Autonomous University of Barcelona and RETICEF, Instituto Carlos III, Barcelona, Spain

Frank H. Ebetino, PhD Chemistry Department, University of Rochester, Rochester, NY, USA

Thomas A. Einhorn, MD Department of Orthopaedic Surgery, Boston University Medical Center, Boston, MA, USA

Erik Fink Eriksen, MD, DMSc Department of Endocrinology, Morbid Obesity and Preventive Medicine, Oslo University Hospital, Oslo, Norway

Libi Z. Galmer, DO Metabolic Bone Diseases Service, Orthopaedics, Hospital for Special Surgery, New York, NY, USA

Joseph C. Giaconi, MD Musculoskeletal Radiology, S. Mark Taper Foundation Imaging Center, Cedars Sinai Medical Center, Los Angeles, CA, USA

Deborah T. Gold, PhD Duke University Medical Center, Durham, NC, USA

Nicholas C. Harvey, MA, MB, BChir, PhD, FRCP MRC Lifecourse Epidemiology Unit, Southampton General Hospital, University of Southampton, Southampton, UK

Jonathan E. Jo, BS Orthopaedic Surgery, Weill Cornell Medical College, New York, NY, USA

Allan C. Jones, DDS, MS A Professional Corporation, Skypark One Professional Building, Torrance, CA, USA

Sarah Karampatos, BASc, MSc(c) Department of Medicine, McMaster University, Hamilton, ON, Canada

Geriatric Education and Research in the Aging Sciences (GERAS) Centre, Hamilton, ON, Canada

Department of Rehabilitation Sciences, McMaster University, Hamilton, ON, Canada

Eli Kupperman, MD Department of Orthopaedics, UCLA, Santa Monica, CA, USA

Joseph M. Lane, MD Metabolic Bone Disease Service, Orthopaedics, Hospital for Special Surgery, New York, NY, USA

William D. Leslie, MD, MSc Department of Medicine, St. Boniface General Hospital, Winnipeg, MB, Canada

Department of Medicine and Radiology, University of Manitoba, Winnipeg, MB, Canada

Michelle A. Lawson, PhD Department of Oncology and Human Metabolism, The Mellanby Centre for Bone Research, The University of Sheffield Medical School, Sheffield, UK

E. Michael Lewiecki, MD New Mexico Clinical Research and Osteoporosis Center, Albuquerque, NM, USA

Department of Medicine, University of New Mexico School of Medicine, Albuquerque, NM, USA

Lisa M. Lix, PhD Department of Community Health Sciences, University of Manitoba, Winnipeg, MB, Canada

Michael R. McClung, MD Oregon Osteoporosis Center, Portland, OR, USA

Rebecca J. Moon, BSc, BM, MRCPCH MRC Lifecourse Epidemiology Unit, Southampton General Hospital, University of Southampton, Southampton, UK

Suzanne N. Morin, MD, MSc Department of Medicine, McGill University Health Center, Montreal, QC, Canada

Jeri W. Nieves, PhD Departments of Epidemiology and Clinical Research Center, Helen Hayes Hospital and Columbia University, West Haverstraw, NY, USA

Alexandra Papaioannou, BScN, MD, MSc, FRCP(C), FACP Department of Medicine, McMaster University, Hamilton, ON, Canada

Geriatric Education and Research in the Aging Sciences (GERAS) Centre, Hamilton, ON, Canada

Department of Biostatistics and Epidemiology, McMaster University, Hamilton, ON, Canada

Socrates E. Papapoulos, MD, PhD Center of Bone Quality, Leiden University Medical Center, Leiden, The Netherlands

Michael Pazianas, MD Nuffield Department of Orthopaedics, Rheumatology and Musculoskeletal Sciences, The Botnar Research Centre and Oxford University Institute of Musculoskeletal Sciences, Oxford, UK

Daniel Prieto-Alhambra, MD, MSc, PhD Botnar Research Centre, Nuffield Department of Orthopaedics, Rheumatology and Musculoskeletal Sciences (NDORMS), University of Oxford, Nuffield Orthopaedics Center, Oxford, UK

Christian Roux, MD, PhD Service de Rhumatologie, Hôpital Cochin, Paris, France

INSERM U1153, Paris-Descartes University, Paris, France

R. Graham G. Russell, MD, PhD, FRS Nuffield Department of Orthopaedics, Rheumatology and Musculoskeletal Sciences, The Botnar Research Centre and Oxford University Institute of Musculoskeletal Sciences, Oxford, UK

Department of Oncology and Human Metabolism, The Mellanby Centre for Bone Research, The University of Sheffield Medical School, Sheffield, UK

Morten Schiødt, DDS, Dr.Odont Department of Oral and Maxillofacial Surgery, Copenhagen University Hospital (Rigshospitalet), Copenhagen, Denmark

Stuart L. Silverman, MD, FACP, FACR Division of Rheumatology, Cedars-Sinai Medical Center, UCLA School of Medicine and the OMC Clinical Research Center, Beverly Hills, CA, USA

Parish P. Sedghizadeh, DDS, MS Ostrow School of Dentistry, Center for Biofilms, University of Southern California, Los Angeles, CA, USA

Joy N. Tsai, MD Endocrine Unit, Massachusetts General Hospital, Boston, MA, USA

Maria K. Tsoumpra, MRes, DPhil Nuffield Department of Orthopaedics, Rheumatology and Musculoskeletal Sciences, The Botnar Research Centre and Oxford University Institute of Musculoskeletal Sciences, Oxford, UK

Marjolein C.H. van der Meulen, PhD Biomedical Engineering and Mechanical & Aerospace Engineering, Cornell University, Ithaca, NY, USA

Peter Vestergaard, MD, PhD, Dr Med Sc Department of Endocrinology, Aalborg University, Aalborg, Denmark

C. Travis Watterson, MD Musculoskeletal Radiology, S. Mark Taper Foundation Imaging Center, Cedars Sinai Medical Center, Los Angeles, CA, USA

David S. Wellman, MD Orthopaedic Surgery, Hospital for Special Surgery, New York Presbyterian Hospital, New York, NY, USA

Orthopaedic Surgery, Weill Cornell Medical College, New York, NY, USA

Osteoporosis: Pathophysiology and Epidemiology

1

Rebecca J. Moon, Cyrus Cooper, and Nicholas C. Harvey

Summary

- Osteoporosis is a common skeletal disorder resulting in increased bone fragility.
- The operational definition of osteoporosis is based on a measurement of bone mineral density (BMD), but changes in bone geometry and bone microarchitecture also contribute to fracture risk.
- Recent work has indicated an important role for bone micro- and nanostructure, with crack propagation observable through shearing of collagen fibrils and disruption of non-collagenous proteins.
- Osteoporotic fracture contributes significantly to functional decline, increased morbidity and mortality, and increased healthcare spending.
- The epidemiology of osteoporotic fractures reflects factors contributing to both reduced bone strength and increased propensity to falls. As such, the risk of fragility fracture increases with age and is greater in women than men. Ethnicity, body habitus, genetic factors, and geographic location also influence an individual's risk.
- Over recent years, in much of the developed world, there has been a plateau or even decrease in age- and sex-specific hip fracture rates; in contrast, many developing nations are experiencing inexorable rises in such adjusted incidence rates. Across the board, populations are aging, increasing the burden of those at risk of fragility fracture.

Definition

Osteoporosis is a skeletal disorder characterized by low bone mass and microarchitectural deterioration of bone tissue, resulting in increased bone fragility [1]. The World Health Organization (WHO) suggests that the operational definition of osteoporosis should be a reduction in bone mineral density (BMD) to more than 2.5 standard deviations below the young (20–29 years) female adult mean (T-score <-2.5) measured at the femoral neck by dual-energy X-ray absorptiometry (DXA). A T-score between -1 and -2.5 SDS is classified as osteopenia. The major clinical consequence of osteoporosis is fracture. However, it is important

R.J. Moon, BSc, BM, MRCPCH
C. Cooper, OBE, FMedSci
N.C. Harvey, MA, MB, BChir, PhD, FRCP (✉)
MRC Lifecourse Epidemiology Unit, Southampton General Hospital, University of Southampton, Southampton SO16 6YD, UK
e-mail: nch@mrc.soton.ac.uk

to recognize that BMD is only one of many factors which determine susceptibility to fracture and many individuals who do sustain a fracture in later life will have a BMD within the osteopenic or normal range [2]. Therefore, as discussed in detail in Chap. 4, BMD is increasingly regarded as a risk factor for fracture and together with other clinical determinants is used in the generation of individualized absolute fracture probabilities, for example, using the online FRAX® calculator.

Pathophysiology of Osteoporotic Fractures

Anatomy of Bone from Organ to Molecule

A fracture will occur when the applied force exceeds bone strength. Theoretically, in order to have maximum strength, a bone needs to be stiff to resist deformation, yet flexible enough to absorb any excess energy transmitted through the bone. This is achieved through the composite nature of bone, comprising both mineral and collagen type I extracellular matrix (osteoid). Thus, individual collagen molecules (a triple-helical structure) weave together to form fibrils which form the basis of cortical osteons and trabecular structures. Collagen fibrils are held together by non-collagenous proteins, acting to prevent shearing of fibrils. The collagen foundation of bone structure allows a degree of flexibility in response to torsion; calcium hydroxyapatite crystals, which deposit on the collagen structure, add strength, particularly to compression forces. Figure 1.1 shows this structure as viewed through an electron microscope and demonstrates the effect of microdamage at the level of collagen fibers [3].

In cortical bone, fibers are arranged longitudinally, and new bone is formed around Haversian canals, which contain the nutrient blood supply and nerve; concentric layers of bone are laid down, yielding cylinders of bone, known as osteons, which are consolidated together by cement lines. These canals are observed in histomorphometric examinations and on images

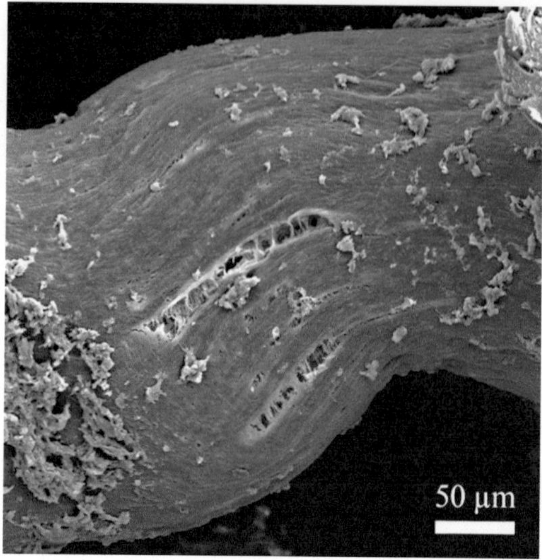

Fig. 1.1 Electron micrograph of damaged trabecula. A microcrack is present. Fibrillar structures can be observed spanning the crack as fibrils have been pulled apart from each other. From Thurner P., et al. Engineering Fracture Mechanics 2007 [3]. Reprinted with permission from Elsevier

obtained from microCT as cortical pores. Their size and number tend to increase with age [4]. The basic structure of trabecular bone, at younger ages, resembles a robust scaffolding, with rods and plates of bone interconnected, around a central repository of marrow tissue. With age, trabeculae tend to thin; a reduction in number and size appears to differ by sex [4]. The combination of the honeycomb trabecular scaffolding with the surrounding dense cortical envelope allows resistance to bending forces, conferred by the cortical bone, and also to compressive forces, contributed by the trabecular bone, while maintaining lightness and so facilitating locomotion.

Natural History of Bone Structure across the Lifecourse

Bone Mass

Bone mineral serves to strengthen the extracellular matrix, increasing bone stiffness and resistance to compression. BMD is measured as the grams of mineral per unit area or volume. Bone mass, a composite of bone mineral content (BMC) and bone size, increases throughout childhood and adolescence to peak in young adulthood (around the end of the second/start of the third decade of life), before a subsequent decline in later life due to bone loss. This bone loss accelerates further after the female menopause. Risk of osteoporosis is therefore determined by both the peak bone mass (PBM) achieved and the rate of bone loss. Attainment of a higher PBM is influenced by nutrition, physical activity, and mechanical loading during growth in addition to genetic variability, and mathematical modeling has suggested that a 10 % higher PBM will delay the onset of osteoporosis by 13 years [5].

Bone Size and Geometry

Macroscopically, the geometric properties of a bone are important. In addition to strength, the skeleton needs to be light to enable locomotion. The bending strength of a tubular structure is determined by the fourth power of its radius, and, as such, the periosteal circumference of a long bone has been demonstrated to predict up to 55 % of the variation in strength [6]. The balance between strength and weight of a bone is achieved through remodeling to increase the periosteal circumference while simultaneously increasing the area of the marrow cavity, resulting in a smaller cortical thickness for the same material weight. A thicker cortex also confers greater strength, although to a lesser extent than total cross-sectional area (CSA) of a bone. Males typically have a larger bone CSA than females, which partly results from the later pubertal growth spurt and hence completion of linear growth in boys [7]. This therefore confers greater bone strength in males compared to females. A reduction in cortical thickness occurs following the menopause, whereas a similar phenomenon is not observed in males [4], which further contributes to the failure load discrepancy between males and females in later life. Furthermore, the macroscopic shape of a bone is also adapted to the direction of normal physiological forces which it experiences. As such, the direction at which an impact force is applied to a bone will determine the likelihood of fracture; for example, a fall sideways rather than forwards is more likely to lead to a hip fracture as the direction of trauma is different to that experience from normal weight-bearing forces.

Bone Microarchitecture

Bone microarchitecture describes the structure of the cortical and trabecular compartments and can be assessed invasively by histomorphometric examination of bone biopsies or noninvasively using high-resolution peripheral quantitative computed tomography (HR-pQCT). Within the trabecular compartment, greater trabecular number confers higher resistance to compressive forces. Trabecular thickness is also an important determinant of deformation. While both trabecular number and trabecular thickness are important determinants of fracture risk, bone loss through trabecular number confers greater structural compromise than bone loss through trabecular thinning [7, 8]. Interconnections between individual trabeculae are important to maintaining the overall structure of the compartment. Greater trabecular separation compromises the integrity and strength of the bone. Sex differences are observed in trabecular arrangement which additionally contribute to the greater fracture risk in women: young women have fewer and thinner trabeculae with higher trabecular separation than young men [4, 9]. With aging, there is greater reduction in trabecular number in women than men [4, 9].

The outer cortex provides a dense outer shell, but increasing porosity and "trabecularization" reduce bone strength. At PBM, females have lower cortical porosity than males; however, this is offset by the greater CSA and cortical thickness in the males, such that strength is not compromised [4]. However, porosity increases with aging in both sexes, and this occurs at a faster rate in women than men, such that at age 80 years, cortical porosity is greater in women [4, 10].

Bone Nanoarchitecture

The importance of the collagen matrix (comprising 90 % of bone tissue) to the mechanical properties of bone is clearly demonstrated by the increased bone fragility observed in patients with osteogenesis imperfecta. This heterogeneous group of diseases illustrates that either qualitative or quantitative reductions in collagen production can lead to increased propensity to fracture. Collagen provides scaffolding on which the mineral can be deposited. The natural history of the collagen content of bone mirrors the pattern observed with bone mass: it reaches a peak in adolescence, with reduction thereafter [11]. Furthermore, cross-linkage of collagen fibrils by non-collagenous proteins confers greater tensile strength, and a reduction in the number of cross-links observed in osteoporotic bone may contribute to increased propensity to fracture [11]. In contrast, the presence of advanced glycation end products (AGE) within the bone matrix and cross-linked with collagen, which occurs as a result of high ambient glucose concentrations as seen in poorly controlled diabetes mellitus (DM), reduces the mechanical strength of bone and might account for the increased fracture risk of individuals with DM [11]. The crystallinity of the bone mineral within the matrix also contributes to bone strength; bones containing large hydroxyapatite crystals are more brittle and therefore more prone to fracture, whereas a greater heterogeneity in crystal size improves bone strength [12] and resistance to crack propagation.

weeks and months. Modeling is defined as the process by which bone mass is acquired during growth, repair, and adaptation to mechanical loading. In contrast, remodeling involves a cycle of resorption and formation of existing bone. Thus the balance between bone formation and resorption has a critical influence on overall bone mass and strength. During growth, formation clearly exceeds resorption, and after the achievement of PBM, the two opposing forces are in relative balance. However, as age increases into later adulthood, resorption begins to outstrip formation, and often the remodeling rate increases, reducing the opportunity for resorption cavities to be filled with new osteoid and for them to undergo a secondary mineralization. Over recent years, it has been recognized that osteocytes, which comprise 90–95 % of the cells within bone, play a key role in the regulation of these processes. The arrangement of the osteocytes within the lacunocanalicular system acts as a mechanosensory system and allows communication both directly and through the release of endocrine, paracrine, and autocrine signaling molecules to the other bone cells. There are a number of pathways which are important to the regulation of osteoblast and osteoclast activity. These are becoming increasingly recognized as targets for anti-osteoporosis agents.

Cellular Basis of Bone Metabolism

At the cellular level, there are three main types of bone cells: osteoblasts, osteocytes, and osteoclasts. In simple terms, osteoblasts are responsible for bone formation and may become embedded within bone mineral as mature osteocytes or remain on the surface of the bone as bone-lining cells. In contrast, multinucleated osteoclasts resorb bone. Osteoblasts and osteoclasts act in a coordinated fashion at specific sites on the surface of trabecular or cortical bone, forming "bone multicellular units" (Fig. 1.2).

After new osteoid collagen matrix is laid down by osteoblasts, crystals of calcium hydroxyapatite form on the collagen fibrils, thus achieving mineralization of the bone tissue over succeeding

Molecular Mechanisms

Osteoblasts are the primary source of receptor activator of nuclear factor κB ligand (RANK-L), which binds to RANK on osteoprogenitor cells, stimulating the differentiation of osteoclasts and activating bone resorption [13, 14]. The production of RANK-L by osteoblasts is increased in response to disuse, estrogen deficiency, and some medications including glucocorticoids and chemotherapeutic agents [15]. The activity of RANK-L is antagonized by osteoprotegerin (OPG), which competitively binds to RANK. This prevents the binding of RANK-L to RANK, and therefore the balance of OPG and RANK-L will determine the extent of bone resorption.

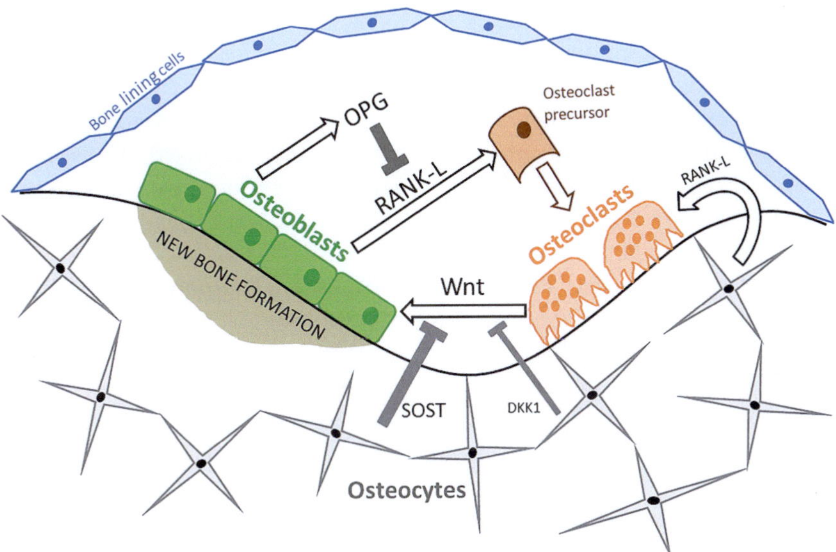

Fig. 1.2 The bone multicellular unit. The bone remodeling unit consists of osteoblasts, osteocytes, and osteoclasts, which operate in a coordinated fashion through the release of stimulatory and inhibitory cytokines. Receptor activator of nuclear factor kB ligand (RANK-L) is released from osteoblasts and osteocytes and stimulates the differentiation and activity of osteoclasts to resorb bone. RANK-L can be antagonized by osteoprotegerin (OPG). Osteoblast differentiation is stimulated by Wnt signaling from osteoclasts, while sclerostin (SOST) and Dickkopf-1 (DKK1) production by osteocytes competitively antagonizes Wnt binding to LRP5 and LRP6 receptors on the osteoblast to reduce bone formation

The Wnt signalingpathway has a key role in osteoblast differentiation, proliferation, and bone mineralization. The activation of this pathway in osteoblasts occurs through the binding of Wnt to a membrane receptor complex comprising Frizzled (Fzd) and either low-density lipoprotein-related protein 5 (LRP5) or 6 (LRP6). This leads to cytoplasmic accumulation of β-catenin, which can subsequently increase osteoblast differentiation. There is simultaneous repression of osteoclast function through increased secretion of OPG by osteoblast and osteocytes in response to Wnt signaling. However, in remodeling, osteoclasts appear to release Wnt ligands to stimulate local differentiation of osteoblasts [16]. The importance of this pathway to bone mineralization is demonstrated clinically by the osteoporosis-pseudoglioma syndrome, which results from loss of function mutations in LRP5. Conversely, gain-of-function mutations in LRP5 can result in a high bone mass phenotype [16]. Osteocytes regulate osteoblast differentiation through secretion of sclerostin (SOST), an antagonist of Wnt signaling which competitively binds to LRP5/6. Thus, lack of sclerostin also results in high bone mass, as observed in van Buchem disease and sclerosteosis [16]. Furthermore, osteocytes also express Dickkopf-1 (DKK1), but to a lesser extent than sclerostin. DKK1 also antagonizes Wnt signaling and thus reduces bone mineralization. No single gene defects in DKK1 associated with alterations in bone mass have been identified, but single nucleotide polymorphism (SNP) in DKK1, in addition to other genes in the Wnt signaling pathway, has been associated with BMD in genome-wide association studies (GWAS) [17].

Factors Influencing Bone Structural Properties

Mechanical Loading

Frost's mechanostat theory recognizes that bone has a homeostatic mechanism which enables BMD and geometric properties of the bone to change in response to mechanical loading or strains [18]. The mechanism through which mechanotransduction of strains to a biological signal occurs is poorly understood, but is likely to involve the osteocyte. Nonetheless, the importance of mechanical loading is clearly demonstrated by deterioration in BMD in astronauts experiencing a period of weightlessness [19] and by the positive effects of exercise. Prior to the attainment of PBM, loading increases BMC and CSA [20]. These changes will confer greater bone strength and may be less marked at older ages. In the adult skeleton, mechanical loading is important for conservation of bone mass, and a recent Cochrane review concluded that exercise can reduce bone loss in postmenopausal women, although the effect size is relatively small [21]. Obese adults tend to have higher BMD than normal weight controls (although not necessarily optimally adapted for their weight), and it is likely that this is due to mechanical loading and a concomitant increase in lean mass, in addition to hormonal influences.

Hormonal Factors

Sex Steroids

Sex steroids are necessary for both linear growth during puberty and maintenance of BMD after PBM. Estrogens are essential for the pubertal growth spurt and closure of the epiphyses in both males and females, whereas the role of androgens in these processes is less clear. Androgens, in addition to estrogens, are however important for periosteal apposition which increases bone width during the pubertal growth spurt. After puberty, sex steroid concentrations affect the rate of bone remodeling, and hypogonadism results in increased osteoclast number and function [22]. Clinically, this is evident in patients with estrogen receptor deficiency and aromatase deficiency, which are monogenic disorders associated with early onset osteoporosis. Furthermore, the importance of estrogen to BMD is also indicated by the rapid increase in the incidence of fragility fractures after the menopause. Early estrogen deficiency in women particularly affects bones with high trabecular content, including vertebral

bodies and the distal radius, and appears to result in a disproportionate loss of connectivity between trabeculae leading to compromised bone strength [7]. A further phase of bone loss in later years affecting both men and women also appears to affect cortical sites, with an increase in cortical porosity and reduction in cortical thickness.

Parathyroid Hormone and Phosphate Metabolism

Bone mineral acts as a reservoir for maintenance of serum calcium; its release into the serum to achieve normocalcemia is tightly regulated by parathyroid hormone (PTH) in combination with vitamin D, calcitonin, and fibroblast growth factor-23 (FGF-23). However, PTH has varied effects on bone metabolism: chronic elevations in PTH, as occurs in primary hyperparathyroidism, can result in mild reductions in BMD. Conversely, intermittent administration of low-dose PTH has anabolic effects on the skeleton [23]. This effect has been utilized in the development of PTH analogues for osteoporosis treatment and will be covered in more detail in Chap. 3.

Adipokines

There is also increasing recognition of the interaction between adipose tissue and bone mineralization, mediated through adipokines and osteocalcin. Leptin is an adipocyte-derived hormone, with key roles in regulation of appetite and body weight. However, ob/ob leptin-deficient mice have high bone mass despite hypogonadism. Furthermore, intracerebroventricular infusion of leptin reverses this high bone mass phenotype in ob/ob mice and in wild-type mice induces bone loss [22], demonstrating that leptin can influence bone metabolism. Leptin inhibits osteoblast differentiation and function via a central pathway mediated through hypothalamic activation of the sympathetic nervous system, which can stimulate $\beta2$ receptors on osteoblasts. While this reduces osteoblastic bone formation, it also increases the release of RANK-L from osteoblasts leading to increased osteoclast activity. In vitro, leptin has also been shown to directly increase osteoblast differentiation from human bone marrow stromal cells [24]. Adiponectin is also secreted by adipose tissue, but inversely to fat mass, and therefore levels are low in obesity. Adiponectin also has an effect on bone remodeling. The exact mechanisms of this action are unclear, and the balance toward formation or resorption may be dependent on the presence or absence of other factors, such as insulin and the source of adiponectin, but the adiponectin receptor has been identified on both osteoblasts and osteoclasts [25].

Epidemiology of Osteoporosis

Prevalence and Burden of Osteoporotic Fractures

In 2010, it was estimated that there were over 5.5 million men and 22 million women with osteoporosis living within the European Union (EU), representing 6.6 % and 22.1 % of the population over 50 years of age, respectively [26]. Worldwide, there are nearly 9 million osteoporotic fractures each year. In the EU, the estimated annual direct cost of 3.5 million fragility fractures in 2010 was approximately €24 billion; however, the total economic cost of osteoporosis management, including pharmacological fracture prevention and long-term fracture care, was estimated at €37 billion per year [26]. Although historically it was thought that the vast majority of this burden could be attributed to hip fracture, more recent data have suggested that just over half (54 %) of the economic cost of fracture is secondary to hip fractures, with non-hip, non-wrist, and non-spine fractures accounting for 39 %, and the remaining 7 % attributable to spine (5 %) and wrist (2 %) [26].

In addition to the economic healthcare costs, osteoporotic fractures lead to a significant individual burden. Excess mortality is a major consequence of fragility fracture, although this varies depending on fracture site and, although highest for hip fracture, has been shown to be elevated for most types of major fracture [27]. There is a five- to eightfold increase in mortality in the first 3 months following a hip fracture, and this is greater in men than women [28]. The excess risk

does decrease with time, although by 10 years postfracture, it has not returned to baseline [28, 29]. Perioperative complications, including cardiovascular events, pulmonary embolism, and respiratory infections, will contribute to the increased short-term mortality [30], but the exact cause for the sustained increase in mortality is unclear. Data relating to the presence of prefracture comorbidities and morality rates are conflicting [29, 31]; however, postfracture frailty is likely to be a significant contributor. Furthermore, individuals who sustain one hip fracture are at higher risk of a second fracture [32, 33], and a second fracture further elevates the 5-year mortality risk [32]. Vertebral fractures are also associated with excess mortality, despite many vertebral fractures not being clinically recognized. Similarly to hip fractures, this increased risk persists for at least 5 years, although the direct fracture-related deaths are fewer. Although earlier data suggested that forearm fractures may not be associated with increased mortality [34], more recent data suggest that all major osteoporotic fractures are linked to reduced survival [27].

Functional decline is common following an osteoporotic fracture; similar to mortality rates, this is greatest for those that sustain a hip fracture, in whom only approximately two-fifths will regain their prefracture ambulatory ability at 2 years [35], and rates of admission to nursing homes in individuals following a hip fracture exceed that of non-fracturing age- and sex-matched controls [36]. Older age at fracture, malignancy, and cognitive impairment are all associated with higher risk of functional decline following a hip fracture [35]. Vertebral fractures are also associated with pain and impaired quality of life [37], whereas forearm fractures are less frequently associated with increased morbidity and demonstrate the least reduction in quality of life [37].

Determinants of Fracture Risk

An osteoporotic bone has reduced strength, but spontaneous fractures remain rare. The epidemiology of osteoporotic fractures therefore reflects both disturbances to the biological processes involved in the balance between bone formation and resorption and also characteristics that lead to an increased propensity to fall, thus applying an impact force.

Age

There is a bimodal distribution of fractures by age; fracture incidence firstly peaks during puberty [38] and secondly in later life [39]. The peak in adolescence tends to coincide with the period of rapid skeletal growth in early to mid-puberty; these fractures are usually associated with substantial trauma and occur in the long bones. In contrast, fractures in later life are often secondary to minimal trauma.

The prevalence of osteoporosis increases significantly with advancing age after 50 years; one study reported an increased prevalence from 4.4 % of individuals aged 50–54 years to 36.8 % of those aged over 80 years [26]. Similarly, the incidence of fragility fractures increases after 50 years of age, as shown in Fig. 1.3 [40], although the absolute number of fractures plateaus in those over 80 years as the size of the at-risk population reduces [26]. The increasing incidence is in part due to age-related reductions in BMD, as the risk of fracture approximately doubles for every standard deviation decrease in BMD [41, 42], but deteriorations in cortical and trabecular structure and an the increasing incidence of falls [42] also contribute. Approximately, one-third of community-dwelling adults over 65 years will fall at least once each year [43], but the incidence is four times greater in 90-year-olds than 60-year-olds and twice as common in women than men [44]. Risk factors for falls include sarcopenia and poor functional mobility, neurocognitive impairment, poor visual acuity, disturbances to balance, cardiovascular instability, and sedative medications [44]. Similarly, the prevalence of these comorbidities tends to increase with age (Fig. 1.3).

Sex

The sex distribution of fractures differs with age. In childhood, fracture rates are higher in boys [38], and this pattern remains until approximately

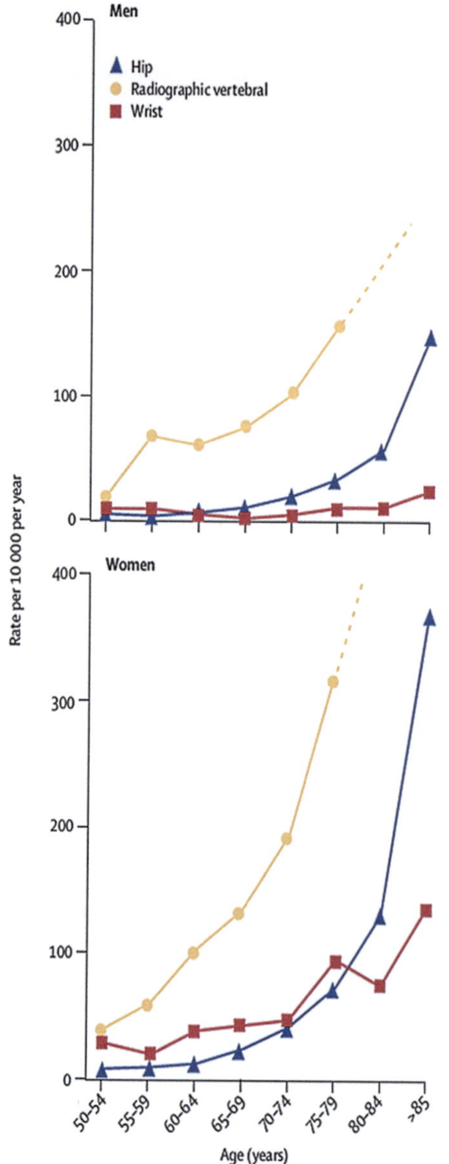

Fig. 1.3 Hip, wrist, and radiographic vertebral fracture incidence by age and gender. From The Lancet, Vol 367 (9527), P Sambrook & C Cooper, Osteoporosis, Pages 2010–18., Copyright 2011 [40]. Reprinted with permission from Elsevier Limited

50–55 years of age when the sex distribution is reversed [45]. After the age of 50 years, women sustain nearly three times as many fractures as men and account for 75 % of the fracture-related costs [46]. This increase in fracture incidence in women coincides with the postmenopausal reductions in bone mass. The gender disparity is particularly marked for forearm fractures, with an age-adjusted female-to-male ratio of 4:1 due to a marked increase in forearm fractures in females with advancing age, but no simultaneous increase in males [45]. Despite the overall incidence of fractures being higher in women than men, hip fractures tend to occur at a younger age, and mortality rates are higher in males [28, 47]. This is likely to reflect higher levels of comorbidity in males than female. However, functional outcome in those that do survive hip fracture is similar between the two sexes [48].

Ethnicity

Fracture rates vary with ethnicity. A recent study of women aged over 65 years living in the USA demonstrated that the incidence of hip fracture was highest in white women, and this was 1.4, 2.0, and 2.3 times higher than that of Hispanic, Asian, and Black American women, respectively [49]. The ethnic variability in fracture rates observed in men is much lower, but white men still have a higher incidence of hip fracture [49]. Some of the variation in fracture rate is due to ethnic differences in BMD: data from the NHANES 1999–2004 cohort demonstrated that at all ages, aBMD is higher in black compared to non-Hispanic white individuals, who had greater aBMD than Mexican Americans [50]. However, the Study of Osteoporotic Fractures demonstrated that even within the same tertile of BMD, black women have a 30–40 % lower risk of fracture than white women [51], indicating that the other factors, for example, skeletal size and microarchitecture, are also likely to contribute to the fracture risk disparity. Even in childhood, African Americans have greater bone area and higher measures of bone strength than Caucasian children [52, 53], and these differences remain apparent in later life [54]. Furthermore, postmenopausal African American women also have increased trabecular thickness, cortical area, and cortical thickness compared to Caucasian women [54], which will also increase resistance to fracture.

Anthropometry, Obesity, and Body Composition

Taller stature [55, 56] and a low body mass index are well-established risk factors for fracture in postmenopausal women, whereas conversely obesity appears to be a protective factor for hip fracture in adults [57, 58]. However, the effect of obesity on the incidence of fractures across skeletal sites is not identical. In the Global Longitudinal Study of Osteoporosis in Women (GLOW), which included 46,443 women from 10 different countries, the overall incidence of fracture did not differ between obese and normal weight women, but the age of reported fracture was significantly younger in obese women than normal or underweight women [59]. Obesity was associated with a higher incidence of ankle and lower leg fractures, but lower incidence of wrist, hip, and pelvic fractures. In contrast, underweight women had a higher incidence of hip and pelvic fractures compared to normal weight and obese women [59]. This variation in fracture site by body weight may be mediated through a combination of mechanical loading resulting in a higher BMD in obese individuals and protective cushioning at some sites, but greater forces applied to other sites, in the event of a fall.

Heritable Influences

The risk of an osteoporotic fracture is greater in individuals who have a parent that suffered a hip fracture. Twin and family studies suggest that a substantial proportion of the variance in bone mass is determined by heritable factors, including intrauterine and shared environmental factors and genetic influences, although this varies by skeletal site, such that the heritance of BMD at the lumbar spine is greater than that at the wrist [60–62]. However, age also influences the heritability of BMD. The heritable component is estimated to be lower in postmenopausal compared with premenopausal women [60, 61], which most likely reflects the additional role of lifestyle-, dietary-, and disease-related factors in the latter group. Genetic determinants of femoral neck geometry [63], markers of bone turnover [64], age at menopause [65], and muscle strength [66] will also contribute to the genetic susceptibility to osteoporotic fracture.

A number of genes have now been identified as possible candidates for the regulation of bone mass and osteoporotic fracture. The majority of these influence the estrogen, Wnt signaling, or RANK-L-RANK-OPG pathways [17, 67]. However, polymorphisms at these loci explain only a small proportion (1–3 %) of the observed variance in BMD in the population, and there is increasing recognition that environmental factors might alter osteoporosis risk directly and through epigenetic mechanisms acting to influence gene expression. These gene-environment interactions might occur either in fetal development, for example, the demonstrated interaction between birth weight and the vitamin D receptor genotype in determining lumbar spine BMD [68], or in later life, for example, in the Framingham Offspring Cohort, genetic variation in the inter-leukin-6 promoter gene was only associated with hip BMD in a subset of women who were not using estrogen replacement and in those who had an inadequate calcium intake [69]. Over recent years, the role of epigenetic processes in mediating such interactions between environmental factors and gene expression has been increasingly recognized as fundamental to the pathogenesis of human disease [70].

Geography

There is a marked variation in hip fracture rates globally. The highest age- standardized annual hip fracture rates, observed in Scandinavia, are tenfold higher than the countries with the lowest incidence, including Tunisia, Ecuador, and Morocco [71]. Generally, hip fracture rates are highest in countries furthest from the equator, and although the underlying mechanisms remain to be elucidated, this variation may be related to differences in vitamin D status. In countries where extensive skin covering due to religious or cultural practices are the norm, such as in many of the Middle Eastern countries [71], higher rates of hip fracture are observed, which further supports lack of sunlight exposure and reduced vitamin D synthesis as contributory factors. Some migration data would suggest that this geographi-

cal variation is the result of environmental, rather than genetic, factors, although not all studies support this. Black Africans residing in the USA have higher incidence of hip fracture than Black Africans in Africa [71], but Japanese women living in Hawaii have a similar incidence of hip fracture to those who have remained in Japan [72]. Clearly any similarities and differences between the current and previous environment have to be borne in mind when interpreting such findings.

Conversely, in Sweden, the overall risk of hip fracture is significantly higher in those who were born in Sweden than for foreign-born individuals [73]. Furthermore, in the foreign-born males, the incidence of hip fracture was highest in those from Norway and Iceland and lower in individuals born in more southern European countries such as Poland and Germany [73]. A number of factors might contribute to these differences in incidence including manual labor intensity in immigrants, anthropometry, and body composition, but these results could also suggest that early life geographical factors, including vitamin D exposure, might be important to determining fracture risk.

Hip fracture rates appear to be higher in more urbanized areas than rural regions [74]. There is much speculation as to the underlying causal factors for this, and proposed factors include physical activity and manual labor, greater sunlight exposure due to occupational and leisure time spent outdoors, and comorbidities leading to relocation for medical or nursing care [74]. Furthermore, some authors suggest that pollution in inner-city areas might have a negative effect on BMD [75].

Seasonal Variation

Some studies have suggested that there is evidence for seasonal variation in osteoporotic fractures [76–78], although this is not supported by all studies [79]. It is likely that environmental factors, such as snow and ice, contribute to the higher winter incidence in some countries; however, many fractures occur indoors [80], and some studies conducted in countries at northern latitudes suggest that the seasonal variation is present only if fractures that occur outdoors are considered [81, 82]. However, seasonal variation is even observed Hong Kong [76] and southern states of the USA [78], where icy winter conditions do not occur, suggesting that other factors, for example, seasonal variation in vitamin D status and bone turnover, might be important.

Secular Trends in Osteoporosis

Improvements in life expectancy and an aging population are resulting in an increasing number of hip fractures worldwide; in 1990, there were estimated to be 1.66 million hip fractures, and in 2050, this figure is predicted to rise to 6.26 million [83]. However, these estimates have assumed a constant age-specific hip fracture incidence, yet marked secular changes have been observed, and these vary across the globe. In Europe, North America, and Oceania, age-specific hip fracture rates increased until the late twentieth century; however, more recently, there is evidence for stabilization or even a decline in the incidences in these countries (Fig. 1.4) [84–86]. In contrast, although there are limited data, the rates of hip fracture in many developing countries continue to increase [84].

The mechanisms underlying these changes in fracture incidence are unclear, but are likely to reflect a combination of factors [84]. It is possible that a change in the prevalence of risk factors which act relatively late in the lifecourse has occurred, and indeed improvements in healthcare

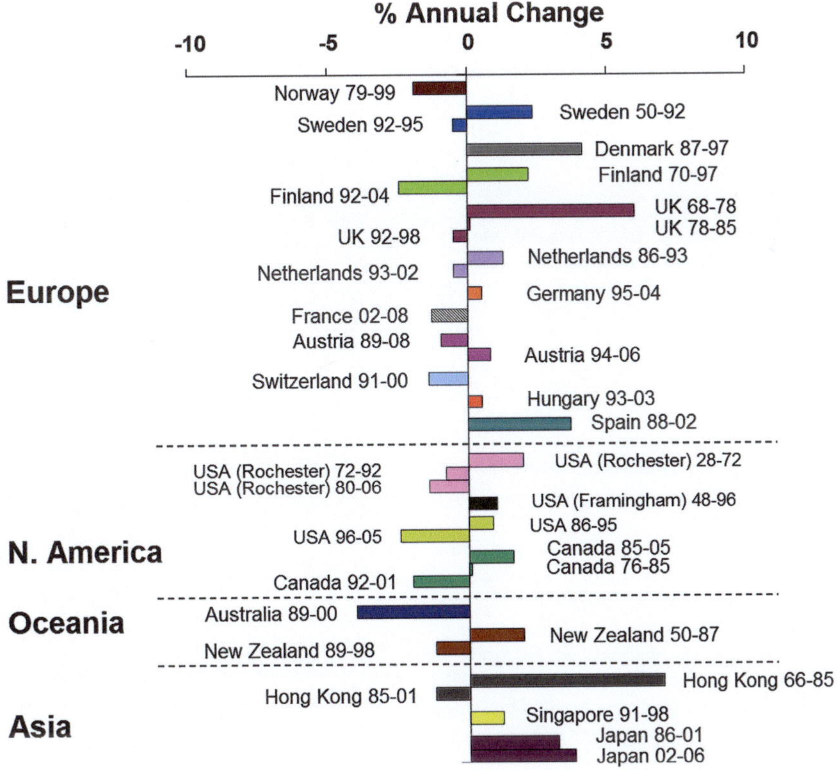

Fig. 1.4 Secular trends in hip fracture incidence. From Cooper C et al., Osteoporosis International 2011 [84]. Reprinted with permission from Springer Science and Business Media

in developed countries leading to improved survival of the frailest elderly would contribute to this. A secular increase in adiposity may also contribute. Bisphosphonates were introduced in fracture prevention in North America and Europe in the mid-1990s. However, the increased use of these agents cannot fully explain the observed reductions in hip fracture incidence [87–89]. Alternatively, a birth cohort effect might arise from a change to risk factor patterns which influence bone development early in the lifecourse.

Conclusions

Osteoporosis and fragility fracture are globally common conditions, which result in huge individual and public health burden and increased mortality. Knowledge of the factors contributing to bone strength, the pathophysiological processes resulting in bone loss and qualitative deteriorations in bone structure, and risk factors for osteoporosis will enable the development of new therapeutic agents and increasing use of individualized treatment programs.

Acknowledgments We would like to thank Medical Research Council (UK), Arthritis Research UK, National Osteoporosis Society (UK), International Osteoporosis Foundation, and NIHR for funding this work.

References[1]

1. Consensus development conference: diagnosis, prophylaxis, and treatment of osteoporosis. Am J Med. 1993;94(6):646–50.
2. Cranney A, Jamal SA, Tsang JF, et al. Low bone mineral density and fracture burden in postmenopausal women. CMAJ. 2007;177(6):575–80. doi:10.1503/cmaj.070234 [published Online First: Epub Date].
3. Thurner PJ, Erickson B, Jungmann R, Schriock Z, Weaver JC, Fantner GE, Schitter G, Morse DE, Hansma PK. High-speed photography of compressed human trabecular bone correlates whitening to microscopic damage. Eng Fract Mech. 2007;74:1928–41. *Elegant biomechanical demonstration of microdamage to bone and associated nano-structural changes consequent on fracture.
4. Hansen S, Shanbhogue V, Folkestad L, et al. Bone microarchitecture and estimated strength in 499 adult Danish women and men: a cross-sectional, population-based high-resolution peripheral quantitative computed tomographic study on peak bone structure. Calcif Tissue Int. 2013. doi:10.1007/s00223-013-9808-5 [published Online First: Epub Date].
5. **Hernandez CJ, Beaupre GS, Carter DR. A theoretical analysis of the relative influences of peak BMD, age-related bone loss and menopause on the development of osteoporosis. Osteoporos Int. 2003;14(10):843–47. **Theoretical analysis demonstrating the importance of peak bone mass, compared with subsequent bone loss, in the determination of osteoporosis.
6. Ammann P, Rizzoli R. Bone strength and its determinants. Osteoporosis Int. 2003;14 Suppl 3:S13–8. doi:10.1007/s00198-002-1345-4 [published Online First: Epub Date].
7. *Seeman E. Bone quality: the material and structural basis of bone strength. J Bone Miner Metab. 2008;26(1):1–8. doi:10.1007/s00774-007-0793-5. [publishedOnline First: Epub Date]. *Excellent introduction to bone biomechanics and structural considerations.
8. Silva MJ, Gibson LJ. Modeling the mechanical behavior of vertebral trabecular bone: effects of age-related changes in microstructure. Bone. 1997;21(2): 191–9.
9. Macdonald HM, Nishiyama KK, Kang J, et al. Age-related patterns of trabecular and cortical bone loss differ between sexes and skeletal sites: a population-based HR-pQCT study. J Bone Miner Res. 2011;26(1):50–62. doi:10.1002/jbmr.171 [published Online First: Epub Date].
10. Zebaze RM, Ghasem-Zadeh A, Bohte A, et al. Intracortical remodelling and porosity in the distal radius and post-mortem femurs of women: a cross-sectional study. Lancet. 2010;375(9727):1729–36. doi:10.1016/s0140-6736(10)60320-0 [published Online First: Epub Date].
11. Saito M, Marumo K. Collagen cross-links as a determinant of bone quality: a possible explanation for bone fragility in aging, osteoporosis, and diabetes mellitus. Osteoporosis Int. 2010;21(2):195–214. doi:10.1007/s00198-009-1066-z [published Online First: Epub Date].
12. Davison KS, Siminoski K, Adachi JD, et al. Bone strength: the whole is greater than the sum of its parts. Semin Arthritis Rheum. 2006;36(1):22–31. doi:10.1016/j.semarthrit.2006.04.002 [published Online First: Epub Date].
13. Xiong J, Onal M, Jilka RL, et al. Matrix-embedded cells control osteoclast formation. Nat Med. 2011;17(10):1235–41. doi:10.1038/nm.2448 [published Online First: Epub Date].

---

[1] *Important References
**Very important References

14. Nakashima T, Hayashi M, Fukunaga T, et al. Evidence for osteocyte regulation of bone homeostasis through RANKL expression. Nat Med. 2011;17(10):1231–4. doi:10.1038/nm.2452 [published Online First: Epub Date].

15. Atkins GJ, Findlay DM. Osteocyte regulation of bone mineral: a little give and take. Osteoporosis Int. 2012;23(8):2067–79. doi:10.1007/s00198-012-1915-z [published Online First: Epub Date].

16. Baron R, Kneissel M. WNT signaling in bone homeostasis and disease: from human mutations to treatments. Nat Med. 2013;19(2):179–92. doi:10.1038/nm.3074 [published Online First: Epub Date].

17. Estrada K, Styrkarsdottir U, Evangelou E, et al. Genome-wide meta-analysis identifies 56 bone mineral density loci and reveals 14 loci associated with risk of fracture. Nat Genet. 2012;44(5):491–501. doi:10.1038/ng.2249 [published Online First: Epub Date].

18. Hughes JM, Petit MA. Biological underpinnings of Frost's mechanostat thresholds: the important role of osteocytes. J Musculoskelet Neuronal Interact. 2010;10(2):128–35.

19. Sibonga JD, Evans HJ, Sung HG, et al. Recovery of spaceflight-induced bone loss: bone mineral density after long-duration missions as fitted with an exponential function. Bone. 2007;41(6):973–8. doi:10.1016/j.bone.2007.08.022 [published Online First: Epub Date].

20. Kannus P, Haapasalo H, Sankelo M, et al. Effect of starting age of physical activity on bone mass in the dominant arm of tennis and squash players. Ann Intern Med. 1995;123(1):27–31.

21. Howe TE, Shea B, Dawson LJ, et al. Exercise for preventing and treating osteoporosis in postmenopausal women. Cochrane Database Syst Rev. 2011;(7): Cd000333. doi:10.1002/14651858.CD000333.pub2. [published Online First: Epub Date].

22. Ducy P, Amling M, Takeda S, et al. Leptin inhibits bone formation through a hypothalamic relay: a central control of bone mass. Cell. 2000;100(2):197–207.

23. Silva BC, Costa AG, Cusano NE, et al. Catabolic and anabolic actions of parathyroid hormone on the skeleton. J Endocrinol Invest. 2011;34(10):801–10. doi:10.3275/7925 [published Online First: Epub Date].

24. Thomas T, Gori F, Khosla S, et al. Leptin acts on human marrow stromal cells to enhance differentiation to osteoblasts and to inhibit differentiation to adipocytes. Endocrinology. 1999;140(4):1630–38.

25. Shinoda Y, Yamaguchi M, Ogata N, et al. Regulation of bone formation by adiponectin through autocrine/paracrine and endocrine pathways. J Cell Biochem. 2006;99(1):196–208. doi:10.1002/jcb.20890 [published Online First: Epub Date].

26. **Hernlund E, Svedbom A, Ivergard M, et al. Osteoporosis in the European Union: medical management, epidemiology and economic burden: a report prepared in collaboration with the International Osteoporosis Foundation (IOF) and the European Federation of Pharmaceutical Industry Associations (EFPIA). Arch Osteoporos. 2013;8(1–2):136. doi:10.1007/s11657-013-0136-1. [published Online First: Epub Date]. **Valuable compendium of osteoporosis epidemiology and burden across Europe.

27. Bliuc D, Nguyen ND, Milch VE, et al. Mortality risk associated with low-trauma osteoporotic fracture and subsequent fracture in men and women. JAMA. 2009;301(5):513–21.

28. Haentjens P, Magaziner J, Colon-Emeric CS, et al. Meta-analysis: excess mortality after hip fracture among older women and men. Ann Intern Med. 2010;152(6);380–90. doi:10.7326/0003-4819-152-6-201003160-00008 [published Online First: Epub Date].

29. Abrahamsen B, van Staa T, Ariely R, et al. Excess mortality following hip fracture: a systematic epidemiological review. Osteoporosis Int. 2009;20(10): 1633–50. doi:10.1007/s00198-009-0920-3 [published Online First: Epub Date].

30. Roche JJ, Wenn RT, Sahota O, et al. Effect of comorbidities and postoperative complications on mortality after hip fracture in elderly people: prospective observational cohort study. BMJ. 2005;331(7529):1374. doi:10.1136/bmj.38643.663843.55 [published Online First: Epub Date].

31. Patel KV, Brennan KL, Brennan ML, et al. Association of a modified frailty index with mortality after femoral neck fracture in patients aged 60 years and older. Clin Orthop Relat Res. 2013. doi:10.1007/s11999-013-3334-7 [published Online First: Epub Date].

32. Ahmed LA, Center JR, Bjornerem A, et al. Progressively increasing fracture risk with advancing age after initial incident fragility fracture: the Tromso study. J Bone Miner Res. 2013;28(10):2214–21. doi:10.1002/jbmr.1952 [published Online First: Epub Date].

33. Berry SD, Samelson EJ, Hannan MT, et al. Second hip fracture in older men and women: the Framingham study. Arch Intern Med. 2007;167(18):1971–6. doi:10.1001/archinte.167.18.1971 [published Online First: Epub Date].

34. Cooper C, Atkinson EJ, Jacobsen SJ, et al. Population-based study of survival after osteoporotic fractures. Am J Epidemiol. 1993;137(9):1001–5.

35. Kim SM, Moon YW, Lim SJ, et al. Prediction of survival, second fracture, and functional recovery following the first hip fracture surgery in elderly patients. Bone. 2012;50(6):1343–50. doi:10.1016/j.bone.2012.02.633 [published Online First: Epub Date].

36. Leibson CL, Tosteson AN, Gabriel SE, et al. Mortality, disability, and nursing home use for persons with and without hip fracture: a population-based study. J Am Geriatr Soc. 2002;50(10):1644–50.

37. Adachi JD, Adami S, Gehlbach S, et al. Impact of prevalent fractures on quality of life: baseline results from the global longitudinal study of osteoporosis in women. Mayo Clin Proc. 2010;85(9):806–13.

doi:10.4065/mcp.2010.0082 [published Online First: Epub Date].

38. Cooper C, Dennison EM, Leufkens HG, et al. Epidemiology of childhood fractures in Britain: a study using the general practice research database. J Bone Miner Res. 2004;19(12):1976–81. doi:10.1359/JBMR.040902 [published Online First: Epub Date].

39. Garraway WM, Stauffer RN, Kurland LT, et al. Limb fractures in a defined population. I. Frequency and distribution. Mayo Clin Proc. 1979;54(11):701–7.

40. Sambrook P, Cooper C. Osteoporosis. Lancet. 2006;367(9527):2010–8. doi:10.1016/s0140-6736(06)68891-0 [published Online First: Epub Date].

41. Marshall D, Johnell O, Wedel H. Meta-analysis of how well measures of bone mineral density predict occurrence of osteoporotic fractures. BMJ. 1996;312(7041):1254–59.

42. Edwards MH, Jameson K, Denison H, et al. Clinical risk factors, bone density and fall history in the prediction of incident fracture among men and women. Bone. 2013;52(2):541–7. doi:10.1016/j.bone.2012.11.006 [published Online First: Epub Date].

43. Gillespie LD, Robertson MC, Gillespie WJ, et al. Interventions for preventing falls in older people living in the community. Cochrane Database Syst Rev. 2012;9:Cd007146. doi:10.1002/14651858.CD007146.pub3 [published Online First: Epub Date].

44. Stenhagen M, Ekstrom H, Nordell E, et al. Falls in the general elderly population: a 3- and 6- year prospective study of risk factors using data from the longitudinal population study 'Good ageing in Skane'. BMC Geriatr. 2013;13:81. doi:10.1186/1471-2318-13-81 [published Online First: Epub Date].

45. **van Staa TP, Dennison EM, Leufkens HG, et al. Epidemiology of fractures in England and Wales. Bone. 2001;29(6):517–22. **Comprehensive description of UK fracture epidemiology.

46. Burge R, Dawson-Hughes B, Solomon DH, et al. Incidence and economic burden of osteoporosis-related fractures in the United States, 2005–2025. J Bone Mineral Res. 2007;22(3):465–75. doi:10.1359/jbmr.061113 [published Online First: Epub Date].

47. Sterling RS. Gender and race/ethnicity differences in hip fracture incidence, morbidity, mortality, and function. Clin Orthop Relat Res. 2011;469(7):1913–8. doi:10.1007/s11999-010-1736-3 [published Online First: Epub Date].

48. Cawthon PM. Gender differences in osteoporosis and fractures. Clin Orthop Relat Res. 2011;469(7):1900–5. doi:10.1007/s11999-011-1780-7 [published Online First: Epub Date].

49. Wright NC, Saag KG, Curtis JR, et al. Recent trends in hip fracture rates by race/ethnicity among older US adults. J Bone Miner Res. 2012;27(11):2325–32. doi:10.1002/jbmr.1684 [published Online First: Epub Date].

50. Looker AC, Melton 3rd LJ, Harris TB, et al. Prevalence and trends in low femur bone density among older US adults: NHANES 2005–2006 compared with NHANES III. J Bone Miner Res. 2010;25(1):64–71. doi:10.1359/jbmr.090706 [published Online First: Epub Date].

51. Cauley JA, Lui LY, Ensrud KE, et al. Bone mineral density and the risk of incident nonspinal fractures in black and white women. JAMA. 2005;293(17):2102–8. doi:10.1001/jama.293.17.2102 [published Online First: Epub Date].

52. Wetzsteon RJ, Hughes JM, Kaufman BC, et al. Ethnic differences in bone geometry and strength are apparent in childhood. Bone. 2009;44(5):970–5. doi:10.1016/j.bone.2009.01.006 [published Online First: Epub Date].

53. Gilsanz V, Skaggs DL, Kovanlikaya A, et al. Differential effect of race on the axial and appendicular skeletons of children. J Clin Endocrinol Metab. 1998;83(5):1420–7. doi:10.1210/jcem.83.5.4765 [published Online First: Epub Date].

54. Putman MS, Yu EW, Lee H, et al. Differences in skeletal microarchitecture and strength in African-American and white women. J Bone Miner Res. 2013;28(10):2177–85. doi:10.1002/jbmr.1953 [published Online First: Epub Date].

55. Benetou V, Orfanos P, Benetos IS, et al. Anthropometry, physical activity and hip fractures in the elderly. Injury. 2011;42(2):188–93. doi:10.1016/j.injury.2010.08.022 [published Online First: Epub Date].

56. Trimpou P, Landin-Wilhelmsen K, Oden A, et al. Male risk factors for hip fracture-a 30-year follow-up study in 7,495 men. Osteoporos Int. 2010;21(3):409–16. doi:10.1007/s00198-009-0961-7 [published Online First: Epub Date].

57. Tang X, Liu G, Kang J, et al. Obesity and risk of hip fracture in adults: a meta-analysis of prospective cohort studies. PLoS One. 2013;8(4), e55077. doi:10.1371/journal.pone.0055077 [published Online First: Epub Date].

58. Johansson H, Kanis JA, Oden A, et al. A meta-analysis of the association of fracture risk and body mass index in women. J Bone Miner Res. 2013. doi:10.1002/jbmr.2017 [published Online First: Epub Date].

59. Compston JE, Watts NB, Chapurlat R, et al. Obesity is not protective against fracture in postmenopausal women: GLOW. Am J Med. 2011;124(11):1043–50. doi:10.1016/j.amjmed.2011.06.013 [published Online First: Epub Date].

60. Pocock NA, Eisman JA, Hopper JL, et al. Genetic determinants of bone mass in adults. A twin study. J Clin Invest. 1987;80(3):706–10. doi:10.1172/jci113125 [published Online First: Epub Date].

61. Slemenda CW, Christian JC, Williams CJ, et al. Genetic determinants of bone mass in adult women: a reevaluation of the twin model and the potential importance of gene interaction on heritability estimates. J Bone Miner Res. 1991;6(6):561–7. doi:10.1002/jbmr.5650060606 [published Online First: Epub Date].

62. Park JH, Song YM, Sung J, et al. Genetic influence on bone mineral density in Korean twins and families: the healthy twin study. Osteoporos Int. 2012; 23(4):1343–9. doi:10.1007/s00198-011-1685-z [published Online First: Epub Date].

63. Arden NK, Baker J, Hogg C, et al. The heritability of bone mineral density, ultrasound of the calcaneus and hip axis length: a study of postmenopausal twins. J Bone Miner Res. 1996;11(4):530–4. doi:10.1002/jbmr.5650110414 [published Online First: Epub Date].

64. Hunter D, De Lange M, Snieder H, et al. Genetic contribution to bone metabolism, calcium excretion, and vitamin D and parathyroid hormone regulation. J Bone Miner Res. 2001;16(2):371–8. doi:10.1359/jbmr.2001.16.2.371 [published Online First: Epub Date].

65. Morris DH, Jones ME, Schoemaker MJ, et al. Familial concordance for age at natural menopause: results from the Breakthrough Generations Study. Menopause. 2011;18(9):956–61. doi:10.1097/gme.0b013e31820ed6d2 [published Online First: Epub Date].

66. Arden NK, Spector TD. Genetic influences on muscle strength, lean body mass, and bone mineral density: a twin study. J Bone Miner Res. 1997;12(12):2076–81. doi:10.1359/jbmr.1997.12.12.2076 [published Online First: Epub Date].

67. Rivadeneira F, Styrkarsdottir U, Estrada K, et al. Twenty bone-mineral-density loci identified by large-scale meta-analysis of genome-wide association studies. Nat Genet. 2009;41(11):1199–206. doi:10.1038/ng.446 [published Online First: Epub Date].

68. Dennison EM, Arden NK, Keen RW, et al. Birthweight, vitamin D receptor genotype and the programming of osteoporosis. Paediatr Perinat Epidemiol. 2001;15(3):211–9.

69. Ferrari SL, Karasik D, Liu J, et al. Interactions of interleukin-6 promoter polymorphisms with dietary and lifestyle factors and their association with bone mass in men and women from the Framingham Osteoporosis Study. J Bone Miner Res. 2004;19(4):552–9. doi:10.1359/jbmr.040103 [published Online First: Epub Date].

70. Holroyd C, Harvey N, Dennison E, et al. Epigenetic influences in the developmental origins of osteoporosis. Osteoporos Int. 2012;23(2):401–10. doi:10.1007/s00198-011-1671-5 [published Online First: Epub Date].

71. Kanis JA, Oden A, McCloskey EV, et al. A systematic review of hip fracture incidence and probability of fracture worldwide. Osteoporos Int. 2012;23(9):2239–56. doi:10.1007/s00198-012-1964-3 [published Online First: Epub Date].

72. Ross PD, Norimatsu H, Davis JW, et al. A comparison of hip fracture incidence among native Japanese, Japanese Americans, and American Caucasians. Am J Epidemiol. 1991;133(8):801–9.

73. Albin B, Hjelm K, Elmstahl S. Lower prevalence of hip fractures in foreign-born individuals than in Swedish-born individuals during the period 1987–1999. BMC Musculoskelet Disord. 2010;11:203. doi:10.1186/1471-2474-11-203 [published Online First: Epub Date].

74. Brennan SL, Pasco JA, Urquhart DM, et al. The association between urban or rural locality and hip fracture in community-based adults: a systematic review. J Epidemiol Community Health. 2010;64(8):656–65. doi:10.1136/jech.2008.085738 [published Online First: Epub Date].

75. Alver K, Meyer HE, Falch JA, et al. Outdoor air pollution, bone density and self-reported forearm fracture: the Oslo Health Study. Osteoporos Int. 2010;21(10):1751–60. doi:10.1007/s00198-009-1130-8 [published Online First: Epub Date].

76. Douglas S, Bunyan A, Chiu KH, et al. Seasonal variation of hip fracture at three latitudes. Injury. 2000;31(1):11–9.

77. Gronskag AB, Forsmo S, Romundstad P, et al. Incidence and seasonal variation in hip fracture incidence among elderly women in Norway. The HUNT Study. Bone. 2010;46(5):1294–8. doi:10.1016/j.bone.2009.11.024 [published Online First: Epub Date].

78. Bischoff-Ferrari HA, Orav JE, Barrett JA, et al. Effect of seasonality and weather on fracture risk in individuals 65 years and older. Osteoporos Int. 2007;18(9):1225–33. doi:10.1007/s00198-007-0364-6 [published Online First: Epub Date].

79. Pedrazzoni M, Alfano FS, Malvi C, et al. Seasonal variation in the incidence of hip fractures in Emilia-Romagna and Parma. Bone. 1993;14 Suppl 1:S57–63.

80. Leavy B, Aberg AC, Melhus H, et al. When and where do hip fractures occur? A population-based study. Osteoporos Int. 2013;24(9):2387–96. doi:10.1007/s00198-013-2333-6 [published Online First: Epub Date].

81. Oyen J, Rohde GE, Hochberg M, et al. Low-energy distal radius fractures in middle-aged and elderly women-seasonal variations, prevalence of osteoporosis, and associates with fractures. Osteoporos Int. 2010;21(7):1247–55. doi:10.1007/s00198-009-1065-0 [published Online First: Epub Date].

82. Emaus N, Olsen LR, Ahmed LA, et al. Hip fractures in a city in Northern Norway over 15 years: time trends, seasonal variation and mortality : the Harstad Injury Prevention Study. Osteoporos Int. 2011;22(10):2603–10. doi:10.1007/s00198-010-1485-x [published Online First: Epub Date].

83. *Cooper C, Campion G, Melton 3rd LJ. Hip fractures in the elderly: a world-wide projection. Osteoporos Int. 1992;2(6):285–9. *Helpful projection of global hip fracture rates accounting for anticipated population changes.

84. **Cooper C, Cole ZA, Holroyd CR, et al. Secular trends in the incidence of hip and other osteoporotic fractures. Osteoporos Int. 2011;22(5):1277–88. doi:10.1007/s00198-011-1601-6. [published Online First: Epub Date]. **Comprehensive assessment of secular trends in hip fracture since the mid 1900s.

85. Amin S, Achenbach SJ, Atkinson EJ, et al. Trends in fracture incidence: a population-based study over 20 years. J Bone Miner Res. 2013. doi:10.1002/jbmr.2072 [published Online First: Epub Date].
86. Rosengren BE, Ahlborg HG, Mellstrom D, et al. Secular trends in Swedish hip fractures 1987–2002: birth cohort and period effects. Epidemiology. 2012;23(4):623–30. doi:10.1097/EDE.0b013e318256982a [published Online First: Epub Date].
87. Hiligsmann M, Bruyere O, Roberfroid D, et al. Trends in hip fracture incidence and in the prescription of antiosteoporosis medications during the same time period in Belgium (2000–2007). Arthritis Care Res. 2012;64(5):744–50. doi:10.1002/acr.21607 [published Online First: Epub Date].
88. Alves SM, Economou T, Oliveira C, et al. Osteoporotic hip fractures: bisphosphonates sales and observed turning point in trend. A population-based retrospective study. Bone. 2013;53(2):430–6. doi:10.1016/j.bone.2012.12.014 [published Online First: Epub Date].
89. Abrahamsen B, Vestergaard P. Declining incidence of hip fractures and the extent of use of anti-osteoporotic therapy in Denmark 1997–2006. Osteoporos Int. 2010;21(3):373–80. doi:10.1007/s00198-009-0957-3 [published Online First: Epub Date].

Antiresorptives

2

R. Graham G. Russell, Maria K. Tsoumpra,
Michelle A. Lawson, Andrew D. Chantry,
Frank H. Ebetino, and Michael Pazianas

Summary

- The term "antiresorptive" is used to refer to drugs that inhibit bone resorption, usually via direct or indirect actions on osteoclast development and function.
- The use of "antiresorptive" drugs continues to dominate the therapy of bone diseases, including osteoporosis.
- Currently, the main group of drugs used worldwide is the bisphosphonates, which have been used clinically for more than 40 years and which can reduce fracture occurrence at vertebral and non-vertebral sites, including hips.
- The remarkable recent advances in understanding the genetic basis of inherited bone disorders have provided a rich source of new targets for therapeutic intervention, notably the RANK-ligand/RANK system and cathepsin K for antiresorptive drugs and the wnt/sclerostin pathway for bone-forming drugs.
- The most recently introduced new drug is the anti-RANK-ligand antibody, denosumab, which is also highly effective against all fracture types, vertebral, non-vertebral, and hips.
- For osteoporosis, older treatments have historically included hormones, such as estrogens as well as calcitonins, but these have been replaced by more selective and effective treatments.
- Other drugs such as strontium salts have been introduced in some but not all countries.
- The development of drugs for treating osteoporosis requires large trials and is expensive. Some drugs fail on grounds of efficacy or safety during development.

R.G.G. Russell, MD, PhD, FRS (✉)
Nuffield Department of Orthopaedics, Rheumatology and Musculoskeletal Sciences, The Botnar Research Centre and Oxford University Institute of Musculoskeletal Sciences, Oxford, UK

Department of Oncology and Human Metabolism, The Mellanby Centre for Bone Research, The University of Sheffield Medical School, Sheffield, UK
e-mail: graham.russell@ndorms.ox.ac.uk; Graham.Russell@sheffield.ac.uk

M.K. Tsoumpra, MRes, DPhil
M. Pazianas, MD
Nuffield Department of Orthopaedics, Rheumatology and Musculoskeletal Sciences, The Botnar Research Centre and Oxford University Institute of Musculoskeletal Sciences, Oxford, UK

M.A. Lawson, PhD • A.D. Chantry, MD, PhD
Department of Oncology and Human Metabolism, The Mellanby Centre for Bone Research, The University of Sheffield Medical School, Sheffield, UK

F.H. Ebetino, PhD
Chemistry Department, University of Rochester, Rochester, NY, USA

© Springer International Publishing Switzerland 2016
S.L. Silverman, B. Abrahamsen (eds.), *The Duration and Safety of Osteoporosis Treatment*, DOI 10.1007/978-3-319-23639-1_2

- Among the several SERMs (selective estrogen receptor modulators) studied, only raloxifene and bazedoxifene have been registered for clinical use.
- Similarly, several cathepsin K inhibitors have been studied, but among these, only odanacatib is close to being likely to be registered for clinical use.
- The pharmacological basis for the action of each of these drug classes is different, but reasonably well understood, and needs to be considered when determining the optimal ways they can be used in clinical practice.

Introduction and Overview

The use of drugs that inhibit bone resorption ("antiresorptives") continues to dominate the therapy of bone diseases, many of which are characterized by enhanced bone destruction. These disorders include not just osteoporosis but also Paget's disease of bone, myeloma, and bone metastases secondary to breast, prostate, and other cancers, as well as many less common acquired or inherited diseases such as osteogenesis imperfecta.

The term "antiresorptive" is used to refer to drugs that inhibit bone resorption, usually via direct or indirect actions on osteoclast development and action. Alternative terms such as "anticatabolic" are sometimes used to contrast with "anabolic" agents that stimulate bone formation [1]. "Anabolic" and "catabolic" can have pejorative meanings. A preferred simple nomenclature would be to talk about "bone resorption inhibitors" and "bone-forming agents."

For osteoporosis, treatments have historically included hormones, such as estrogens as well as calcitonins, which have been replaced by more effective treatments. Several SERMs (selective estrogen receptor modulators) such as raloxifene and bazedoxifene continue to be used. Other drugs such as strontium salts have been introduced in some but not all countries. Currently, the mainstay of treatment worldwide is still with bisphosphonates, which have been used clinically for more than 40 years and which can reduce fracture occurrence at vertebral and nonvertebral sites, including hips.

The most recently introduced new drug is the anti-RANK-ligand antibody, denosumab, which is also effective against these fractures. Several cathepsin K inhibitors have also been studied, but among these, only odanacatib is close to being likely to be registered for clinical use.

In this chapter, the pharmacological basis for the action of each of these drug classes will be briefly described, pointing out the similarities and differences among them. These properties need to be considered when determining the optimal ways they can be used in clinical practice.

There is a vast published literature about osteoporosis and its treatment, and many good reviews are available [2, 3]. For example, a search in PubMed using the term "bisphosphonates" reveals over 20,000 references. This chapter will provide only a few key references to the pharmacology and clinical results obtained with the various classes of drugs, which will be dealt with in a sequence that reflects their history and current scale of use.

How Drugs Are Discovered and Developed. The Role of Serendipity and Lessons from Rare Diseases

Drug discovery is an interesting process. The rewards of success can be great, but sadly more drugs fail than succeed during clinical development. The costs of developing drugs for osteoporosis are particularly high and may approach $1 billion to successfully complete the necessary phase 3 studies and to show fracture reduction in populations of 10,000–20,000 patients studied over several years.

Even though promising drugs such as estrogens, calcitonins, and bisphosphonates were emerging in the 1960s, large-scale trials were only contemplated and became feasible after the development of robust techniques for measuring bone mass. The development of bone densitometry (DXA) was therefore a critical step, enabling better diagnosis and assessment of response to treatment. The pharmaceutical industry only became seriously interested in osteoporosis as a therapeutic objective in the 1980s when medicinal chemists began to work on improving bisphosphonates and synthetic estrogens and also to design other small molecules such as protease inhibitors. The current approach to drug development is to start with defined molecular targets, many of them identified from the genetics of inherited skeletal disorders.

It is fascinating to note how the study of rare diseases has led us to many of the drugs now used for or being developed for treating skeletal diseases. Even the bisphosphonates, as stable chemical analogues of pyrophosphate, can be traced back to studies on the inherited disorder hypophosphatasia. In hypophosphatasia, the enzyme, alkaline phosphatase, is deficient, and the resulting increased levels of pyrophosphate, the body's natural water softener, contribute to the defective skeletal mineralization. Altered pyrophosphate metabolism also occurs in other calcification disorders, such as chondrocalcinosis and infantile vascular calcification. The bisphosphonates were first studied as analogues of pyrophosphate for their inhibitory effects on mineralization. Only when it was realized that they could also affect mineral dissolution were their effects on bone resorption evaluated, illustrating that serendipity has also played a role in drug discovery.

The development of denosumab and cathepsin K inhibitors can also both be traced back to the study of rare diseases. Among other potential antiresorptives derived from studies of various osteopetrotic disorders are src inhibitors, chloride channel blockers, and ATP proton pump inhibitors, but to date only denosumab, as an anti-RANK-ligand antibody, has been registered for clinical use. Similarly new bone-forming agents such as anti-sclerostin antibodies and dkk antagonists have their origin in studies of the genetics of wnt pathway modulators.

Although the many genetic discoveries underlying the osteopetroses and other high-bone-mass disorders have inspired many pharmacological approaches, the treatment of osteopetrotic syndromes themselves remains challenging, but marrow transplantation, or interferons, can be helpful in selected cases [4].

Bisphosphonates

The bisphosphonates (BPs) were originally called diphosphonates, and their biological effects were first reported in 1969 [5–7]. Their early use was for bone scintigraphy and the treatment of Paget's disease. Starting in the 1970s, this was extended to hypercalcemia of malignancy and then to the prevention of skeletal-related events in patients with myeloma or bone metastases. It was only much later in the 1990s, when bone densitometry became widely available and enabled quantitative diagnosis and evaluation of osteoporosis, that bisphosphonates (BPs) became firmly established as the leading drugs for the treatment of osteoporosis.

Over the years, many hundreds of BPs have been made, and more than a dozen have been studied in man. Although BPs share several common properties as a drug class, there are obvious chemical, biochemical, and pharmacological differences among the individual BPs that may help to explain observed clinical differences (Fig. 2.1).

Bisphosphonates have been used since the 1970s across the whole spectrum of bone resorption disorders, including Paget's disease and cancer-related bone destruction. Their exact molecular mechanisms of action are now better understood. Within bone, bisphosphonates are internalized selectively by osteoclasts and interfere with specific biochemical processes. The antiresorptive effects on osteoclasts of the nitrogen-containing BPs (including alendronate, risedronate, ibandronate, minodronate, and zoledronate) appear to result principally from their strong and selective inhibition of farnesyl pyrophosphate synthase (FPPS), a key enzyme in the mevalonate pathway of cholesterol biosynthesis. This pathway generates isoprenoid lipids utilized for the posttranslational modification (prenylation) of small GTP-binding proteins that are essential for osteoclast function.

The inhibition of farnesyl pyrophosphate synthase (FPPS) in the mevalonate pathway results in the accumulation of the upstream metabolite, isopentenyl pyrophosphate (IPP), that may be responsible for immunomodulatory effects on gamma delta ($\gamma\delta$) T cells. Accumulation of IPP can also lead to production of another ATP

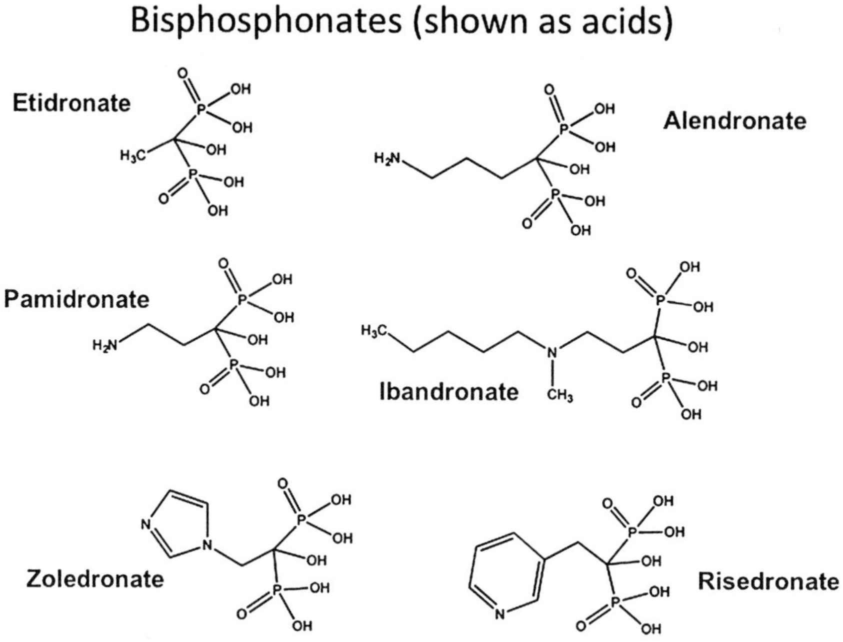

Fig. 2.1 Structures of major bisphosphonates used clinically

metabolite called ApppI, which has intracellular actions, including induction of apoptosis in osteoclasts. BPs may have other biologically important cellular effects on inhibiting osteoclast differentiation, on decreasing tumor cell viability, and on preventing osteocyte apoptosis, the latter possibly through other pathways, e.g., connexin channels [8].

The pharmacological effects of BPs as inhibitors of bone resorption appear to depend upon two key properties: their affinity for bone mineral and their inhibitory effects on osteoclasts [9]. There are differences in binding affinities for bone mineral among the clinically used BPs, which may influence their distribution within bone, their biological potency, and their duration of action. Although it is obvious that different BPs share many pharmacological properties, it is also obvious that every BP has a specific and often unique profile. Clinicians may understandably question whether these pharmacological differences are of practical importance. Based on the available data, we have proposed that these differences may be clinically relevant [10]. Thus, there is evidence to indicate that there may be differences among the BPs in terms of the speed of onset of fracture reduction, efficacy at different skeletal sites, and the degree and duration of reduction of bone turnover, which may influence how long to treat patients with individual drugs (Fig. 2.2).

Bisphosphonates are currently the leading drugs used worldwide for the treatment of osteoporosis. In randomized controlled trials (RCTs), alendronate, risedronate, and zoledronate have shown to reduce the risk of vertebral, nonvertebral, and hip fractures, whereas RCTs with ibandronate show anti-fracture efficacy at vertebral sites. The clinical effects of bisphosphonates on fracture reduction derived from RCTs and other studies are reviewed by Papapoulos in Chap. 15.

There are however difficulties with comparing the clinical effects of individual bisphosphonates with each other and with other antiresorptive drugs, because of the lack of direct comparisons in head-to-head clinical trials with appropriate endpoints (e.g., fracture). Despite this, using the

Explaining How Bisphosphonates Work
Each BP has a distinct profile

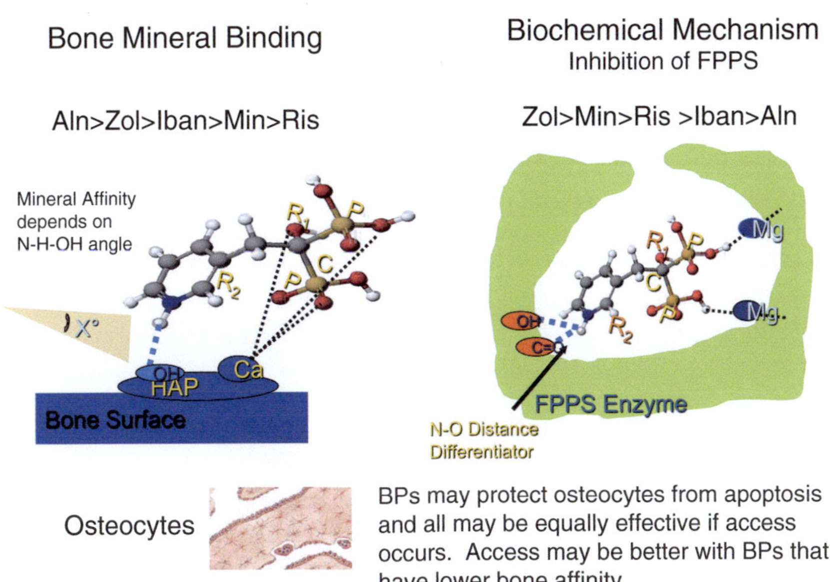

Fig. 2.2 Explaining how bisphosphonates work. They differ in their binding affinity for bone mineral and their inhibitory activity on farnesyl pyrophosphate synthase (FPPS). These properties contribute to the pharmacological potency and differences among the bisphosphonates

data generated from individual clinical studies, there is evidence for potential differences among BPs in terms of their clinical effects on speed of onset of fracture protection, sites of anti-fracture efficacy, and duration of effect. This may reflect their different profiles in terms of mineral binding properties and biochemical actions within cells.

Apart from the "big" four (alendronate, risedronate, zoledronate, ibandronate), other bisphosphonates also have been used in osteoporosis but have not achieved broad indications and been licensed for this indication. These include clodronate, pamidronate, tiludronate, neridronate, minodronate, and olpadronate. Etidronate was approved in most countries in the early 1990s. Pamidronate has been extensively used off-label for osteoporosis as it was the only intravenous bisphosphonate available before zoledronate. It is still used in the management of osteogenesis imperfecta [11].

In the case of osteoporosis, some of the currently debated topical issues include deciding whom to treat and for how long, which BP to use, and how to manage poor compliance [12]. In general, BPs have proved to be not only highly effective but also very safe drugs. Nonetheless, issues of side effects and adverse events attract often disproportionate attention, as with osteonecrosis of the jaw (ONJ) and atypical femoral (subtrochanteric) fractures (AFFs), where the nature of any association with BPs remains unclear [13]. This is discussed in other chapters in this book.

Bisphosphonates have now become largely generic drugs, as key patents have expired, but are likely to remain major drugs for treating bone diseases for some time to come. Advances continue to be made, such as producing formulations to overcome interference of intestinal absorption by food [14]. Novel bisphosphonates have been made with even greater potency and selectivity, but they will have to have added benefits if they are to compete with cheaper generics. In looking ahead, there are obvious opportunities for extending the use of BPs to other areas of medicine. Several recent studies suggest that BPs may be associated with other clinical benefits outside the field of bone diseases, e.g., on mortality, cardiovascular disease, and reduction of colon cancer. The pharmacology underlying these potential effects needs to be understood. Further intriguing examples of non-skeletal effects include inhibition of several protozoan parasites, increasing longevity in animal progeroid models, and enhancing human stem cell life span, DNA repair, and tissue regeneration. Several of these effects may be explained by modulation of the isoprenylation of proteins that have regulatory functions in many cell types. We may be entering an era in which BPs are viewed as modulators of mevalonate metabolism ("MMMs"), rather than as bone-active drugs. This research is opening up a wide range of new potential medical uses of bisphosphonates, including effects on T cells, tissue regeneration, radioprotection, and extension of life span.

Denosumab

Denosumab is a fully human monoclonal antibody against RANK ligand (RANKL) marketed under the name of Prolia® (Pralia® in Japan) for osteoporosis and Xgeva® for the prevention of skeletal complications in oncology. The discovery of the essential role of RANK ligand and of RANK signaling in osteoclast differentiation, activity, and survival led the way to developing denosumab. Denosumab acts by binding to and inhibiting RANKL from binding to RANK, leading to the loss of osteoclasts from bone surfaces.

RANK ligand is one of the two cytokines that are essential and sufficient to induce osteoclast differentiation. The other is the macrophage colony-stimulating factor (M-CSF). M-CSF binds to c-Fms, a single transmembrane domain receptor of the tyrosine kinase family, and RANKL binds to RANK, a single transmembrane receptor of the tumor necrosis factor (TNF) receptor family, which forms trimers upon ligand binding. The role of M-CSF is to first activate the proliferation and survival of cells of the monocyte–macrophage lineage and the expression of RANK, allowing the action of RANKL, which, together with M-CSF, constitutes an absolute requirement for commitment to and progression of early precursors along the osteoclast lineage. The differentiation step from osteoclast precursors to multinucleated osteoclasts is then induced by RANKL, again through the M-CSF-dependent expression of RANK at the cell surface of these early precursors. M-CSF and RANKL are both secreted by bone marrow stromal cells and osteoblasts, whereas RANKL is also secreted by T cells and to a lesser extent by B cells. The other component of the RANKL/RANK system is osteoprotegerin (OPG), which is a shed extracellular portion of the RANK receptor. Most of the cells producing RANKL also produce this decoy RANK receptor, OPG, which acts as an antagonist to RANK signaling and osteoclastogenesis by scavenging RANKL in the extracellular environment. OPG is also a regulated molecule, and it is the ratio between RANKL and OPG which determines the level of activation of RANK and therefore the extent to which osteoclast production and function is activated. All these molecules are thought to act in a paracrine manner and to regulate bone resorption locally. The overall endocrine regulation of skeletal homeostasis involves interactions between systemic hormones and the RANKL/RANK/OPG system. The expression and secretion of both RANKL and OPG are regulated by several calcium-regulating hormones, including estrogens, parathyroid hormone (PTH), and vitamin D3.

The first attempts to develop therapeutics based on these pathways utilized a chimeric OPG-Fc fusion protein to antagonize RANKL. However, the formation of neutralizing antibodies against OPG after administration of the fusion protein and its potential cross-reactivity with tumor necrosis factor-related apoptosis-inducing ligand (TRAIL) led to the more attractive strategy of inhibiting RANKL directly using denosumab.

The key pharmacological differences between denosumab and the bisphosphonates reside in the distribution of the drugs within bone and their effects on precursors and mature osteoclasts [15]. This may explain differences in the degree and rapidity of reduction of bone resorption, their potential differential effects on trabecular and cortical bone, and the reversibility of their actions.

In the FREEDOM pivotal phase 3 clinical trial, denosumab was shown to significantly reduce vertebral, non-vertebral, and hip fractures by 68 %, 20 %, and 40 %, respectively, compared with placebo. In the FREEDOM study, 7808 women with postmenopausal osteoporosis were randomized to receive denosumab 60 mg subcutaneously once every 6 months or placebo [16]. FREEDOM is the acronym for the Fracture Reduction Evaluation of Denosumab in Osteoporosis every 6 Months study.

These and further studies involving over 12,000 patients have confirmed the efficacy and overall safety of denosumab [17–20], out to 8 years of treatment in the ongoing extension studies. Denosumab treatment increased BMD at the total hip, lumbar spine, and/or femoral neck and reduced markers of bone turnover to a significantly greater extent than oral bisphosphonates in women who had not received bisphosphonates at all or in the recent past or in those who had switched from alendronate to denosumab treatment.

There are several respects in which the differences between bisphosphonates and denosumab have practical consequences. It appears that the effects of denosumab to increase BMD continue on prolonged treatment, whereas they may plateau earlier on bisphosphonates.

Denosumab may also have a greater impact on protecting cortical bone than bisphosphonates, which is likely to contribute to its efficacy in reducing fractures.

However, the effects of denosumab rapidly reverse when treatment stops which means that ensuring compliance is even more important if potential benefits are to be sustained. Another difference is the potential use of denosumab in patients with impaired renal function, in whom use of bisphosphonates is contraindicated.

Estrogens: Background and Current Status

The recognition that the decline in estrogen production at the menopause was associated with bone loss dates back to the time of Albright more than half a century ago. The use of estrogens as HRT (ERT or hormone replacement therapy) in postmenopausal women was therefore a logical approach toward alleviating the symptoms and consequences of the menopause. After the link between menopause and osteoporosis was first identified, estrogen treatment became the standard means for preventing bone loss, even though there was no fracture data. This changed dramatically when results from the Women's Health Initiative (WHI) study were published, which showed an increase in heart attacks and breast cancer [21]. Even though the risks were small, this prompted a large drop off in estrogen use. In later analyses, the WHI study showed that estrogen reduced fractures and actually prevented heart attacks in the 50–60-year age group. Estrogen alone appeared to be safer to use than estrogen plus the progestin medroxyprogesterone acetate and actually reduced breast cancer. The overall benefits and risks of estrogens are now better appreciated and are being continuously reappraised [22, 23]. In one analysis of hysterectomized women, it was estimated that by avoiding estrogen, there had been ~50,000 extra deaths from 2002 to 2011 [24]. Currently, it is widely accepted that estrogens are effective in relieving menopausal symptoms and in preventing perimenopausal bone loss, as well as having other potential benefits, but their use as first-line therapy in osteoporosis is no longer appropriate.

The way in which estrogens act on bone and indeed on other tissues is complex. Estrogens may have direct effects on bone cells, but many of their effects may be indirect, mediated, for example, by reducing the actions of the RANK-ligand system on osteoclast differentiation. Estrogens exert their cellular effects mainly by binding to estrogen receptors (α & β), which are members of the large family of nuclear hormone receptors that regulate the transcription of specific genes. The different cofactors present in various tissues result in differential effects of individual ER ligands in key target tissues [25].

Estrogens can also exert rapid cellular responses by non-genomic mechanisms by binding to another type of receptor, called the G protein-coupled estrogen receptor 1 (GPER), formerly referred to as G protein-coupled receptor 30 (GPR30). GPER is an integral membrane protein with high affinity for estradiol and is a member of the rhodopsin-like family of G protein-coupled receptors.

Selective Estrogen Receptor Modulators

Selective estrogen receptor modulators (SERMs) are a diverse group of naturally occurring or synthetic nonsteroidal compounds that exhibit tissue-specific estrogen receptor (ER) agonist or antagonist activity, i.e., they can act as estrogens on some tissues but antiestrogens on others. The biochemical basis for differential actions on various target tissues is most likely to be due to the different conformation changes induced in the receptor after binding to individual ligands. These conformational changes in the ER in turn result in different patterns of binding to various coactivators and corepressor molecules, thereby leading to distinctive patterns of gene transcription and protein expression in the various target tissues.

The pharmacological profile of individual SERMs is therefore determined by the effects observed on the key target tissues that are important for human health. An ideal SERM would therefore have positive effects on the cardiovascular system and bone, without stimulating breast or endometrial tissue and raising the risk of cancer. Attempts to meet this ideal profile have been partially successful with currently approved SERMs such as raloxifene and bazedoxifene. However, it has so far proved impossible to wean out the adverse effects of provoking hot flushes or venous thrombosis from any of the individual SERMs in current clinical use. There are several comprehensive reviews of estrogens and SERMs available [26, 27].

Many different molecules with estrogen agonist or antagonist activity have been synthesized and evaluated experimentally. Several have been examined for their clinical potential. Some have failed to progress on account of unacceptable side effects or lack of desired efficacy. These include droloxifene, idoxifene, and arzoxifene. Overall, there have been more failures than successes in clinical development. There are currently only two SERMs approved for use of osteoporosis, namely, raloxifene and bazedoxifene (Fig. 2.3).

Estradiol & Different Classes of SERM Structures

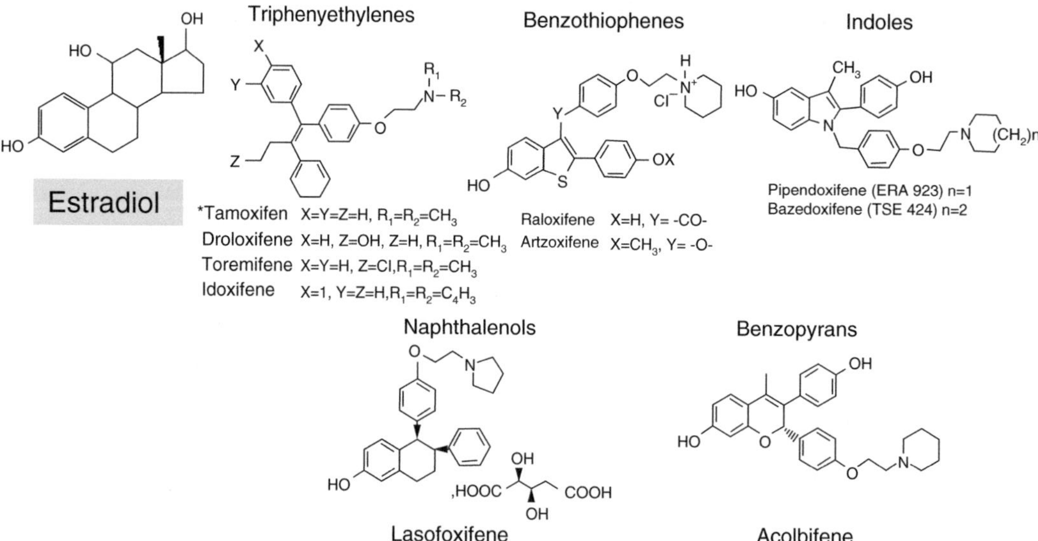

Fig. 2.3 Structures of estradiol and of various SERMs. It is interesting to note how many of the SERMs have two –OH groups separated by a similar distance to that found in estradiol, which contributes to their binding to the estrogen receptor (ER)

The earliest SERMs developed for clinical use were agents such as clomiphene, still used for induction of ovulation, and tamoxifen used as an antiestrogen in the management of breast cancer. Currently, other FDA-approved SERMs include toremifene, also used for prevention and treatment of breast cancer, and ospemifene approved for treatment of dyspareunia from menopausal vaginal atrophy. Raloxifene is approved for the prevention and treatment of osteoporosis and prevention of invasive breast cancer. Bazedoxifene is also approved in many countries either as a single agent but interestingly also as a combined preparation with estrogen. This tissue-selective estrogen complex (TSEC) involves a pairing of conjugated equine estrogens with bazedoxifene and is approved by the FDA. This pairing is designed to reduce the risk of endometrial hyperplasia that can occur with the estrogenic component of the TSEC without the need for a progestogen in women with a uterus. The combination also allows for the estrogen to control hot flushes and to prevent bone loss without stimulating the breast or the endometrium.

Although bisphosphonates remain first-line therapy for most patients, SERMs such as raloxifene and bazedoxifene provide a safe and effective alternative to bisphosphonates for women who are unable to tolerate bisphosphonates and for younger women with an increased risk of fracture who may remain on therapy for many years [28, 29].

Raloxifene

The first SERM developed specifically for use in osteoporosis was raloxifene, which interestingly had also being previously studied by Lilly but discontinued for its potential as an anti-breast cancer agent. Raloxifene is an estrogen agonist in bone and the liver. It increases BMD and reduces LDL cholesterol. It does not stimulate the endometrium and is a potent antiestrogen in the breast. There have been many clinical studies with raloxifene. In the large Multiple Outcomes of Raloxifene Evaluation (MORE) trial, a total of 7705 women who had a mean age of 65 years (low bone mass group) and 68 years (osteoporosis group) were randomly assigned to raloxifene (60 or 120 mg) or placebo daily and were followed up for a total of 8 years. There were significant increases in BMD at the spine and hip, and the risk of vertebral fracture was significantly reduced by 30 and 50 %, respectively, with raloxifene at 60 or 120 mg/day compared with placebo. There was no effect on non-vertebral fractures, but importantly treatment with raloxifene reduced the incidence of invasive and invasive estrogen receptor-positive breast cancers by more than 60 %

Bazedoxifene

Bazedoxifene is a novel synthetic "third-generation" estrogen agonist–antagonist, with an attractive experimental and clinical profile, with apparent added advantages when used in combination with conjugated estrogen (20 mg bazedoxifene plus 0.45 mg CE).

Several clinical studies have been reported, showing increases in BMD at the spine and also at the hip. In the pivotal phase III treatment study of bazedoxifene, 7492 healthy postmenopausal women (average age, 66 year) were randomly assigned to daily oral doses of bazedoxifene 20 or 40 mg, raloxifene 60 mg, or placebo. There was a reduction in spine fractures on all doses at 3 years of 42 % for bazedoxifene at 20 mg, 37 % for the 40 mg dose, and 42 % for raloxifene at 60 mg [30]. The efficacy of bazedoxifene was sustained through 5 and 7 years of treatment as observed in the extensions of the core trial [31].

Bazedoxifene reduced non-vertebral fractures when results from both doses were combined, and this became more evident when higher-risk groups were studied. A recent analysis of the data using FRAX® indicates that reductions in non-vertebral fractures appear to be greater than with raloxifene in the higher-risk groups [32].

Bazedoxifene treatment was not associated with detectable effects on risk of breast cancer, or cardiovascular outcomes, but had positive effects on lipid profiles. Bazedoxifene had neutral effects on the reproductive tract and was not associated with increases in endometrial thickness or increases in the rate of endometrial hyperplasia or carcinoma. Increases in venous thrombosis events were noted, which were not unexpected, since they were already well known to occur with estrogens and other SERMs.

Lasofoxifene

Lasofoxifene is another synthetic estrogen agonist–antagonist (SERM). It has a high affinity for both ERs, in a similar range to estradiol, and an order of magnitude higher than raloxifene, tamoxifen, or droloxifene. It has better oral bioavailability than several other SERMs.

Two doses of lasofoxifene 0.25 and 0.5 mg daily were evaluated in a large phase 3 double-blind, randomized trial, denoted as the PEARL (Postmenopausal Evaluation and Risk Reduction with Lasofoxifene) trial. A total of 8556 women were initially enrolled, and assessment of outcomes at 5 years was completed for 6614 (~77 %) of these [33]. There were significant increases in both lumbar spine and femoral neck BMD relative to placebo. There was a reduction in the risk of vertebral fractures by 31 % and 42 % with lasofoxifene given at 0.25 mg and 0.5 mg/day, respectively, while non-vertebral fractures were significantly reduced by 22 % with the 0.5 mg/day dose. The higher dose of lasofoxifene reduced the risk of total breast cancer by 79 % and of ER-positive invasive breast cancer by 83 % and the lower dose by 49 %.

Treatment with 0.5 mg of lasofoxifene per day was also associated with a reduction in major coronary heart disease events and stroke and was not associated with an increase in the risk of endometrial cancer or endometrial hyperplasia. However, reports of leg cramps, hot flushes, endometrial hypertrophy, uterine polyps, and vaginal candidiasis were significantly more common in women assigned to lasofoxifene than in those assigned to placebo.

Although lasofoxifene received approval for use in the European Union countries, it has never been marketed, despite the encouraging clinical results and fracture data compared with other SERMs.

Strontium

Strontium ranelate emerged in the 1990s as a potential treatment for osteoporosis. It was initially portrayed as an uncoupling agent, which stimulated bone formation while decreasing bone resorption. This was an attractive profile for a new drug for osteoporosis. The proposed dual mechanism of action even led to the introduction of the term "DABA" (dual-acting bone agent).

Two large pivotal phase 3 trials (Spinal Osteoporosis Therapeutic Intervention (SOTI) and Treatment of Peripheral Osteoporosis (TROPOS)) were conducted within a total of 6740 Caucasian women with postmenopausal osteoporosis. In these trials, strontium ranelate showed efficacy in reducing fractures [34].

Strontium is the active component, while ranelate is an anion that enabled patent protection. Despite its apparent efficacy in reducing fractures, the mechanism by which this is achieved remains unclear [35]. The effects on bone resorption and formation are small, but there are substantial changes in BMD measurements largely due to substitution of strontium for calcium in bone mineral. It is known that strontium apatites have different solubility and physical characteristics than the calcium-containing hydroxyapatites and related minerals normally present in bone. Strontium salts have been used in the dental field as toothpaste additives for their protective effects on mineral dissolution. The simple classification of strontium as a dual-acting agent or an antiresorptive drug does not properly reflect these other properties on the physicochemical behavior of bone mineral, which may be an important part of its pharmacological actions.

Strontium ranelate has been quite widely used in osteoporosis treatment in several countries particularly in the elderly. Safety concerns about sensitivity reactions, venous thrombosis, and adverse cardiovascular effects are now limiting its use.

Calcitonins

Calcitonin is a peptide hormone secreted by the C-cells of the thyroid gland, which lowers blood calcium by inhibiting bone resorption. It acts directly on osteoclasts to produce a temporary cessation of their resorptive activity. Calcitonins were first used therapeutically in the 1970s for Paget's disease of bone, in which they were moderately active. The potencies of calcitonins vary according to the species of origin, and porcine, human, and salmon calcitonins have all been used to varying extents in clinical practice. Salmon calcitonin emerged as the preferred of these, predominantly and curiously because it is more potent than human. It was eventually developed as a nasal inhalation rather than being given by injection. Studies with salmon calcitonin in osteoporosis only showed weak anti-fracture effects, and its use has been superseded by more effective treatments. Recent studies with oral calcitonin have also proved disappointing.

Calcitonin is still sometimes used for pain relief after vertebral fracture. The nasal forms of calcitonin have been recently withdrawn by the CHMP because of concerns about cancer risk.

Cathepsin K Protease Inhibitors

Cathepsin K (Cat K) is one of the primary enzymes involved in degrading type I collagen, the major component of the organic bone matrix. Cathepsin K is a member of the papain family of cysteine proteases and is highly expressed by activated osteoclasts but also in other cell types, giving rise to potential off-target effects (the skin, lungs, etc.). Cathepsins are lysosomal proteases that belong to the papain-like cysteine protease family. There are 11 different types (B, C, F, H, K, L, O, S, V, X, and W). There is incomplete homology of these enzymes among animal species, making animal experiments sometimes misleading. Making selective inhibitors is difficult but key to success. There has been intense activity in the pharmaceutical industry to create inhibitors as illustrated by the many patents that have been issued [36] (Fig. 2.4).

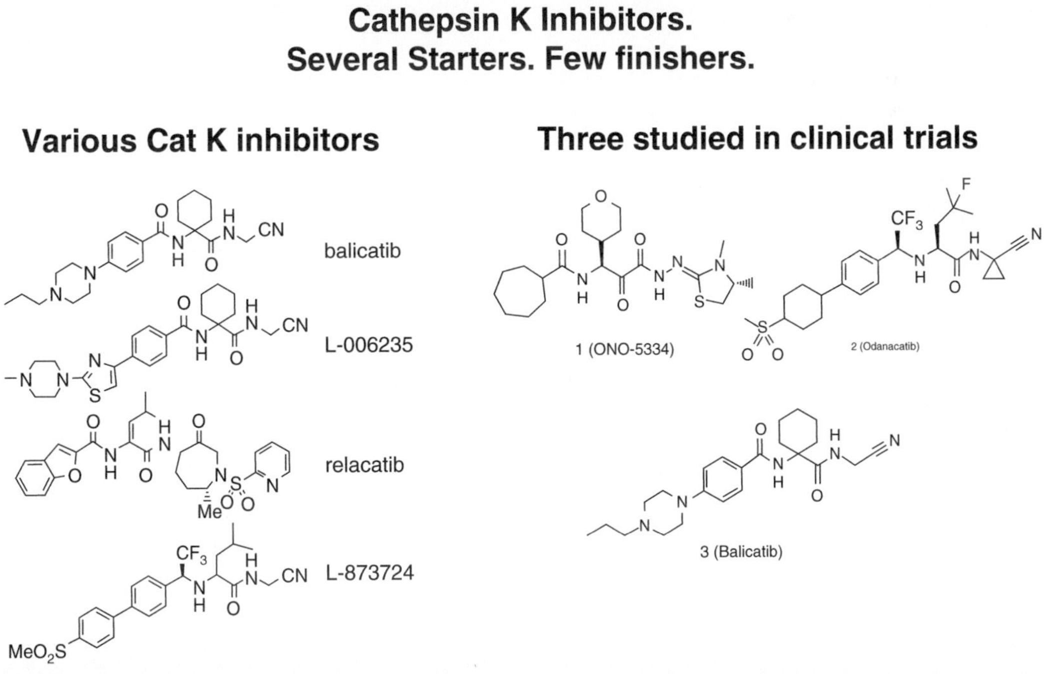

Fig. 2.4 Structures of various cathepsin K inhibitors. As discussed in the text, only odanacatib has been shown to reduce fractures in a phase 3 trial

Loss-of-function mutations in the cathepsin K gene lead to pycnodysostosis, a disorder characterized by osteosclerosis, bone fragility, and decreased bone turnover. This discovery led to a flurry of research activity especially in the mid-1990s. Cathepsin K therefore became an attractive therapeutic target in osteoporosis and also potentially in osteoarthritis and bone cancers. The concept is scientifically interesting and illustrates the process of modern drug design and development, based on identifying a target (cathepsin K) and then using medicinal chemistry to design and synthesize selective inhibitors [37]. Key components of a clinically viable inhibitor are oral bioavailability, high selectivity over related cathepsins, and a covalent, reversible warhead to bind to the active-site cysteine of the enzyme.

There have been many hurdles encountered during the discovery and development of cathepsin K inhibitors as drugs. These include species differences in amino acid sequences in the critical site of the target enzyme, species differences in bone metabolism, and also discrepancies between pharmacokinetic and pharmacodynamic (PK/PD) profiles due to unique tissue distribution of the inhibitor affecting both efficacy and side effects, originating from idiosyncratic intracellular or tissue distribution of some classes of compounds [38]. The antiresorptive properties of several cathepsin K inhibitors have been studied in phase I and phase II clinical trials. Phase III studies have recently been completed for odanacatib, the only cathepsin K inhibitor for which fracture reduction has been shown. Overall and despite the involvement of "big Pharma," there have been more failures than successes in this field so far, with several "failures" in the development of Cat K inhibitors (e.g., balicatib, relacatib; see below).

The impetus to develop a new class of antiresorptives has been further driven by the fact that they are not bisphosphonates, which now carry a burden of perceived but exaggerated safety issues (ONJ, AFF, etc.). The development of cathepsin K inhibitors has been further encouraged by the notion that inhibition of cathepsin K may partially uncouple the link between reduction in bone resorption and bone formation, allowing bone formation to continue while bone resorption is reduced [39]. This may lead to greater increases in bone mass (BMD) including at cortical sites.

Whether these theoretical benefits will eventually translate into a greater reduction of fractures and long-term benefits is still uncertain, even after the outcome of the trials with odanacatib have been announced.

Balicatib

Balicatib (AAE-581) was one of the early inhibitors, investigated by Novartis, but has now been abandoned. It is a nitrile-based compound and was a highly selective inhibitor of cathepsin K in enzyme assays, but not so selective in living cells, an effect attributed to lysosomotropism. Thus, it accumulates in lysosomes and can reach inhibitory levels against other cathepsins that are present in these compartments.

Two phase II trials (in osteoarthritis and osteopenia/osteoporosis), designed as multicenter, randomized, double-blind, placebo-controlled studies, were completed, using daily oral doses of balicatib (5, 10, 25, or 50 mg for 12 months).

Although the oral daily doses were generally well tolerated, there were a greater number of skin reactions, mainly reported as pruritus, in patients taking the study medication (particularly the 50 mg dose) compared with the placebo group. Despite the favorable skeletal endpoints, balicatib trials were discontinued due to dermatologic adverse effects, including a morphea-like syndrome. These off-target dermatologic events might be explained by the lysosomotropism of this basic compound, potentially leading to inhibition of cathepsins B, L, and S expressed in skin fibroblasts.

Relacatib

Relacatib (SB-462795) is a monobasic, α-heteroatom cyclic ketone that nonselectively acts on cathepsins K, L, and V and was initially developed for oral use by SKB and subsequently by GlaxoSmithKline after the companies merged [40].

Clinical studies were discontinued after a phase I osteoporosis/osteoarthritis trial showed possible drug–drug interactions with paracetamol (acetaminophen), ibuprofen, and atorvastatin. This adverse profile with medications that are commonly prescribed to patients with osteoporosis and osteoarthritis led to the decision to halt the further development of this compound.

ONO-5334

ONO-5334 is a hydrazine-based cathepsin K inhibitor originally developed by Ono Pharmaceuticals in Japan [41]. Phase II results have shown efficacy on BMD and biomarkers, when dosed daily up to 300 mg [42]. Overall, all doses of ONO-5334 were well tolerated, and no differences in the rate of dermal or subcutaneous adverse events were observed across study groups. Despite these potentially encouraging results, the company announced in May 2012 that it was discontinuing development "taking into consideration competitiveness as well as marketing conditions in osteoporosis area."

Odanacatib

Odanacatib (MK-0822), a non-basic and non-lysosomotropic nitrile-based molecule, is currently under development by Merck. It is highly selective for cathepsin K, compared with other cathepsins (B, L, and S) that are widely expressed, particularly in the skin. Odanacatib is cleverly designed to avoid uptake by lysosomes, thereby hopefully also minimizing off-target effects [43]. The non-lysosomotropic property is probably very important, as is the long half-life (>60 h) in humans, which enables once-weekly treatment.

Phase 2 results have been published and are encouraging up to 5 years using once-weekly dosing [44]. Overall, all doses were well tolerated and adverse events, with special attention to the skin and pulmonary events, were similar in the treatment and placebo groups.

The pivotal phase 3 fracture trial was called LOFT (the Long-Term Odanacatib Fracture Trial). LOFT is a randomized, double-blind, placebo-controlled, event-driven trial. LOFT enrolled 16,713 women with osteoporosis, 65 years of age or older (mean age 73), from 40 countries, and had been in progress for 5 years before the results were presented in 2014 [45]. Treatment was with odanacatib 50 mg once a week or placebo, and the mean duration of therapy was 34 months. All patients received vitamin D (5600 IU/week) and calcium up to 1200 mg/day, if required.

The LOFT trial met its primary endpoints and demonstrated a significant reduction in the risk of three types of osteoporotic fracture (hip, spine, and non-vertebral fractures) compared to placebo in the primary efficacy analysis and also reduced the risk of the secondary endpoint of clinical vertebral fractures by 72 %. Specifically, there was a 54 % relative risk reduction of new and worsening morphometric (radiographically assessed) vertebral fractures and a reduction of 23 % in non-vertebral fractures. A total of 237 hip fractures occurred in this event-driven trial, and odanacatib produced a 47 % reduction in hip fractures compared with placebo.

In addition, treatment with odanacatib led to progressive increases over 5 years in bone mineral density (BMD) at the lumbar spine and total hip, compared to placebo. The change in BMD from baseline at 5 years with odanacatib for lumbar spine was 11.2 % and for total hip was 9.5 %.

The rates of adverse events overall in LOFT were generally balanced between patients taking odanacatib and placebo. Adjudicated events of morphea-like skin lesions and atypical femoral fractures occurred more often in the odanacatib group than in the placebo group. Adjudicated major adverse cardiovascular events were generally balanced overall between the treatment groups. There were numerically more adjudicated stroke events with odanacatib than with placebo. Adjudicated atypical femoral shaft fractures were reported for 5 patients in the odanacatib group (incidence of 0.1 %) and not reported in patients in the placebo group. There were no adjudicated cases of osteonecrosis of the jaw.

There has been an expectation that the responses to a cathepsin K inhibitor might be

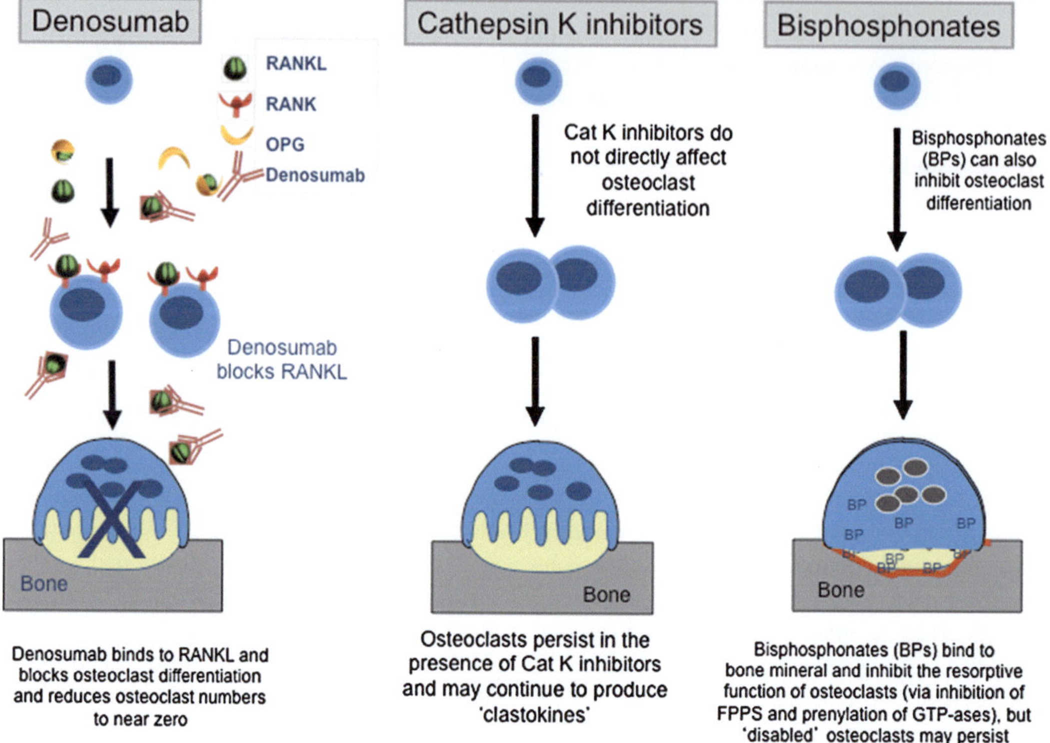

Fig. 2.5 Scheme to illustrate differences in the way denosumab, cathepsin K inhibitors, and bisphosphonates act on osteoclast differentiation and function. Denosumab inhibits osteoclast production, whereas cathepsin K inhibitors do not. Bisphosphonates act both on osteoclast differentiation and function, resulting in impaired resorptive activity and persistence of "crippled" osteoclasts

different from other antiresorptive drugs. In the early preclinical and clinical studies with odanacatib, the extent of reduction in biochemical markers of bone resorption was dose-dependent, but the effects on bone formation biomarkers seemed less than with other drugs such as bisphosphonates or denosumab. This suggested that it might be possible to dissociate inhibition of bone resorption from a reduction in bone formation favoring a better response in terms of potential fracture reduction (Fig. 2.5).

The underlying pharmacology and cellular actions of cathepsin K inhibitors differ from other bone-active drugs. Because these inhibitors act on a protease and affect matrix degradation rather than osteoclast differentiation or apoptosis, the number of osteoclasts and their function should not be reduced. This may allow osteoclast to osteoblast communication, e.g., via "clasto-kine" signaling, that contributes to maintaining bone formation while suppressing bone resorption. It may also explain why the rebound bone loss seems to be rapid and possibly excessive, when a patient discontinues treatment.

If successfully registered, odanacatib will be the first cathepsin K inhibitor to enter the market, but will have to compete with cheap generic drugs especially bisphosphonates, as well as with denosumab.

Other Pharmacological Agents That May Act as Resorption Inhibitors

There are a number of other drugs that are being explored as resorption inhibitors. Most of these are being derived from knowledge of the genetic basis of osteoclast dysfunction in animal models and inherited human diseases. Those mentioned below are examples where there is data from clinical studies, but none of these are yet approved for treating osteoporosis or other bone diseases.

Saracatinib

The impairment of osteoclast function in src-deficient mice provided the rationale for exploring the skeletal effects of src kinase inhibitors. The src kinase inhibitor saracatinib (AZD0530) was shown to inhibit bone resorption in a phase 1 clinical trial. Despite some side effects, saracatinib is still being explored in phase 2 studies for osteosarcoma and bone metastases, but not osteoporosis.

Glucagon-Like Peptide (GLP)-2

It is known that bone resorption biomarkers fall after feeding and there is a circadian pattern in bone remodeling which increases at night. One of the underlying mechanisms involves the release of glucagon-like peptide (GLP)-2, in response to food. Administration of GLP-2 is an experimental clinical approach to modifying bone loss at night.

Other Osteoclast Functional Targets

One approach to inhibiting bone resorption has been to target the $\alpha v \beta 3$ integrin involved in the attachment of the osteoclast to bone and the formation of the sealing zone. Antibodies and peptide inhibitors have been evaluated, but seem no longer to be being pursued as serious drug candidates. Other experimental strategies involve inhibition of Atp6v0d2, a subunit of v-ATPase that is required for acidification by the osteoclast, and the voltage-gated chloride channel ClC-7, for which an inhibitor NS3736 has been shown to prevent bone loss in ovariectomized rats. These are all theoretical targets for osteoporosis and other disorders of bone resorption, but it is not clear whether any of them will be developed further for clinical use.

Nitrates

Several organic nitrates, which can act as nitric oxide donors, have been used in medicine for many years for the treatment of angina. There are several studies showing that nitric oxide may be one of the many locally active mediators produced endogenously in bone that can modulate bone resorption and formation.

This has led to an interest in whether nitrates might be used in osteoporosis, and this has been studied by epidemiological approaches as well as in clinical trials [46]. Nitrates appear to increase BMD, but effects on fractures are so far inconclusive.

Headaches are a common adverse event among women taking nitrates, and this may limit their attractiveness as a potential therapy.

Vitamin D and Calcium

The importance of vitamin D and calcium for bone health is well known. Any deficiencies or insufficiencies of either should be corrected prior to giving specific treatments for osteoporosis. In addition, the adjustment of the daily calcium intake to 1200 mg using diet or supplements and ensuring adequate vitamin D (~800 IU/day) to maintain a serum 25-hydroxyvitamin D level greater than 20 ng/mL (50 nmol/L) are still recommended as part of routine management during therapy. In many placebo-controlled trials, there is evidence from changes in BMD and bone markers that this type of supplementation with vitamin D and calcium reduces bone turnover in its own right. There is also reasonably good evidence that vitamin D and calcium supplementation may reduce fractures on their own, particularly when given to elderly populations who may be deficient.

In most of the pivotal clinical trials of anti-osteoporotic treatments with fracture endpoints, all patients receive vitamin D and calcium supplements, so any effects of pharmacological interventions on fracture prevention are over and above those that can be obtained with vitamin D and calcium alone.

The routine use of vitamin D and calcium supplementation has recently been questioned as a result of studies suggesting that there may be an increased risk of cardiovascular and other adverse events in patients receiving high intakes of calcium [47]. This topic remains controversial but is already having an impact on recommendations about how patients should be managed.

Combination and Sequential Treatments

There are steadily increasing numbers of drugs available for the treatment of osteoporosis, which increases the number of choices available to individual patients. This raises a number of questions. One is which drugs should be used first for treatment and if there is any preferred sequence. Will any of the drugs interfere with the action of the next? Furthermore, can drugs be used concurrently?

A full discussion is beyond the scope of this chapter, but a few examples will illustrate some of the issues. Several clinical studies indicate that prior or concurrent treatment with raloxifene or with bisphosphonates such as alendronate may interfere with the subsequent anabolic response to parathyroid hormone (PTH). Interestingly, this seems not to occur with zoledronate. Although it seems illogical to give two antiresorptive drugs concurrently, it does seem that additional reduction of bone turnover can be attained when denosumab is given after a bisphosphonate. Combining an antiresorptive drug with a bone-forming agent has attractions, and several examples of success with such combinations include the combinations of estrogens with PTH and also of zoledronate or denosumab with PTH [48]. Such combinations can achieve greater changes in BMD than with either drug alone but remain experimental and have not so far been shown to produce added reductions in fractures. Another important example of drug combinations is the use of bone resorption inhibitors to preserve the bone gain achieved during finite courses of treatment with bone-forming agents such as teriparatide or PTH analogues and possibly in the future with anti-sclerostin treatment.

Here, the drugs are used in sequence with, for example, bisphosphonates or denosumab being used to follow a course of teriparatide [49].

Effects of Antiresorptive Drugs on Bone Repair Mechanisms and Fracture Healing

There is a widespread assumption that antiresorptive drugs might impair fracture healing. This has not been borne out in practice. From the earliest days of bisphosphonate research, this issue has been explored experimentally and clinically. There are reassuring reports that show this is not a problem in several animal models unless very high doses of BPs are used. Furthermore, in the major clinical studies with the antiresorptive drugs, there has been no evidence of delayed fracture healing or malunion.

The biology of fracture healing is now well understood [50], and there is great interest in finding therapeutic strategies to improve the process [51]. The temporal sequence of events involves vascular invasion, production of a cartilaginous callus, and its subsequent ossification. There is no early stage in this process at which antiresorptive drugs would be expected to impair the process. It is only during the latter stages of remodeling of the calcified callus that one would expect antiresorptive drugs to have an impact.

In contrast to these concerns, there are now several reports suggesting that BPs may actually enhance fracture repair [52], probably by stabilizing the fracture callus [53].

Other Uses of Antiresorptive Drugs

There are in fact many potential applications of BPs in orthopedics [54]. These include protection against loosening of prostheses [55], better integration of biomaterials and implants [56], improved healing in distraction osteogenesis, and conserving bone architecture in hips affected by Perthes disease or osteonecrosis [57].

Another potential application of antiresorptive drugs is in osteoarthritis. The underlying rationale includes modulating the excessive subchondral bone remodeling and perhaps preventing cartilage damage directly. Several studies have been conducted with bisphosphonates and also with strontium. A reduction in the cartilage resorption marker, CTX-II derived from type 2 collagen, has been seen with several bone antiresorptives, including bisphosphonates, calcitonin, and even strontium. This probably represents blocking of osteoclast-mediated resorption of calcified cartilage. Whether this type of therapy is likely to be clinically beneficial in OA is still unclear.

Conclusions and Future Prospects

Despite the impressive advances that have taken place in the past 20 years in the diagnosis and management of osteoporosis, we are still a long way from being able to offer a "cure" to patients. Antiresorptive agents are still the predominant therapeutic means we have for preventing bone loss and fractures, and reductions of 40–70 % can be achieved for vertebral fractures and up to ~40 % for non-vertebral fractures. The ability of current treatments to reduce hip fractures by 40 % or more in certain groups of patients is encouraging in terms of its impact on individuals and on health-care costs.

Is it possible to do better? Clearly improved identification of patients at risk and ensuring compliance should reduce fractures at a population level. However, it may be hard to achieve better anti-fracture efficacy than already reported for the bisphosphonates or denosumab. Several drugs intended for osteoporosis have failed during clinical development, notably several SERMs including lasofoxifene despite favorable effects on fractures. Others such as the cathepsin K inhibitor, Ono 5334, were suspended from further study, not because of safety or efficacy issues but apparently for commercial reasons.

Will the current efforts being devoted to developing new drugs overcome these obstacles [58]? It has long been hoped that bone-forming drugs would eventually outperform antiresorptives and achieving that aspiration now depends on the outcome of trials with anti-sclerostin antibodies [59, 60]. Sclerostin is an inhibitor of the wnt signaling pathway [61] and is a physiological regulator of bone formation. Genetic deficiencies in sclerostin lead to marked increases in bone mass in the inherited disorders of van Buchem's disease and sclerosteosis. Romosozumab and blosozumab are anti-sclerostin antibodies, which produce rapid and marked increases in BMD. These biologics are being evaluated in clinical trials, and early data looks promising [62, 63].

We have to hope that these new approaches to promote endogenous wnt signaling plus the creative use of drug combinations will change the landscape and encourage further innovation. But will the pharmaceutical industry have the appetite for clinical development programs that would take at least 5 years to complete and incur huge costs? A glimmer of hope resides on the possibility of new drugs having additional applications in the management of bone diseases. It should be remembered that for preventing skeletal-related events in cancer indications, zoledronate and denosumab represent the "standard of care" for many patients with cancer. There are many other unmet medical needs, not only in cancer but also including fracture healing, implant fixation, and osteoarthritis to name just a few.

References[1]

1. Riggs BL, Parfitt AM. Drugs used to treat osteoporosis: the critical need for a uniform nomenclature based on their action on bone remodeling. J Bone Miner Res. 2005;20(2):177–84.
2. Appelman-Dijkstra NM, Papapoulos SE. Prevention of incident fractures in patients with prevalent fragility fractures: current and future approaches. Best Pract Res Clin Rheumatol. 2013;27(6):805–20.
3. Lems WF, Geusens P. Established and forthcoming drugs for the treatment of osteoporosis. Curr Opin Rheumatol. 2014;26(3):245–51.
4. *Sobacchi C, Schulz A, Coxon FP, Villa A, Helfrich MH. Osteopetrosis: genetics, treatment and new insights into osteoclast function. Nat Rev Endocrinol. 2013;9(9):522–36. *An excellent review of the multiple genetic mechanisms underlying human osteopetrotic syndromes.

[1] *Important References

5. Fleisch H, Russell RGG, Francis MD. Diphosphonates inhibit hydroxyapatite dissolution in vitro and bone resorption in tissue culture and in vivo. Science. 1969;165:1262–4.

6. *Russell RG. Bisphosphonates: the first 40 years. Bone. 2011;49(1):2–19. *A review of the history of bisphosphonates from bench to bedside.

7. Burr D, Russell RG. Special issue of bone to mark the 40th anniversary of bisphosphonates. Bone. 2011; 49(1):1.

8. Plotkin LI, Bellido T. Beyond gap junctions: connexin43 and bone cell signaling. Bone. 2013;52(1): 157–66.

9. Ebetino FH, Hogan AM, Sun S, Tsoumpra MK, Duan X, Triffitt JT, Kwaasi AA, Dunford JE, Barnett BL, Oppermann U, Lundy MW, Boyde A, Kashemirov BA, McKenna CE, Russell RG. The relationship between the chemistry and biological activity of the bisphosphonates. Bone. 2011;49:20–33.

10. Russell RG, Watts NB, Ebetino FH, Rogers MJ. Mechanisms of action of bisphosphonates: similarities and differences and their potential influence on clinical efficacy. Osteoporos Int. 2008;19:733–59.

11. Shapiro JR, Byers PH. Osteogenesis imperfecta. A translational approach to Brittle Bone Disease. In: Glorieux FH, Sponseller PD, editors. Elsevier Publishers USA; 2014. ISBN: 978-0-12-397165-4.

12. *McClung M, Harris ST, Miller PD, Bauer DC, Davison KS, Dian L, Hanley DA, Kendler DL, Yuen CK, Lewiecki EM. Bisphosphonate therapy for osteoporosis: benefits, risks, and drug holiday. Am J Med. 2013;126(1):13–20. *A good discussion of bisphosphonate therapy.

13. Pazianas M, Cooper C, Ebetino FH, Russell RG. Long-term treatment with bisphosphonates and their safety in postmenopausal osteoporosis. Ther Clin Risk Manag. 2010;6:325–43.

14. Pazianas M, Abrahamsen B, Ferrari S, Russell RG. Eliminating the need for fasting with oral administration of bisphosphonates. Ther Clin Risk Manag. 2013;9:395–402.

15. *Baron R, Ferrari S, Russell RG. Denosumab and bisphosphonates: different mechanisms of action and effects. Bone. 2011;48(4):677–92. *A review of the differential effects of denosumab compared with bisphosphonates.

16. Cummings SR, San Martin J, McClung MR, Siris ES, Eastell R, Reid IR, Delmas P, Zoog HB, Austin M, Wang A, Kutilek S, Adami S, Zanchetta J, Libanati C, Siddhanti S, Christiansen C; FREEDOM Trial. Denosumab for prevention of fractures in postmenopausal women with osteoporosis. N Engl J Med. 2009;361:756–65.

17. Boonen S, Adachi JD, Man Z, Cummings SR, Lippuner K, Törring O, Gallagher JC, Farrerons J, Wang A, Franchimont N, San Martin J, Grauer A, McClung M. Treatment with denosumab reduces the incidence of new vertebral and hip fractures in post-menopausal women at high risk. J Clin Endocrinol Metab. 2011;96(6):1727–36.

18. Papapoulos S, Chapurlat R, Libanati C, Brandi ML, Brown JP, Czerwiński E, Krieg MA, Man Z, Mellström D, Radominski SC, Reginster JY, Resch H, Román Ivorra JA, Roux C, Vittinghoff E, Austin M, Daizadeh N, Bradley MN, Grauer A, Cummings SR, Bone HG. Five years of denosumab exposure in women with postmenopausal osteoporosis: results from the first two years of the FREEDOM extension. J Bone Miner Res. 2012;27(3):694–701.

19. Scott LJ. Denosumab: a review of its use in postmenopausal women with osteoporosis. Drugs Aging. 2014;31(7):555–76.

20. *Bone HG, Chapurlat R, Brandi ML, Brown JP, Czerwinski E, Krieg MA, Mellström D, Radominski SC, Reginster JY, Resch H, Ivorra JA, Roux C, Vittinghoff E, Daizadeh NS, Wang A, Bradley MN, Franchimont N, Geller ML, Wagman RB, Cummings SR, Papapoulos S. The effect of three or six years of denosumab exposure in women with postmenopausal osteoporosis: results from the FREEDOM extension. J Clin Endocrinol Metab. 2013;98(11):4483–92. *Important follow up study of denosumab from the FREEDOM trial.

21. Rossouw JE, Anderson GL, Prentice RL, LaCroix AZ, Kooperberg C, Stefanick ML, Jackson RD, Beresford SA, Howard BV, Johnson KC, Kotchen JM, Ockene J, Writing Group for the Women's Health Initiative Investigators. Risks and benefits of estrogen plus progestin in healthy postmenopausal women: principal results from the Women's Health Initiative randomized controlled trial. JAMA. 2002;288(3):321–33.

22. Wells G, Tugwell P, Shea B, Guyatt G, Peterson J, Zytaruk N, Robinson V, Henry D, O'Connell D, Cranney A, Osteoporosis Methodology Group and The Osteoporosis Research Advisory Group. Meta-analyses of therapies for postmenopausal osteoporosis. V. Meta-analysis of the efficacy of hormone replacement therapy in treating and preventing osteoporosis in postmenopausal women. Endocr Rev. 2002;23(4):529–39.

23. Santen RJ, Allred DC, Ardoin SP, Archer DF, Boyd N, Braunstein GD, Burger HG, Colditz GA, Davis SR, Gambacciani M, Gower BA, Henderson VW, Jarjour WN, Karas RH, Kleerekoper M, Lobo RA, Manson JE, Marsden J, Martin KA, Martin L, Pinkerton JV, Rubinow DR, Teede H, Thiboutot DM, Utian WH, Endocrine Society. Postmenopausal hormone therapy: an Endocrine Society scientific statement. J Clin Endocrinol Metab. 2010;95(7 Suppl 1):s1–66.

24. Sarrel PM, Njike VY, Vinante V, Katz DL. The mortality toll of estrogen avoidance: an analysis of excess deaths among hysterectomized women aged 50 to 59 years. Am J Public Health. 2013;103(9):1583–8.

25. Nelson ER, Wardell SE, McDonnell DP. The molecular mechanisms underlying the pharmacological actions of estrogens, SERMs and oxysterols: implications for

the treatment and prevention of osteoporosis. Bone. 2013;53(1):42–50.

26. Komm BS, Chines AA. An update on selective estrogen receptor modulators for the prevention and treatment of osteoporosis. Maturitas. 2012;71(3):221–6.

27. *Komm BS, Mirkin S. An overview of current and emerging SERMs. J Steroid Biochem Mol Biol. 2014;143:207–22. *An excellent review of SERMS and their actions.

28. Pinkerton JV, Thomas S. Use of SERMs for treatment in postmenopausal women. J Steroid Biochem Mol Biol. 2014;142:142–54.

29. Santen RJ, Kagan R, Altomare CJ, Komm B, Mirkin S, Taylor HS. Current and evolving approaches to individualizing estrogen receptor-based therapy for menopausal women. J Clin Endocrinol Metab. 2014;99(3):733–47.

30. Silverman SL, Christiansen C, Genant HK, Vukicevic S, Zanchetta JR, de Villiers TJ, Constantine GD, Chines AA. Efficacy of bazedoxifene in reducing new vertebral fracture risk in postmenopausal women with osteoporosis: results from a 3-year, randomized, placebo-, and active-controlled clinical trial. J Bone Miner Res. 2008;23(12):1923–34.

31. Silverman SL, Chines AA, Kendler DL, Kung AW, Teglbjærg CS, Felsenberg D, Mairon N, Constantine GD, Adachi JD, Bazedoxifene Study Group. Sustained efficacy and safety of bazedoxifene in preventing fractures in postmenopausal women with osteoporosis: results of a 5-year, randomized, placebo-controlled study. Osteoporos Int. 2012;23(1): 351–63.

32. Kaufman JM, Palacios S, Silverman S, Sutradhar S, Chines A. An evaluation of the Fracture Risk Assessment Tool (FRAX®) as an indicator of treatment efficacy: the effects of bazedoxifene and raloxifene on vertebral, nonvertebral, and all clinical fractures as a function of baseline fracture risk assessed by FRAX®. Osteoporos Int. 2013;24(10): 2561–9.

33. Cummings SR, Ensrud K, Delmas PD, LaCroix AZ, Vukicevic S, Reid DM, Goldstein S, Sriram U, Lee A, Thompson J, Armstrong RA, Thompson DD, Powles T, Zanchetta J, Kendler D, Neven P, Eastell R, PEARL Study Investigators. Lasofoxifene in postmenopausal women with osteoporosis. N Engl J Med. 2010;362(8):686–96. Erratum in: N Engl J Med. 2011 Jan 20;364(3):290. Kucukdeveci A [corrected to Kucukdeveci, A].

34. Bolland MJ, Grey A. A comparison of adverse event and fracture efficacy data for strontium ranelate in regulatory documents and the publication record. BMJ Open. 2014;7:4(10).

35. Stepan JJ. Strontium ranelate: in search for the mechanism of action. J Bone Miner Metab. 2013;31(6): 606–12.

36. Wijkmans J, Gossen J. Inhibitors of cathepsin K: a patent review (2004–2010). Expert Opin Ther Pat. 2011;21(10):1611–29.

37. Black WC. Peptidomimetic inhibitors of cathepsin K. Curr Top Med Chem. 2010;10(7):745–51.

38. Kometani M, Nonomura K, Tomoo T, Niwa S. Hurdles in the drug discovery of cathepsin K inhibitors. Curr Top Med Chem. 2010;10(7):733–44.

39. Costa AG, Cusano NE, Silva BC, Cremers S, Bilezikian JP. Cathepsin K: its skeletal actions and role as a therapeutic target in osteoporosis. Nat Rev Rheumatol. 2011;7(8):447–56.

40. Kumar S, Dare L, Vasko-Moser JA, James IE, Blake SM, Rickard DJ, Hwang SM, Tomaszek T, Yamashita DS, Marquis RW, Oh H, Jeong JU, Veber DF, Gowen M, Lark MW, Stroup G. A highly potent inhibitor of cathepsin K (relacatib) reduces biomarkers of bone resorption both in vitro and in an acute model of elevated bone turnover in vivo in monkeys. Bone. 2007;40(1):122–31.

41. Ochi Y, Yamada H, Mori H, Nakanishi Y, Nishikawa S, Kayasuga R, Kawada N, Kunishige A, Hashimoto Y, Tanaka M, Sugitani M, Kawabata K. Effects of ONO-5334, a novel orally-active inhibitor of cathepsin K, on bone metabolism. Bone. 2011;49(6):1351–6.

42. Eastell R, Nagase S, Ohyama M, Small M, Sawyer J, Boonen S, Spector T, Kuwayama T, Deacon S. Safety and efficacy of the cathepsin K inhibitor ONO-5334 in postmenopausal osteoporosis: the OCEAN study. J Bone Miner Res. 2011;26(6):1303–12.

43. Gauthier JY, Chauret N, Cromlish W, Desmarais S, le Duong T, Falgueyret JP, Kimmel DB, Lamontagne S, Léger S, LeRiche T, Li CS, Massé F, McKay DJ, Nicoll-Griffith DA, Oballa RM, Palmer JT, Percival MD, Riendeau D, Robichaud J, Rodan GA, Rodan SB, Seto C, Thérien M, Truong VL, Venuti MC, Wesolowski G, Young RN, Zamboni R, Black WC. The discovery of odanacatib (MK-0822), a selective inhibitor of cathepsin K. Bioorg Med Chem Lett. 2008;18(3):923–8.

44. Langdahl B, Binkley N, Bone H, Gilchrist N, Resch H, Rodriguez Portales J, Denker A, Lombardi A, Le Bailly De Tilleghem C, Dasilva C, Rosenberg E, Leung A. Odanacatib in the treatment of postmenopausal women with low bone mineral density: five years of continued therapy in a phase 2 study. J Bone Miner Res. 2012;27(11):2251–8.

45. *http://www.mercknewsroom.com/news-release/research-and-development-news/merck-announces-data-pivotal-phase-3-fracture-outcomes-st. *Press release announcing outcome of LOFT trial with odanacatib.

46. Jamal SA, Reid LS, Hamilton CJ. The effects of organic nitrates on osteoporosis: a systematic review. Osteoporos Int. 2013;24(3):763–70.

47. Bolland MJ, Grey A, Reid IR. Calcium supplements and cardiovascular risk: 5 years on. Ther Adv Drug Saf. 2013;4(5):199–210.

48. *Tella SH, Gallagher JC. Prevention and treatment of postmenopausal osteoporosis. J Steroid Biochem Mol Biol. 2014;142:155–70. *An excellent review of the current and future treatments.

49. Cosman F. Anabolic and antiresorptive therapy for osteoporosis: combination and sequential approaches. Curr Osteoporos Rep. 2014;12(4):385–95.
50. Einhorn TA, Gerstenfeld LC. Fracture healing: mechanisms and interventions. Nat Rev Rheumatol. 2014 Sep 30.
51. Aspenberg P. Special review: accelerating fracture repair in humans: a reading of old experiments and recent clinical trials. Bonekey Rep. 2013;2:244.
52. Rao SK, Rao AP. A literature review and case series of accelerating fracture healing in postmenopausal osteoporotic working women. J Orthop. 2014;11(3):150–2.
53. Little DG, McDonald M, Bransford R, Godfrey CB, Amanat N. Manipulation of the anabolic and catabolic responses with OP-1 and zoledronic acid in a rat critical defect model. J Bone Miner Res. 2005;20:2044–52.
54. Wilkinson JM, Little DG. Bisphosphonates in orthopedic applications. Bone. 2011;49(1):95–102.
55. Wilkinson JM, Eagleton AC, Stockley I, Peel NF, Hamer AJ, Eastell R. Effect of pamidronate on bone turnover and implant migration after total hip arthroplasty: a randomized trial. J Orthop Res. 2005;23:1–8.
56. Aspenberg P. Bisphosphonates and implants: an overview. Acta Orthop. 2009;80(1):119–23.
57. Lai KA, Shen WJ, Yang CY, Shao CJ, Hsu JT, Lin RM. The use of alendronate to prevent early collapse of the femoral head in patients with nontraumatic osteonecrosis. A randomized clinical study. J Bone Joint Surg Am. 2005;87(10):2155–9.
58. Reginster JY, Neuprez A, Beaudart C, Lecart MP, Sarlet N, Bernard D, Disteche S, Bruyere O. Antiresorptive drugs beyond bisphosphonates and selective oestrogen receptor modulators for the management of postmenopausal osteoporosis. Drugs Aging. 2014;31(6):413–24.
59. Costa AG, Bilezikian JP. Sclerostin: therapeutic horizons based upon its actions. Curr Osteoporos Rep. 2012;10(1):64–72.
60. Ke HZ, Richards WG, Li X, Ominsky MS. Sclerostin and Dickkopf-1 as therapeutic targets in bone diseases. Endocr Rev. 2012;33(5):747–83.
61. *Kahn M. Can we safely target the WNT pathway? Nat Rev Drug Discov. 2014;13(7):513–32. *An excellent review of the wnt pathway.
62. *McClung MR, Grauer A, Boonen S, Bolognese MA, Brown JP, Diez-Perez A, Langdahl BL, Reginster JY, Zanchetta JR, Wasserman SM, Katz L, Maddox J, Yang YC, Libanati C, Bone HG. Romosozumab in postmenopausal women with low bone mineral density. N Engl J Med. 2014;370(5):412–20. *The first report of the clinical effects of the anti-sclerostin antibody romosozumab on bone density and turnover.
63. Tella SH, Gallagher JC. Biological agents in management of osteoporosis. Eur J Clin Pharmacol. 2014;70(11):1291–301.

Anabolics

3

Erik Fink Eriksen

Summary

- The only osteoanabolic therapy currently available is PTH, but new agents based on PTHrp and anti-sclerostin monoclonal antibodies are being developed.
- PTH given by once-daily subcutaneous injection increases bone mass, improves architecture of both trabecular and cortical bone, and increases bony dimensions, thus reducing vertebral and non-vertebral fractures significantly.
- Treatment duration exceeding 2 years provides little extra benefit, because bone over time becomes refractory to PTH.
- Due to hypomineralization of newly formed bone, DXA will underestimate the amount of bone formed when performed early during therapy. The bone marker PINP provides a better assessment of the amount of new bone formed.
- The main side effects are nausea, headache, and vertigo during the first 2–3 weeks following injections. Hypercalcemia, usually very marginal, and hypercalciuria may occur, and later during therapy, transient extremity pain may ensue. The risk of osteosarcoma is not increased.
- Concomitant use of PTH + antiresorptive drugs provides little extra benefit in most cases. Sequential administration with antiresorptive drugs is, however, needed after discontinuation of PTH in order to consolidate bone mass.
- Anti-sclerostin monoclonal antibodies hold a lot of promise as future anabolic agents. They seem to provide more pronounced increases in BMD than PTH and achieve these increases within a shorter period of 6–12 months.
- PTHrP analogues (e.g. abaloparatide) may also provide an alternative to PTH as a future anabolic treatment regimen.

Introduction

Contrary to antiresorptive agents, which reduce fracture incidence by reducing bone turnover, thereby reducing bone loss and deterioration of cancellous and cortical bone structure, anabolic treatments stimulate net accrual of new bone into the skeleton and repair deficiencies in cancellous and cortical bone architecture. In contrast to the antiresorptive drugs, which mainly target osteoclasts and removal of bone, anabolic agents target the osteoblast and formation of new bone. By stimulating bone formation to a greater extent and earlier than bone resorption, creating the so-called

E.F. Eriksen, MD, DMSc (✉)
Department of Endocrinology, Morbid Obesity
and Preventive Medicine, Oslo University Hospital,
Pb 4959 Bydalen, Oslo 0424, Norway
e-mail: e.f.eriksen@medisin.uio.no

© Springer International Publishing Switzerland 2016
S.L. Silverman, B. Abrahamsen (eds.), *The Duration and Safety
of Osteoporosis Treatment*, DOI 10.1007/978-3-319-23639-1_3

anabolic window, anabolic agents have the potential to positively affect a number of skeletal properties besides bone density. These include increased bone size, improved microarchitecture, and changes in bone matrix calcification and collagen cross-linking. They therefore improve bone architecture at both the cancellous and cortical envelope of the skeleton, an endpoint not shared by any of the antiresorptive (anti-catabolic) agents. The anabolic agents to be discussed in this review include the recombinant PTH(1–34), which is currently available in most countries as teriparatide (TPTD); recombinant intact PTH(1–84), which is not approved in the USA; PTHrP, which is still undergoing clinical testing; and anti-sclerostin monoclonal antibody, which is currently undergoing phase 3 testing. As the majority of clinical data are available for TPTD, the emphasis of this review will be on this compound. It has to be remembered, however, that the clinical trial securing approval of TPTD in 2002 (The Fracture Prevention Trial) was stopped prematurely due to osteosarcoma findings in a concurrent long-term rat toxicology study. This is important because later post hoc subanalyses have demonstrated that TPTD further improved both vertebral and non-vertebral anti-fracture efficacy, when treated for more than 18 months [1].

Parathyroid Hormone as an Anabolic Agent

In primary hyperparathyroidism (PHPT), characterized by chronic, continuous excessive secretion of PTH, catabolic effects, primarily at cortical sites such as the distal 1/3 radius, are common in the more severe cases. In milder cases, however, cortical bone loss is low, and trabecular bone architecture is actually preserved [2]. The pronounced anabolism of intermittent administration of the hormone hinges on the attainment of a narrow peak of PTH in the circulation. The peak should not exceed 3 h in width; otherwise, the catabolic effects seen in chronic hypersecretion tend to predominate [3].

When comparing the bone response to intermittent versus chronically elevated levels of PTH, several significant differences emerge at the cellular, tissue and organ levels.

Effects of PTH at the Cellular Level

The effects of PTH are mediated via binding to the PTH/PTH-related protein (PTHrP) receptor [4]. The genes that are turned on differ profoundly with little overlap between intermittent and chronic excess [5]. Postreceptor effects include activation of the cAMP-dependent protein kinase (PK)A and calcium-dependent protein kinase C (PKC), the former pathway accounting for most of the anabolic action. Studies conducted in rodents suggest that the anabolic activity of PTH also depends on intact $\beta 2$ adrenergic receptors—a G-protein-coupled receptor just like the PTH/PTHrP receptor [6]. Generally, G-protein-coupled receptors seem intimately associated with bone anabolism [7].

Intermittent administration of PTH causes upregulation of osteoprotegerin (OPG) and downregulation of RANK ligand which promotes a reduction in osteoclastic activity, while chronic elevated levels of PTH induce the opposite changes, thus favoring bone resorption [8].

Intermittent administration of PTH enhances bone formation through the suppression of sclerostin, dickkopf protein 1 (DKK1), and sFRP1, all inhibitors of canonical Wnt-β signaling. As osteocytes contain the highest levels of SOST/sclerostin, they have been implicated as important participants in this pathway [9]. Moreover, recent data suggest that a newly identified osteoblast differentiation factor, Tmem119, may be mediating PTH-induced increases in osteoblastic β-catenin levels [10, 11].

Additional cellular effects, which have been identified, include increased osteoblast proliferation and differentiation, decreased osteoblast apoptosis, and blunting the negative effects of peroxisome proliferator activator (PPARγ) receptor on osteoblast differentiation [12].

Effects of PTH at the Tissue Level

Intermittent administration causes increased osteoblastic activity without increasing cell proliferation, which likely results from dedifferentiation of bone lining cells into a more active bone-forming phenotype. This leads to deposition of bone without previous resorption and the formation of smooth cement lines [9, 13, 14]. These changes are not seen with continuously elevated PTH levels (Fig. 3.1).

While remodeling balance in moderate primary hyperparathyroidism is neutral [15], intermittent administration of PTH causes overfilling of resorption lacunae (Fig. 3.1). Based on the histological studies conducted so far, the remodeling-based bone accretion seems to supersede modeling-based accretion [16, 17].

Intermittent administration of PTH also induces increases in IGFs and other anabolic growth factors (BMPs, cbfa1), and the increased IGF-1 levels have been implicated in PTH-induced stimulation of hematopoiesis [18]. A similar role has also been proposed for the newly discovered nuclear matrix protein 4/cas interacting zinc finger protein (Nmp4/CIZ) [19]. Immunohistochemical studies on human bone biopsies have demonstrated increased levels of IGF-2 in the bone matrix after PTH treatment [5, 17].

Recent data suggest that bone formation induced by osteocytic PTH receptor signaling on the periosteal surface depends on Wnt signaling but not on resorption, while bone formation on the endocortical surface results from a combination of Wnt-driven increased osteoblast number and modulation of osteoclast–osteoblast cross talk [20].

Bone histomorphometry studies after therapy with PTH reveal increased remodeling as reflected in increased osteoid synthesis, mineralization of bone surfaces, and increased osteoblastic vigor as reflected by an increased distance between double tetracycline labels [21]. The increased bone formation eventually results in pronounced improvements in cancellous and cortical bone. Cancellous bone volume increases by an average of 35 %, and trabecular connectivity, which is reduced in osteoporosis, is improving as well. Also, trabecular number increases, and trabecular morphology returns to a more platelike appearance as seen in younger individuals and different from the more rodlike shape of osteoporotic bone. Cortical thickness and cortical cross-sectional area also increase, which is an effect not seen with antiresorptive treatments [22]. Quantitative CT (QCT) has also corroborated these improvements in cancellous and cortical bone structure in vivo [23, 24].

Bone matrix formed during PTH treatment exhibits less mineralization and less collagen cross-links typical of more immature bone [25]. Albeit the impact of microcrack accumulation

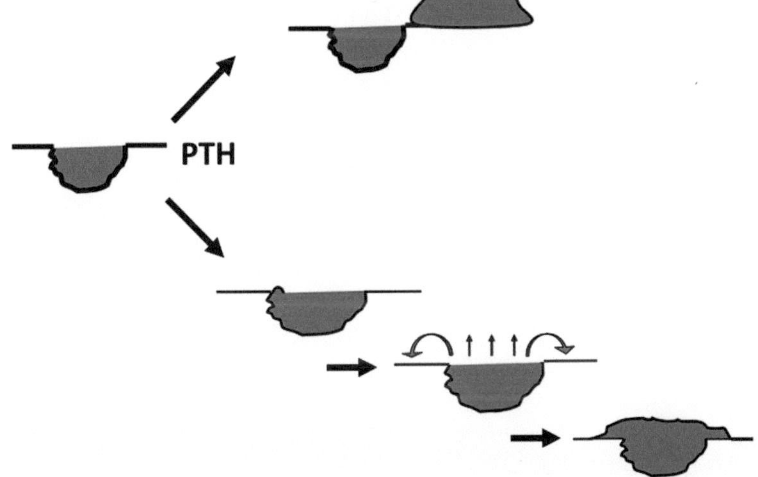

Fig. 3.1 PTH causes accrual of new bone by mainly remodeling-based "overfilling" of resorption pits (*lower panel*), but a certain degree of modeling-based accrual of bone on surfaces without preceding resorption is taking place (*upper panel*)

after antiresorptive treatment on bone quality still remains obscure, PTH treatment has been shown to reduce microcracks in patients pretreated with alendronate [26].

Effects of PTH at the Organ Level

In humans, intermittent administration of teriparatide leads to a rapid increase in bone formation markers followed sometime (usually about 2–3 months later) by increases in bone resorption markers. This sequence of events has led to the concept of the "anabolic window," a period of time when the actions of PTH are maximally anabolic. Bone formation markers peak at 6 months, and then they gradually return toward baseline over a period of 2–3 years with some interindividual variation (Fig. 3.2) [27]. The reasons behind this apparent refractory response of human bone is largely still unknown, but a treatment period of more than 14 months seems important to maximize anti-fracture efficacy [1].

Quantitative radionuclide imaging studies using technetium-99m methylene diphosphonate [(99m)Tc-MDP] have demonstrated accumulation of isotope in the calvarium, mandible, spine, pelvis, and upper and lower extremities [28]. Median increases from baseline in bone turnover as assessed with this technique were 22 % at 3 months and 34 % at 18 months. All subregions exhibited increased an accumulation at both time points except for the pelvis, and these increases at organ level revealed significant positive correlations to markers of bone formation (BAP and PINP). Another study from the same group using PET technology demonstrated that the increase in bone turnover was more pronounced in cortical than trabecular bone [29].

Another effect seen after treatment with PTH, which has not been reported for antiresorptive agents, is an increase in bony dimensions. Peripheral QC measurements and analyses of hip DXA scans have demonstrated a dose-dependent increase in cortical thickness, bone perimeter, and bending strength in the forearm and hip after PTH treatment [30, 31]. Other studies were, however, unable to corroborate such increases [24]. For vertebral bodies, two studies have reported increases in vertebral cross-sectional area (CSA), which would potentially lower fracture risk further, but the estimates differ widely ranging between 4.8 % [32] and 0.7 % [33].

The stimulation of bone formation causes a dose-dependent increase in BMD amounting to 6–9 % over placebo in the spine and 3–6 % at the hip with 20 and 40 µg daily dosing after a median treatment period of 21 months [34]. At certain

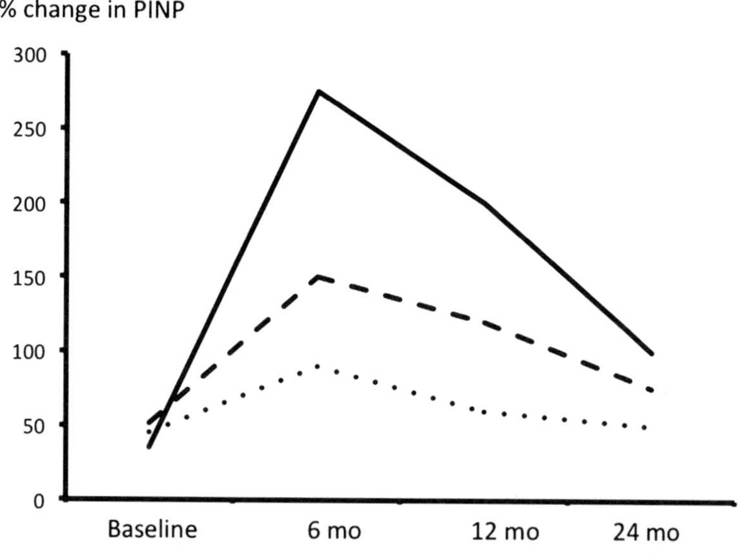

Fig. 3.2 Changes in a marker of bone formation (PINP) after initiation of therapy with PTH(1–34) in 3 patients. Note the peak at 6 months

sites rich in cortical bone, such as the distal 1/3 of the radius, PTH typically does not increase bone density. In fact, there may be a small decline in BMD. Early BMD assessment at the hip usually reveals a decrease too, which then gradually reverses into an increase. This is mainly caused by an increase in cortical porosity accompanying the increase in overall bone turn-over and to a lesser extent the formation of new, less mineralized bone together with dimensional changes. This notion is further corroborated by the fact that the maximal decrease in porosity is seen after 6 month treatment duration where the activation of bone remodeling is at its highest [21]. The transient reduction of BMD does not translate into decreased bone strength, however, because the increased porosity occurs only in the inner one third of bone, where the mechanical effect is minimal. Moreover, the changes in bone geometry and microarchitecture (increased cortical thickness) more than compensate for any potential adverse effects of increased cortical porosity on bone strength [35].

Effects on Vertebral Strength

Using FE modeling on QCT imaging from patients treated with either PTH(1–34) or alendronate, Keaveny et al. [36] reported that both treatments induced positive effects on vertebral strength characteristics (Fig. 3.3). At least 75 % of the patients in each treatment group had increased strength of the vertebra at 6 months compared with baseline. Patients in both treatment groups had increased average volumetric density and increased strength in the trabecular bone, but the median percentage increases for these parameters were 5- to 12-fold greater for TPTD.

Graef et al. [23] studied postmenopausal women with established osteoporosis participating treatment with TPTD for 12 and 24 months in the EUROFORS study. After 12 months, they found an increase in apparent BV/TV (app. BV/TV) by QCT of 30.6 ± 4.4 % (SE), which was paralleled by an increase in apparent trabecular number (app. Tb.N.) by 19.0 ± 3.2 %. These increases were much bigger than those recorded

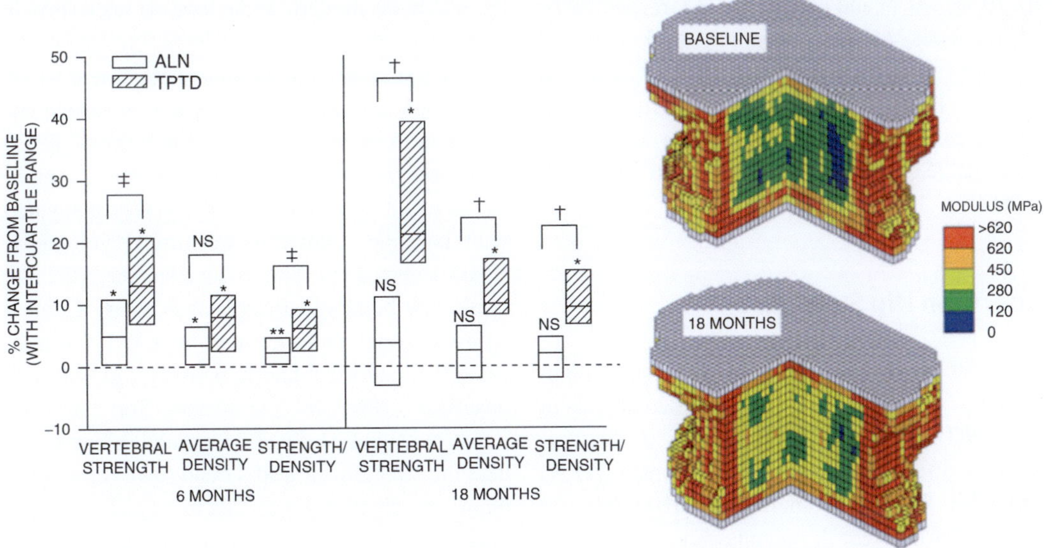

Fig. 3.3 The *right panel* shows increases in vertebral body compressive strength calculated from finite element analysis (FEA) in patients treated with alendronate (*white bars*) and teriparatide (*hatched bars*). *Left panel* shows the improvements in modulus derived from FEA in a patient at baseline after being treated with TPTD for 18 months. From Keaveny TM et al. Journal of Bone and Mineral Research 2007;22(1):149-57. Reprinted with permission from John Wiley and Sons

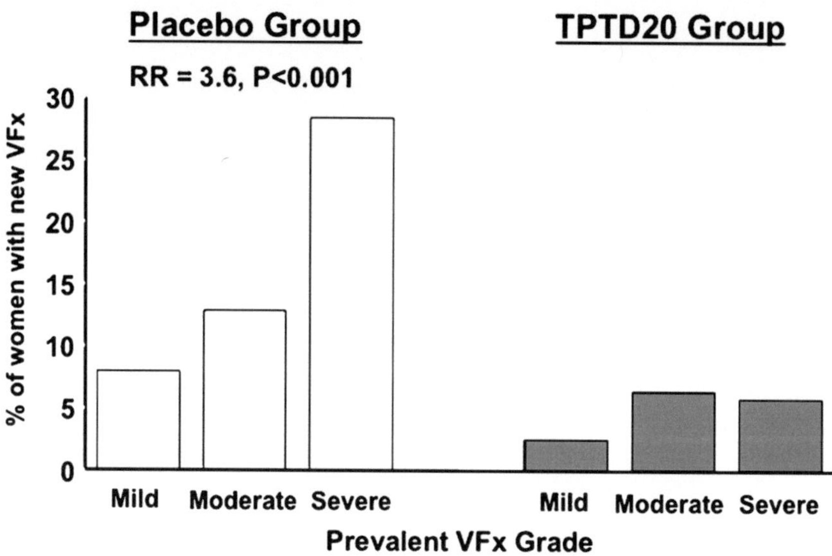

Fig. 3.4 Distribution of vertebral compression fractures classified as either mild (20–25 % compression [SQ1]), moderate (25–40 % compression [SQ2]), and severe (>40 % compression [SQ3]). Based on data from the pivotal PTH(1–34) trial [34]

for areal and volumetric BMD—6.4 % and 19.3 %, respectively. After 24 months, they found an increase of app BV/TV by 54.7 ± 8.8 %, while volumetric BMD and areal BMD increased by 19.1 ± 4.0 % and (10.2 ± 1.2 %), respectively. FE analysis of the 24-month data revealed increases in bone strength by 28 % in compression and bending. These results are further corroborated by the virtual absence of severe vertebral (SQ3) fractures in patients treated with PTH (Fig. 3.4).

Effects on Hip Strength

Keaveny et al. [37] performed finite element analysis on the Hip QCT scans of 162 subjects in the PATH trial to assess changes in femoral strength after treatment with alendronate (ALN) or PTH(1–84) or combinations (CMB) thereof in year 1. During year 2, patients were switched to either ALN or placebo (PLC) in the following groups: PTH–PLC, PTH–ALN, CMB–ALN, and ALN–ALN (year 1–year 2) treatments. After year 1, femoral strength increased significantly for both PTH and ALN, and after year 2, significant changes were seen for all groups except

PTH–PLC, with the most pronounced increase seen in patients treated with PTH–ALN (7.7 %).

In the EUROFORS study, Borgrefe et al. [24] studied the changes in bone distribution, geometry, and bone strength of the femoral neck (FN) in 52 postmenopausal women with severe osteoporosis. They studied three subgroups: treatment-naïve, pretreated, and pretreated showing an inadequate response to treatment. After 24 months of TPTD treatment, volumetric FN BMD increased significantly by 4.0 % and 3.0 %, respectively, compared with baseline. Decreases in cortical volumetric BMD occurred in locations not adversely affecting minimum bending strength indicators. Cortical cross-sectional area increased by 4.3 % and indicated that endosteal but no periosteal growth was observed. Strength parameters for buckling improved significantly at 24 months. Measures of bending strength showed a trend toward improvement, and the changes tended to be larger in individuals at higher risk of buckling failure. In this study, prior antiresorptive treatment was not found to affect treatment results significantly.

In another analysis of the same EUROFORS cohort, Poole et al. [38] mapped small changes in cortical bone distribution in 69 women with severe osteoporosis after treatment with TPTD for 2 years.

Changes in cortical thickness were recorded in each subject by subtracting the baseline thickness distributions from the distributions obtained at 24 months. Interestingly, the analyses demonstrated that new bone was being targeted to regions, which encounter high stress during normal locomotion (i.e., the inferomedial junction of the cortex with the load-bearing calcar femorale and the head–neck junction of the superior cortex)—both sites commonly involved in hip fracture. These findings suggest that mechanical stimulation may enhance local actions of PTH and are in keeping with PTH acting as a modulator of osteocytic mechanosensing and sclerostin secretion as outlined above,

Effects of PTH(1–34) (Teriparatide [TPTD]) in Postmenopausal Osteoporosis

In the pivotal PTH trial by Neer et al., women with severe osteoporosis were treated with subcutaneous injections of placebo or 20 or 40 µg of teriparatide (TPTD) [17]. The average number of fragility fractures per patient was over 2, defining the population as high risk. Over a follow-up period of 21 months, BMD increased by an average of 10–14 %. Femoral neck BMD also improved, but more slowly and to a lesser extent (approximately 3 %). The incidence of new vertebral fractures was reduced by 65 % with the 20 µg dose. The overall incidence of new non-vertebral fractures was reduced by 35 % with the 20 µg dose. When examining non-vertebral low trauma fragility fractures separately, a reduction of 53 % was demonstrable. The higher, 40 µg dose, used in the trial did not further enhance the anti-fracture efficacy. Hip fracture incidence was not analyzed separately because the study was not sufficiently powered to examine this endpoint [34]. When evaluating these results, it is worth noting, however, that the effect sizes emerging were the result of an incomplete trial as the trial was stopped abruptly due to an increased risk of osteosarcoma identified in a long-term toxicology study in rats. This means that the results were obtained in patients with huge variations in treatment duration. The potential anti-fracture efficacy of TPTD in patients treated was shown in a post hoc analysis by Lindsay et al. [1], where patients receiving more than 18 months of treatment with teriparatide revealed a 90 % relative risk reduction in vertebral fractures and a 75–80 % relative risk reduction in non-vertebral fractures (Fig. 3.5).

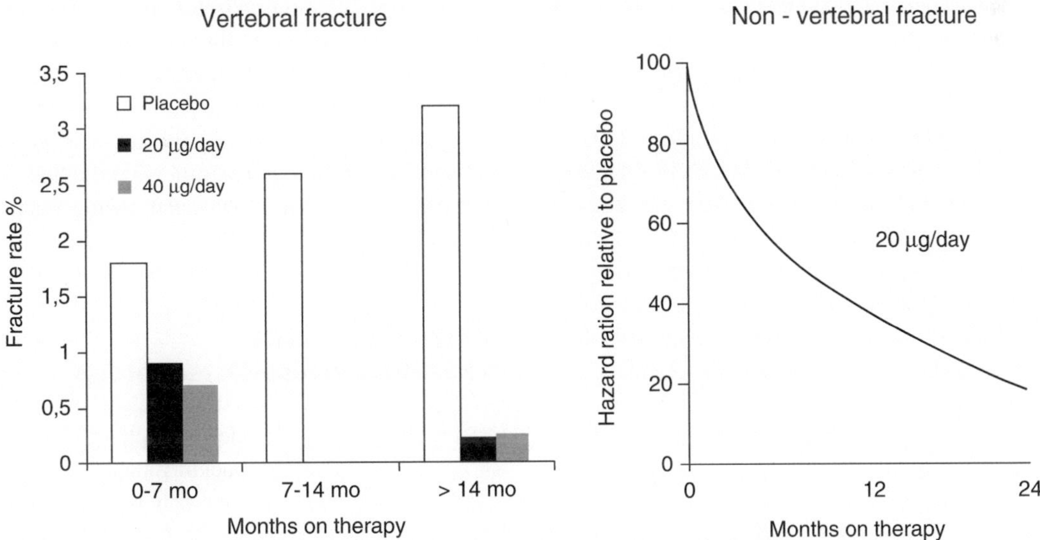

Fig. 3.5 Post hoc analysis of fracture data obtained in the pivotal PTH(1–34) trial by Neer et al. [34]. Vertebral (*left panel*) and non-vertebral (*right panel*) fracture incidences in patients treated with the marketed 20 µg dose were analyzed according to duration of treatment in the trial. With increasing duration, a progressive reduction of both fractures was observed. From Lindsay R et al. Osteoporos Int. 2009; 20(6):943–8. Reprinted with permission from Springer

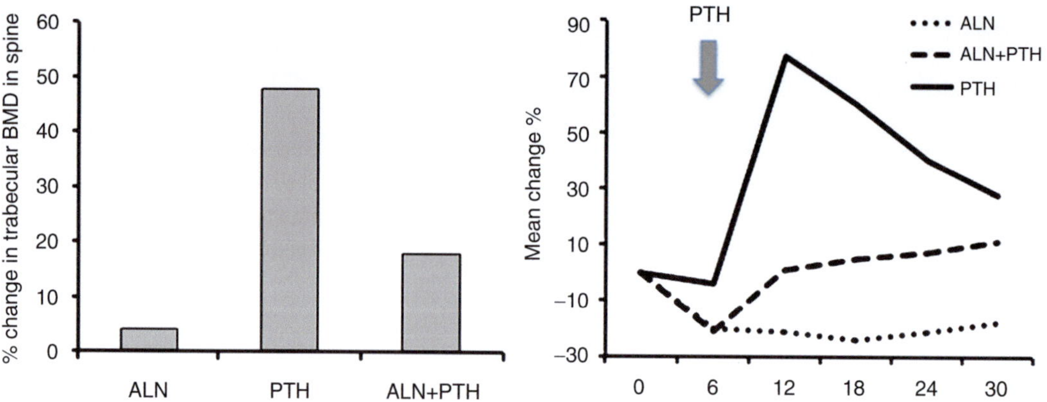

Fig. 3.6 Trabecular bone density of lumbar vertebrae as assessed by quantitative computerized tomography (QCT) and bone formation as reflected in serum levels of bone-specific alkaline phosphatase in men treated with alendronate and PTH as monotherapy or combination of the two.

Note the reduced BMD and the blunted marker response in the combination group treated with PTH + alendronate. From Finkelstein JS et al. The New England Journal of Medicine. 2003;349(13):1216-26. Reprinted with permission from Massachusetts Medical Society

The latter effect should be compared to the 20–25 % reduction seen in the trials using the newer parenteral antiresorptives like zoledronic acid and denosumab [39, 40]. The pronounced effects of TPTD on severe vertebral compression fractures (Fig. 3.6) are probably the main reason behind the significant reduction in back pain demonstrated in several studies [34]. Further post hoc analyses revealed that the reduction in fracture incidence due to teriparatide was not related to the number, severity, or site of previous fractures [41] and was largely independent of age and initial BMD [42].

Two observational studies in Europe, EFOS and EUROFORS, have studied effects of TPTD on back pain and quality of life. With the necessary reservations related to the design of both studies (observational and open label, respectively), significant improvements in bone mass, reductions in back pain, and improvements of quality of life after 18 and up to 36 months of treatment were reported.

The European Forsteo Observational Study (EFOS) enrolled 1648 women with postmenopausal osteoporosis in order to examine the effectiveness of teriparatide. The women were treated for up to 18 months in clinical centers in eight European countries. All participants were TPTD treatment-naïve, but 91.0 % of them had previously received other anti-osteoporosis drugs. After both 18 and 36 months of treatment, significant reduction in back pain and improvements in quality of life were demonstrable [43, 44].

EUROFORS was a prospective, controlled, randomized, open-label, 2-year study, which enrolled 868 postmenopausal women with osteoporosis and a recent fragility fracture. The women were treated at clinical centers around Europe. After 12 months of teriparatide (20 µg/day), 507 patients were randomized to another 12 months with either teriparatide ($n=305$) or raloxifene 60 mg/day ($n=100$). After 2 years of treatment, TPTD caused a significant increase in BMD of 10.5 % [45] and significant reduction in back pain as assessed with visual analog scales (VAS) [46].

Effects of PTH(1–84) in Postmenopausal Osteoporosis

PTH(1–84) has been the object of a limited number of studies. In a preliminary clinical trial, preparatory to the definitive clinical trial, subjects were administered placebo or 1 of 3 doses of PTH(1–84): 50, 75, or 100 µg for 12 months [47]. These data demonstrated both time- and dose-related increases in lumbar spine BMD. Similar to the teriparatide studies, bone turnover markers rose quickly. Histomorphometric analyses of bone biopsy specimens confirmed an anabolic response to PTH(1–84) with an increase in bone formation and improvements in cancellous bone architecture [48]. PTH(1–84) was found to reduce the risk for new or worsening vertebral fractures by 40 % [49]. Contrary to the results obtained in the teriparatide trial, no reduction of non-vertebral fractures was seen with PTH(1–84), however. This study used a higher overall dose of PTH [100 µg PTH(1–84)], which on a molar basis is equivalent to 40 µg of PTH(1–34). Not surprisingly, this higher dose also resulted in far more adverse events and discontinuations due to hypercalcemia [49]. Moreover, the population tested in this study also had a lower overall risk of osteoporotic fracture. In contrast to the study by Neer et al. in which the average number of fragility fractures in subjects at baseline was >2, the incidence in the PTH(1–84) study was only 19 %. This difference in baseline fracture status, together with the higher dose, may have contributed to the lack of demonstrable effects on non-vertebral fractures.

Teriparatide in Men with Osteoporosis

For most osteoporosis agents, the studies on men are smaller and mainly rely on bridging from studies on changes in bone mineral density in women. In the first study that evaluated the effects of PTH in men, Kurland et al. randomized 23 men to 400 U/day of teriparatide (equivalent to 25 µg/day) or placebo for 18 months [50]. The men treated with teriparatide demonstrated a 13.5 % increase in lumbar spine BMD and a 2.9 % increase in femoral neck BMD. Cortical bone density at the distal radius did not change as compared to placebo. In a larger trial of 437 men by Orwoll et al. [51], BMD increased significantly in the 20 µg treatment group by 5.9 % at the lumbar spine and by 1.5 % at the femoral neck independent of gonadal status. This study was shortened to 11 months due to emergence of osteosarcoma data in rats, but the magnitude and

time course of BMD increases at the lumbar spine and hip over the 11 months of the study, were superimposable on the time course seen in the postmenopausal women studied by Neer et al. in the pivotal study [34]. In a follow-up observational period of 30 months, 279 men from the original cohort had lateral spine X-rays 18 months after the treatment was stopped. When combining fracture assessment in the combined treatment groups (20 µg and 40 µg), the risk of vertebral fracture was reduced nonsignificantly by 51 % ($P=0.07$), but when only moderate or severe fractures were considered, significant 83 % fracture risk reductions were found (6.8 % vs. 1.1 %; $P<0.02$) [52]. When evaluating these fracture reductions, one has to keep in mind that a substantial number (25–30 %) of study subjects reported use of antiresorptive agents during the follow-up period.

PTH in Secondary Osteoporosis

In secondary osteoporosis characterized by severe impairment of bone formation such as in glucocorticoid-induced osteoporosis (GIO), PTH should theoretically be more effective than antiresorptive agents, because it more specifically affects the primary defect of these diseases being impaired bone formation. This was indeed shown to be the case in a recent study. Saag et al. [53] compared teriparatide with alendronate in 428 women and men with GIO (22–89 years of age) and glucocorticoid treatment for at least 3 months (dose $\geq$5 mg prednisolone equivalents daily or more). Patients received either teriparatide (20 µg/ day) or alendronate (10 mg/day) for 18 months. In the teriparatide group, the increase in BMD was higher than in the alendronate group (7.2 ± 0.7 % vs. 3.4 ± 0.7 %, $P<0.001$). Although the trial was not powered to assess differences in fracture rates, pronounced differences in vertebral fractures were demonstrable, however. Patients in the teriparatide group suffered fewer vertebral fractures than patients treated with alendronate (0.6 % vs. 6.1 %, $P=0.004$), while the incidence of non-vertebral fractures was similar in the two groups (5.6 % vs. 3.7 %, $P=0.36$). In the 18-month extension study, the difference in fracture risk between the two groups was maintained.

The EuroGIOPs trial [54] compared changes in BMD in 92 men (mean age 56 years) who had been treated with glucocorticoids (GC) for ≥3 months and a T-score ≤ −1.5 standard deviations at baseline. Subjects were then randomized to receive either teriparatide or risedronate for 18 months. At endpoint, trabecular BMD by QCT increased by 16.3 % in the TPTD group vs. 3.8 % in subjects treated with risedronate ($P=0.004$). High-resolution QCT analyses revealed improvements in both trabecular and cortical structural indices, and finite element analyses showed larger improvements in vertebral strength. Although this study, like the Saag study [55], was insufficiently powered for evaluation of fracture incidence studies, it is noteworthy that none of the patients on teriparatide but five on risedronate developed new clinical fractures ($P=0.056$).

Indications for PTH

Teriparatide is used in postmenopausal women and men with osteoporosis who are at high risk for fracture. It is an injectable drug, so patients have to be able to self-administer a daily subcutaneous pen injection. However, the technique of administration of teriparatide has been successfully taught to very old patients. Patients with prevalent osteoporotic fractures before treatment are good candidates for therapy as they carry a much higher risk of fracture as compared to patients without fractures and a T-score below −2.5. Moreover, this risk increases progressively with both the number and severity of fractures. Thus, teriparatide is clearly indicated in severe manifest osteoporosis with multiple prevalent low energy fractures. A very low T-score on its own (e.g., < −3.5), even without an osteoporotic fracture, also confers a high risk for fracture. Patient age is also important as for any T-score, the older the patient, the greater the risk. Due to the high risk of subsequent fracture in patients with multiple (> 3–4) or severe (> 40 % compression) vertebral fractures, PTH should also be considered in these groups. Certainly, patients who fracture while on antiresorptive therapy are good candidates for teriparatide. Other potential candidates for teriparatide include patients for whom one might consider a bisphosphonate, but who cannot tolerate the drug, and finally, severe osteoporosis in younger individuals in the thirties or forties also may constitute an indication for PTH therapy. These individuals have a long life ahead of them, and it seems logical to add bone to the skeleton to reduce their future risk of fracture, instead of just preserving bone mass and stabilizing the skeleton with antiresorptive regimens.

Monitoring PTH Therapy

Assessment of bone mass by DXA in the early phases generally leads to underestimation of new bone formed due to the relative hypomineralization of newly formed bone [21, 56]. The increase in turnover and porosity, which reaches its maximum at 6 months [21], will also contribute to a decreased DXA response early on. Therefore, DXA measurements will tend to underestimate skeletal responses during early phases of PTH therapy. Later DXA measurements will suffer less from the biases associated with the early phases of PTH therapy and are therefore useful after 1 year of therapy as well as during sequential treatment with antiresorptive agents.

Assessment of bone markers is more informative than DXA in the early phases of PTH therapy. PINP (Type I procollagen N-terminal propeptide) has emerged as the most dynamic and specific bone turnover marker for monitoring PTH effects in vivo, but markers like bone-specific alkaline phosphatase and osteocalcin will also increase significantly [57]. Further supporting the use of bone markers is the fact the initial increases between 1 and 6 months in bone markers, in particular PICP and PINP, predict subsequent improvements in bone structure [58] and BMD increases [59, 60].

In the EUROFORS study, Stepan et al. demonstrated significant correlations between 3-month increases in PINP and 24-month increases in Ac.F. Following 3 months of treatment, increases in PINP predicted the increase in Ac.F. ($r=0.52$, $P<0.01$) and OS ($r=0.54$, $P<0.01$) after 24 months [61].

Sequential and Combination Therapy with Teriparatide and Antiresorptive Agents

Prior Use of Antiresorptive Drugs

As candidates for anabolic treatment often have been treated with bisphosphonates or other antiresorptive agents, it is important to consider whether such treatment affects the bone-forming effects of PTH.

Prior treatment with raloxifene has been shown to leave the BMD response to TPTD unperturbed, and markers of bone formation increased to a similar extent in patients treated with raloxifene + TPTD and TPTD alone [62, 63].

Cosman et al. treated postmenopausal women, previously given estrogen for at least 1 year, with teriparatide (25 µg) [64]. Lumbar spine BMD increased in a linear fashion during the entire 3-year study and reached a maximum of 13.4 % after 2 years. Moreover, solid stimulation of bone markers was demonstrable. Thus, no blunting of TPTD anabolism was demonstrable.

Pretreatment with alendronate has, however, been shown to blunt PTH anabolism. This is reflected in an inferior BMD response and reduced stimulation of markers of bone formation [63]. Another study, however, showed a good response to teriparatide with rapid increases in BMD [65]. These results imply that the potency of the antiresorptive regimen to control bone turnover can determine the early response to teriparatide. To account for these differences, it is important to note that the baseline bone turnover markers prior to the initiation of teriparatide therapy were markedly different in the two studies. In the study by Ettinger et al., bone turnover markers were almost completely suppressed, while the women in the study by Cosman et al. exhibited less suppression. Thus, it may not be the specific antiresorptive agent used prior to teriparatide, which determines the subsequent skeletal response but rather the extent to which bone turnover is reduced by this agent. To support this idea, the response to teriparatide has been shown to be a function of the level of baseline bone turnover, with higher turnover levels achieving more robust densitometric responses [50].

In the EUROFORS trial, postmenopausal women with established osteoporosis were randomized to receive open-label teriparatide 20 µg/day for the first year. In a post hoc analysis, their BMD response was assessed according to previous osteoporosis treatment as follows: (a) treatment-naïve, (b) prior treatment with an antiresorptive drug with adequate response, and (c) prior antiresorptive treatment with inadequate response (inadequate AR-responders) ($n=421$). In all three groups, BMD increased significantly from baseline, but differed slightly between treatment-naïve patients (8.4 %), patients treated adequately with antiresorptive drug (7.1 %), and inadequate responders to antiresorptive therapy (6.2 %). The same trend was seen for total hip BMD, which increased only in treatment-naive patients (1.8 %), while remaining unchanged in the two other groups [66].

Histomorphometric analysis of a subgroup of women in this trial revealed that the stimulation of bone formation was similar in alendronate pretreated and treatment-naive women. Women pretreated with alendronate exhibited increases in activation frequency from 0.11 (cycles/year) at baseline to 0.34 cycles/year after 24 months, while women who were treatment-naïve exhibited increases from 0.19 to 0.33 cycles/year [61].

Thus, the blunting after prior alendronate therapy previously observed in other trials was demonstrable in an open-label study, but less pronounced. This discrepancy may be due to variations in compliance.

Concomitant Use of Anabolic and Antiresorptive Therapy

The initial decreases in BMD seen early after the initiation of PTH therapy at sites rich in cortical have not been associated with increased skeletal fragility at these sites [67]. Nevertheless, some clinicians have considered combination therapy with antiresorptive agents as more beneficial than monotherapy in high-risk patients. Several trials exploring this concept have, however, yielded important data pertaining to this concept [68, 69]. Several groups have published trials using a form of PTH(1–34) or PTH(1–84) alone, alendronate alone, or the combination of PTH and alendronate. Black et al. studied postmenopausal women treated with 100 µg of PTH(1–84)/day [68]. The study by Finkelstein et al. treated men with 40 µg/day of teriparatide [69]. Both studies used both DXA and QCT to measure areal and volumetric BMD. Much to the surprise of proponents of combination therapy, the gains in BMD in patients treated with PTH alone exceeded densitometric gains seen with combination therapy at the lumbar spine and to a lesser degree at the hip (Fig. 3.6). Measurement by QCT, in fact, showed that combination therapy was associated with substantially smaller increases in cancellous bone BMD as compared to monotherapy with PTH. Bone turnover markers exhibited the expected increases and decreases for PTH and alendronate, respectively. Subjects treated with combination therapy, however, revealed bone marker levels in between the two other regimens, indicating a blunting stimulation of bone formation by PTH.

It seems, however, that the mode of administration of the bisphosphonate also plays a role. Cosman et al. compared the BMD and bone marker response to combined therapy with once-yearly zoledronic acid (5 mg) and daily PTH(1–34) with the response seen in patients treated with either agent alone [70]. Contrary to the findings of the studies using orally administered bisphosphonate, the combination of intravenous bisphosphonate and PTH yielded superior BMD responses at the hip and spine over those seen in patients treated with either agent alone (Fig. 3.7). Bone markers revealed an initial reduction of formation markers as seen with oral bisphosphonates, but over time these markers increased and approached markers levels in patients treated with PTH alone within a year, much different from the constant suppression of bone formation seen in the combination group with PTH and alendronate.

Recent data testing the combination of TPTD and denosumab show data similar to those

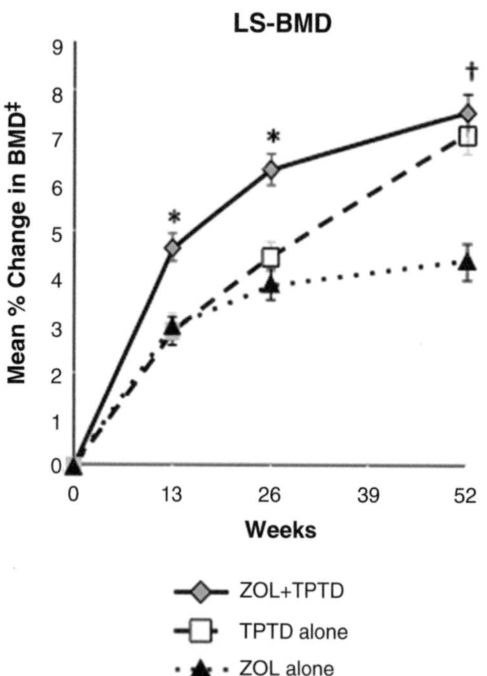

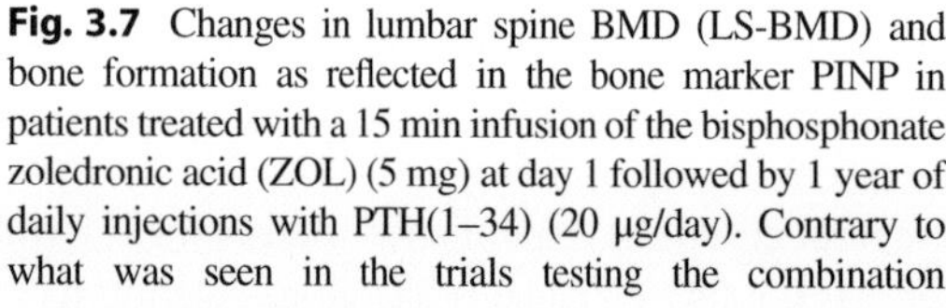

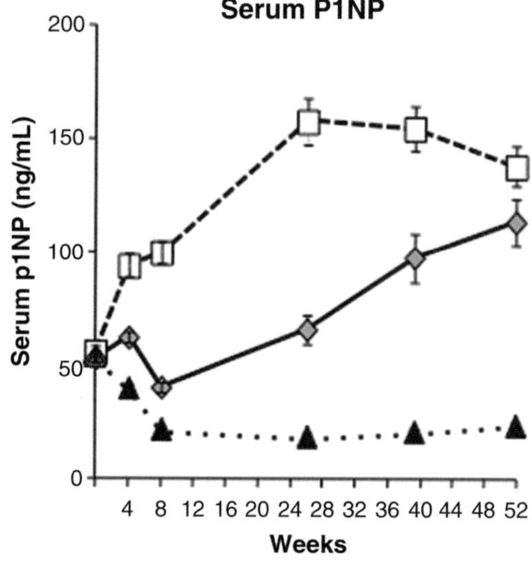

*P<0.001 vs TPTD alone + ZOL alone

†P<0.001 vs ZOL alone

Fig. 3.7 Changes in lumbar spine BMD (LS-BMD) and bone formation as reflected in the bone marker PINP in patients treated with a 15 min infusion of the bisphosphonate zoledronic acid (ZOL) (5 mg) at day 1 followed by 1 year of daily injections with PTH(1–34) (20 µg/day). Contrary to what was seen in the trials testing the combination PTH+alendronate, ZOL did not blunt the BMD response in the combination group (PTH+ZOL). After an initial decrease, bone formation in the combination group picked up and reached the level seen in patients treated with PTH alone. From Cosman F J Bone Miner Res. 2011;26(3):503-11. Reprinted with permission from John Wiley and Sons

obtained for IV zoledronic acid with the best BMD response in patients treated with the combination of TPTD and denosumab [71]. PINP, however, remained suppressed throughput the treatment period.

Sequential Use of Anabolic and Antiresorptive Therapy

Several different sequential regimens using PTH and bisphosphonates have been published. Cosman et al. studied adding (i.e., concomitant treatment) vs. switching (i.e., sequential treatment) in women either treated with alendronate or raloxifene. They reported that the BMD responses were superior in women where PTH was added, while the biochemical response was better in the switch group. Similarly, Black et al. reported the results of a 2-year study where ibandronate was either given together with PTH for 6 months followed by monthly ibandronate alone for 18 months or PTH was given 3 months every year, followed sequentially by monthly ibandronate. In this study, concomitant therapy led to impaired bone marker responses, while the BMD response was similar in the two groups.

In conclusion, it seems that treatment with weak antiresorptives (raloxifene and estrogen) does not significantly blunt the anabolic effect of PTH. Concomitant and to a lesser degree sequential administration of potent antiresorptive drugs, however, reduces the osteoanabolic action of PTH as reflected in inferior PINP responses. The BMD response is highly variable, with alendronate + PTH showing inferior responses to PTH alone, ibandronate being neutral, while zoledronic acid and denosumab show improvements in BMD response over PTH alone. The improvements in BMD responses seen for the two latter drugs cannot be ascribed to increased anabolism, as PINP is down. Thus, the most likely explanation is a reduction in remodeling space induced by the two drugs. Concomitant treatment with PTH and antiresorptive drugs should therefore be reserved to extreme cases of secondary osteoporosis, where the underlying disease may blunt PTH action (e.g., severe inflammation).

Consequences of Discontinuing PTH Therapy

After discontinuation of PTH, bone mass will return to levels close to baseline within a 2-year period (Fig. 3.8) [67, 72]. Several studies have suggested that this loss of bone mass after discontinuation can be offset by antiresorptive treatment with either bisphosphonate [72, 73], estrogen [74], or raloxifene [45, 62].

The PATH study provided further prospective data to address this issue [75]. In this study, postmenopausal women who had received PTH(1–84) for 12 months were randomly assigned to 12 additional months of therapy with 10 mg of alendronate daily or placebo. In subjects who received alendronate, BMD at the lumbar spine increased further by 4.9 %, while those who received placebo experienced a substantial decline in BMD. By QCT analysis, the net increase over 24 months in cancellous bone BMD among those treated with alendronate after PTH(1–84) was 30 %. In those who received placebo after PTH(1–84), the net change was only 13 %. There were similar differences in hip BMD, with patients treated with alendronate exhibiting 13 % increase vs. 5 % increase in patients on placebo.

Prince et al. studied a cohort of patients for 30 months following the pivotal PTH trial. After discontinuation of PTH(1–34), subjects were given the option of switching to a bisphosphonate or not taking any further medications following teriparatide. A majority (60 %) of patients was treated with antiresorptive therapy after PTH discontinuation [72]. Gains in bone density were maintained in those who chose to begin antiresorptive therapy immediately after teriparatide (Fig. 3.8). Reductions in BMD were progressive throughout the 30-month observational period in subjects who elected not to follow teriparatide with any therapy. In a group who did not begin antiresorptive therapy until 6 months after discontinuation of teriparatide (Fig. 3.8), major reductions in BMD were seen during these first 6 months, but no further reductions were observed after initiation of antiresorptive regimens [67]. Despite the loss of bone mass in a substantial proportion of patients after

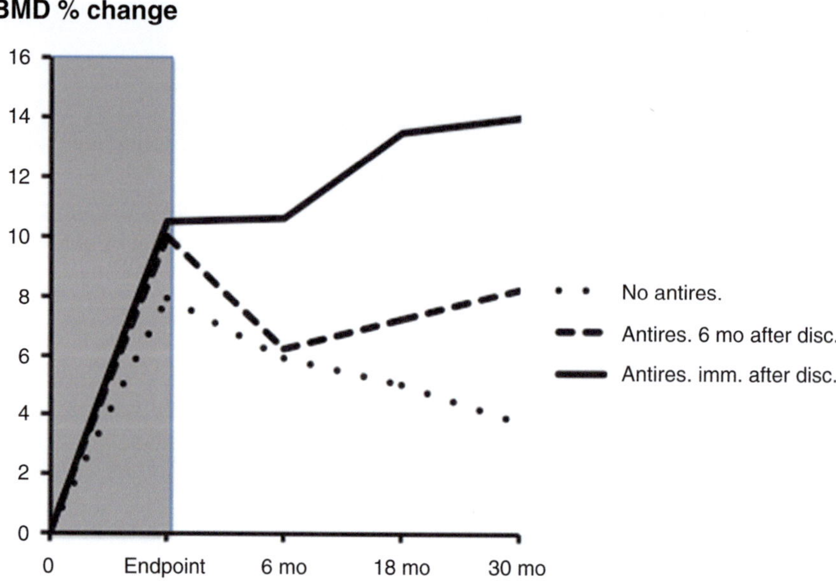

Fig. 3.8 Changes in bone mineral density (BMD) in three groups after discontinuation following therapy with teriparatide (*shaded area*): (1) no antiresorptive after discontinuation (*dotted line*), (2) initiation of antiresorptive treatment 6 months after discontinuation (*broken line*), (3) initiation of antiresorptive immediately after discontinuation (continuous line). Note the additional increase in BMD after antiresorptive treatment. Sixty percent received some kind of osteoporosis treatment after discontinuation, mainly bisphosphonates. From Prince R et al. Journal of Bone and Mineral Research 2005;20(9):1507–13. Reprinted with permission from John Wiley and Sons

the discontinuation of teriparatide, vertebral and non-vertebral fracture rates remained reduced for as long as 31 months after discontinuation in women previously treated with PTH (with or without a bisphosphonate) as compared with those treated with placebo (with or without a bisphosphonate; $P<0.03$).

Following the initial trial testing of the effect of PTH(1–34) in estrogen-treated postmenopausal women, 52 women were randomly assigned to remain on hormone therapy (HT) alone or continue PTH + HT. Women continuing PTH + HT showed an increase in bone mass over baseline after 3 years by 13.4 % in the spine and by 4.4 % in the total hip. In women discontinuing PTH, but continuing HT, bone density did not increase but remained stable for 1 year after discontinuation without any significant loss, as did bone markers. PTH + HT reduced vertebral fractures from 37.5 % to 8.3 % ($P<0.02$).

Raloxifene and estrogen also preserve bone mass after discontinuation of PTH. In the EUROFORS study, Eastell et al. reported a preservation of bone mass after discontinuation of PTH therapy for 1 year, while patients receiving calcium + D supplementation alone lost 2.8 % at the spine and 2 % at the hip in year 2 [45]. The study compared changes in BMD obtained in three groups of postmenopausal women with osteoporosis randomized to (1) continue teriparatide for another year, (2) switch to raloxifene 60 mg/day, or (3) receive no active treatment for the second year. Two years of teriparatide increased LS-BMD by 10.7 %. Patients receiving raloxifene in year 2 had no further change in LS-BMD from year 1, while patients receiving no active treatment exhibited a decrease of 2.5 %.

Based on these results, it has become routine to institute treatment with antiresorptive drugs, mainly bisphosphonates, after discontinuation of PTH after 2 years [45].

Safety of PTH

Overall, PTH is well tolerated. The main side effects of PTH(1–34) and PTH(1–84) are usually mild nausea, vertigo, and headache, which appear early after initiation of treatment and usually resolve over a few weeks [34]. These effects are mostly caused by PTH-induced vasodilation.

Effects on Calcium Metabolism and Serum Biochemistry

Hypercalcemia occurred in 11 % of patients in the pivotal teriparatide trial 4–6 h after injection, but long-standing hypercalcemia was rare. Hypercalciuria was seen in 4.8 to 11 % of women during the first 12 months [34]. Hypercalcemia and hypercalciuria were more prevalent in the PTH(1–84) study affecting 27.8 % and 46 % of women, respectively [49]. This difference is explained by several factors: (1) inclusion of patients with preexisting hypercalcemia and hypercalciuria, (2) use of a higher dose (100 µg PTH(1–84) is equal to 40 µg of TPTD on a molar basis), and (3) the longer serum half-life of PTH(1–84). Serum calcium should be measured early after initiation of PTH therapy and at regular intervals. In clinical practice, using 20 µg TPTD hypercalcemia is usually mild and transient, but if it persists, the first intervention should be discontinuation of calcium supplements, and if that does not lead to resolution of the condition, PTH should be discontinued for a period of time. Progressive hypercalcemia during PTH therapy should be considered a sign of other underlying disease, in particular malignancy.

PTH treatment also increased uric acid concentrations, and 3 % of patients exhibited hyperuricemia in the pivotal teriparatide trial [34]. Neither the hypercalciuria nor the elevations in uric acid, however, lead to an increased risk of kidney stones, even in patients with renal impairment [76].

Osteosarcoma

A safety signal, which appears to be unique to rodents, is osteosarcoma. The pivotal trial of PTH(1–34) was terminated early by the finding of increased risk osteosarcoma in Fisher rats given very high doses of PTH(1–34) with a treatment duration close to the lifespan of a rat (2 years) [77]. It is unlikely that this animal toxicity is related to human skeletal physiology [78], and no increased risk has ever been demonstrable in humans. Growing rats, which were used in the toxicology studies, seem severalfold more sensitive to PTH than monkeys or humans [78]. This is also reflected in the fact that continuous treatment with PTH in rats leads to osteopetrosis [77], which is never seen in monkeys or humans, where the skeleton gradually becomes refractory to PTH over a period of 2–3 years [27, 34]. The risk of osteosarcoma after treatment of more than one million patients with PTH remains at the background level of 1/250,000 [79].

Use of PTH in Patients with Previous or Current Malignancies

Increased bone turnover seems to increase the risk of bone metastasis from cancers like breast and prostate cancer [80], while a decrease in bone turnover protects against bone metastasis, which is the main underlying cause for the protective effects of bisphosphonates in breast and prostate cancer [81]. As PTH increases bone turnover, it is therefore contraindicated in patients with cancers causing bone metastases. Moreover, as PTH stimulates Wnt signaling, which is also involved in malignant transformation [82], stimulates hematopoiesis [83], and because certain solid tumors may express PTH/PTHrP receptors, caution is also warranted in patients suffering from other cancers [84]. It has to be emphasized, however, that neither the rat toxicology studies nor the clinical studies' data as well as post-marketing surveillance have been able to demonstrate any increase in non-osseous cancer risk in animals or patients treated with PTH [34, 51, 77].

Concerns have been raised with respect to the PTH-induced increase in bone formation which might worsen compression symptoms due to narrowing of the spinal canal or cranial nerve canals. The clinical studies as well as later adverse event reporting have not revealed any significant issues pertaining to these issues, and in the EUROFORS study, actual increases in spinal canal cross-sectional area were reported [33].

PTH and the Future

Less frequent administration of PTH, such as once weekly, has been considered as a treatment option, but the skeletal response is generally inferior, and whether the excellent vertebral and non-vertebral anti-fracture efficacy is preserved with this regimen remains unclear [85, 86].

Other modes of administration such as nasal and transdermal administration have also been considered, but large-scale clinical trials that evaluate these options have not emerged.

Cyclical 3-month courses of teriparatide during continued alendronate use have been reported by Cosman et al. [65]. In comparison to regular, uninterrupted teriparatide use, the cyclic administration of teriparatide was associated with similar densitometric gains. Due to the small size of these studies, no fracture endpoints were assessed.

Calcilytics, which induce increases in short-term boosts of endogenous PTH from the parathyroids by interacting with the calcium receptor, have also been subjected to early phase testing [87]. However, no phase 3 trials have been performed using these agents.

Parathyroid Hormone-Related Peptide

Parathyroid hormone-related peptide (PTHrP) was initially cloned as the dominating agent causing humoral hypercalcemia of malignancy [88]. It is, however, expressed in a wide variety of tissues including the skin, blood vessels, mammary epithelium, kidney, bone, and cartilage. PTHrP is involved in transcellular calcium transport, but is also pivotal for cartilage development and skeletal growth, development of mammary epithelium, tooth eruption, and regulation of keratinocyte differentiation [88].

Horwitz et al. showed anabolic properties of PTHrP(1–36) in 2003 in a 3-month trial [89]. They reported a 4.7 % increase in BMD in patients treated with PTHrP vs. 1.3 % in controls on placebo (Ca+D). They also reported an increase in osteocalcin, but no significant changes in other markers of bone formation or resorption, albeit deoxypyridinoline cross-links showed a trend toward increase toward the end of the trial. A later small-scale, 3-week, dose-finding study [90] reported PTHrP to be safe up to doses of 625 µg/day, while slight hypercalcemia was seen at doses of 750 µg/day. Using newer markers of bone remodeling including PINP and CTS, the study showed the expected increase in PINP, the most specific bone marker for assessing PTH effects on osteoblasts. Contrary to PTH(1–34) and PTH(1–84), however, bone resorption was unperturbed, actually slightly reduced. Thus, the hypercalcemia seen was ascribed to increased $1,25(OH)_2D$ levels.

A larger, more recent dose-finding study in 105 postmenopausal women with low bone density or osteoporosis [91] compared daily subcutaneous injections of two doses of PTHrP(1–36) (400 and 600 µg/day) to PTH(1–34) (20 µg/day). Patients on PTH(1–34) exhibited an increase in bone resorption of 90 % over baseline compared to 30 % for PTHrP(1–36). The stimulation of bone formation as reflected in PINP was, however, more pronounced for patients treated with PTH(1–34) (171 %) than for the two doses of PTHrP(1–36) (46 % and 87 %). No significant differences in lumbar spine or hip BMD were demonstrable between groups. Patients treated with PTHrP exhibited more hypercalcemia events than patients treated with PTH(1–34), and 3 patients treated with 600 µg/day had to have the dose reduced. Other adverse events were similar between the three regimens. No studies involving fracture data have been published for PTHrP yet.

A novel PTHrP(1–34) analog, abaloparatide (BA058), is currently being tested in a phase 3 study [92]. Previous phase 2 data demonstrated increases of 5.2 % and 6.7 % at doses of 40 and 80 µg, respectively, after 24 weeks. These increases were similar to those seen with teriparatide (5.5 %). Further increases in a further 24-week extension study were also reported. As with PTH, the most common adverse events were influenza and headaches, while serum calcium levels were reported to be higher with teriparatide [93]. Separately, positive results using a transdermal approach were recently reported.

Anti-sclerostin Monoclonal Antibody

Sclerostin is produced by osteocytes and acts as an inhibitor of osteoblastic bone formation. It is thought to modulate bone formation in response to mechanosensation by osteocytes, and PTH exerts part of its anabolic effects via reducing SOST expression [10]. Two diseases characterized by pronounced increases in bone mass and sometimes nerve compression symptoms, sclerosteosis and van Buchem disease, are both associated with alterations in SOST expression. While sclerosteosis is associated with mutations in the SOST gene, van Buchem disease is caused by a 52 kb deletion downstream of the SOST gene that probably affects transcription of the gene. Sclerostin inhibits BMP-stimulated bone formation, but does not antagonize all BMP responses [94]. Two different diseases causing increased bone mass, osteopetrosis, and pycnodysostosis are characterized by disordered deposition of bone matrix and subsequent mineralization, offsetting the beneficial effects of increased bone mass, causing increased fracture propensity [95, 96]. In sclerosteosis and van Buchem disease, matrix deposition and mineralization seem well regulated, causing very solid bone that does not break even after major trauma [97].

Anti-sclerostin monoclonal antibody has proven to be very effective in increasing bone mass and improves cortical and cancellous bone quality in rodent [98] and primate models [99] as well as in humans [100]. In primates, administration of anti-sclerostin increases bone mass more to levels exceeding those previously seen with PTH. Moreover, it seems that modeling and periosteal bone formation show more pronounced stimulation than that seen with PTH, and the increases are achieved over a shorter time span [99, 101]. Contrary to PTH which gradually over time stimulates bone resorption, anti-sclerostin actually inhibits bone resorption further amplifying net accrual of bone mass. Currently, anti-sclerostin antibody is being tested in a phase 3 trial comprising more than 5000 postmenopausal women with osteoporosis being treated for 12 months. The primary endpoint will evaluate the incidence of new vertebral fractures at 12 months [102].

The most extensive data pertaining to effects of anti-sclerostin antibody on human bone were recently reported by McClung et al. [100], who tested the efficacy and safety of anti-sclerostin monoclonal antibody developed by Amgen (romosozumab) in 419 postmenopausal women (55–85 years) with a score of −2.0 or less at the lumbar spine, total hip, or femoral neck and −3.5 or more at each of the three sites). Participants were administered monthly doses of romosozumab (70 mg, 140 mg, or 210 mg) or every 3 months (140 mg or 210 mg) or placebo. For comparison, two groups received either open-label oral alendronate (70 mg weekly) or subcutaneous teriparatide (20 μg daily). Patients given 210 mg monthly exhibited the biggest increases in lumbar spine BMD (11.3 %), compared with a decrease of 0.1 % with placebo and increases of 4.1 % with alendronate and 7.1 % with teriparatide (Fig. 3.9). Romosozumab was also associated with significant increases in total hip and femoral neck BMD. Bone markers revealed stimulation of bone formation and concomitant reduction of bone resorption (Fig. 3.9). Thus, anti-sclerostin antibody does not cause increased cortical porosity reducing increases in BMD stemming from increases in cancellous bone mass and increased cortical thickness. The antibody would rather be expected to reduce porosity, further amplifying BMD increases. This may be partly responsible for the larger increases in BMD compared to PTH in this study. In keeping with this notion, the relative difference in BMD between PTH and romosozumab was more pronounced in the hip, which has a larger cortical component than the spine. Elevated PINP levels reflecting stimulation of bone formation persisted longer in patients treated with PTH than in patients treated

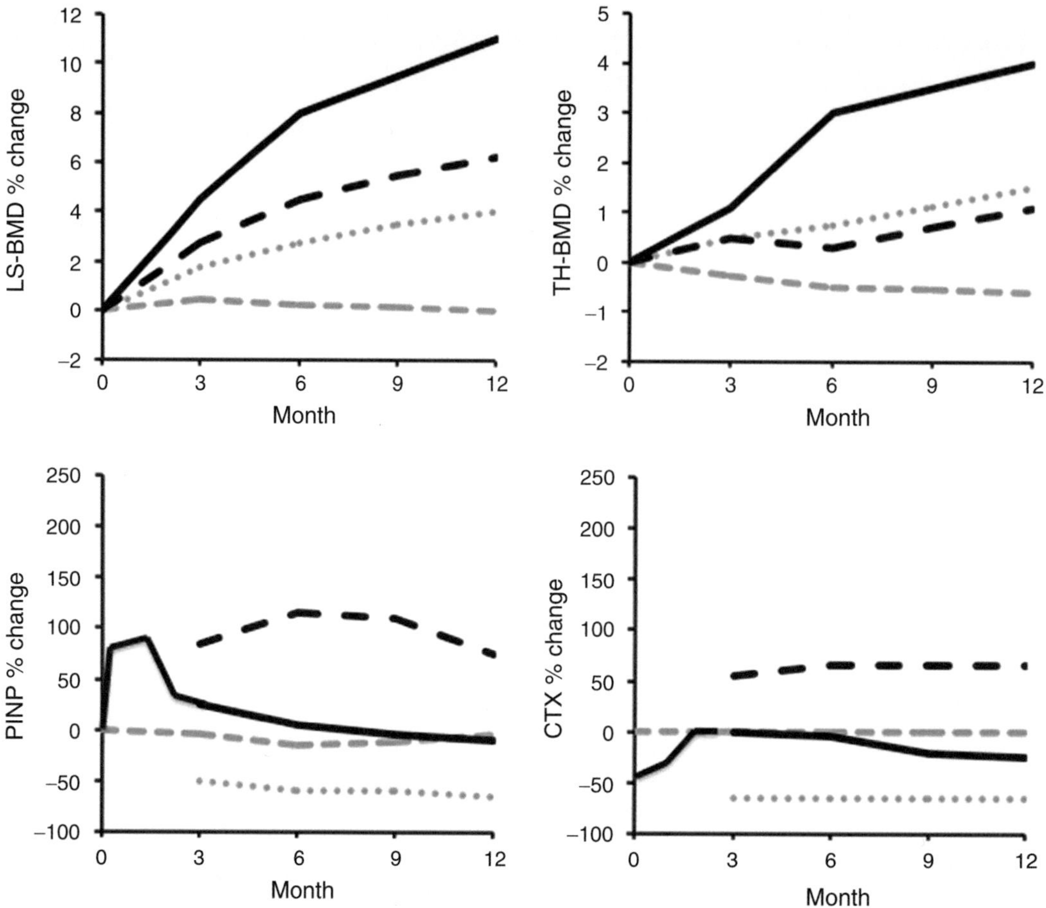

Fig. 3.9 Changes in lumbar spine BMD (LS-BMD) (**a**) and total hip BMD (TH-BMD) (**b**) in patients treated with anti-sclerostin (*continuous line*), PTH (*broken line*), alendronate (*dotted line*), and placebo (*dotted-broken line*). The *lower panels* show changes in PINP (**a**) and CTX (**b**). Adapted from McClung MR et al. The New England Journal of Medicine. 2014;370(5):412–20 with permission from Massachusetts Medical Society

with romosozumab, where PINP levels returned to baseline within 6–7 months. Except for mild injection site reactions with romosozumab, adverse events were similar among groups [100]. No evidence of neutralizing antibodies was seen. Side effects due to bony overgrowth, characteristic for van Buchem disease, are unlikely due to the short treatment period.

Using a different anti-sclerostin antibody developed by Eli Lilly (blosozumab), McClung et al. [103] investigated the effects of a wide variety of dosing regimens using doses ranging from 7.5 to 750 mg. Dose-dependent increases in biochemical markers of bone formation were demonstrable. Single dosing of 750 mg elicited a 3.1 % increase in lumbar spine BMD. A maximal increase of 7.7 % was, however, recorded after administration of 750 mg every 2 weeks over an 8-week period. These increases in bone mass were paralleled by increases in bone-specific alkaline phosphatase and PINP of 200 and 300 %, respectively. Previous treatment with bisphosphonate did not seem to inhibit stimulation of bone formation. Antibodies against blosozumab were detected but did not seem to affect efficacy.

Conclusion

Intermittent administration of PTH elicits pronounced improvements in bone structure in patients with osteoporosis and constitutes the only anabolic regimen currently approved for the treatment of osteoporosis. The severely impaired quality of osteoporotic bone characterized by reduced cortical thickness, disrupted cancellous bone structure, and reduced mass is reversed by PTH therapy, and a significant, albeit variable, amount of new bone is added to the skeleton. These changes result in a pronounced reduction in the risk of vertebral and in particular non-vertebral fractures. PTH treatment also significantly reduces back pain. Due to price and mode of administration, PTH is generally reserved for patients with the most severe osteoporosis including those with multiple or severe fractures and very low bone mass, but a more widespread use in certain conditions, e.g., GIO, is warranted. While sequential therapy with antiresorptive drugs following discontinuation of PTH is considered necessary to preserve bone mass, concomitant therapy is rarely indicated. Moreover, if oral bisphosphonates are administered concomitantly, varying degrees of blunting of the anabolic effect may occur. This blunting seems less pronounced with IV bisphosphonate like zoledronic acid and denosumab.

References[1]

1. *Lindsay R, Miller P, Pohl G, Glass EV, Chen P, Krege JH. Relationship between duration of teriparatide therapy and clinical outcomes in postmenopausal women with osteoporosis. Osteoporos Int. 2009;20(6):943–8. *Post hoc analysis on long term effects on teriparatide.
2. Dempster DW, Parisien M, Silverberg SJ, Liang XG, Schnitzer M, Shen V, et al. On the mechanism of cancellous bone preservation in postmenopausal women with mild primary hyperparathyroidism. J Clin Endocrinol Metab. 1999;84(5):1562–6.
3. *Dobnig H, Turner RT. The effects of programmed administration of human parathyroid hormone fragment (1-34) on bone histomorphometry and serum chemistry in rats. Endocrinology. 1997;138(11):4607–12. *Important data on effects of intermittens vs. continuous administration of PTH.
4. Bedi B, Li JY, Tawfeek H, Baek KH, Adams J, Vangara SS, et al. Silencing of parathyroid hormone (PTH) receptor 1 in T cells blunts the bone anabolic activity of PTH. Proc Natl Acad Sci USA. 2012;109(12):E725–33.
5. Onyia JE, Helvering LM, Gelbert L, Wei T, Huang S, Chen P, et al. Molecular profile of catabolic versus anabolic treatment regimens of parathyroid hormone (PTH) in rat bone: an analysis by DNA microarray. J Cell Biochem. 2005;95(2):403–18.
6. Hanyu R, Wehbi VL, Hayata T, Moriya S, Feinstein TN, Ezura Y, et al. Anabolic action of parathyroid hormone regulated by the beta2-adrenergic receptor. Proc Natl Acad Sci USA. 2012;109(19):7433–8.
7. Spurney RF, Flannery PJ, Garner SC, Athirakul K, Liu S, Guilak F, et al. Anabolic effects of a G protein-coupled receptor kinase inhibitor expressed in osteoblasts. J Clin Invest. 2002;109(10):1361–71.
8. Ma YL, Cain RL, Halladay DL, Yang X, Zeng Q, Miles RR, et al. Catabolic effects of continuous human PTH (1-38) in vivo is associated with sustained stimulation of RANKL and inhibition of osteoprotegerin and gene-associated bone formation. Endocrinology. 2001;142(9):4047–54.
9. Bellido T, Saini V, Pajevic PD. Effects of PTH on osteocyte function. Bone. 2013;54(2):250–7.
10. Keller H, Kneissel M. SOST is a target gene for PTH in bone. Bone. 2005;37(2):148–58.
11. Tamura Y, Kaji H. Parathyroid hormone and Wnt signaling. Clin Calcium. 2013;23(6):847–52.
12. Lombardi G, Di Somma C, Rubino M, Faggiano A, Vuolo L, Guerra E, et al. The roles of parathyroid hormone in bone remodeling: prospects for novel therapeutics. J Endocrinol Invest. 2011;34(7 Suppl):18–22.
13. *Dobnig H, Turner RT. Evidence that intermittent treatment with parathyroid hormone increases bone formation in adult rats by activation of bone lining cells. Endocrinology. 1995;136(8):3632–8. *First paper proposing the lining cell hypothesis.
14. Kim SW, Pajevic PD, Selig M, Barry KJ, Yang JY, Shin CS, et al. Intermittent parathyroid hormone administration converts quiescent lining cells to active osteoblasts. J Bone Miner Res. 2012;27(10):2075–84.
15. Eriksen EF, Mosekilde L, Melsen F. Trabecular bone remodeling and balance in primary hyperparathyroidism. Bone. 1986;7(3):213–21.
16. Dempster DW, Cosman F, Kurland ES, Zhou H, Nieves J, Woelfert L, et al. Effects of daily treatment with parathyroid hormone on bone microarchitecture and turnover in patients with osteoporosis: a paired biopsy study. J Bone Miner Res. 2001;16(10):1846–53.
17. Ma YL, Zeng Q, Donley DW, Ste-Marie LG, Gallagher JC, Dalsky GP, et al. Teriparatide increases bone formation in modeling and remodeling osteons and enhances IGF-II immunoreactivity in postmenopausal women with osteoporosis. J Bone Miner Res. 2006;21(6):855–64.
18. Lee JH, Hwang KJ, Kim MY, Lim YJ, Seol IJ, Jin HJ, et al. Human parathyroid hormone increases the mRNA expression of the IGF system and hematopoietic growth factors in osteoblasts, but does not

[1] *Important References

influence expression in mesenchymal stem cells. J Pediatr Hematol Oncol. 2012;34(7):491–6.

19. Bidwell JP, Childress P, Alvarez MB, Hood Jr M, He Y, Pavalko FM, et al. Nmp4/CIZ closes the parathyroid hormone anabolic window. Crit Rev Eukaryot Gene Expr. 2012;22(3):205–18.

20. Rhee Y, Lee EY, Lezcano V, Ronda AC, Condon KW, Allen MR, et al. Resorption controls bone anabolism driven by parathyroid hormone (PTH) receptor signaling in osteocytes. J Biol Chem. 2013;288(41):29809–20.

21. Arlot M, Meunier PJ, Boivin G, Haddock L, Tamayo J, Correa-Rotter R, et al. Differential effects of teriparatide and alendronate on bone remodeling in postmenopausal women assessed by histomorphometric parameters. J Bone Miner Res. 2005;20(7):1244–53.

22. Jiang Y, Zhao JJ, Mitlak BH, Wang O, Genant HK, Eriksen EF. Recombinant human parathyroid hormone (1-34) [teriparatide] improves both cortical and cancellous bone structure. J Bone Miner Res. 2003;18(11):1932–41.

23. Graeff C, Timm W, Nickelsen TN, Farrerons J, Marin F, Barker C, et al. Monitoring teriparatide-associated changes in vertebral microstructure by high-resolution CT in vivo: results from the EUROFORS study. J Bone Miner Res. 2007;22(9):1426–33.

24. Borggrefe J, Graeff C, Nickelsen TN, Marin F, Gluer CC. Quantitative computed tomographic assessment of the effects of 24 months of teriparatide treatment on 3D femoral neck bone distribution, geometry, and bone strength: results from the EUROFORS study. J Bone Miner Res. 2010;25(3):472–81.

25. *Paschalis EP, Glass EV, Donley DW, Eriksen EF. Bone mineral and collagen quality in iliac crest biopsies of patients given teriparatide: new results from the fracture prevention trial. J Clin Endocrinol Metab. 2005;90(8):4644–9. *Characterization of changes in bone matrix and mineralization after PTH.

26. Dobnig H, Stepan JJ, Burr DB, Li J, Michalska D, Sipos A, et al. Teriparatide reduces bone microdamage accumulation in postmenopausal women previously treated with alendronate. J Bone Miner Res. 2009;24(12):1998–2006.

27. Lindsay R, Nieves J, Formica C, Henneman E, Woelfert L, Shen V, et al. Randomised controlled study of effect of parathyroid hormone on vertebral-bone mass and fracture incidence among postmenopausal women on oestrogen with osteoporosis. Lancet. 1997;350(9077):550–5.

28. Moore AE, Blake GM, Taylor KA, Rana AE, Wong M, Chen P, et al. Assessment of regional changes in skeletal metabolism following 3 and 18 months of teriparatide treatment. J Bone Miner Res. 2010;25(5):960–7.

29. Frost ML, Siddique M, Blake GM, Moore AE, Schleyer PJ, Dunn JT, et al. Differential effects of teriparatide on regional bone formation using (18)

F-fluoride positron emission tomography. J Bone Miner Res. 2011;26(5):1002–11.

30. Uusi-Rasi K, Semanick LM, Zanchetta JR, Bogado CE, Eriksen EF, Sato M, et al. Effects of teriparatide [rhPTH (1-34)] treatment on structural geometry of the proximal femur in elderly osteoporotic women. Bone. 2005;36(6):948–58.

31. Zanchetta JR, Bogado CE, Ferretti JL, Wang O, Wilson MG, Sato M, et al. Effects of teriparatide [recombinant human parathyroid hormone (1-34)] on cortical bone in postmenopausal women with osteoporosis. J Bone Miner Res. 2003;18(3):539–43.

32. Rehman Q, Lang TF, Arnaud CD, Modin GW, Lane NE. Daily treatment with parathyroid hormone is associated with an increase in vertebral cross-sectional area in postmenopausal women with glucocorticoid-induced osteoporosis. Osteoporos Int. 2003;14(1):77–81.

33. Schnell R, Graeff C, Krebs A, Oertel H, Gluer CC. Changes in cross-sectional area of spinal canal and vertebral body under 2 years of teriparatide treatment: results from the EUROFORS study. Calcif Tissue Int. 2010;87(2):130–6.

34. *Neer RM, Arnaud CD, Zanchetta JR, Prince R, Gaich GA, Reginster JY, et al. Effect of parathyroid hormone (1-34) on fractures and bone mineral density in postmenopausal women with osteoporosis. N Engl J Med. 2001;344(19):1434–41. *Pivotal efficacy and safety data.

35. Burr DB, Hirano T, Turner CH, Hotchkiss C, Brommage R, Hock JM. Intermittently administered human parathyroid hormone(1-34) treatment increases intracortical bone turnover and porosity without reducing bone strength in the humerus of ovariectomized cynomolgus monkeys. J Bone Miner Res. 2001;16(1):157–65.

36. *Keaveny TM, Donley DW, Hoffmann PF, Mitlak BH, Glass EV, San Martin JA. Effects of teriparatide and alendronate on vertebral strength as assessed by finite element modeling of QCT scans in women with osteoporosis. J Bone Miner Res. 2007;22(1):149–57. *Finite element analysis of bone strength after PTH compared to Alendronate.

37. Keaveny TM, Hoffmann PF, Singh M, Palermo L, Bilezikian JP, Greenspan SL, et al. Femoral bone strength and its relation to cortical and trabecular changes after treatment with PTH, alendronate, and their combination as assessed by finite element analysis of quantitative CT scans. J Bone Miner Res. 2008;23(12):1974–82.

38. Poole KE, Treece GM, Ridgway GR, Mayhew PM, Borggrefe J, Gee AH. Targeted regeneration of bone in the osteoporotic human femur. PloS one. 2011;6(1):e16190.

39. Black DM, Delmas PD, Eastell R, Reid IR, Boonen S, Cauley JA, et al. Once-yearly zoledronic acid for treatment of postmenopausal osteoporosis. N Engl J Med. 2007;356(18):1809–22.

40. Cummings SR, San MJ, McClung MR, Siris ES, Eastell R, Reid IR, et al. Denosumab for prevention

of fractures in postmenopausal women with osteoporosis. N Engl J Med. 2009;361(8):756–65.

41. Gallagher JC, Genant HK, Crans GG, Vargas SJ, Krege JH. Teriparatide reduces the fracture risk associated with increasing number and severity of osteoporotic fractures. J Clin Endocrinol Metab. 2005;90(3):1583–7.

42. Marcus R, Wang O, Satterwhite J, Mitlak B. The skeletal response to teriparatide is largely independent of age, initial bone mineral density, and prevalent vertebral fractures in postmenopausal women with osteoporosis. J Bone Miner Res. 2003;18(1):18–23.

43. *Langdahl BL, Rajzbaum G, Jakob F, Karras D, Ljunggren O, Lems WF, et al. Reduction in fracture rate and back pain and increased quality of life in postmenopausal women treated with teriparatide: 18-month data from the European Forsteo Observational Study (EFOS). Calcif Tissue Int. 2009;85(6):484–93. *Important data on real life clinical use of PTH.

44. Ljunggren O, Barrett A, Stoykov I, Langdahl BL, Lems WF, Walsh JB, et al. Effective osteoporosis treatment with teriparatide is associated with enhanced quality of life in postmenopausal women with osteoporosis: the European Forsteo Observational Study. BMC Musculoskelet Disord. 2013;14:251.

45. Eastell R, Nickelsen T, Marin F, Barker C, Hadji P, Farrerons J, et al. Sequential treatment of severe postmenopausal osteoporosis after teriparatide: final results of the randomized, controlled European Study of Forsteo (EUROFORS). J Bone Miner Res. 2009;24(4):726–36.

46. Lyritis G, Marin F, Barker C, Pfeifer M, Farrerons J, Brixen K, et al. Back pain during different sequential treatment regimens of teriparatide: results from EUROFORS. Curr Med Res Opin. 2010;26(8):1799–807.

47. Hodsman AB, Hanley DA, Ettinger MP, Bolognese MA, Fox J, Metcalfe AJ, et al. Efficacy and safety of human parathyroid hormone-(1-84) in increasing bone mineral density in postmenopausal osteoporosis. J Clin Endocrinol Metab. 2003;88(11):5212–20.

48. Fox J, Miller MA, Recker RR, Bare SP, Smith SY, Moreau I. Treatment of postmenopausal osteoporotic women with parathyroid hormone 1-84 for 18 months increases cancellous bone formation and improves cancellous architecture: a study of iliac crest biopsies using histomorphometry and micro computed tomography. J Musculoskelet Neuronal Interact. 2005;5(4):356–7.

49. Greenspan SL, Bone HG, Ettinger MP, Hanley DA, Lindsay R, Zanchetta JR, et al. Effect of recombinant human parathyroid hormone (1-84) on vertebral fracture and bone mineral density in postmenopausal women with osteoporosis: a randomized trial. Ann Intern Med. 2007;146(5):326–39.

50. Kurland ES, Cosman F, McMahon DJ, Rosen CJ, Lindsay R, Bilezikian JP. Parathyroid hormone as a therapy for idiopathic osteoporosis in men: effects on bone mineral density and bone markers. J Clin Endocrinol Metab. 2000;85(9):3069–76.

51. Orwoll ES, Scheele WH, Paul S, Adami S, Syversen U, Diez-Perez A, et al. The effect of teriparatide [human parathyroid hormone (1-34)] therapy on bone density in men with osteoporosis. J Bone Miner Res. 2003;18(1):9–17.

52. Kaufman JM, Orwoll E, Goemaere S, San Martin J, Hossain A, Dalsky GP, et al. Teriparatide effects on vertebral fractures and bone mineral density in men with osteoporosis: treatment and discontinuation of therapy. Osteoporos Int. 2005;16(5):510–6.

53. Saag KG, Shane E, Boonen S, Marin F, Donley DW, Taylor KA, et al. Teriparatide or alendronate in glucocorticoid-induced osteoporosis. N Engl J Med. 2007;357(20):2028–39.

54. Gluer CC, Marin F, Ringe JD, Hawkins F, Moricke R, Papaioannu N, et al. Comparative effects of teriparatide and risedronate in glucocorticoid-induced osteoporosis in men: 18-month results of the EuroGIOPs trial. J Bone Miner Res. 2013;28(6):1355–68.

55. *Saag KG, Zanchetta JR, Devogelaer JP, Adler RA, Eastell R, See K, et al. Effects of teriparatide versus alendronate for treating glucocorticoid-induced osteoporosis: thirty-six-month results of a randomized, double-blind, controlled trial. Arthritis Rheum. 2009;60(11):3346–55. *Use of PTH in GIO.

56. Misof BM, Roschger P, Cosman F, Kurland ES, Tesch W, Messmer P, et al. Effects of intermittent parathyroid hormone administration on bone mineralization density in iliac crest biopsies from patients with osteoporosis: a paired study before and after treatment. J Clin Endocrinol Metab. 2003;88(3):1150–6.

57. *McClung MR, San MJ, Miller PD, Civitelli R, Bandeira F, Omizo M, et al. Opposite bone remodeling effects of teriparatide and alendronate in increasing bone mass. Arch Intern Med. 2005;165(15):1762–8. *Contrasting effects of anabolics vs. antiresorptives.

58. *Dobnig H, Sipos A, Jiang Y, Fahrleitner-Pammer A, Ste-Marie LG, Gallagher JC, et al. Early changes in biochemical markers of bone formation correlate with improvements in bone structure during teriparatide therapy. J Clin Endocrinol Metab. 2005;90(7):3970–7. *Predictive value of early changes of bone markers.

59. Chen P, Miller PD, Recker R, Resch H, Rana A, Pavo I, et al. Increases in BMD correlate with improvements in bone microarchitecture with teriparatide treatment in postmenopausal women with osteoporosis. J Bone Miner Res. 2007;22(8):1173–80.

60. Blumsohn A, Marin F, Nickelsen T, Brixen K, Sigurdsson G, Gonzalez de la Vera J, et al. Early changes in biochemical markers of bone turnover and their relationship with bone mineral density changes after 24 months of treatment with teriparatide. Osteoporos Int. 2011;22(6):1935–46.

61. Stepan JJ, Burr DB, Li J, Ma YL, Petto H, Sipos A, et al. Histomorphometric changes by teriparatide in alendronate-pretreated women with osteoporosis. Osteoporos Int. 2010;21(12):2027–36.

62. Deal C, Omizo M, Schwartz EN, Eriksen EF, Cantor P, Wang J, et al. Combination teriparatide and raloxifene therapy for postmenopausal osteoporosis: results from a 6-month double-blind placebo-controlled trial. J Bone Miner Res. 2005;20(11):1905–11.

63. Ettinger B, San Martin J, Crans G, Pavo I. Differential effects of teriparatide on BMD after treatment with raloxifene or alendronate. J Bone Miner Res. 2004;19(5):745–51.

64. *Cosman F, Nieves J, Woelfert L, Formica C, Gordon S, Shen V, et al. Parathyroid hormone added to established hormone therapy: effects on vertebral fracture and maintenance of bone mass after parathyroid hormone withdrawal. J Bone Miner Res. 2001;16(5):925–31.

65. Cosman F, Nieves J, Zion M, Woelfert L, Luckey M, Lindsay R. Daily and cyclic parathyroid hormone in women receiving alendronate. N Engl J Med. 2005;353(6):566–75.

66. Obermayer-Pietsch BM, Marin F, McCloskey EV, Hadji P, Farrerons J, Boonen S, et al. Effects of two years of daily teriparatide treatment on BMD in postmenopausal women with severe osteoporosis with and without prior antiresorptive treatment. J Bone Miner Res. 2008;23(10):1591–600.

67. Lindsay R, Scheele WH, Neer R, Pohl G, Adami S, Mautalen C, et al. Sustained vertebral fracture risk reduction after withdrawal of teriparatide in postmenopausal women with osteoporosis. Arch Intern Med. 2004;164(18):2024–30.

68. *Black DM, Greenspan SL, Ensrud KE, Palermo L, McGowan JA, Lang TF, et al. The effects of parathyroid hormone and alendronate alone or in combination in postmenopausal osteoporosis. N Engl J Med. 2003;349(13):1207–15. *Blunting of PTH effects by Alendronate.

69. Finkelstein JS, Hayes A, Hunzelman JL, Wyland JJ, Lee H, Neer RM. The effects of parathyroid hormone, alendronate, or both in men with osteoporosis. N Engl J Med. 2003;349(13):1216–26.

70. Cosman F, Eriksen EF, Recknor C, Miller PD, Guanabens N, Kasperk C, et al. Effects of intravenous zoledronic acid plus subcutaneous teriparatide [rhPTH(1-34)] in postmenopausal osteoporosis. J Bone Miner Res. 2011;26(3):503–11.

71. Tsai JN, Uihlein AV, Lee H, Kumbhani R, Siwila-Sackman E, McKay EA, et al. Teriparatide and denosumab, alone or combined, in women with postmenopausal osteoporosis: the DATA study randomised trial. Lancet. 2013;382(9886):50–6.

72. *Prince R, Sipos A, Hossain A, Syversen U, Ish-Shalom S, Marcinowska E, et al. Sustained nonvertebral fragility fracture risk reduction after discontinuation of teriparatide treatment. J Bone Miner Res. 2005;20(9):1507–13. *Preservation of antifracture efficacy after discontinuation.

73. Kurland ES, Heller SL, Diamond B, McMahon DJ, Cosman F, Bilezikian JP. The importance of bisphosphonate therapy in maintaining bone mass in men after therapy with teriparatide [human parathyroid hormone(1-34)]. Osteoporos Int. 2004;15(12):992–7.

74. Lane NE, Sanchez S, Modin GW, Genant HK, Pierini E, Arnaud CD. Bone mass continues to increase at the hip after parathyroid hormone treatment is discontinued in glucocorticoid-induced osteoporosis: results of a randomized controlled clinical trial. J Bone Miner Res. 2000;15(5):944–51.

75. Black DM, Bilezikian JP, Ensrud KE, Greenspan SL, Palermo L, Hue T, et al. One year of alendronate after one year of parathyroid hormone (1-84) for osteoporosis. N Engl J Med. 2005;353(6):555–65.

76. Miller PD, Schwartz EN, Chen P, Misurski DA, Krege JH. Teriparatide in postmenopausal women with osteoporosis and mild or moderate renal impairment. Osteoporos Int. 2007;18(1):59–68.

77. Vahle JL, Long GG, Sandusky G, Westmore M, Ma YL, Sato M. Bone neoplasms in F344 rats given teriparatide [rhPTH(1-34)] are dependent on duration of treatment and dose. Toxicol Pathol. 2004;32(4):426–38.

78. Tashjian Jr AH, Gagel RF. Teriparatide [human PTH(1-34)]: 2.5 years of experience on the use and safety of the drug for the treatment of osteoporosis. J Bone Miner Res. 2006;21(3):354–65.

79. Harper KD, Krege JH, Marcus R, Mitlak BH. Osteosarcoma and teriparatide? J Bone Miner Res. 2007;22(2):334.

80. Lipton A, Chapman JA, Demers L, Shepherd LE, Han L, Wilson CF, et al. Elevated bone turnover predicts for bone metastasis in postmenopausal breast cancer: results of NCIC CTG MA.14. J Clin Oncol. 2011;29(27):3605–10.

81. Lipton A. Zoledronic acid: multiplicity of use across the cancer continuum. Expert Rev Anticancer Ther. 2011;11(7):999–1012.

82. Hall CL, Kang S, MacDougald OA, Keller ET. Role of Wnts in prostate cancer bone metastases. J Cell Biochem. 2006;97(4):661–72.

83. Whitfield JF. Parathyroid hormone: a novel tool for treating bone marrow depletion in cancer patients caused by chemotherapeutic drugs and ionizing radiation. Cancer Lett. 2006;244(1):8–15.

84. Hodsman AB, Bauer DC, Dempster DW, Dian L, Hanley DA, Harris ST, et al. Parathyroid hormone and teriparatide for the treatment of osteoporosis: a review of the evidence and suggested guidelines for its use. Endocr Rev. 2005;26(5):688–703.

85. Nakamura Y. Parathyroid hormone as a bone anabolic agent. Evidence of osteoporosis treatment with weekly teriparatide injection. Clin Calcium. 2012;22(3):407–13.

86. Fujita T, Inoue T, Morii H, Morita R, Norimatsu H, Orimo H, et al. Effect of an intermittent weekly dose of human parathyroid hormone (1-34) on osteoporosis: a randomized double-masked prospective study using three dose levels. Osteoporos Int. 1999;9(4):296–306.

87. Gowen M, Stroup GB, Dodds RA, James IE, Votta BJ, Smith BR, et al. Antagonizing the parathyroid calcium receptor stimulates parathyroid hormone secretion and bone formation in osteopenic rats. J Clin Invest. 2000;105(11):1595–604.

88. McCauley LK, Martin TJ. Twenty-five years of PTHrP progress: from cancer hormone to multifunctional cytokine. J Bone Miner Res. 2012;27(6): 1231–9.

89. Horwitz MJ, Tedesco MB, Gundberg C, Garcia-Ocana A, Stewart AF. Short-term, high-dose parathyroid hormone-related protein as a skeletal anabolic agent for the treatment of postmenopausal osteoporosis. J Clin Endocrinol Metab. 2003;88(2): 569–75.

90. Horwitz MJ, Tedesco MB, Garcia-Ocana A, Sereika SM, Prebehala L, Bisello A, et al. Parathyroid hormone-related protein for the treatment of postmenopausal osteoporosis: defining the maximal tolerable dose. J Clin Endocrinol Metab. 2010;95(3):1279–87.

91. Horwitz MJ, Augustine M, Kahn L, Martin E, Oakley CC, Carneiro RM, et al. A comparison of parathyroid hormone-related protein (1-36) and parathyroid hormone (1-34) on markers of bone turnover and bone density in postmenopausal women: the PrOP study. J Bone Miner Res. 2013;28(11):2266–76.

92. http://www.clinicaltrials.gov/ct2/show/study/NCT0 1343004?term=ba058&rank=3.

93. *Hattersley GBJ, Guerriero J, et al. Bone anabolic efficacy and safety of BA058, a novel analog of hPTHrP: results from a phase 2 clinical trial in postmenopausal women with osteoporosis. The Endocrine Society's 94th Annual Meeting; Houston 2012. *Important PTHrp paper.

94. van Bezooijen RL, Papapoulos SE, Lowik CW. Bone morphogenetic proteins and their antagonists: the sclerostin paradigm. J Endocrinol Invest. 2005;28 (8 Suppl):15–7.

95. Helfrich MH, Aronson DC, Everts V, Mieremet RH, Gerritsen EJ, Eckhardt PG, et al. Morphologic features of bone in human osteopetrosis. Bone. 1991;12(6):411–9.

96. Fratzl-Zelman N, Valenta A, Roschger P, Nader A, Gelb BD, Fratzl P, et al. Decreased bone turnover and deterioration of bone structure in two cases of pycnodysostosis. J Clin Endocrinol Metab. 2004;89(4):1538–47.

97. Hassler N, Roschger A, Gamsjaeger S, Kramer I, Lueger S, van Lierop A, et al. Sclerostin deficiency is linked to altered bone composition. J Bone Miner Res. 2014;29:2144–51.

98. Li C, Ominsky MS, Tan HL, Barrero M, Niu QT, Asuncion FJ, et al. Increased callus mass and enhanced strength during fracture healing in mice lacking the sclerostin gene. Bone. 2011;49(6):1178–85.

99. Ominsky MS, Vlasseros F, Jolette J, Smith SY, Stouch B, Doellgast G, et al. Two doses of sclerostin antibody in cynomolgus monkeys increases bone formation, bone mineral density, and bone strength. J Bone Miner Res. 2010;25(5):948–59.

100. *McClung MR, Grauer A, Boonen S, Bolognese MA, Brown JP, Diez-Perez A, et al. Romosozumab in postmenopausal women with low bone mineral density. N Engl J Med. 2014;370(5):412–20. *Important comparative data pertaining to antisclerostin and PTH.

101. Ominsky MS, Niu QT, Li C, Li X, Ke HZ. Tissue-level mechanisms responsible for the increase in bone formation and bone volume by sclerostin antibody. J Bone Miner Res. 2014;29(6):1424–30.

102. http://www.amgen.com/media/media_pr_detail. jsp?releaseID=1679935.

103. McColm J, Hu L, Womack T, Tang CC, Chiang AY. Single- and multiple-dose randomized studies of blosozumab, a monoclonal antibody against sclerostin, in healthy postmenopausal women. J Bone Miner Res. 2014;29(4):935–43.

Tools for Assessing Fracture Risk and for Treatment Monitoring

4

William D. Leslie, Lisa M. Lix, and Suzanne N. Morin

Summary

- Validated prognostic models for fracture risk assessment can guide clinicians and individuals in appreciating the risk of having an osteoporosis-related fracture and can inform decision-making to mitigate these risks.
- Fracture probability algorithms that have been independently evaluated in at least one cohort other than the derivation population include the World Health Organization FRAX® tool, the Garvan Fracture Risk Calculator, and the QResearch Database's QFracture®.
- The use of fracture risk prediction tools is expanding beyond their role in treatment initiation, but data are still limited. For example, FRAX appears to be useful in assessing individuals on treatment. However, FRAX-derived fracture probability is not particularly responsive to osteoporosis treatments and cannot be recommended as a target for goal-directed therapy.
- Treatment-responsive measures need to be identified that can better inform the osteoporosis management paradigm.

W.D. Leslie, MD, MSc (✉)
Department of Medicine, St. Boniface General
Hospital, C5121-409 Tache Ave., Winnipeg, MB,
Canada, R2H 2A6

Departments of Medicine and Radiology, University
of Manitoba, Winnipeg, MB, Canada
e-mail: bleslie@sbgh.mb.ca

L.M. Lix, PhD
Department of Community Health Sciences,
University of Manitoba, Winnipeg, MB, Canada

S.N. Morin, MD, MSc
Department of Medicine, McGill University Health
Center, Montreal, QC, Canada

Introduction

Osteoporosis is a major risk factor for the development of fractures of the hip, proximal humerus, vertebra, and forearm (often termed the "major osteoporotic fracture" sites), though other skeletal sites contribute to the global fracture burden in osteoporosis [1]. In the absence of a fragility fracture, osteoporosis is typically diagnosed from bone mineral density (BMD) measured with dual X-ray absorptiometry (DXA). The World Health Organization operational definition of osteoporosis is a BMD that lies 2.5 standard deviations (SD) or more below the average mean value for young healthy women (T-Score ≤ -2.5) based upon a standardized reference site (the femoral neck) and reference population (National Health and Nutrition Examination Survey [NHANES] III data for White women aged 20–29 years) [2–4].

© Springer International Publishing Switzerland 2016
S.L. Silverman, B. Abrahamsen (eds.), *The Duration and Safety
of Osteoporosis Treatment*, DOI 10.1007/978-3-319-23639-1_4

BMD measurement from DXA provides a relative estimate of fracture risk, increasing 1.4- to 2.6-fold for every SD decrease in BMD [5, 6]. Despite the deceptive simplicity of a BMD-based approach to osteoporosis management, many studies show that most fractures occur in individuals who have a BMD T-score above the defining cutoff for osteoporosis [1, 7–9]. The suboptimal performance of BMD alone for fracture prediction has led to the development of new risk prediction algorithms that estimate fracture probability using additional risk factors for fracture, including demographic and physical characteristics, personal and family history, other health conditions, and medication use. This chapter reviews selected risk assessment tools, based upon absolute fracture probability, and their value in the decision for treatment initiation and monitoring.

Overview of Fracture Prediction Tools

Development of fracture prediction tools should ideally follow a systematic and rigorous methodology involving variable selection, model fit evaluation, performance evaluation, and both internal and external validation. Procedures for development and validation of fracture prediction models are reviewed elsewhere [10–14]. Discrimination (the model's ability to distinguish between individuals who do or do not experience the event of interest) and calibration (agreement between observed and predicted event rates for groups of individuals) are key performance aspects in risk prediction. The ability of the model to discriminate between individuals with and without the outcome is commonly assessed using the c-statistic [15, 16], which corresponds to the area under the receiver operation characteristic (ROC) curve for binary outcomes. The c-statistic ranges from zero to one, with a value of one representing perfect prediction and a value of 0.5 representing chance prediction. A value between 0.7 and 0.8 is typically considered to demonstrate acceptable performance, while a value greater than 0.8 is indicative of excellent performance. ROC analy-

ses are relatively insensitive to additional risk information even when the presence (or absence) of that information can make a difference in determining whether an individual patient lies below or above an intervention threshold. For example, the addition of a strong but uncommon new risk factor (hazard ratio 3.0 with prevalence 1 %) would only increase the c-statistic from 0.7 to 0.703, but could easily alter the decision to treat an individual with that risk factor [17]. Reclassification tables and net reclassification improvement statistics help to explore the effect of a novel risk factor on performance by describing how much more frequently appropriate reclassification occurs versus inappropriate reclassification [18, 19]. This underscores the importance of examining multiple measures of discrimination and classification for a fracture prediction tool [20, 21]. Both conventional and newer methods for assessing discrimination and calibration should be considered. External validation samples must have sufficiently large sample size to assess performance, with data collected using the same method as for the original model derivation.

This chapter focuses on model-based algorithms that have been validated in at least one cohort independent from the original derivation population: the World Health Organization FRAX tool, the Garvan Fracture Risk Calculator, and the QResearch Database's QFracture. The basic components of these tools are summarized in Table 4.1. Tools developed to identify individuals with low BMD (e.g., SCORE, OST, ORAI) do not provide a direct estimate of fracture probability and are not discussed further, although it is worth noting that some of these have also been shown to stratify fracture risk [22–24].

FRAX (www.shef.ac.uk/FRAX)

FRAX was developed by the WHO Collaborating Centre for Metabolic Bone Diseases to estimate an individual's 10-year probability of major osteoporotic fracture (composite of the clinical spine, hip, forearm, and proximal humerus) and hip fracture [25]. The input variables were

Table 4.1 Fracture risk prediction tools and their potential for intervention or pharmacologic response

Prediction tool, URL	Risk factors	Outputs	Risk factors amenable to intervention	Risk factors responsive to anti-osteoporosis treatment
FRAX (Fracture Risk Assessment Tool) [26] www.shef.ac.uk/FRAX	• Age, sex, BMI • Prior fragility fracture, glucocorticoid use ≥3 months, secondary osteoporosis, rheumatoid arthritis, parental hip fracture, current cigarette smoking, alcohol intake of ≥3 units/day (yes/no) • Femoral neck BMD or T-score (optional)	• 10-year major osteoporotic fracture (clinical vertebrae, hip, forearm, proximal humerus) • 10-year hip fracture	• BMI • Glucocorticoid use • Smoking • Alcohol intake • Femoral neck BMD	• Femoral neck BMD
Garvan Fracture Risk Calculator (Dubbo nomogram) [54, 55] www.garvan.org.au/ bone-fracture-risk	• Age, sex • Fractures after age 50 (none, 0, 1, 2, >3) • History of falls in the previous 12 months (none, 0, 1, 2, ≥3) • Femoral neck BMD (or T-score) or weight	• 5 or 10 years of any osteoporotic fracture (hip, clinical vertebrae, wrist, metacarpal, humerus, scapula, clavicle, distal femur, proximal tibia, patella, pelvis, and sternum) • 5- or 10-year hip fracture	• Falls in the previous 12 months • Weight • Femoral neck BMD	• Femoral neck BMD
QFracture [57, 58] www.qfracture.org	• Age, sex, 10 ethnic origins • Height, weight • Smoking (4 levels), alcohol intake (5 levels), diabetes (type 1, type 2), previous fracture, parental osteoporosis or hip fracture, living in a nursing or care home, history of falls, dementia, cancer, asthma/COPD, cardiovascular disease, chronic liver disease, chronic kidney disease, Parkinson's disease, rheumatoid arthritis/SLE, malabsorption, endocrine problems, epilepsy or anticonvulsant use, antidepressant use, steroid use, HRT use	• 1- to 10-year osteoporotic fracture (clinical spine, hip, distal forearm; humerus fracture was included with the 2012 version) • 1- to 10-year hip fracture	• Weight • Smoking • Alcohol intake • Anticonvulsant use • Antidepressant use • Steroid use • HRT use	• None

BMI body mass index, *BMD* bone mineral density, *HRT* hormone replacement therapy, *COPD* chronic obstructive pulmonary disease

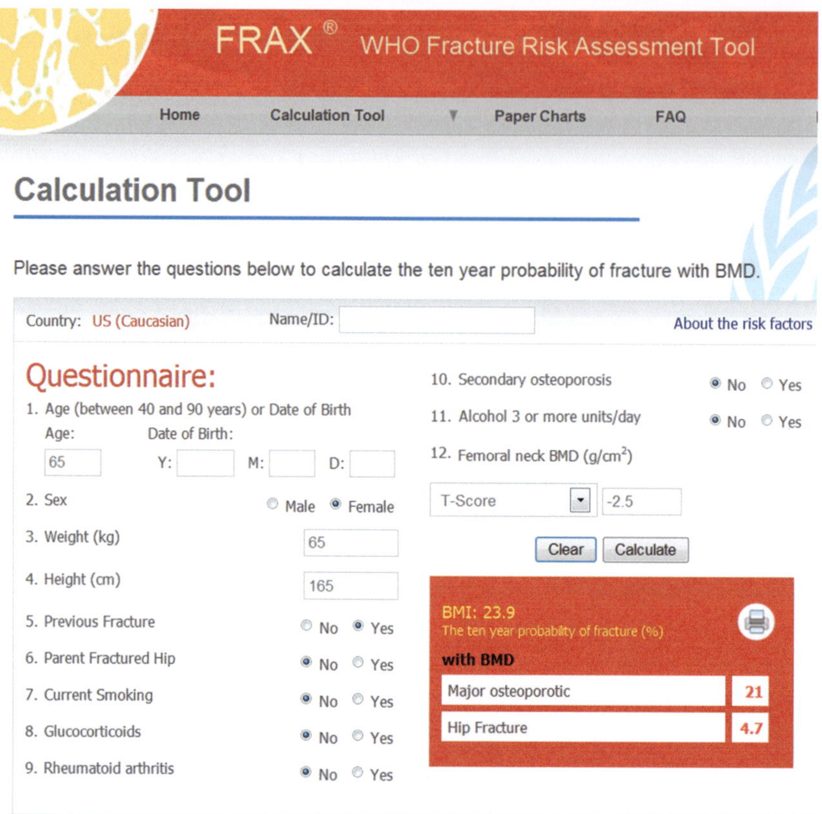

Fig. 4.1 Sample screenshot for FRAX® (US Caucasian tool). 10-year probability for major osteoporotic fracture is 21 % and for hip fracture is 4.7 % in a woman age 65 years, weight 65 kg, height 165 cm, previous fracture and femoral neck T-score −2.5. (Note that more than one fracture, type 2 diabetes, or fall in the prior year do not affect the calculation)

selected following a series of meta-analyses using data from nine prospective international population-based cohorts [26]. In addition to age, sex, and body mass index (BMI), additional clinical risk factors (CRFs) for fractures include prior fragility fracture, a parental history of hip fracture, prolonged use of glucocorticoids, rheumatoid arthritis, current cigarette smoking, alcohol intake of 3 or more units/day, and secondary osteoporosis (Fig. 4.1). Femoral neck BMD is an optional input that can refine the risk estimate, though even in its absence FRAX performs very well [27, 28]. Interactions among CRFs are also incorporated into the FRAX algorithm.

In survival analysis, the time at which a subject experiences an event of interest may be altered by another event, known as competing risk events [29]. For fracture, competing death is particularly important to consider in order to produce unbiased estimates of fracture risk since, following death, fracture is no longer possible. FRAX adjusts for competing mortality, and the competing mortality approach used by FRAX is unique among the risk prediction models. Individuals may have equivalent hazards for fracture, but if they differ in terms of hazard for death, then this will affect the 10-year fracture probability. For example, smoking is a risk factor for fracture but also increases the risk for death. Thus, the increased mortality associated with smoking reduces the importance of smoking as a risk factor for fracture. The 10-year major fracture probability tends to increase with age to peak around 80–85 years and then declines as the death hazard rises faster than the fracture hazard. Failure to account for competing mortality has been shown to overestimate major fracture probability by 15–56 % and hip fracture probability by 17–36 % in those with high mortality: men, age >80 years, high fracture probability, and diagnosed diabetes [30].

In recognition of the large international variability in fracture and mortality rates [31], population-specific FRAX tools are customized to the fracture and mortality epidemiology in a specific region [25]. The initial release of FRAX in 2008 covered nine countries (including four ethnic calculators for the USA), while the most recent version (3.8) includes over 50 countries. Minimum data requirements for constructing a new FRAX tool are sex- and age-specific mortality and hip fracture rates (5-year subgroups). In many countries, such data are relatively easy to obtain. In contrast, non-hip fracture data considered by FRAX (the clinical spine, distal forearm, proximal humerus) are difficult to accurately collect at the population level. Where high-quality data are not available, country-specific FRAX tools can be calibrated under the assumption that the ratio of these non-hip to hip fracture rates is similar to that observed in historical Swedish data (1987–1996) [32, 33]. Whether these ratios are universally applicable in all populations has been questioned. Population-based data from Canada suggest that these ratios may underestimate the rate of major osteoporotic fractures, possibly due to recent declines in hip fracture rates [34]. Although Swedish vertebral to hip fracture ratios were similar to Canadian ratios, those for other skeletal fracture sites were significantly lower (in men and women, respectively: 46 % and 35 % lower for forearm/hip ratios, 19 % and 15 % lower for humerus/hip ratios, and 19 % and 23 % lower for any MOF/hip ratio).

Fracture discrimination with FRAX was initially assessed in 9 primary derivation cohorts (46,340 subjects with 189,852 person-years follow-up) and then in 11 additional validation cohorts (230,486 persons with 1,208,528 person-years of follow-up) [35]. Risk stratification with FRAX including BMD was superior to FRAX without BMD or to BMD alone. In the primary derivation cohorts, the gradient of risk for hip fracture increased from 1.84 to 2.91 (area under

the curve [AUC] from 0.67 to 0.78) with the inclusion of BMD and for major osteoporotic fractures increased from 1.55 to 1.61 (AUC from 0.62 to 0.63) with the inclusion of BMD. In the validation cohorts, the averaged hip fracture gradient of risk (1.83 without BMD and 2.52 with BMD) and AUC (0.66 without BMD and 0.74 with BMD) was similar to that of the derivation cohorts, but the gradient of risk for other osteoporotic fractures (1.53 without BMD, 1.57 with BMD) and AUC (0.60 without BMD and 0.62 with BMD) was slightly lower.

A potential explanation for the lower AUC measurements for major osteoporotic versus hip fractures was described in a recent publication from the Global Longitudinal Study of Osteoporosis in Postmenopausal Women (GLOW) [36]. Varying associations with age were seen for 10 different bone fracture sites in 53,896 women age 55 years and older, with clinical fractures of the hip, pelvis, upper leg, clavicle, and spine (designed the F5 sites) each exhibiting a strong association with advanced age. In contrast, five other fracture sites, which include the upper arm/shoulder and wrist, had much weaker associations with age. As a result, an age-related fracture prediction model for the F5 sites performed better than FRAX for all major osteoporotic fractures (Harrell's c-index 0.75 and 0.67, respectively).

A number of studies have performed independent assessments of FRAX to predict subsequent fracture, but they differ widely in sample size, methodology (particularly incorporation of competing mortality risk), and techniques used to assess the performance of the fracture prediction tool (discrimination versus calibration) [10], which can affect the validity of these validation studies [17]. In 2010, Sornay-Rendu et al. [37] examined 867 French women age 40 years and over from the OFELY (Os des Femmes de Lyon) cohort which included 95 incident major osteoporotic fractures. Predicted probabilities of fracture were considerably greater in women with incident fractures than in women without incident fractures. The observed incidence of major osteoporotic fractures was found to be higher than the predicted FRAX probability, but the analysis did not account for the effect of competing mortality. Fracture discrimination for major osteoporotic fractures was good (AUC 0.75 [95 % CI 0.71–0.79] without BMD, 0.78 [95 % CI 0.72–0.82] with BMD). Trémollieres et al. [38] examined a separate group of 2651 French women from the MENOS (Menopause et Os) cohort who sustained 145 major osteoporotic fractures (13 hip fractures) during the follow-up period. Once again, fracture discrimination was good for major osteoporotic fractures, but the study was underpowered to show an improvement in risk assessment with FRAX (AUC 0.63, 95 % CI 0.56–0.69) over BMD alone (AUC 0.66, 95 % CI 0.60–0.73).

A FRAX tool for Canada was developed from national hip fracture and mortality data [39]. The accuracy of fracture predictions was assessed in two large, independent cohorts: the Canadian Multicentre Osteoporosis Study (CaMos) (one of the population-based FRAX derivation cohorts) and the Manitoba Bone Density Program (a long-term observational clinical cohort not included in FRAX derivation cohorts) [40, 41]. Analyses for the Manitoba BMD cohort (36,730 women and 2873 men) and CaMos cohort (4778 women and 1919 men) were similar and showed that the Canadian FRAX tool generated fracture risk predictions that were consistent with observed fracture rates across a wide range of risk categories in both clinical and average populations. In the Manitoba cohort [40], discrimination for incident hip fracture (AUC 0.83, 95 % CI 0.82–0.85) and major osteoporosis-related fractures (AUC 0.69, 95 % CI 0.68–0.71) was similar to the derivation and validation cohorts studied by the WHO Collaborating Centre [35]. Fracture discrimination using FRAX with BMD was better than FRAX without BMD (hip fracture AUC 0.79, major osteoporosis fracture AUC 0.66) or femoral neck BMD alone (hip fracture AUC 0.80, major osteoporosis fracture AUC 0.68). In CaMos [41], results were similar with the FRAX estimates using BMD and CRFs superior to BMD alone or CRFs alone for both major osteoporotic fractures and hip fractures. For major osteoporotic fractures, FRAX with BMD gave an AUC 0.69 (95 % CI 0.67–0.71) vs. FRAX without BMD 0.66 (95 % CI 0.63–0.68) versus femoral

neck T-score alone 0.66 (95 % CI 0.64–69). For hip fractures, FRAX with BMD gave AUC 0.80 (95 % CI 0.77–0.83) vs. FRAX without BMD 0.77 (95 % CI 0.73–0.80). The average 10-year probability for major osteoporotic fractures, with BMD, was not significantly different from the observed value in men [predicted 5.4 % vs. observed 6.4 % (95 % CI 5.2–7.5 %)] and only slightly lower in women [predicted 10.8 % vs. observed 12.0 % (95 % CI 11.0–12.9 %)]. FRAX with BMD was well calibrated for hip fracture assessment in women [predicted 2.7 % vs. observed 2.7 % (95 % CI 2.2–3.2 %)] but underestimated risk in men [predicted 1.3 % vs. observed 2.4 % (95 % CI 1.7–3.1 %)].

The importance of correct calibration was noted when the UK FRAX tool was used to assess fracture risk in a convenience sample of 501 Polish women referred for BMD testing [42]. Self-reported incident fractures 9–12 years later were assessed by telephone interview. The observed/expected ratio for fracture was 1.79 (95 % CI 1.44–2.21) without BMD and 1.94 (95 % CI 1.45–2.54) with BMD suggesting that the UK model significantly underestimated fracture risk in Polish women. However, fractures could only be assessed in long-term survivors, a factor which likely contributed to biased results due to failure to account for competing mortality.

A small Japanese study (43 self-reported major osteoporotic fractures and 4 hip fractures) was reported by Tamaki et al. [43] using the Japanese Population-Based Osteoporosis Study (JPOS) cohort. The numbers of observed major osteoporotic or hip fracture events were found to be consistent with FRAX predictions, with significant stratification in fracture risk (major osteoporotic fracture AUC without BMD 0.67, 95 % CI 0.59–0.75; AUC with BMD 0.69, 95 % CI 0.61–0.76).

Rubin et al. [44] performed a registry linkage study using baseline questionnaire data from 3636 Danish women with FRAX hip fracture probabilities calculated from the Swedish tool. Predicted and observed risk estimates incorporated adjustment for 10-year survival rates. The predicted 10-year hip fracture risk was 7.6 % overall with observed risk also 7.6 %, with similarly good results from age 41–50 years (predicted 0.3 %, observed 0.4 %) to age 81–90 years (predicted 25.0 %, observed 24.0 %).

Premaor et al. [45] examined the question of whether FRAX was applicable to obese older women using 6049 white women from the US Study of Osteoporotic Fractures (SOF) cohort. Fracture discrimination from AUC was similar in obese and nonobese women. Calibration was good in both groups for prediction of major osteoporotic fractures using FRAX with BMD, but hip fracture risk was found to be underestimated, most marked among obese women in the lowest category for FRAX probability with BMD (though only based on a small number of 4 predicted vs. 9 observed hip fractures).

Ettinger et al. [46] examined 5891 men age 65 years and older (374 with incident major osteoporotic fractures, 161 incident hip fractures). Hip fracture discrimination (AUC 0.77 with BMD vs. 0.69 without BMD) was better than for major osteoporotic fractures (AUC 0.67 with BMD vs. 0.63 without BMD). Inclusion of BMD improved the overall net reclassification index for major osteoporotic fractures and hip fractures. Observed to predicted fracture ratios according to probability quintiles showed good calibration for hip fracture prediction without BMD (ratios 0.9–1.1), but hip fracture risk was significantly underestimated in the highest risk quintile when BMD was used in the calculation. Conversely, major osteoporotic fracture risk was underestimated without BMD (predicted ratio 0.7–0.9), and addition of BMD did not significantly affect the results (predicted ratio 0.7–1.1).

Byberg et al. [47] examined 5921 men age 50 years and older from Sweden in the Uppsala Longitudinal Study of Adult Men (ULSAM) in which 585 individuals sustained fracture (189 with hip fractures). FRAX explained 7–17 % of all fractures and 41–60 % of hip fractures. Including comorbidity, medications and behavioral factors improved overall fracture prediction. However, femoral neck BMD was only available in a small subset of those aged 82 years and older.

Gonzalez-Macias et al. [48] examined 5201 women age 65 years and older in a 3-year prospective follow-up study in Spain (201 with major osteoporotic fractures, 50 with incident hip fractures) using data from the Ecografía Osea en Atención Primaria (ECOSAP) study. AUC for FRAX without BMD was 0.62 for major osteoporotic fractures and 0.64 for hip fractures. Estimated to observed fracture ratios of 0.66 and 1.10, respectively, were likely influenced by the limited 3-year study duration of the follow-up, lack of data on clinical vertebral fractures, and lack of adjustment for competing mortality risk. Another Spanish study from Tebe Cordomi et al. [49] conducted a retrospective cohort study of 1231 women aged 40–90 years (222 with at least 1 self-reported fracture after baseline assessment). AUC for major osteoporotic fracture estimated with BMD was 0.61 (95 % CI 0.57–0.65). The number of observed fractures was 3.9 times higher than the expected number. Fractures were self-reported at a follow-up survey at least 10 years after baseline assessment, but there was a large rate of non-response/nonparticipation (855 of 2086). Fractures could only be assessed in long-term survivors, and excluding individuals who died prior to 10 years could bias results.

On balance, these studies confirm the validity of FRAX for fracture risk assessment but highlight the importance of using high-quality fracture data to ensure accurate calibration of the FRAX tool. A set of 28 jointly endorsed positions were developed by the International Society of Clinical Densitometry (ISCD) and International Osteoporosis Foundation (IOF) to facilitate the use of FRAX in clinical practice and provide guidance on its application in specific and challenging circumstances [50, 51]. Specific adjustments can be applied to FRAX-derived risk scores to accommodate discordantly lower or higher lumbar spine BMD (more than 1 SD difference from femoral neck BMD) or glucocorticoid doses that are above or below average (average use defined as daily 2.5–7.5 mg prednisone equivalent) [52, 53].

Garvan Fracture Risk Calculator (www.garvan.org.au/ bone-fracture-risk)

The Dubbo Osteoporosis Epidemiology Study (DOES) was initiated in 1989 and involves follow-up of over 3500 participants. Using information on 426 clinical fractures in women (96 hip) and 149 clinical fractures in men (31 hip) excluding digits, 5- and 10-year fracture probability nomograms were constructed [54, 55]. Inputs include age, sex, femoral neck BMD (optional), history of prior fractures after age 50 years (none, 0, 1, 2, 3 or more), and history of falls in the previous 12 months (none, 0, 1, 2, 3 or more) (Fig. 4.2). If femoral neck BMD is not available, then weight is used as a surrogate. Risk factors that are relatively uncommon in the general population (e.g., glucocorticoid use and specific medical conditions) are not included. The model has only been calibrated for the Australian population and does not include an explicit competing mortality risk adjustment.

The Garvan algorithm has been independently evaluated in the Canadian population (4152 women and 1606 men age 55–95 years at baseline) with 8.6 years of follow-up (699 low-trauma fractures including 97 hip fractures) [56]. Fracture discrimination and calibration were found to be generally good in both women and men. For low-trauma fractures, the concordance between predicted risk and fracture events (Harrell's C which is similar to AUC) was 0.69 among women and 0.70 among men. For hip fractures, the concordance was 0.80 among women and 0.85 among men. Observed 10-year low-trauma fracture risk agreed with the predicted risk for all risk subgroups except in the highest risk quintile in men and women where observed risk was lower than predicted. Observed 10-year hip fracture risk agreed with the predicted risk for all risk subgroups except in the highest quintile of risk for women (observed risk lower than predicted).

QFracture (www.qfracture.org)

The largest prospective database for osteoporotic fracture prediction is from England and Wales using patients from 357 general practices for derivation and patients from 178 practices for validation in the initial analysis (QResearch Database) [57]. This provided more than one million women and more than one million men age 30–85 years in the derivation cohort with 24,350 incident osteoporotic fractures in women (9302 hip fractures) and 7934 osteoporotic fractures in men (5424 hip fractures). The risk calculator includes numerous CRFs, but not BMD (Fig. 4.3). It provides outputs of any osteoporotic fracture (hip, wrist, or spine) and hip fracture over a user-selected follow-up period from 1 year to 10 years. The QFracture algorithm was updated in 2012, with inclusion of a number of new CRFs, removal of several others, and the addition of humerus fractures as one of the osteoporotic fractures [58]. In addition to age, sex, and ethnicity (10 different ethnic origins), the algorithm includes smoking status (4 levels), alcohol consumption (5 levels), diabetes (type 1 and type 2), previous fracture, parental osteoporosis or hip fracture, living in a nursing or care home, history of falls, dementia, cancer, asthma/COPD, cardiovascular disease, chronic liver disease, chronic kidney disease, Parkinson's disease, rheumatoid arthritis/SLE, malabsorption, endocrine problems, epilepsy or anticonvulsant use, antidepressant use, steroid use, HRT use, height, and weight.

The 2012 version reported very good performance for osteoporotic fracture prediction (AUC 0.79 in women and 0.71 in men) and excellent performance for hip fracture prediction (AUC 0.89 in women and 0.88 in men). An independent validation study was performed using patients from 364 general practices in The Health Improvement Network (THIN) (UK) database (2.2 million adults aged 30–85 years with 25,208 osteoporotic and 12,188 hip fractures) [59]. The validation cohort gave AUC discrimination for osteoporotic fracture of 0.82 in women and 0.74 in men and for hip fracture of 0.89 in women and 0.86 in men. Calibration plots adhered closely to the line of identity. QFracture explained 63 % of the variation in hip fracture risk in women and 60 % of the variation in men (49 % and 38 % for osteoporotic fracture risk).

A small retrospective comparison of FRAX and QFracture was conducted in 246 postmenopausal women aged 50–85 years with recent low-trauma fracture and 338 non-fracture control women from 6 centers in Ireland and the UK [60]. AUC for fracture discrimination were similar in QFracture and FRAX (0.668 vs. 0.665) and also for hip fractures (0.637 vs. 0.710). The striking difference with AUC measures from the THIN database validation study is unexplained.

The broad age range used in the initial validation work may have inflated the performance measures since osteoporotic fractures are unlikely before age 50. Additional assessments of QFracture in older women and men are needed.

Comparative Performance

Figures 4.1, 4.2, and 4.3 illustrate some of the differences between the fracture prediction systems discussed above for a 65-year-old woman of average height and weight with femoral neck T-score at the osteoporotic threshold of −2.5 and having the following CRFs: two previous fragility fractures (distal radius and humerus), type 2 diabetes, and one fall in the prior year. None of the systems uses all of the available information, and this contributes to the range in fracture predictions. For example, 10-year hip fracture probability varies from 4.7 % for FRAX, to 5.3 % for QFracture-2013, to 28.4 % for the Garvan calculator. It is clear that where an important CRF is not captured by a tool, clinical judgment

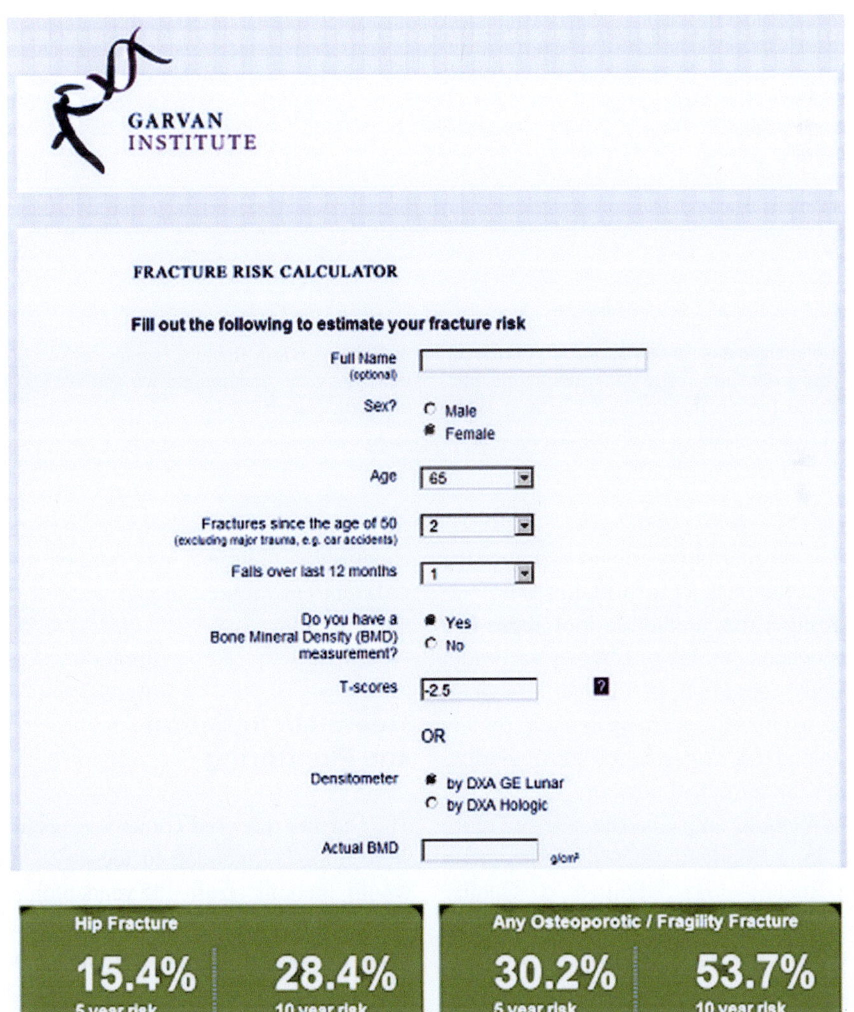

Fig. 4.2 Sample screenshot for Garvan fracture risk calculator. 10-year probability for major osteoporotic fracture is 53.7 % and for hip fracture is 28.4 % in a woman age 65 years, two previous fractures, one previous fall, and femoral neck T-score −2.5. (Note that weight 65 kg, height 165 cm, and type 2 diabetes do not affect the calculation)

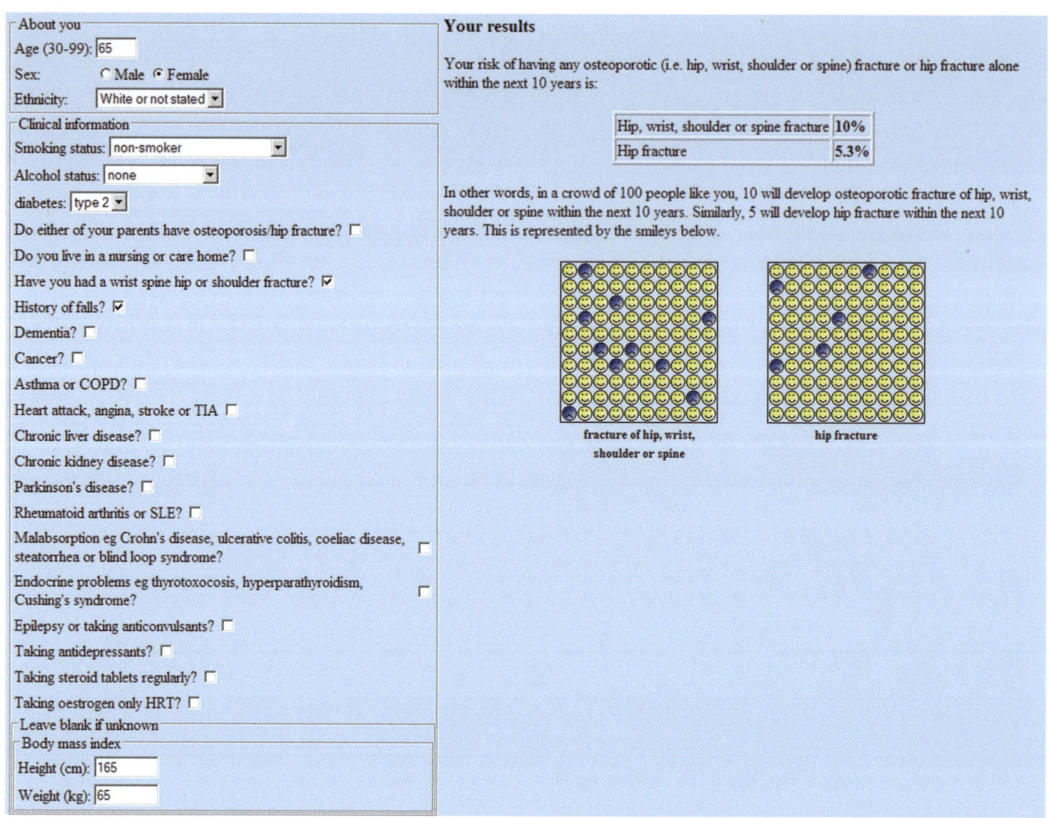

Fig. 4.3 Sample screenshot for QFracture®-2013 risk calculator. 10-year probability for major osteoporotic fracture is 10 % and for hip fracture is 5.3 % in a White woman age 65 years, weight 65 kg, height 165 cm, type 2 diabetes, previous fracture, and history of falls. (Note that more than one fracture and femoral neck T-score do not affect the calculation)

must make some qualitative consideration of the importance of the missing information.

In designing a risk prediction tool, there is a trade-off between complexity (greater accuracy) and simplicity (adoption in clinical practice). Rubin et al. [61] performed a systematic review of screening and risk assessment tools (including FRAX, the Garvan calculator, and QFracture). Of a total of 48 tools, only 6 had been tested more than once in a population-based setting with acceptable methodology (defined a Quality Assessment Tool for Diagnostic Accuracy Studies [QUADAS] score above 60 %) [62]. There was no consistent evidence that more complex tools had better performance characteristics than simpler tools; however, the paucity of head-to-head comparisons limits any definitive conclusions. Larger, high-quality studies with different case mixes should address this important question.

Treatment Initiation and Monitoring

The fracture risk prediction tools described above were initially intended to identify patients who would benefit from pharmacologic therapy. Increasingly, there is interest in whether these tools can be used in treated individuals to (re) assess fracture risk and detect treatment-related reduction in fracture risk. These concepts and evolving clinical applications are explored in the following sections.

Treatment Decision-Making in the Untreated Individual

To date, only the FRAX tool has been integrated into national clinical practice guidelines [63–71], though a recent review of updated guidelines around the world found a wide diversity of approaches [72]. Some guidelines have embraced fracture risk as the preferred decision-making approach, and others are still largely dictated by BMD, whereas others are a hybrid. The National Osteoporosis Foundation (NOF) guidelines are an example of the latter, where treatment is recommended for individuals with an osteoporotic T-score, clinical osteoporosis based upon low-trauma spine or hip fracture, or in individuals with low bone mass (osteopenia) where fracture risk under the US FRAX tools exceeds 20 % for major osteoporotic fractures or 3 % for hip fractures [63, 64]. The NOF intervention thresholds were based on a cost-effectiveness analysis [73]. The Taiwanese guidelines are similar to the NOF guidelines but do not differentiate between those with osteoporosis or osteopenia or treat based upon BMD alone; treatment is suggested for postmenopausal women with osteoporotic fracture after 50 years of age or when FRAX with BMD reveals a 10-year major osteoporotic fracture risk ≥20 % or hip fracture risk ≥3 % [74]. Canadian guidelines recommend treatment initiation based upon high-risk fracture events (hip fracture, spine fracture, or multiple fragility fractures) or where major osteoporotic fracture probability exceeds 20 % [71]. The National Osteoporosis Guideline Group (NOGG), working in collaboration with many other societies from the UK, has fully embraced fracture risk in guiding therapy and recommends that treatment be considered in women with a prior fragility fracture (BMD measurement is optional) or when fracture probability with FRAX exceeds an age-specific intervention threshold [66, 75]. The intervention threshold at each age is set at a risk equivalent to that associated with a prior fracture, resulting in a lower threshold in younger individuals and a higher threshold in older individuals. NOGG restricts BMD to individuals whose fracture risk is close to the intervention threshold: individuals with fracture risk sufficiently below or above the intervention threshold are not recommended for BMD testing. The NOGG guidelines suggested treatment if the chance of fracture in a given individual exceeded that of a subject at a similar age with a prior fragility fracture [66, 75]. A similar approach has been advocated for the European setting by the European Society for Clinical and Economic Aspects of Osteoporosis and Osteoarthritis (ESCEO) and International Osteoporosis Foundation (IOF) [76]. The UK National Clinical Guideline Centre has provided guidance on the selection and use of FRAX UK and QFracture in the care of people who may be at risk of fragility fractures [77]. The diversity of guideline approaches in part reflects regional variations in population disease burden, practice patterns, health-care priorities, and economic considerations.

Reversibility of Fracture Risk with Treatment

The use of risk factors for case finding requires that the risk so identified is responsive to a therapeutic intervention. Table 4.1 indicates potentially reversible risk factors for each of the fracture prediction tools that are amenable to intervention, as well as those expected to be responsive to pharmacologic treatment. Some risk factors (e.g., age, sex, parental hip fracture) are clearly not amenable to intervention. Others could be specifically targeted (e.g., optimizing nutritional status and lifestyle factors, avoidance of high-risk medications, fall prevention) independent of pharmacotherapy for osteoporosis. Finally, pharmacologic intervention for osteoporosis targets one risk factor alone (e.g., femoral neck BMD) and would not affect other risk factors or fracture probability estimated in the absence of a BMD measurement.

The distinction between a reversible risk factor and reversibility of risk associated with that risk factor is important to highlight. Age is an example of an irreversible risk factor, but the fracture risk associated with older age has reversibility, i.e., the risk identified by age is amenable to therapeutic intervention. Most clinical trials that have shown efficacy recruited subjects on the basis of low BMD, but some trials have recruited patients on the basis of age, sex, a prior vertebral or hip fracture, and exposure to glucocorticoids [27, 78–81].

In the absence of a specific clinical trial, an alternative approach is to demonstrate through post hoc analyses that the presence (or absence) of a risk factor does not adversely influence therapeutic efficacy. The presence or absence of an interaction between treatment benefit and specific risk factors can help to inform the expectation of reversibility of risk. Lack of interaction implies that groups with or without the risk factors respond similarly. Therefore, even for irreversible risk factors, as long as there is no negative interaction, then this implies that the risk factor will not adversely affect treatment response. Alternatively, where a significant interaction exists, it may help to identify groups in whom greater (or lesser) benefit may be expected. These types of post hoc analyses conducted as part of pivotal clinical trials have generally not shown major interactions with the clinical risk factors used in FRAX [27]. Conversely, patients selected solely on the basis of risk factors for falling may respond less well to agents that preserve bone mass than those selected on the basis of low BMD [82]. In some cases, test for interaction may be nonsignificant due to limited power to detect such effects. Conversely, caution also needs to be exercised in interpreting results from multiple post hoc analyses due to the potential for false-positive findings [83]. For example, post hoc analyses from the FREEDOM study evaluating denosumab examined nine subgroups (age, BMI, femoral neck BMD T-score, prevalent vertebral fracture, prior non-vertebral fracture, estimated creatinine clearance, geographic region, race, and prior use of osteoporosis medications) [84]. No significant treatment interactions were observed on vertebral fracture prevention, but vertebral fracture prevention showed nominally significant interactions with BMI (treatment effective for BMI <25 kg/m^2 but not for higher BMI; P-interaction 0.0135), baseline femoral neck T-score (treatment effective for T-score <

−2.5 but not for higher BMD; P-interaction 0.0229), and prevalent vertebral fracture (treatment effective for those without but not with fracture; P-interaction 0.0377). In contrast, the HORIZON-PFT trial found greater intravenous zoledronic acid effects on vertebral fracture risk in younger women (P-interaction 0.05), normal creatinine clearance (P-interaction 0.04), and body mass index $\geq$25 kg/m^2 (P-interaction 0.02), without significant treatment interactions for hip or non-vertebral fracture [85]. A meta-analysis found that the efficacy or raloxifene on vertebral fracture risk was significantly greater at lower ages [86]. Consistency of treatment effect among subgroups has been observed with alendronate, risedronate, and strontium ranelate [87–90].

Anti-fracture effect of several therapeutic agents has been analyzed based on initial FRAX fracture probabilities. Results have not been consistent between or even within classes of therapeutic agents. Greater relative risk reduction (beyond absolute risk reduction) has been observed with higher FRAX probability measurements with clodronate [91], bazedoxifene [92], and denosumab [93], but not with alendronate [94], raloxifene [86], or strontium ranelate [95]. For example, the FREEDOM study found that denosumab reduced fracture risk to a greater extent in those at moderate to high risk (Fig. 4.4) [93]. For example, at 10 % probability, denosumab decreased fracture risk by 11 % ($P=0.629$), whereas at 30 % probability (90th percentile of study population), the reduction was 50 % ($P=0.001$). It remains uncertain why differences would exist for some antiresorptive agents and not others. Similar type analyses with the Garvan calculator and QFracture have not yet been performed.

There is an implicit assumption that fracture prediction tools demonstrating increased fracture probability should identify individuals who will benefit from treatment with a reduction in fracture risk. If the relative risk reduction is relatively constant, then greater absolute fracture risk would imply a greater absolute benefit (equivalent to a lower number needed to treat [NNT]). Although intuitive, this is an area of controversy as no clinical trials have prospectively recruited

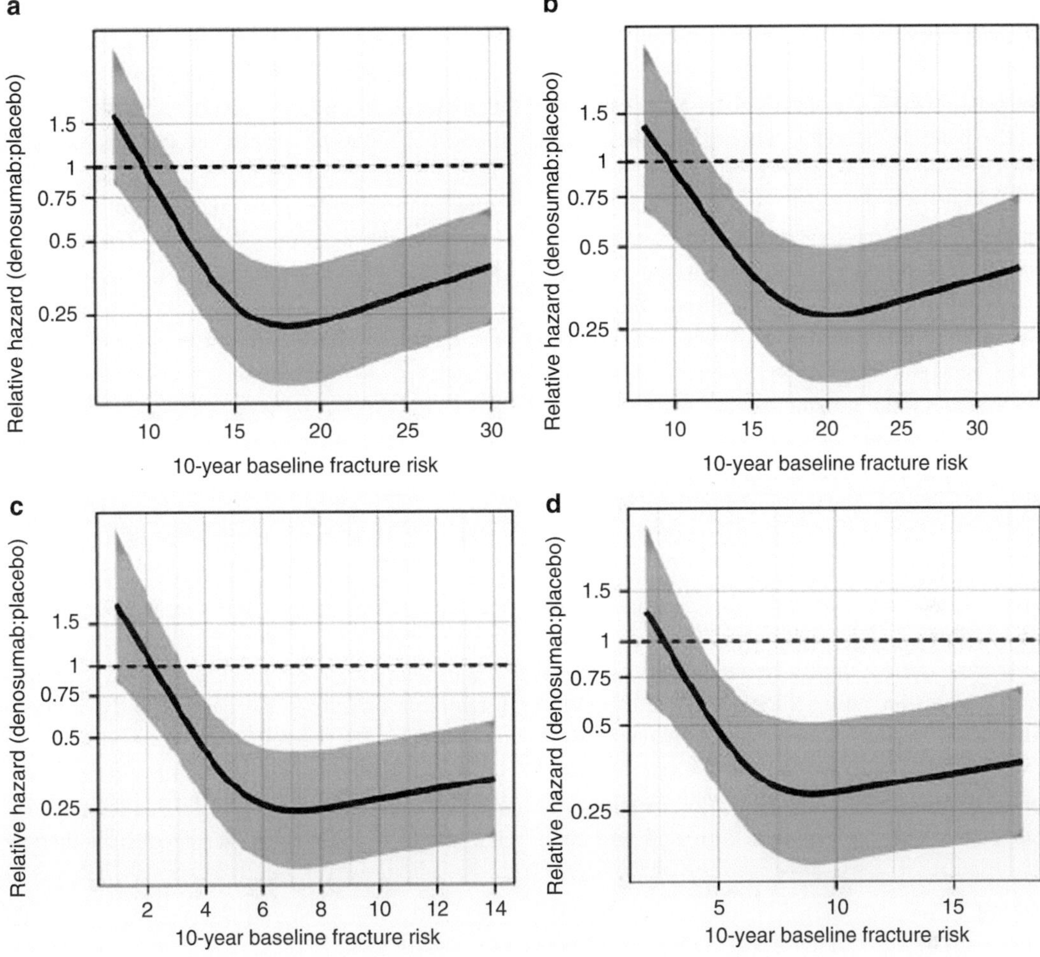

Fig. 4.4 Relationship between denosumab efficacy on clinical osteoporotic fractures and baseline FRAX probability of major osteoporotic fracture calculated with (**a**) or without (**b**) femoral neck bone mineral density (**c**, **d**). The efficacy on clinical osteoporotic fractures against baseline FRAX probability of hip fracture is shown. The extremes of the baseline probabilities represent the 10th and 90th percentile values. From McCloskey et al. [93]. Reprinted with permission from the American Society for Bone and Mineral Research

on the basis of fracture probability. Subgroup analyses from two pivotal clinical trials, the Fracture Intervention Trial (alendronate) and the Hip Intervention Program Study Group (risedronate), showed little or no benefit from bisphosphonate therapy in subjects without low BMD [82, 94, 96].

Ultimately, if it were possible to identify factors robustly predicting greater anti-fracture effect, then this might allow for the construction of prediction tools for treatment benefit (as opposed to baseline fracture risk which may or may not always be reversible). The construct of such a tool might be quite different from the fracture probability tool used to identify baseline fracture risk and, as noted above, must consider differences between therapeutic agents. In some studies, change in BMD on therapy [97–99], bone turnover markers [100, 101], and measures of compliance/persistence on therapy have shown an association with treatment response [102]. Whether any such tool would explain sufficient variation in treatment response to be of clinical value would need to be established.

Effect of Treatment on Fracture Risk Prediction

Whether FRAX can be used to assess fracture risk in patients receiving concurrent treatment for osteoporosis has been uncertain since treatment effects are not explicitly accommodated in the model [50]. However, since many individuals were initiated on treatment prior to the availability of FRAX, this potentially limits the use of important information for advising patients on their need for continued treatment or whether treatment could potentially be withdrawn. To address this issue, a large clinical cohort was linked to population-based databases to determine medication prescriptions and fracture outcomes in 35,764 women (age ≥50 years) and baseline BMD testing and FRAX probabilities [103]. A pharmacy database was used to categorize women using osteoporosis medication as untreated, current high adherence users (medication possession ratio [MPR] ≥0.80 in the year after BMD testing), current low adherence users (MPR < 0.80), and past users. FRAX and femoral neck BMD alone stratified major osteoporotic and hip fracture risk within untreated and each treated subgroup (all P-values <0.001) with similar area under the receiver operating characteristic curve (Table 4.2). Hazard ratios for prediction of major osteoporotic fractures and hip fracture using FRAX were equally strong regardless of treatment status. In untreated and in each treated subgroup, a stepwise gradient in observed 10-year major osteoporotic and hip fracture incidence was seen as a function of the predicted probability tertile (all p-values <0.001 for linear trend). Concordance (calibration) plots for major osteoporotic fractures and hip fractures showed good agreement between the predicted and observed 10-year fracture incidence in untreated women and each treated subgroup (Fig. 4.5). Only in the highest risk tertile of women highly adherent to at least 5 years of bisphosphonate use was the observed hip fracture risk significantly less than predicted, while major osteoporotic fracture risk was similar to predicted. These data suggest that the FRAX tool can be used to predict fracture probability in women currently or previously treated for osteoporosis.

The same data source also confirmed that repeat BMD measurements were useful for fracture risk assessment in individuals on osteoporosis therapy

Table 4.2 Area under the receiver operating characteristic curve (AUROC) for fracture prediction and adjusted hazard ratios (HR) for fracture per standard deviation decrease in femoral neck T-score

	Untreated	High adherence current treatment (MPR≥0.8)	Low adherence current treatment (MPR<0.8)	Past treatment
Prediction of major osteoporotic fractures				
AUROC major fracture probability without BMD	0.63 (0.61–0.65)	0.67 (0.65–0.69)	0.69 (0.67–0.71)	0.67 (0.62–0.72)
AUROC major fracture probability with BMD	0.66 (0.64–0.68)	0.64 (0.62–0.66)	0.71 (0.70–0.73)	0.69 (0.64–0.74)
AUROC femoral neck BMD	0.65 (0.62–0.67)	0.65 (0.63–0.67)	0.69 (0.67–0.71)	0.66 (0.61–0.71)
HR per SD decrease in BMD	1.53 (1.43–1.65)	1.52 (1.34–1.72)	1.64 (1.50–1.79)	1.53 (1.40–1.67)
Prediction of hip fractures				
AUROC hip fracture probability without BMD	0.78 (0.74–0.82)	0.76 (0.72–0.79)	0.83 (0.80–0.86)	0.83 (0.80–0.86)
AUROC hip fracture probability with BMD	0.82 (0.79–0.85)	0.80 (0.77–0.83)	0.85 (0.83–0.88)	0.85 (0.83–0.88)
AUROC femoral neck BMD	0.78 (0.74–0.83)	0.77 (0.73–0.8)	0.82 (0.79–0.85)	0.79 (0.70–0.88)
HR per SD decrease in BMD	2.33 (1.99–2.72)	2.26 (1.74–2.93)	2.32 (1.93–2.79)	2.18 (1.81–2.62)

Adapted with permission from Leslie et al. [103]
Data are AUROC (95 % CI). *MPR* medication possession ratio, *BMD* bone mineral density. Data are HR (95 % CI) from Cox proportional hazards' models adjusted for age, BMI, prior fragility fracture, rheumatoid arthritis, recent corticosteroid use, COPD diagnosis, and substance abuse diagnosis. *P*-interaction for BMD*treatment status nonsignificant (>0.1)

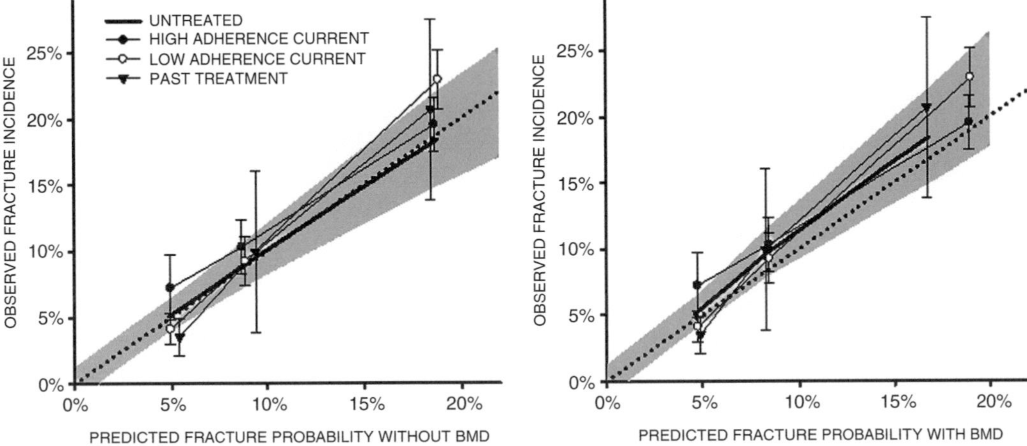

Fig. 4.5 Predicted 10-year major osteoporotic fracture probability from FRAX versus observed fracture incidence estimated to 10 years according to risk tertile. Results are stratified by osteoporosis treatment status with the reference group being untreated women (*heavy solid line* with 95 % CI *shaded area*). 95 % CI bars are shown for the treated subgroups. The *dotted line* indicates the line of identity (perfect concordance between observed and predicted fracture incidence). Reprinted with permission from the American Society for Bone and Mineral Research (Leslie et al. [103])

[104]. Baseline BMD results were available in 50,215 women over age 50 years, among whom repeat BMD testing occurred in 14,619. Total hip BMD (adjusted for FRAX variables) was similarly predictive of major osteoporotic fractures on first or second scans (adjusted HR per SD 1.45 [95 % CI 1.34–1.56] vs. 1.64 [1.48–1.81]). No significant differences were seen whether second scans were stratified by osteoporosis therapy use over the prior year (HRs 1.50 [1.28–1.76] for MPR=0, 1.46 [1.09–1.96] for MPR <0.5, 1.83 [1.30–2.58] for MPR 0.5–0.8, 2.08 [1.72–2.51] for MPR >0.8; *P*-interaction nonsignificant) or by BMD change (HR for 1.58 [1.37–1.82] for no change, 1.50 [1.09–2.06] for significant increase, 1.66 [1.30–2.13] for significant decrease; *P*-interaction nonsignificant). Similar results were seen for hip fracture prediction or when lumbar spine and femoral neck BMD were analyzed. Therefore, BMD is a robust predictor of fractures, and this does not diminish if it is a repeat measurement or if individuals are receiving osteoporosis therapy.

QFracture considers current use of estrogen replacement therapy. Coding estrogen use lowers the calculated fracture probability (from 10 % to 8.6 % for 10-year MOF and from 5.3 % to 4.1 % for 10-year hip fracture for the case in Fig. 4.3). However, there are likely to be major limitations to this approach as it is now recommended that women use hormone replacement therapy for shorter time periods and at the lowest dose that will relieve menopausal symptoms [105]. Non-estrogen based anti-osteoporosis therapies, which are most frequently prescribed to reduce fracture risk in postmenopausal women, are not considered nor is adherence/persistence or duration of therapy.

Responsiveness to Treatment

Available treatments for osteoporosis are very effective, with several agents safely yielding 40–60 % reductions in the risk of fracture [71, 106]. In general, absence of fracture and lack of BMD loss are considered treatment success (i.e., "goal achieved"), while fracture and loss of BMD are considered treatment failures [107, 108]. The anti-fracture benefit from osteoporosis therapy is consistently greater than can be explained from the increase in BMD alone, and the latter typically accounts for only a minority of the anti-fracture benefits seen in clinical trials [109, 110]. As a result, BMD change alone cannot be considered an adequate surrogate measure of treatment effectiveness [111]. Furthermore, BMD is only one of the risk factors included in the FRAX and

Garvan risk assessment models and does not appear in the QFracture model. Other risk factors used in these tools would not be expected to change as a result of osteoporosis therapy.

This situation is different than for many other chronic conditions—such as hypertension, dyslipidemia, or diabetes—where validated surrogate measures exist [112, 113]. That is, systolic blood pressure, LDL cholesterol, and hemoglobin A1c are quantifiable parameters that change with treatment and for which there are specific targets to guide therapy [112, 113]. The goals are evidence-based, and it is well documented that changes in these surrogate measures are tightly linked with clinical endpoints [112–114]. Because of this, goals such as systolic blood pressure <140 mmHg, LDL cholesterol <2.0 mmol/L, or hemoglobin A1c<7 % guide the primary care physicians in the treatment of these conditions [114]. The use of well-defined treatment targets to assist physicians in disease management is a strategy often called "treat to target." Establishing treatment targets is intended to simplify clinical decision-making, improve clinical outcomes, and permit comparative performance measurement, but this all presupposes the existence of a suitably responsive biomarker that also accurately predicts clinical outcomes. Since BMD by itself is inadequate in this regard, it has been proposed that change in estimated fracture probability might well serve the purpose for osteoporosis [107, 115]. Fracture probability tools can already be used to predict fracture risk in the general population and (in the case of FRAX) in those on treatment, but to attain the status of a treatment goal, it would need to be responsive to changes in risk factors and osteoporosis treatments. The need to develop more responsive methods for monitoring drug treatment in osteoporosis was highlighted in an initiative to develop goal-directed treatment "treat-to-target" guidelines for osteoporosis [107].

However, FRAX was not found to be sufficiently responsive to anti-osteoporosis treatment for "treat to target" in an analysis of 11,049 previously untreated women age 50 years and older from a large BMD registry with paired FRAX estimates (median interval 4 years) [116]. 6534 women initiated treatment after the initial assessment (40 % were highly adherent with medication possession ratio of 80 % or greater). BMD decreased in untreated women and showed expected gains in adherent women (5.6–7.8 % for the lumbar spine, 2.8–3.0 % for the femoral neck, $P<0.001$ for linear trend). Despite this, median FRAX probability still increased, predominantly due to increasing age (Fig. 4.6). Only 2.2 % of women had a clinically important decrease in major osteoporotic fracture probability (4 % or greater), and only 1.2 % had an important decrease in hip fracture probability (1 % or greater). Baseline FRAX probability was strongly predictive of incident major osteoporotic fractures (hazard ratio 1.8 per SD; 95 % CI 1.7:1.9) and hip fractures (hazard ratio 4.5 per SD, 95 % CI 3.7:5.7), but change in FRAX score was not an independent predictor of fractures.

Despite the intuitive appeal of monitoring change in fracture probability, it has proven very challenging to identify suitably responsive indices and treatment targets. Currently, only BMD and bone turnover markers appear to be sufficiently responsive to pharmacologic therapy to serve as possible targets [97–101].

Posttreatment Monitoring

Drugs with persistent skeletal effects after discontinuation (such as the bisphosphonates) raise the possibility of intermittent cycles of treatment and "drug holiday." To date, no fracture prediction tools have been studied in relation to posttreatment monitoring during the "drug holiday" in order to identify when treatment should be reinitiated. Based upon the limited responsiveness of FRAX to treatment noted earlier, this is unlikely to be a good candidate for posttreatment monitoring. Similar limitations are likely to apply to the Garvan calculator and QFracture scores which share many similar characteristics and inputs. Once again, prediction tools that would be useful in this context would almost certainly be very different than those used for initial treatment selection.

Posttreatment BMD loss was studied in 406 women enrolled in the Fracture Intervention Trial (FIT) who had taken alendronate for a mean of

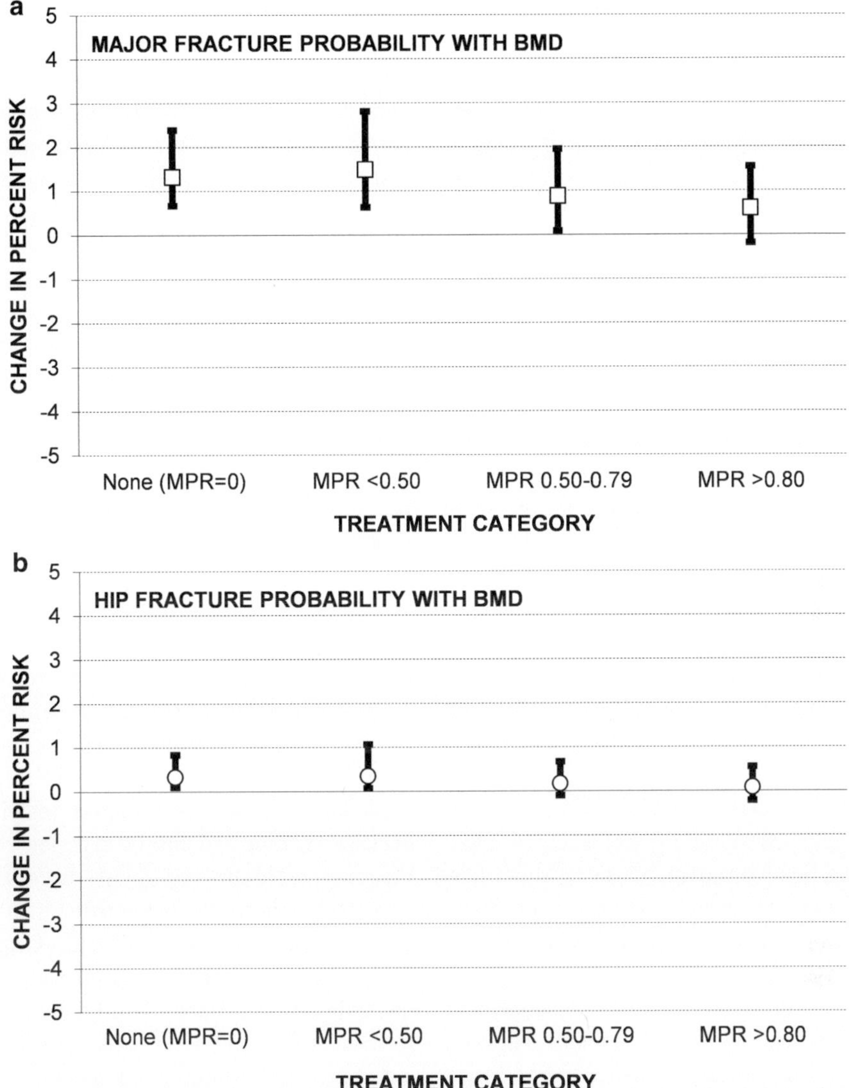

Fig. 4.6 Change in FRAX score between DXA scans according to osteoporosis treatment. (**a**) Major fractures and (**b**) hip fractures. Data are median values with inter-quartile range. *MPR* medication possession ratio. Reprinted with permission from the American Society for Bone and Mineral Research (Leslie et al. [116])

5 years and were then randomized to the placebo arm of the FIT Long-Term Extension (FLEX) trial for an additional 5 years [117]. Mean 5-year BMD changes during the treatment-free period were −3.6 % at the total hip, −1.7 % at the femoral neck, and +1.3 % at the lumbar spine (BMD losses exceeded 5 % observed in 29 % at the total hip, 11 % at the femoral neck, 1 % of subjects at the lumbar spine). Although some risk factors (such as age and BMI) were associated with greater BMD loss, the effects were relatively weak, and predicting which women will lose at a higher rate was not possible (models explained less than 15 % of the variability in the 5-year percent changes in BMD). Bone turnover markers were only assessed in 76 women but did not significantly improve prediction. Although about one-third of women who discontinued alendronate experienced >5 % bone loss at the total hip after 5 years, it was not possible to identify good predictors of this loss.

Future Directions

It is evident that no risk prediction model can include all possible risk factors for fracture; even if such a model could be constructed, it would be impossibly detailed and might not perform better than a more parsimonious model. More than 80 secondary causes of osteoporosis were specified in the US Surgeon General's report on osteoporosis [118]. Moreover, not all risk factors can be easily or reliably measured. Several studies have reported that very simple prediction models (e.g., age, BMD, and prior fracture) can discriminate fractures as well as more complex models [61, 119–122], but it is not altogether surprising that various models provide similar results given the insensitivity of global measures of test performance (e.g., ROC) to detect incremental improvement in risk classification from additional risk factors [13, 17]. For example, the prevalence of high-dose glucocorticoid use in the general population is very low (~1 %), and excluding this risk factor from the assessment is barely noticeable at the population level despite the importance it has for the individual risk prediction. Inclusion of additional skeletal measures (e.g., bone turnover markers, trabecular bone score) or sites of BMD measurement (e.g., lumbar spine) adds to the complexity with uncertain benefit in terms of the classification and improvement in overall patient management [50–52]. Finding the "right" balance between complexity and simplicity will require broad stakeholder input.

More studies evaluating the effect of osteoporosis treatment on risk assessment tools are needed. FRAX (and even BMD alone) appears to be useful in assessing individuals on treatment in one large historical cohort study [103, 104], but this needs to be confirmed in other cohorts, with the newer and more potent therapies, and with the other risk prediction tools. While FRAX scores are strongly predictive of incident major fractures and of hip fractures, they are not particularly responsive to osteoporosis treatments [116]. Directly modeling the effect of specific osteoporosis therapies is likely to be very challenging as there are significant between-agent differences in terms of antiresorptive potency, effect on BMD, effect on vertebral vs. non-vertebral fractures, and adherence/persistence. An unanswered question is whether patients differ in terms of their anti-fracture response when selected for treatment based upon a risk prediction model, and why reported treatment interactions are inconsistent between and within classes of agents. Formal clinical trials to evaluate anti-fracture efficacy in patients selected for treatment based upon fracture probability would be ideal but may not be feasible, but post hoc analyses of large clinical trials should be a priority.

Conclusions

Validated prognostic models for fracture risk assessment can guide clinicians and individuals in understanding the risk of suffering an osteoporosis-related fracture and inform their decision-making to mitigate this risk. Integration of risk prediction tools into clinical practice guidelines can in turn support better clinical decision-making and improved patient outcomes. Fracture probability algorithms discussed earlier have been independently validated in at least one other cohort: the World Health Organization FRAX, the Garvan Fracture Risk Calculator, and the QResearch Database's QFracture. The role for risk prediction tools is expanding beyond the initial decision regarding treatment initiation, but data are limited. Change in fracture probability is a poor surrogate measure for treatment response and cannot be recommended as a target for goal-directed therapy. More treatment-responsive measures are needed to better inform osteoporosis management paradigms.

Sources of Support LML is supported by a Manitoba Research Chair. SNM is Chercheur-clinicien Boursier des Fonds de la Recherche en Santé du Quebec.

Disclosures WDL (all fees paid to facility). Speaker bureau: Amgen, Eli Lilly, and Novartis. Research grants: Amgen and Genzyme. SNM: Consultant to Amgen, Novartis, Eli Lilly, and Merck. Speaker bureau: Amgen and Novartis. Research grant: Amgen.

References[1]

1. Stone KL, Seeley DG, Lui LY, Cauley JA, Ensrud K, Browner WS, et al. BMD at multiple sites and risk of fracture of multiple types: long-term results from the Study of Osteoporotic Fractures. J Bone Miner Res. 2003;18(11):1947–54.

2. Kanis JA, Melton III LJ, Christiansen C, Johnston CC, Khaltaev N. The diagnosis of osteoporosis. J Bone Miner Res. 1994;9(8):1137–41.

3. Looker AC, Wahner HW, Dunn WL, Calvo MS, Harris TB, Heyse SP, et al. Updated data on proximal femur bone mineral levels of US adults. Osteoporos Int. 1998;8(5):468–89.

4. Kanis JA, McCloskey EV, Johansson H, Oden A, Melton III LJ, Khaltaev N. A reference standard for the description of osteoporosis. Bone. 2008;42(3):467–75.

5. Johnell O, Kanis JA, Oden A, Johansson H, De Laet C, Delmas P, et al. Predictive value of BMD for hip and other fractures. J Bone Miner Res. 2005;20(7):1185–94.

6. Marshall D, Johnell O, Wedel H. Meta-analysis of how well measures of bone mineral density predict occurrence of osteoporotic fractures. BMJ. 1996;312(7041):1254–9.

7. Siris ES, Chen YT, Abbott TA, Barrett-Connor E, Miller PD, Wehren LE, et al. Bone mineral density thresholds for pharmacological intervention to prevent fractures. Arch Intern Med. 2004;164(10):1108–12.

8. Schuit SC, Van der KM, Weel AE, De Laet CE, Burger H, Seeman E, et al. Fracture incidence and association with bone mineral density in elderly men and women: the Rotterdam Study. Bone. 2004;34(1):195–202.

9. Cranney A, Jamal SA, Tsang JF, Josse RG, Leslie WD. Low bone mineral density and fracture burden in postmenopausal women. CMAJ. 2007;177(6):575–80.

10. Steyerberg EW. Clinical prediction models: a practical approach to development, validation, and updating. New York: Springer; 2008.

11. Altman DG, Vergouwe Y, Royston P, Moons KG. Prognosis and prognostic research: validating a prognostic model. BMJ. 2009;338:1432–5.

12. Royston P, Moons KG, Altman DG, Vergouwe Y. Prognosis and prognostic research: developing a prognostic model. BMJ. 2009;338:1373–7.

13. Steyerberg EW, Vickers AJ, Cook NR, Gerds T, Gonen M, Obuchowski N, et al. Assessing the performance of prediction models: a framework for traditional and novel measures. Epidemiology. 2010;21(1):128–38.

14. Leslie WD, Lix LM. Comparison between various fracture risk assessment tools. Osteoporos Int. 2014;25(1):1–21.

15. Ikeda M, Ishigaki T, Yamauchi K. Relationship between Brier score and area under the binormal ROC curve. Comput Methods Programs Biomed. 2002;67(3):187–94.

16. Harrell Jr FE, Lee KL, Mark DB. Multivariable prognostic models: issues in developing models, evaluating assumptions and adequacy, and measuring and reducing errors. Stat Med. 1996;15(4):361–87.

17. Kanis JA, Oden A, Johansson H, McCloskey E. Pitfalls in the external validation of FRAX. Osteoporos Int. 2012;23(2):423–31.

18. Pencina MJ, D'Agostino Sr RB, D'Agostino Jr RB, Vasan RS. Evaluating the added predictive ability of a new marker: from area under the ROC curve to reclassification and beyond. Stat Med. 2008;27(2):157–72.

19. Leening MJ, Vedder MM, Witteman JC, Pencina MJ, Steyerberg EW. Net reclassification improvement: computation, interpretation, and controversies: a literature review and clinician's guide. Ann Intern Med. 2014;160(2):122–31.

20. Pressman AR, Lo JC, Chandra M, Ettinger B. Methods for assessing fracture risk prediction models: experience with FRAX in a large integrated health care delivery system. J Clin Densitom. 2011;14(4):407–15.

21. Leslie WD, Lix LM. Absolute fracture risk assessment using lumbar spine and femoral neck bone density measurements: derivation and validation of a hybrid system. J Bone Miner Res. 2011;26(3):460–7.

22. Gourlay ML, Powers JM, Lui LY, Ensrud KE. Clinical performance of osteoporosis risk assessment tools in women aged 67 years and older. Osteoporos Int. 2008;19(8):1175–83.

23. Rud B, Hilden J, Hyldstrup L, Hrobjartsson A. The Osteoporosis Self-Assessment Tool versus alternative tests for selecting postmenopausal women for bone mineral density assessment: a comparative systematic review of accuracy. Osteoporos Int. 2009;20(4):599–607.

24. Schwartz EN, Steinberg DM. Prescreening tools to determine who needs DXA. Curr Osteoporos Rep. 2006;4(4):148–52.

25. Kanis JA, Oden A, Johansson H, Borgstrom F, Strom O, McCloskey E. FRAX and its applications to clinical practice. Bone. 2009;44(5):734–43.

26. Kanis JA, on behalf of the World Health Organization Scientific Group. Assessment of osteoporosis at the primary health-care level. Technical Report. Accessible at: http://www.shef.ac.uk/FRAX/pdfs/WHO_Technical_Report.pdf. Sheffield: University of Sheffield; 2007.

27. Kanis JA, McCloskey E, Johansson H, Oden A, Leslie WD. FRAX((R)) with and without bone mineral density. Calcif Tissue Int. 2012;90(1):1–13.

---

[1] *Important References

**Very Important References

28. Leslie WD, Morin S, Lix LM, Johansson H, Oden A, McCloskey E, et al. Fracture risk assessment without bone density measurement in routine clinical practice. Osteoporos Int. 2012;23(1):75–85.

29. Satagopan JM, Ben-Porat L, Berwick M, Robson M, Kutler D, Auerbach AD. A note on competing risks in survival data analysis. Br J Cancer. 2004;91(7): 1229–35.

30. Leslie WD, Lix LM, Wu X. Competing mortality and fracture risk assessment. Osteoporos Int. 2013;24(2):681–8.

31. Kanis JA, Oden A, McCloskey EV, Johansson H, Wahl DA, Cooper C. A systematic review of hip fracture incidence and probability of fracture worldwide. Osteoporos Int. 2012;23(9):2239–56.

32. Kanis JA, Johnell O, Oden A, Sembo I, Redlund-Johnell I, Dawson A, et al. Long-term risk of osteoporotic fracture in Malmo. Osteoporos Int. 2000;11(8):669–74.

33. Kanis JA, Oden A, Johnell O, Jonsson B, De Laet C, Dawson A. The burden of osteoporotic fractures: a method for setting intervention thresholds. Osteoporos Int. 2001;12(5):417–27.

34. Lam A, Leslie WD, Lix LM, Yogendran M, Morin SN, Majumdar SR. Major osteoporotic to hip fracture ratios in Canadian men and women with Swedish comparisons: a population based analysis. J Bone Miner Res. 2013;29(5):1067–73.

35. **Kanis JA, Oden A, Johnell O, Johansson H, De Laet C, Brown J, et al. The use of clinical risk factors enhances the performance of BMD in the prediction of hip and osteoporotic fractures in men and women. Osteoporos Int. 2007;18(8):1033–46. **This seminal report from the WHO Collaborating Centre for Metabolic Bone Diseases evaluated the performance characteristics of clinical risk factors with and without BMD in eleven independent population-based cohorts. The models developed provide the basis for the integrated use of validated clinical risk factors in men and women to aid in fracture risk prediction.

36. Fitzgerald G, Compston JE, Chapurlat RD, Pfeilschifter J, Cooper C, Hosmer Jr DW, et al. Empirically based composite fracture prediction model from the Global Longitudinal Study of Osteoporosis in Postmenopausal Women (GLOW). J Clin Endocrinol Metab. 2014;99(3):817–26.

37. Sornay-Rendu E, Munoz F, Delmas PD, Chapurlat RD. The FRAX tool in French women: how well does it describe the real incidence of fracture in the OFELY cohort? J Bone Miner Res. 2010;25(10): 2101–7.

38. Tremollieres FA, Pouilles JM, Drewniak N, Laparra J, Ribot CA, Dargent-Molina P. Fracture risk prediction using BMD and clinical risk factors in early postmenopausal women: sensitivity of the WHO FRAX tool. J Bone Miner Res. 2010;25(5):1002–9.

39. Leslie WD, Lix LM, Langsetmo L, Berger C, Goltzman D, Hanley DA, et al. Construction of a FRAX((R)) model for the assessment of fracture probability in Canada and implications for treatment. Osteoporos Int. 2011;22(3):817–27.

40. Leslie WD, Lix LM, Johansson H, Oden A, McCloskey E, Kanis JA. Independent clinical validation of a Canadian FRAX tool: fracture prediction and model calibration. J Bone Miner Res. 2010;25(11):2350–8.

41. Fraser LA, Langsetmo L, Berger C, Ioannidis G, Goltzman D, Adachi JD, et al. Fracture prediction and calibration of a Canadian FRAX(R) tool: a population-based report from CaMos. Osteoporos Int. 2011;22(3):829–37.

42. Czerwinski E, Kanis JA, Osieleniec J, Kumorek A, Milert A, Johansson H, et al. Evaluation of FRAX to characterise fracture risk in Poland. Osteoporos Int. 2011;22(9):2507–12.

43. Tamaki J, Iki M, Kadowaki E, Sato Y, Kajita E, Kagamimori S, et al. Fracture risk prediction using FRAX(R): a 10-year follow-up survey of the Japanese Population-Based Osteoporosis (JPOS) Cohort Study. Osteoporos Int. 2011;22(12): 3037–45.

44. Rubin KH, Abrahamsen B, Hermann AP, Bech M, Gram J, Brixen K. Fracture risk assessed by Fracture Risk Assessment Tool (FRAX) compared with fracture risk derived from population fracture rates. Scand J Public Health. 2011;39(3):312–8.

45. Premaor M, Parker RA, Cummings S, Ensrud K, Cauley JA, Lui LY, et al. Predictive value of FRAX for fracture in obese older women. J Bone Miner Res. 2013;28(1):188–95.

46. Ettinger B, Ensrud KE, Blackwell T, Curtis JR, Lapidus JA, Orwoll ES. Performance of FRAX in a cohort of community-dwelling, ambulatory older men: the Osteoporotic Fractures in Men (MrOS) study. Osteoporos Int. 2013;24(4):1185–93.

47. Byberg L, Gedeborg R, Cars T, Sundstrom J, Berglund L, Kilander L, et al. Prediction of fracture risk in men: a cohort study. J Bone Miner Res. 2012;27(4):797–807.

48. Gonzalez-Macias J, Marin F, Vila J, Diez-Perez A. Probability of fractures predicted by FRAX(R) and observed incidence in the Spanish ECOSAP Study cohort. Bone. 2012;50(1):373–7.

49. Tebe Cordomi C, Del Rio LM, Di GS, Casas L, Estrada MD, Kotzeva A, et al. Validation of the FRAX predictive model for major osteoporotic fracture in a historical cohort of Spanish women. J Clin Densitom. 2013;16(2):231–7.

50. **Kanis JA, Hans D, Cooper C, Baim S, Bilezikian JP, Binkley N, et al. Interpretation and use of FRAX in clinical practice. Osteoporos Int. 2011;22(9):2395–411. **The joint Official Positions of the ISCD and IOF are the most updated and accepted guidelines for quantitatively or qualitatively adjusting FRAX clinical risk factors and subsequent fracture probabilities for the individual patient.

51. Hans DB, Kanis JA, Baim S, Bilezikian JP, Binkley N, Cauley JA, et al. Joint Official Positions of the

International Society for Clinical Densitometry and International Osteoporosis Foundation on FRAX((R)) Executive Summary of the 2010 Position Development Conference on Interpretation and Use of FRAX((R)) in Clinical Practice. J Clin Densitom. 2011;14(3):171–80.

52. Leslie WD, Lix LM, Johansson H, Oden A, McCloskey E, Kanis JA. Spine-hip discordance and fracture risk assessment: a physician-friendly FRAX enhancement. Osteoporos Int. 2011;22(3):839–47.

53. Kanis JA, Johansson H, Oden A, McCloskey EV. Guidance for the adjustment of FRAX according to the dose of glucocorticoids. Osteoporos Int. 2011;22(3):809–16.

54. Nguyen ND, Frost SA, Center JR, Eisman JA, Nguyen TV, Nguyen ND, et al. Development of a nomogram for individualizing hip fracture risk in men and women. Osteoporos Int. 2007;18(8):1109–17.

55. Nguyen ND, Frost SA, Center JR, Eisman JA, Nguyen TV, Nguyen ND, et al. Development of prognostic nomograms for individualizing 5-year and 10-year fracture risks. Osteoporos Int. 2008; 19(10):1431–44.

56. Langsetmo L, Nguyen TV, Nguyen ND, Kovacs CS, Prior JC, Center JR, et al. Independent external validation of nomograms for predicting risk of low-trauma fracture and hip fracture. CMAJ. 2011;183(2):E107–14.

57. Hippisley-Cox J, Coupland C. Predicting risk of osteoporotic fracture in men and women in England and Wales: prospective derivation and validation of QFractureScores. BMJ. 2009;339:b4229.

58. Hippisley-Cox J, Coupland C. Derivation and validation of updated QFracture algorithm to predict risk of osteoporotic fracture in primary care in the United Kingdom: prospective open cohort study. BMJ. 2012;344:e3427.

59. Collins GS, Mallett S, Altman DG. Predicting risk of osteoporotic and hip fracture in the United Kingdom: prospective independent and external validation of QFractureScores. BMJ. 2011;342:d3651.

60. Cummins NM, Poku EK, Towler MR, O'Driscoll OM, Ralston SH. Clinical risk factors for osteoporosis in Ireland and the UK: a comparison of FRAX and QFractureScores. Calcif Tissue Int. 2011;89(2): 172–7.

61. Rubin KH, Friis-Holmberg T, Hermann AP, Abrahamsen B, Brixen K. Risk assessment tools to identify women with increased risk of osteoporotic fracture: complexity or simplicity? A systematic review. J Bone Miner Res. 2013;28(8):1701–17.

62. Whiting P, Rutjes AW, Reitsma JB, Bossuyt PM, Kleijnen J. The development of QUADAS: a tool for the quality assessment of studies of diagnostic accuracy included in systematic reviews. BMC Med Res Methodol. 2003;3:25.

63. Dawson-Hughes B. A revised clinician's guide to the prevention and treatment of osteoporosis. J Clin Endocrinol Metab. 2008;93(7):2463–5.

64. Dawson-Hughes B, Tosteson AN, Melton III LJ, Baim S, Favus MJ, Khosla S, et al. Implications of absolute fracture risk assessment for osteoporosis practice guidelines in the USA. Osteoporos Int. 2008;19(4):449–58.

65. Kanis JA, Johnell O, Oden A, Johansson H, McCloskey E. FRAX and the assessment of fracture probability in men and women from the UK. Osteoporos Int. 2008;19(4):385–97.

66. Kanis JA, McCloskey EV, Johansson H, Strom O, Borgstrom F, Oden A. Case finding for the management of osteoporosis with FRAX((R))-assessment and intervention thresholds for the UK. Osteoporos Int. 2008;19(10):1395–408.

67. Lippuner K, Johansson H, Kanis JA, Rizzoli R. FRAX assessment of osteoporotic fracture probability in Switzerland. Osteoporos Int. 2010;21(3):381–9.

68. Kanis JA, Burlet N, Cooper C, Delmas PD, Reginster JY, Borgstrom F, et al. European guidance for the diagnosis and management of osteoporosis in postmenopausal women. Osteoporos Int. 2008;19(4):399–428.

69. Fujiwara S, Kasagi F, Masunari N, Naito K, Suzuki G, Fukunaga M. Fracture prediction from bone mineral density in Japanese men and women. J Bone Miner Res. 2003;18(8):1547–53.

70. Neuprez A, Johansson H, Kanis JA, McCloskey EV, Oden A, Bruyere O, et al. A FRAX model for the assessment of fracture probability in Belgium. Rev Med Liege. 2009;64(12):612–9.

71. Papaioannou A, Morin S, Cheung AM, Atkinson S, Brown JP, Feldman S, et al. 2010 clinical practice guidelines for the diagnosis and management of osteoporosis in Canada: summary. CMAJ. 2010;182(17):1864–73.

72. Leslie WD, Schousboe JT. A review of osteoporosis diagnosis and treatment options in new and recently updated guidelines on case finding around the world. Curr Osteoporos Rep. 2011;9(3):129–40.

73. Tosteson AN, Melton III LJ, Dawson-Hughes B, Baim S, Favus MJ, Khosla S, et al. Cost-effective osteoporosis treatment thresholds: the United States perspective. Osteoporos Int. 2008;19(4):437–47.

74. Cheung E, Kung AW, Tan KC. Outcomes of applying the NOF, NOGG and Taiwanese guidelines to a cohort of Chinese early postmenopausal women. Clin Endocrinol (Oxf). 2014;80(2):200–7.

75. Compston J, Cooper A, Cooper C, Francis R, Kanis JA, Marsh D, et al. Guidelines for the diagnosis and management of osteoporosis in postmenopausal women and men from the age of 50 years in the UK. Maturitas. 2009;62(2):105–8.

76. Kanis JA, McCloskey EV, Johansson H, Cooper C, Rizzoli R, Reginster JY. European guidance for the diagnosis and management of osteoporosis in postmenopausal women. Osteoporos Int. 2013;24(1): 23–57.

77. NICE National Institute for Health and Clinical Excellence. Osteoporosis: assessing the risk of fragility fracture. http://www.nice.org.uk/guidance/

cg146/resources/guidance-osteoporosis-assessing-the-risk-of-fragility-fracture-pdf. Accessed on March 4, 2015.

78. McCloskey EV, Beneton M, Charlesworth D, Kayan K, de Takats D, Dey A, et al. Clodronate reduces the incidence of fractures in community-dwelling elderly women unselected for osteoporosis: results of a double-blind, placebo-controlled randomized study. J Bone Miner Res. 2007;22(1):135–41.

79. Kanis JA, Barton IP, Johnell O. Risedronate decreases fracture risk in patients selected solely on the basis of prior vertebral fracture. Osteoporos Int. 2005;16(5):475–82.

80. Lyles KW, Colon-Emeric CS, Magaziner JS, Adachi JD, Pieper CF, Mautalen C, et al. Zoledronic acid and clinical fractures and mortality after hip fracture. N Engl J Med. 2007;357(18):1799–809.

81. Ryder KM, Cummings SR, Palermo L, Satterfield S, Bauer DC, Feldstein AC, et al. Does a history of non-vertebral fracture identify women without osteoporosis for treatment? J Gen Intern Med. 2008;23(8):1177–81.

82. McClung MR, Geusens P, Miller PD, Zippel H, Bensen WG, Roux C, et al. Effect of risedronate on the risk of hip fracture in elderly women. Hip Intervention Program Study Group. N Engl J Med. 2001;344(5):333–40.

83. Sun X, Ioannidis JP, Agoritsas T, Alba AC, Guyatt G. How to use a subgroup analysis: users' guide to the medical literature. JAMA. 2014;311(4):405–11.

84. McClung MR, Boonen S, Torring O, Roux C, Rizzoli R, Bone HG, et al. Effect of denosumab treatment on the risk of fractures in subgroups of women with postmenopausal osteoporosis. J Bone Miner Res. 2012;27(1):211–8.

85. Eastell R, Black DM, Boonen S, Adami S, Felsenberg D, Lippuner K, et al. Effect of once-yearly zoledronic acid five milligrams on fracture risk and change in femoral neck bone mineral density. J Clin Endocrinol Metab. 2009;94(9):3215–25.

86. Kanis JA, Johansson H, Oden A, McCloskey EV. A meta-analysis of the efficacy of raloxifene on all clinical and vertebral fractures and its dependency on FRAX. Bone. 2010;47(4):729–35.

87. Boonen S, McClung MR, Eastell R, El-Hajj FG, Barton IP, Delmas P. Safety and efficacy of risedronate in reducing fracture risk in osteoporotic women aged 80 and older: implications for the use of antiresorptive agents in the old and oldest old. J Am Geriatr Soc. 2004;52(11):1832–9.

88. Ensrud KE, Black DM, Palermo L, Bauer DC, Barrett-Connor E, Quandt SA, et al. Treatment with alendronate prevents fractures in women at highest risk: results from the Fracture Intervention Trial. Arch Intern Med. 1997;157(22):2617–24.

89. Roux C, Reginster JY, Fechtenbaum J, Kolta S, Sawicki A, Tulassay Z, et al. Vertebral fracture risk reduction with strontium ranelate in women with postmenopausal osteoporosis is independent of baseline risk factors. J Bone Miner Res. 2006;21(4):536–42.

90. Watts NB, Josse RG, Hamdy RC, Hughes RA, Manhart MD, Barton I, et al. Risedronate prevents new vertebral fractures in postmenopausal women at high risk. J Clin Endocrinol Metab. 2003;88(2):542–9.

91. McCloskey EV, Johansson H, Oden A, Vasireddy S, Kayan K, Pande K, et al. Ten-year fracture probability identifies women who will benefit from clodronate therapy–additional results from a double-blind, placebo-controlled randomised study. Osteoporos Int. 2009;20(5):811–7.

92. Kanis JA, Johansson H, Oden A, McCloskey EV. Bazedoxifene reduces vertebral and clinical fractures in postmenopausal women at high risk assessed with FRAX. Bone. 2009;44(6):1049–54.

93. *McCloskey EV, Johansson H, Oden A, Austin M, Siris E, Wang A, et al. Denosumab reduces the risk of osteoporotic fractures in postmenopausal women, particularly in those with moderate to high fracture risk as assessed with FRAX. J Bone Miner Res. 2012;27(7):1480–6. *Compelling evidence of a treatment-risk reduction interaction. Denosumab reduced fracture risk to a greater extent in those at moderate to high risk. For example, at 10% probability, denosumab decreased fracture risk by 11% (p = 0.629), whereas at 30% probability (90th percentile of study population) the reduction was 50% (p = 0.001).

94. Donaldson MG, Palermo L, Ensrud KE, Hochberg MC, Schousboe JT, Cummings SR. Effect of alendronate for reducing fracture by FRAX score and femoral neck bone mineral density: the Fracture Intervention Trial. J Bone Miner Res. 2012;27(8):1804–10.

95. Kanis JA, Johansson H, Oden A, McCloskey EV. A meta-analysis of the effect of strontium ranelate on the risk of vertebral and non-vertebral fracture in postmenopausal osteoporosis and the interaction with FRAX((R)). Osteoporos Int. 2011;22(8):2347–55.

96. Cummings SR, Black DM, Thompson DE, Applegate WB, Barrett-Connor E, Musliner TA, et al. Effect of alendronate on risk of fracture in women with low bone density but without vertebral fractures: results from the Fracture Intervention Trial. JAMA. 1998;280(24):2077–82.

97. Hochberg MC, Ross PD, Black D, Cummings SR, Genant HK, Nevitt MC, et al. Larger increases in bone mineral density during alendronate therapy are associated with a lower risk of new vertebral fractures in women with postmenopausal osteoporosis. Fracture Intervention Trial Research Group. Arthritis Rheum. 1999;42(6):1246–54.

98. Hochberg MC, Greenspan S, Wasnich RD, Miller P, Thompson DE, Ross PD. Changes in bone density and turnover explain the reductions in incidence of nonverterbal fractures that occur during treatment with antiresorptive agents. J Clin Endocrinol Metab. 2002;87(4):1586–92.

99. Jacques RM, Boonen S, Cosman F, Reid IR, Bauer DC, Black DM, et al. Relationship of changes in total hip bone mineral density to vertebral and nonvertebral

fracture risk in women with postmenopausal osteoporosis treated with once-yearly zoledronic acid 5 mg: the HORIZON-Pivotal Fracture Trial (PFT). J Bone Miner Res. 2012;27(8):1627–34.

100. Brown JP, Albert C, Nassar BA, Adachi JD, Cole D, Davison KS, et al. Bone turnover markers in the management of postmenopausal osteoporosis. Clin Biochem. 2009;42(10-11):929–42.

101. Szulc P. The role of bone turnover markers in monitoring treatment in postmenopausal osteoporosis. Clin Biochem. 2012;45(12):907–19.

102. Silverman S. Adherence to medications for the treatment of osteoporosis. Rheum Dis Clin North Am. 2006;32(4):721–31.

103. Leslie WD, Lix LM, Johansson H, Oden A, McCloskey E, Kanis JA. Does osteoporosis therapy invalidate FRAX for fracture prediction? J Bone Miner Res. 2012;27(6):1243–51.

104. Leslie WD, Morin SN, Lix LM. Fracture prediction from repeat BMD measurements in routine clinical practice for: the Manitoba BMD Cohort. J Bone Miner Res. 2011;26 Suppl 1:S78.

105. The 2012 hormone therapy position statement of: The North American Menopause Society. Menopause 2012;19(3):257–71.

106. MacLean C, Newberry S, Maglione M, McMahon M, Ranganath V, Suttorp M, et al. Systematic review: comparative effectiveness of treatments to prevent fractures in men and women with low bone density or osteoporosis. Ann Intern Med. 2008;148(3):197–213.

107. **Cummings SR, Cosman F, Eastell R, Reid IR, Mehta M, Lewiecki EM. Goal-directed treatment of osteoporosis. J Bone Miner Res. 2013;28(3):433–8. **This paper proposes a bold new way of looking at the initiation and monitoring of osteoporosis treatment. The idea is to follow the example of other conditions, such as hypertension, where treatment is based on achieving a goal. Although there are many obstacles in setting treatment goals, the result could be more rational and effective use of the expanding array of treatments for osteoporosis.

108. Diez-Perez A, Adachi JD, Agnusdei D, Bilezikian JP, Compston JE, Cummings SR, et al. Treatment failure in osteoporosis. Osteoporos Int. 2012;23(12):2769–74.

109. Cummings SR, Karpf DB, Harris F, Genant HK, Ensrud K, LaCroix AZ, et al. Improvement in spine bone density and reduction in risk of vertebral fractures during treatment with antiresorptive drugs. Am J Med. 2002;112(4):281–9.

110. Seeman E. Is a change in bone mineral density a sensitive and specific surrogate of anti-fracture efficacy? Bone. 2007;41(3):308–17.

111. Khosla S. Surrogates for fracture endpoints in clinical trials. J Bone Miner Res. 2003;18(6):1146–9.

112. Fleming TR, DeMets DL. Surrogate end points in clinical trials: are we being misled? Ann Intern Med. 1996;125(7):605–13.

113. Bucher HC, Guyatt GH, Cook DJ, Holbrook A, McAlister FA. Users' guides to the medical literature: XIX. Applying clinical trial results. A. How to use an article measuring the effect of an intervention on surrogate end points. Evidence-Based Medicine Working Group. JAMA. 1999;282(8):771–8.

114. McAlister FA, van DS, Padawal RS, Johnson JA, Majumdar SR. How evidence-based are the recommendations in evidence-based guidelines? PLoS Med. 2007;4(8):e250.

115. McCloskey E, Leslie WD. Goal-directed therapy in osteoporosis. J Bone Miner Res. 2013;28(3):439–41.

116. **Leslie WD, Majumdar SR, Lix LM, Morin SN, Johansson H, Oden A, et al. Can change in FRAX score be used to "treat-to-target"? A population-based cohort study. J Bone Miner Res. 2014;29(5):1074–80. **This study in 11,049 previously untreated women age >50 years undergoing baseline and follow-up DXA examinations and FRAX probability calculations provided a clear answer to the question - "No". FRAX scores increased over time and this increase was attenuated but not prevented by treatment. Few women had meaningful reductions in FRAX scores. FRAX with BMD is not responsive enough to be used as a target for goal-directed treatment.

117. McNabb BL, Vittinghoff E, Schwartz AV, Eastell R, Bauer DC, Ensrud K, et al. BMD changes and predictors of increased bone loss in postmenopausal women after a 5-year course of alendronate. J Bone Miner Res. 2013;28(6):1319–27.

118. Office of the Surgeon General (US). Bone health and osteoporosis: a report of the Surgeon General. Rockville (MD): Office of the Surgeon General (US). Available from: http://www.ncbinlmnihgov/books/NBK45513/2004

119. Bolland MJ, Siu AT, Mason BH, Horne AM, Ames RW, Grey AB, et al. Evaluation of the FRAX and Garvan fracture risk calculators in older women. J Bone Miner Res. 2011;26(2):420–7.

120. Chen P, Krege JH, Adachi JD, Prior JC, Tenenhouse A, Brown JP, et al. Vertebral fracture status and the World Health Organization risk factors for predicting osteoporotic fracture risk. J Bone Miner Res. 2009;24(3):495–502.

121. Donaldson M, Palermo L, Schousboe JT, Ensrud K, Hochberg MC, Cummings SR. FRAX and risk of vertebral fractures: The Fracture Intervention Trial (FIT). J Bone Miner.Res. in press. 2009.

122. Ensrud KE, Lui LY, Taylor BC, Schousboe JT, Donaldson MG, Fink HA, et al. A comparison of prediction models for fractures in older women: is more better? Arch Intern Med. 2009;169(22):2087–94.

Elisa Torres del Pliego, Daniel Prieto-Alhambra, and Adolfo Díez-Perez

Summary

- Some patients, even with optimal adherence to treatment, do not respond adequately to treatment.
- Incident fractures, decrease in BMD, and lack of variation in turnover markers are the clinical tools for evaluating the response to treatments.
- Two incident fractures while on drug therapy indicate treatment failure.
- Two of the following indicate treatment fracture: one incident fracture, BMD loss, and no variation in markers.
- Comorbidities, concomitant treatments, and an advanced degree of bone deterioration are risk factors for treatment failure.

E. Torres del Pliego, MD
A. Díez-Perez, MD, PhD (✉)
Department of Internal Medicine, Hospital del Mar-IMIM, Autonomous University of Barcelona and RETICEF, Instituto Carlos III,
P Maritim 25-29, 08003 Barcelona, Spain
e-mail: ADiez@parcdesalutmar.cat

D. Prieto-Alhambra, MD, MSc, PhD
Botnar Research Centre, Nuffield Department of Orthopaedics, Rheumatology and Musculoskeletal Sciences (NDORMS), University of Oxford, Nuffield Orthopaedics Center, Oxford, UK

Introduction: The Response in Osteoporosis

A number of drugs for the treatment of osteoporosis have been developed in the last four decades. Calcitonin was the first available agent specifically [1–4] developed for osteoporosis treatment and widely employed. Other options like hormone replacement therapy (both estrogens and androgens) had been used before but sporadically and in isolated trials. The effects on bone mineral density, as the first radiological and isotopic methods became available, were used for monitoring drug response. However, as research in the field progressed and new drugs were incorporated into the clinical armamentarium, the evaluation of the efficacy of these treatments became increasingly complex.

A hallmark in the evaluation of the efficacy of the treatments for osteoporosis was the design of the trials with alendronate, and Gideon Rodan was the key figure that settled up what still today are the standard criteria for measuring the effect of drug interventions in osteoporosis. The design of the FIT trial [5] established the reduction of fracture incidence as the main outcome for the first time. This criterion required a large sample size and a long period of follow-up to achieve enough statistical power for detecting differences

© Springer International Publishing Switzerland 2016
S.L. Silverman, B. Abrahamsen (eds.), *The Duration and Safety of Osteoporosis Treatment*, DOI 10.1007/978-3-319-23639-1_5

between arms. Moreover, like in other areas of medicine, FIT focused on a final endpoint representing the pathological event in clinics, fracture; additionally, intermediate endpoints, basically bone mineral density (BMD) variation and bone turnover markers (BTM), were used as surrogates of the efficacy. This scheme has been persisting, and therefore, efficacy estimates have relied in these three pillars.

Regulatory agencies and evidence evaluation have been working on these grounds. Pivotal trials have been carried out in a highly controlled setting, with excellent follow-up and adherence, in populations with selected clinical profile where strict inclusion and exclusion criteria were applied. However, for the practicing clinician using these drugs, two problems immediately came out. First, patients attending clinics in real-life environment often do not match with the ideal patients included in clinical trials, raising potential issues of applicability (external validity) of the results to the "common patient." It has been estimated that up to 80 % of patients attending an osteoporosis clinics would have been excluded from participation in the pivotal trials [6]. Second, adherence to osteoporosis medications is poor, and this is associated with a reduction in effectiveness [7–9]. Therefore, a gap between evidence gathered under ideal conditions and daily practice was an element of uncertainty for the clinician.

Furthermore, even under ideal controlled conditions, some patients in the pivotal trials [10–18] still suffered fractures in the treatment arm. The consequence for the clinician is the lack of firm basis for making decisions in the individual patient.

Clinical Elements for the Evaluation of Response

Bone mineral density is a common element for the clinical evaluation of a treatment response, and it is well known that BMD levels are a good predictor of fracture risk [19, 20], although the risk modification associated to treatment is less well captured [21–23] or even misleading [24]

except, perhaps, for denosumab [25]. When a patient shows a decrease in bone density in spite of taking the treatment with reasonably good adherence, it can well be that he/she is not responding to treatment. However, the repeated measurement of BMD has limitations in the assessment of response to treatment because the variations require prolonged periods of time to be valued [26–28] and must be greater than the least significant change for the technique [29–31]. Moreover, even in cases where the BMD declines, there is a reduction in fracture risk in comparison with the group without treatment [32, 33]. However, in spite of all these limitations, the clinician in care of a patient that shows a decrease (or even no increase) in the BMD levels has trouble in explaining to the patient that the treatment is working appropriately and he/she can ask the clinician for an alternative. Similarly, patients with a good densitometric response who experience fractures while on treatment pose a significant challenge to our clinical skills.

Biochemical markers of bone turnover are another available clinical variable. The effect of the drugs at a cellular level can be tracked by these elements of collagen degradation, regulating enzymes, or other products of the remodeling cycle. Variations in turnover markers reflect very accurately decreases in fracture risk in treated populations [34–39]. However, the practical use of these markers for routine monitoring still faces several limitations as is, although greatly improved, the precision error of the technique [40] or the problems in establishing a reference range for a given laboratory [41] and the important within-laboratory variability [40], let alone the costs of testing. A recent recommendation by two official societies intends to standardize the laboratory assessment of biochemical markers of bone turnover endorsing the measurement of P1NP and sCTX [42]. However, the real-life practice is still far from what can be achieved in first-level sophisticated laboratories and induces significant limitations for a reliable widespread use of this tool for monitoring the response to anti-osteoporosis drugs.

But, with no doubt, the cornerstone in the evaluation of the performance of anti-osteoporosis drugs is the occurrence of fracture/s. Fractures are the pathological event of the disease and responsible for the impact in morbidity and mortality as well as the strongest predictor for future fractures [43]. This predictive value increases with the recentness of the index fracture [44, 45]. Both clinicians and patients perceive a fracture occurring during a treatment with good adherence as a fact that opens a big deal of doubts about the efficacy of the drug. However, no drug reduces the excess risk of fracture to zero. Patients in the treatment arm of the pivotal trials still suffered a significant number of fractures, with a cumulative rate that ranged approximately from 5 to 18 % for vertebral fractures and from 6 to almost 18 % for non-vertebral after 3–5 years of treatment [10, 12–14, 16–18]. Therefore, sustaining a fragility fracture can occur without this event, meaning that the treatment is not working at a tissue level and reducing somehow the fracture risk with respect to placebo-treated individuals as shown by analysis of surrogate markers of efficacy [32, 33]. In spite of that, sometimes patients ask for a change in treatment, and the clinician can also make this decision without a firm basis. But if a single fracture can purely be a chance event, the occurrence of a second fragility fracture is highly unlikely as the risk reduction observed in trials for a second fracture was in the order of 80–90 % [46–49].

One element to take into account is that any drug requires a given period of time before reaching any antifracture efficacy. Given that the currently available drugs base their action on a remodeling–modification effect, we might expect that at least the period required for one or two remodeling cycles would be required. However, the data from clinical trials suggest an initiation in fracture reduction in a period between 6 months and 1 year [50, 51]. Therefore, any fracture occurring before 12 months on treatment, in a conservative estimate, cannot be judged as a failure in the response to the drug. Moreover, fractures occurring after the treatment period in the pivotal trials (5 years for most drugs) cannot be ascertained with enough confidence given that the antifracture efficacy beyond this period is not firmly demonstrated. Furthermore, all the trials have supplemented the participants with calcium and, often, vitamin D. Therefore, in some degree, all the registered drugs are part of a regimen that includes these two supplements. Another consideration is that not all the fractures have been associated with osteoporosis. Specifically, fractures of the skull, digits, hand, foot, and ankle are considered as non-osteoporotic [52, 53].

Definition of Treatment Failure

For years, the concept of *treatment failure*, or its equivalent, *inadequate response*, has been included in some publications [54–60]. Lack of increase in bone density, no change in bone markers, and incident fractures during treatment have been, not surprisingly, the variables considered. In an attempt to set up a standard common ground, an operative definition based also on incident fractures and BMD was proposed [61]. Following on this point, the International Osteoporosis Foundation assembled a working group of the Committee of Scientific Advisors that proposed a definition of treatment failure.

The available evidence for defining the concept was minimal, and, as a consequence, an important part of the conclusions was based on expert opinion. However, the reasons for moving ahead with such a definition were several. Common criteria would be desirable to be used by the clinicians given the absence of a standard, widely accepted definition to allow the clinicians to make decisions in a consistent manner. Moreover, in some areas, the reimbursement of second-line drugs is limited to a demonstrated lack of efficacy of the first-option treatments, with great variability and criteria sometimes arbitrary. Furthermore, the concept itself deserved further investigation given the fact that not all the cases of osteoporosis are expected to respond in the same way.

The reason for a heterogeneous response is the heterogeneity of osteoporosis itself. Osteoporosis is a common end, of bone loss and architecture deterioration, that can be reached by a wide number of pathophysiological ways and clinical conditions. Moreover, the patients usually take multiple drugs that, eventually, might interfere with the efficacy of anti-osteoporosis medications. By defining the concept of treatment failure, factors involved in their development might be identified and corrected when starting a drug. Finally, and importantly enough, if some factors of failure to treatment are associated to a very advanced stage of the disease, with deep bone loss and quality deterioration, this would be a clear indication of a therapeutic ceiling for the available drugs and raise the need for developing more potent drugs or combination regimens.

With all these elements in mind, a position paper of the working group of the IOF proposed the following criteria of treatment failure in osteoporosis [62]:

1. Two or more incident fragility fractures
2. One incident fracture and elevated serum βCTX or PINP at baseline with no significant reduction during treatment, a significant decrease in BMD or both
3. Both no significant decrease in serum βCTX or PINP and a significant decrease in BMD

A simplified description of these criteria is depicted in Textbox 5.1. Additional elements to be taken into account are the following:

- At least 1 year on treatment is required before considering a possible failure to treatment.
- Changes to be expected in BMD and bone markers can vary for different drugs.
- Adherence should be evaluated and has to be good for a clinician to consider treatment failure.
- Hidden secondary causes of osteoporosis should be ruled out.
- Fractures of the hand, skull, digits, feet, and ankle are not considered as fragility fractures.
- The overall decline in BMD should be in the order of 5 % or more in at least two serial BMD measurements at the lumbar spine or 4 % at the proximal femur.
- Sequential measurements of markers of bone turnover should use the same assay. A significant response is a decline of 25 % from baseline levels for antiresorptive treatments and a

Textbox 5.1. Criteria for defining a treatment failure [62]

Twoor more incident fragility fractures
Or
Two of the following:

- **One incident fragility fracture**
- **A decline in BMD ≥ 5 % (lumbar spine) or 4 % (proximal femur) in at least two measurements**
- **A decline ≤ 25 % (for antiresorptives) or an increase ≤ 25 % (for anabolics) after 6 months**

Additional elements

- At least 1 year on treatment
- Changes in BMD and bone markers vary for different drugs
- Adherence should be good
- Rule out secondary osteoporosis
- Do not consider fractures of the hand, skull, digits, feet and ankle
- Measurements of markers of bone turnover should use the same assay
- Always consider falls

25 % increase for anabolic agents (PTH) after 6 months.
- If baseline levels of bone turnover markers are not known, a positive response is a decrease below the average value of young healthy adults.
- Falls are an important driver of fracture.

Risk Factors for Treatment Failure

After defining the criteria for considering that a treatment is failing, the next step is to investigate which factors are associated with the problem. The potential reasons are numerous and can be due to external factors, intrinsic characteristics of the patient or element/s that interfere with the bioavailability or the effectiveness of the drugs. Hereby, we report three studies specifically designed to answer this question.

A first approach has been a case–control study in women with postmenopausal osteoporosis, on treatment with antiresorptives [63] carried out in 12 tertiary-care hospitals in Spain. Cases were included if an incident fracture occurred after 1 year and before completing 5 years on a stable treatment, with good adherence. Controls were patients that completed 5 years of treatment without incident fractures. Treatments for diseases with potential effect on bone were part of exclusion criteria. Clinical variables, DXA, bone turnover markers, 25-OH vitamin D, PTH, spinal radiographs, hip structural analysis of the hip (Imaging Therapeutics Inc. ImaTx OsDx™), and fractal analysis of the distal radius (Trabeculae Q-Bone®) were measured.

Seventy-six cases of inadequate response and 103 with adequate response were included. The mean age was 68, and in the univariate analysis, having a fracture before starting the treatment, two or more falls in the previous year, BMD level at the spine, plasma levels of 25-OH vitamin D, and the bone microstructure at the proximal femur were associated with fracture in spite of being on therapy. In the multivariable-adjusted logistic regression, two falls in the previous year and 25-OH vitamin D levels below 20 ng/ml were associated with an increased risk, while having a better fracture load index was protective. The results of this study are summarized in Table 5.1.

A second opportunity for assessing predictive elements of treatment failure was offered by the GLOW study [64]. This is a prospective cohort study of more than 60,000 women from ten countries recruited from 723 primary care

Table 5.1 Factors associated to treatment failure/inadequate response

Year [ref.]	Design	Subjects	Measurements	Factors identified	Odds ratio/ subhazard ratio (95 % CI)
2012 [63]	Cross-sectional study	179 postmenopausal women	Bone turnover markers DXA Femur structure Fractal analysis	Prior fracture 25-OHD < 20 ng/ml Fracture load[a] × 100 U	OR 3.89 (1.47–8.82) OR 3.89 (1.55–9.77) OR 0.96 (0.93–0.99)
2014 [64]	Prospective cohort study (GLOW)	26,918 women, 5550 on treatment. Follow-up 3 years	Yearly questionnaire (self-administered)	SF-36 vitality × 10 points 2 or more falls[b] Prior fracture	OR 0.85 (0.76–0.95) OR 2.40 (1.34–4.29) OR 2.93 (1.81–4.75)
2014 [65]	Nationwide health database (retrospective cohort)	5 million, 21,385 treated with BP	GP e-records + hospital admissions (ICD fracture codes), specialists referrals, pharmacy invoicing (BP (bisphosponates) use, MPR)	Age > 80 vs. 60 Previous fracture Underweight Inflammatory arthritis PPIs use Vitamin D deficiency	SHR 2.18 (1.70–2.80) SHR 1.75 (1.39–1.20) SHR 2.11 (1.14–3.92) SHR 1.46 (1.02–2.10) SHR 1.22 (1.02–1.46) SHR 2.69 (1.27–5.72)

BP bisphosphonates, *PPIs* proton pump inhibitors
[a]Fracture load = proximal femur structure index (ImaTx™)
[b]In the previous year

practices in 17 sites. These centers were located in six European countries, Canada, the USA, and Australia. Women received a self-administered posted questionnaire including personal characteristics, diagnostics, and treatments received, quality of life, and fracture history. The results of this analysis were those from baseline to the end of the third year of observation. According to the definition of the IOF working group [62], treatment failure was defined as the occurrence of two incident fractures after being on therapy for at least 1 year. During the 3-year study period, 6.5 % of women on continuous therapy with the same drug sustained one fracture, while 1.3 % suffered two or more. The variables associated with treatment failure (≥ 2 incident fractures) in univariate analyses were a lower score in the SF-36 scale (physical function and vitality) at baseline, higher FRAX© score, falls in the past 12 months, having more comorbid conditions, prior fracture, current use of glucocorticoids, need of arms to assist when standing, and unexplained weight loss. After multivariate analysis, a worse SF-36 vitality score, prior fracture, and two or more falls in the previous year remained as independent predictors. These results are summarized in Table 5.1 and Fig. 5.1.

A third recent investigation has been carried out using the SIDIAP database in Catalonia, Spain [65]. SIDIAP gathers clinical information from electronic records of primary care health providers, prescription and pharmacy invoices, laboratory tests, and hospital admissions. The ICD-10 coding system is used, and the database includes data of more than five million people (over 80 % of the population of Catalonia). The cases analyzed were those patients suffering incident fractures in spite of being persistent for at least 6 months and with a medication possession ratio of 80 % or above. Only 35 % of patients among the 21,385 got a prescription completed at least 6 months of treatment. In this subgroup of persistent individuals, the incidence of fractures while on treatment was of 3.4 per 100 person-years. The predictors of these fractures were older age, previous fracture, underweight, inflammatory arthritis, use of proton pump inhibitors, and vitamin D deficiency (Table 5.1). To note that when starting bisphosphonates, the time elapsed between a prior fracture and the date of treatment initiation was relevant in these data. When the fracture was recent (less than 6 months before starting therapy), the risk was higher than for "older" fractures (those that had occurred more than 6 months before starting the drugs) (Fig. 5.2).

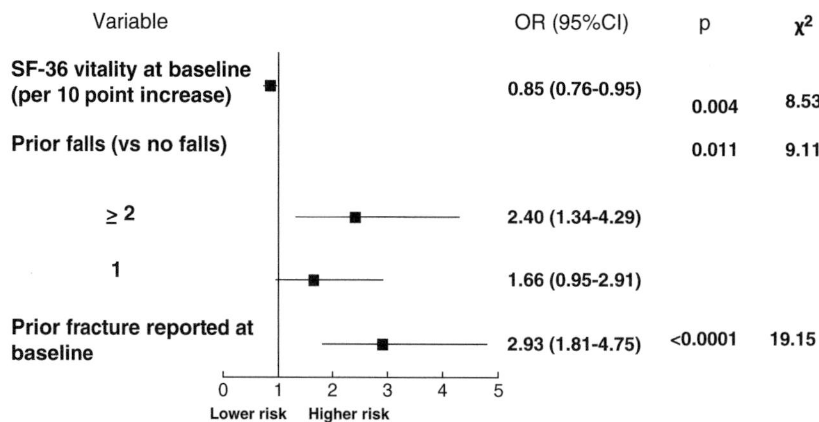

Fig. 5.1 Predictors of risk of treatment failure in the GLOW study [64]. Patients sustaining two or more incident fractures [65]

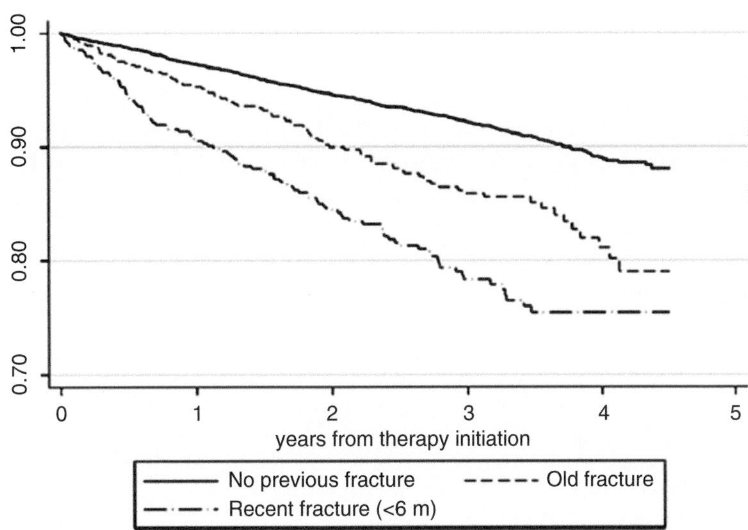

Fig. 5.2 Cumulative incidence of fracture in patients taking bisphosphonates in the SIDIAP database. Kaplan–Meier estimates of cumulative incidence of fracture while on treatment among incident users of bisphosphonates for patients with no previous fracture, recent fracture (in the past 6 months), and an old fracture (more than 6 months prior to therapy initiation)

Concluding Remarks

Patients on treatment with the drugs used in osteoporosis still are at risk of suffering fractures, and the rate observed is around 2–3 % per year. However, not every incident fracture while on treatment indicates a failure of the drug. When a second incident fracture occurs or when, in addition to one fracture, surrogate markers (BMD and/or bone turnover markers) also show a negative evolution, the likelihood for that particular individual of being a nonresponder is high.

A very appealing concept, treatment-to-target, is currently being developed [66]. In fact, the treatment-to-target strategy is symmetrical to treatment failure since it aims to establish when a treatment has obtained a desired effect, that is, the cure or control of the disease. Both together promise to be of great help to the clinician in making decisions on when a treatment can be stopped (target reached) or has to be modified (treatment failed). Again, the available evidence is terribly scarce, and the best clinical judgment in the evaluation of an individual patient is, as of today, the only way to decide when the target has been attained.

Several clinical variables can predict this incident fracture in spite of receiving an active drug with good compliance, in the vast majority of cases for oral bisphosphonates. In general, predictors of fracture while on treatment can be grouped in (1) elements showing an advanced stage of the disease, (2) with a degree of deterioration in bone strength too important to be compensated by the drug effects, or (3) in extra-skeletal elements that can jeopardize the risk reduction obtained by a given drug in the clinical trials. Often, both groups of elements merge in the same individual, and perhaps the most common example is the frail elderly, with several concomitant diseases and taking a number of medications, with deficiency in vitamin D, sarcopenia, and frequent falls potentiated by sedatives, anti hypertensive drugs, and taking regularly proton pump inhibitors to make a multi-pill regime tolerable.

Besides maximizing the effectiveness of currently available therapies by improving treatment adherence and avoiding, where possible, the previously described risk factors (e.g., ensuring vitamin D repletion concomitant or previous to anti-osteoporosis therapy), specific strategies to overcome the therapeutic ceiling of these medications, by developing new molecules or combining the ones we have today, are advisable. Parenteral administration can represent a progress for ensuring full adherence and bioavailability of drugs that have no need to be absorbed.

But, with no doubt, medical care has to be more comprehensive than merely prescribing a good drug for bones. Other health problems and medications should be reviewed, and rehabilitation, psychosocial support, and integral care are key for extracting from our drugs the maximal benefit.

References[1]

1. Bloch-Michel H, Milhaud G, Coutris G, Waltzing P, Charret A, Morin Y, et al. [Long term treatment of osteoporosis with thyrocalcitonin. Apropos of 7 cases]. Revue du rhumatisme et des maladies osteo-articulaires. 1970;37(10):629–38.

2. Dambacher MA, Olah AJ, Guncaga J, Lentner C, Haas HG. [Metabolic rates and histological-morphometrical investigations in bones of patients with osteoporosis subjected to long-term application of calcitonin]. Acta endocrinologica Supplementum. 1971;152:87.

3. Jowsey J, Riggs BL, Goldsmith RS, Kelly PJ, Arnaud CD. Effects of prolonged administration of porcine calcitonin in postmenopausal osteoporosis. J Clin Endocrinol Metab. 1971;33(5):752–8.

4. Wallach S, Aloia J, Cohn S. Treatment of osteoporosis with calcitonin. Semin Drug Treat. 1972;2(1):21–5.

5. Black DM, Reiss TF, Nevitt MC, Cauley J, Karpf D, Cummings SR. Design of the fracture intervention trial. Osteoporos Int. 1993;3 Suppl 3:S29–39.

6. *Dowd R, Recker RR, Heaney RP. Study subjects and ordinary patients. Osteoporos Int. 2000;11(6):533–6. *This paper shows how ordinary patients in every-day's practice do not fulfill inclusion criteria or have major exclusion criteria when compared with the cases included in the pivotal trials for osteoporosis treatment.

7. Cramer JA, Gold DT, Silverman SL, Lewiecki EM. A systematic review of persistence and compliance with bisphosphonates for osteoporosis. Osteoporos Int. 2007;18(8):1023–31.

8. Caro JJ, Ishak KJ, Huybrechts KF, Raggio G, Naujoks C. The impact of compliance with osteoporosis therapy on fracture rates in actual practice. Osteoporos Int. 2004;15(12):1003–8.

9. *Siris ES, Harris ST, Rosen CJ, Barr CE, Arvesen JN, Abbott TA, et al. Adherence to bisphosphonate therapy and fracture rates in osteoporotic women: relationship to vertebral and nonvertebral fractures from 2 US claims databases. Mayo Clin Proc. 2006;81(8):1013–22. *When adherence to treatment decreases, so does the antifracture efficacy. Below 80% adherence efficacy declines and for adherence rates of 50% & or less, the treatment efficacy totally vanishes.

10. Black DM, Cummings SR, Karpf DB, Cauley JA, Thompson DE, Nevitt MC, et al. Randomised trial of effect of alendronate on risk of fracture in women with existing vertebral fractures. Fracture Intervention Trial Research Group. Lancet. 1996;348(9041):1535–41.

11. Reginster J, Minne HW, Sorensen OH, Hooper M, Roux C, Brandi ML, et al. Randomized trial of the effects of risedronate on vertebral fractures in women with established postmenopausal osteoporosis. Vertebral Efficacy with Risedronate Therapy (VERT) Study Group. Osteoporos Int. 2000;11(1):83–91.

12. Harris ST, Watts NB, Genant HK, McKeever CD, Hangartner T, Keller M, et al. Effects of risedronate treatment on vertebral and nonvertebral fractures in women with postmenopausal osteoporosis: a randomized controlled trial. Vertebral Efficacy With Risedronate Therapy (VERT) Study Group. JAMA. 1999;282(14):1344–52.

13. Ettinger B, Black DM, Mitlak BH, Knickerbocker RK, Nickelsen T, Genant HK, et al. Reduction of vertebral fracture risk in postmenopausal women with osteoporosis treated with raloxifene: results from a 3-year randomized clinical trial. Multiple Outcomes of Raloxifene Evaluation (MORE) Investigators. JAMA. 1999;282(7):637–45.

14. Chesnut 3rd CH, Silverman S, Andriano K, Genant H, Gimona A, Harris S, et al. A randomized trial of nasal spray salmon calcitonin in postmenopausal women with established osteoporosis: the prevent recurrence of osteoporotic fractures study. PROOF Study Group. Am J Med. 2000;109(4):267–76.

15. Meunier PJ, Roux C, Seeman E, Ortolani S, Badurski JE, Spector TD, et al. The effects of strontium ranelate on the risk of vertebral fracture in women with postmenopausal osteoporosis. N Engl J Med. 2004;350(5):459–68.

16. Neer RM, Arnaud CD, Zanchetta JR, Prince R, Gaich GA, Reginster JY, et al. Effect of parathyroid hormone (1-34) on fractures and bone mineral density in postmenopausal women with osteoporosis. N Engl J Med. 2001;344(19):1434–41.

17. Cummings SR, San Martin J, McClung MR, Siris ES, Eastell R, Reid IR, et al. Denosumab for prevention of fractures in postmenopausal women with osteoporosis. N Engl J Med. 2009;361(8):756–65.

18. Black DM, Delmas PD, Eastell R, Reid IR, Boonen S, Cauley JA, et al. Once-yearly zoledronic acid for treatment of postmenopausal osteoporosis. N Engl J Med. 2007;356(18):1809–22.

19. Marshall D, Johnell O, Wedel H. Meta-analysis of how well measures of bone mineral density predict occurrence of osteoporotic fractures. BMJ. 1996;312(7041):1254–9.

20. Johnell O, Kanis JA, Oden A, Johansson H, De Laet C, Delmas P, et al. Predictive value of BMD for hip and other fractures. J Bone Miner Res. 2005;20(7):1185–94.

21. *Delmas PD, Li Z, Cooper C. Relationship between changes in bone mineral density and fracture risk reduction with antiresorptive drugs: some issues with

---

[1] *Important References

meta-analyses. J Bone Miner Res. 2004;19(2):330–7. *Methodological approach to discuss the caveats in the relationship established between BMD variations in response to treatment and fracture risk reduction.

22. Delmas PD, Seeman E. Changes in bone mineral density explain little of the reduction in vertebral or non-vertebral fracture risk with anti-resorptive therapy. Bone. 2004;34(4):599–604.

23. *Cummings SR, Karpf DB, Harris F, Genant HK, Ensrud K, LaCroix AZ, et al. Improvement in spine bone density and reduction in risk of vertebral fractures during treatment with antiresorptive drugs. Am J Med. 2002;112(4):281–9. *Analysis of the fracture risk reduction proportion that is explained by the modifications in bone density in response to treatment.

24. Bell KJ, Hayen A, Macaskill P, Irwig L, Craig JC, Ensrud K, et al. Value of routine monitoring of bone mineral density after starting bisphosphonate treatment: secondary analysis of trial data. BMJ. 2009;338:b2266.

25. *Austin M, Yang YC, Vittinghoff E, Adami S, Boonen S, Bauer DC, et al. Relationship between bone mineral density changes with denosumab treatment and risk reduction for vertebral and nonvertebral fractures. J Bone Miner Res. 2012;27(3):687–93. *Analysis of the fracture risk reduction proportion that is explained by the modifications in bone density in response to treatment with osumab, the drug where this relationship is the strongest among the currently available drugs.

26. Khosla S. Surrogates for fracture endpoints in clinical trials. J Bone Miner Res. 2003;18(6):1146–9.

27. Compston J. Monitoring bone mineral density during antiresorptive treatment for osteoporosis. BMJ. 2009;338:b1276.

28. Lenchik L, Kiebzak GM, Blunt BA. What is the role of serial bone mineral density measurements in patient management? J Clin Densitom. 2002;5(Suppl):S29–38.

29. Baim S, Wilson CR, Lewiecki EM, Luckey MM, Downs Jr RW, Lentle BC. Precision assessment and radiation safety for dual-energy X-ray absorptiometry: position paper of the International Society for Clinical Densitometry. J Clin Densitom. 2005;8(4):371–8.

30. Gluer CC. Monitoring skeletal changes by radiological techniques. J Bone Miner Res. 1999;14(11):1952–62.

31. Lodder MC, Lems WF, Ader HJ, Marthinsen AE, van Coeverden SC, Lips P, et al. Reproducibility of bone mineral density measurement in daily practice. Ann Rheum Dis. 2004;63(3):285–9.

32. *Chapurlat RD, Palermo L, Ramsay P, Cummings SR. Risk of fracture among women who lose bone density during treatment with alendronate. The Fracture Intervention Trial. Osteoporos Int. 2005;16(7):842–8. *Demonstration of the anti fracture benefit even in patients that loose BMD on treatment when compared with not-treated individuals in the placebo arm.

33. Sarkar S, Mitlak BH, Wong M, Stock JL, Black DM, Harper KD. Relationships between bone mineral density and incident vertebral fracture risk with raloxifene therapy. J Bone Miner Res. 2002;17(1):1–10.

34. Eastell R, Barton I, Hannon RA, Chines A, Garnero P, Delmas PD. Relationship of early changes in bone resorption to the reduction in fracture risk with risedronate. J Bone Miner Res. 2003;18(6):1051–6.

35. Eastell R, Hannon RA, Garnero P, Campbell MJ, Delmas PD. Relationship of early changes in bone resorption to the reduction in fracture risk with risedronate: review of statistical analysis. J Bone Miner Res. 2007;22(11):1656–60.

36. Sarkar S, Reginster JY, Crans GG, Diez-Perez A, Pinette KV, Delmas PD. Relationship between changes in biochemical markers of bone turnover and BMD to predict vertebral fracture risk. J Bone Miner Res. 2004;19(3):394–401.

37. Reginster JY, Sarkar S, Zegels B, Henrotin Y, Bruyere O, Agnusdei D, et al. Reduction in PINP, a marker of bone metabolism, with raloxifene treatment and its relationship with vertebral fracture risk. Bone. 2004;34(2):344–51.

38. Bauer DC, Black DM, Garnero P, Hochberg M, Ott S, Orloff J, et al. Change in bone turnover and hip, non-spine, and vertebral fracture in alendronate-treated women: the fracture intervention trial. J Bone Miner Res. 2004;19(8):1250–8.

39. Delmas PD, Munoz F, Black DM, Cosman F, Boonen S, Watts NB, et al. Effects of yearly zoledronic acid 5 mg on bone turnover markers and relation of PINP with fracture reduction in postmenopausal women with osteoporosis. J Bone Miner Res. 2009;24(9):1544–51.

40. *Meier C, Seibel MJ, Kraenzlin ME. Use of bone turnover markers in the real world: are we there yet? J Bone Miner Res. 2009;24(3):386–8. *Review of the strengths and weakness of the bone turnover markers, in special with respect to their use in clinical practice.

41. Glover SJ, Gall M, Schoenborn-Kellenberger O, Wagener M, Garnero P, Boonen S, et al. Establishing a reference interval for bone turnover markers in 637 healthy, young, premenopausal women from the United Kingdom, France, Belgium, and the United States. J Bone Miner Res. 2009;24(3):389–97.

42. *Vasikaran S, Eastell R, Bruyere O, Foldes AJ, Garnero P, Griesmacher A, et al. Markers of bone turnover for the prediction of fracture risk and monitoring of osteoporosis treatment: a need for international reference standards. Osteoporos Int. 2011;22(2):391–420. *Position paper on the practical use of bone turnover markers.

43. Diez-Perez A, Gonzalez-Macias J, Marin F, Abizanda M, Alvarez R, Gimeno A, et al. Prediction of absolute risk of non-spinal fractures using clinical risk factors and heel quantitative ultrasound. Osteoporos Int. 2007;18(5):629–39.

44. Johnell O, Oden A, Caulin F, Kanis JA. Acute and long-term increase in fracture risk after hospitalization for vertebral fracture. Osteoporos Int. 2001;12(3):207–14.

45. Johnell O, Kanis JA, Oden A, Sernbo I, Redlund-Johnell I, Petterson C, et al. Fracture risk following an osteoporotic fracture. Osteoporos Int. 2004;15(3):175–9.

46. Levis S, Quandt SA, Thompson D, Scott J, Schneider DL, Ross PD, et al. Alendronate reduces the risk of

multiple symptomatic fractures: results from the fracture intervention trial. J Am Geriatr Soc. 2002;50(3):409–15.

47. Watts NB, Josse RG, Hamdy RC, Hughes RA, Manhart MD, Barton I, et al. Risedronate prevents new vertebral fractures in postmenopausal women at high risk. J Clin Endocrinol Metab. 2003;88(2):542–9.

48. Barrett-Connor E, Nielson CM, Orwoll E, Bauer DC, Cauley JA. Epidemiology of rib fractures in older men: osteoporotic fractures in men (MrOS) prospective cohort study. BMJ. 2010;340:c1069.

49. *van Staa TP, Leufkens HG, Cooper C. Does a fracture at one site predict later fractures at other sites? A British cohort study. Osteoporos Int. 2002;13(8):624–9. *Analysis of how much a previous fracture predicts the occurrence of new fragility fractures in other anatomical locations.

50. Harrington JT, Ste-Marie LG, Brandi ML, Civitelli R, Fardellone P, Grauer A, et al. Risedronate rapidly reduces the risk for nonvertebral fractures in women with postmenopausal osteoporosis. Calcif Tissue Int. 2004;74(2):129–35.

51. Pols HA, Felsenberg D, Hanley DA, Stepan J, Munoz-Torres M, Wilkin TJ, et al. Multinational, placebo-controlled, randomized trial of the effects of alendronate on bone density and fracture risk in postmenopausal women with low bone mass: results of the FOSIT study. Fosamax International Trial Study Group. Osteoporos Int. 1999;9(5):461–8.

52. Seeley DG, Browner WS, Nevitt MC, Genant HK, Scott JC, Cummings SR. Which fractures are associated with low appendicular bone mass in elderly women? The Study of Osteoporotic Fractures Research Group. Ann Intern Med. 1991;115(11):837–42.

53. Mackey DC, Black DM, Bauer DC, McCloskey EV, Eastell R, Mesenbrink P, et al. Effects of antiresorptive treatment on nonvertebral fracture outcomes. J Bone Miner Res. 2011;26(10):2411–8.

54. Adami S, Isaia G, Luisetto G, Minisola S, Sinigaglia L, Gentilella R, et al. Fracture incidence and characterization in patients on osteoporosis treatment: the ICARO study. J Bone Miner Res. 2006;21(10):1565–70.

55. del Puente A, Scognamiglio A, Itto E, Ferrara G, Oriente P. Intramuscular clodronate in nonresponders to oral alendronate therapy for osteoporosis. J Rheumatol. 2000;27(8):1980–3.

56. Heckman GA, Papaioannou A, Sebaldt RJ, Ioannidis G, Petrie A, Goldsmith C, et al. Effect of vitamin D on bone mineral density of elderly patients with osteoporosis responding poorly to bisphosphonates. BMC Musculoskelet Disord. 2002;3:6.

57. Sawka AM, Adachi JD, Ioannidis G, Olszynski WP, Brown JP, Hanley DA, et al. What predicts early fracture or bone loss on bisphosphonate therapy? J Clin Densitom. 2003;6(4):315–22.

58. Lewiecki EM. Nonresponders to osteoporosis therapy. J Clin Densitom. 2003;6(4):307–14.

59. Jakob F, Marin F, Martin-Mola E, Torgerson D, Fardellone P, Adami S, et al. Characterization of patients with an inadequate clinical outcome from osteoporosis therapy: the Observational Study of Severe Osteoporosis (OSSO). QJM. 2006;99(8):531–43.

60. Obermayer-Pietsch BM, Marin F, McCloskey EV, Hadji P, Farrerons J, Boonen S, et al. Effects of two years of daily teriparatide treatment on BMD in postmenopausal women with severe osteoporosis with and without prior antiresorptive treatment. J Bone Miner Res. 2008;23(10):1591–600.

61. Diez-Perez A, Gonzalez-Macias J. Inadequate responders to osteoporosis treatment: proposal for an operational definition. Osteoporos Int. 2008;19(11):1511–6.

62. *Diez-Perez A, Adachi JD, Agnusdei D, Bilezikian JP, Compston JE, Cummings SR, et al. Treatment failure in osteoporosis. Osteoporos Int. 2012;23(12):2769–74. *Position paper establishing the criteria for considering failure in patients receiving antiosteoporosis medications.

63. Diez-Perez A, Olmos JM, Nogues X, Sosa M, Diaz-Curiel M, Perez-Castrillon JL, et al. Risk factors for prediction of inadequate response to antiresorptives. J Bone Miner Res. 2012;27(4):817–24.

64. Diez-Perez A, Adachi JD, Adami S, Anderson Jr FA, Boonen S, Chapurlat R, et al. Risk factors for treatment failure with antiosteoporosis medication: the global longitudinal study of osteoporosis in women (GLOW). J Bone Miner Res. 2014;29(1):260–7.

65. Prieto-Alhambra D, Pages-Castella A, Wallace G, Javaid MK, Judge A, Nogues X, et al. Predictors of fracture while on treatment with oral bisphosphonates: a population-based cohort study. J Bone Miner Res. 2014;29(1):268–74.

66. *Lewiecki EM, Cummings SR, Cosman F. Treat-to-target for osteoporosis: is now the time? J Clin Endocrinol Metab. 2013;98(3):946–53. *Article on the importance and future prospects for setting standard targets to be achieved when treating patients with osteoporosis.

Epidemiology of Atypical Subtrochanteric and Femoral Shaft Fractures

Jeri W. Nieves

Summary

- Atypical femoral fractures (AFFs) are located along the femoral diaphysis from just distal to the lesser trochanter to just proximal to the supracondylar flare and must meet certain criteria to be considered atypical.
- AFF are rare, and the absolute risk of these fractures ranges from 3.2 to 50 cases per 100,000 person-years.
- Risk factors include prodromal pain (70 %), Asian race, and several comorbid conditions and use of medications.
- AFFs appear to be more frequent among individuals who are being treated with bisphosphonates, and longer duration of use may further increase risk; however, the benefits of bisphosphonates have been estimated to be 100-fold greater than the risk of AFF.
- After bisphosphonates are stopped, the risk of AFF is reduced by 70 % per year.

J.W. Nieves, PhD (✉)
Department of Epidemiology and Clinical Research Center, Helen Hayes Hospital and Columbia University, 55 Route 9W, West Haverstraw, NY, 10993, USA
e-mail: Jwn5@columbia.edu

Definition of Atypical Femoral Fracture

The most recent American Society for Bone and Mineral Research (ASBMR) Task Force on Atypical Fractures [1] has defined an atypical femoral fracture (AFF) as located along the femoral diaphysis from just distal to the lesser trochanter to just proximal to the supracondylar flare. In addition, there are specific features listed below that should help to separate out AFFs from ordinary osteoporosis-related femur fractures. The ASBMR published a list of five major features of which four must be present [1]. Briefly, these features include minimal or no trauma, a predominately transverse or short oblique fracture line originating at lateral cortex, complete fractures extending through both cortices (incomplete only lateral), minimal or non-comminuted fracture, and localized periosteal or endosteal thickening of the lateral cortex ("beaking" or "flaring"). There are also several minor features that have been associated with atypical fractures, although none of these are required. Minor features include cortical thickening of the femoral shaft, prodromal pain prior to the fracture, bilateral incomplete or complete femoral diaphysis fractures, and delayed healing. AFFs are rare, and the absolute risk of these fractures ranges from 3.2 to 50 cases per 100,000 person-years [1].

© Springer International Publishing Switzerland 2016
S.L. Silverman, B. Abrahamsen (eds.), *The Duration and Safety of Osteoporosis Treatment*, DOI 10.1007/978-3-319-23639-1_6

Fig. 6.1 Classification of subtrochanteric and femoral shaft fractures

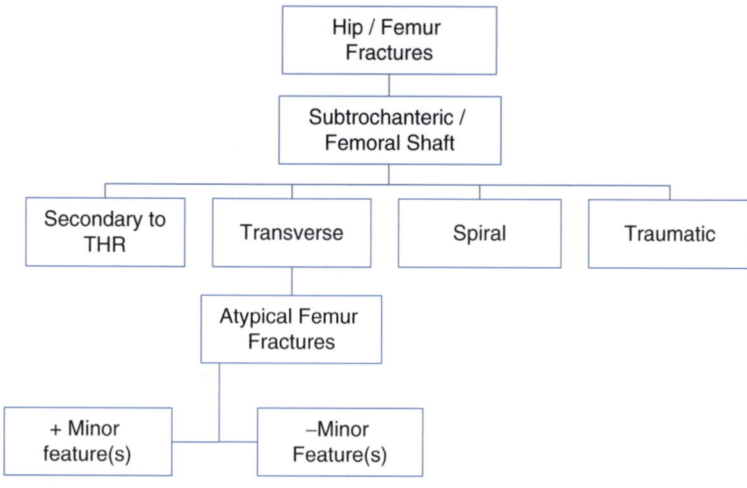

Classification of Subtrochanteric and Femoral Shaft Fractures

Subtrochanteric or femoral shaft fractures represent a small subset (10–30 %) of all hip/femur fractures [2]. Stress fractures occur in this region in athletes [3], and many of these fractures (~75 %) are associated with major trauma such as motor vehicle accidents, regardless of age [2]. Femoral shaft fractures may also occur after total hip replacement adjacent to the stem of the prosthesis [4]. In adult femoral shaft fractures, spiral fractures account for about 50 %, transverse fractures approximately 20 %, oblique transverse fractures 14 %, and oblique fractures 8 % of total femoral shaft fractures [2, 5]. The categorization of these fractures is noted in Fig. 6.1. It has been suggested that there may be differences in the clinical characteristics between subtrochanteric and femoral shaft fractures [6]. Furthermore, there may be important clinical differences between the AFFs that have minor features present as compared to those that only meet the major features of AFF [7].

The Use of Large Datasets in the Study of AFF

There are several studies that have evaluated subtrochanteric and femoral shaft (ST/FS) by the International Classification of Disease (ICD) codes, which have allowed large-scale studies of numerous data sources. These data can be used to determine the potential impact of these fractures in terms of providing an upper limit of the number of atypical fractures to expect, since only a small fraction of ST/FS fractures are atypical. However, with this type of database study, it is impossible to determine if the fractures are atypical since there is no radiographic adjudication. In addition, when these databases are used, the results can be impacted by the source of the data, whether there was a restriction on age, exclusion of trauma or other diseases, as well as which ICD codes were used in the analysis. For example, a comparison of 3 studies [8–10] used to evaluate trends in hip fracture rates and ST/FS fractures is found in Table 6.1. Ng used a subanalysis to determine that ST/FS fractures are increasing in women age 60 and older who sustained a fracture with moderate trauma, and this includes falls from standing height [10]. There are differences noted in terms of the database evaluated, age studied, ICD-9 codes utilized, and the exclusions applied as well as the results. An additional problem in studies that use ICD-9 codes for finding fracture cases is that the fracture location could be misclassified. In fact, only 36 % of femoral shaft fractures were correctly identified for their location [11]. However, despite these limitations, many studies have found that the rate of ST/FS fractures have increased recently [10, 12, 13].

Several studies have found that subtrochanteric and diaphyseal femur fractures share the

Table 6.1 Characteristics of studies evaluating trends in rates of hip fracture and ST/FS fractures

Study author	Age	Data source	ICD 9 codes used	Exclusions	Results
Wang	50+	Nationwide inpatient sample (NIS) developed from HCUP by AHRQ Represents 20 % discharges from community hospitals in the USA 1996–2007 (~90 million)	Only subtrochanteric ICD-9-CM: 820.22 primary surgical or replacement	Open fracture also excluded discharges for follow-up visits, procedures for peri-prosthetic fractures, and revision procedures	31.2 per 100,000 in 1996 to 34.2 per 100,000 in 2007 for only subtrochanteric (9.6 % increase)
Nieves	65+	National Center for Health Statistics 1996–2006 ~2.7 million records over 10 years and MarketScan 2002–2006 (~15 million)	Subtrochanteric (820.22), femoral shaft (including 821.00, unspecified part of femur; 821.01, shaft), and lower femur (including 821.20, lower end, unspecified; 821.21, condyle; 821.22, epiphysis, lower; 821.23, supracondylar; and 821.29, other)	Open fracture and Paget's disease (ICD-9 731.0) and malignancy (ICD-9 140-208)	Incidence of subtrochanteric and femoral shaft fractures combined was <25/100,000 person-years Stable over time evaluated
Ng	All ages	Olmsted County	ICD-9 codes 820–821 X-ray or report reviewed for location and level of trauma but not for atypia	Subanalysis based on age, level of trauma, or pathologic causes, and location—distal femur, diaphyseal, and subtrochanteric fractures	In women age 60+, moderate and no trauma fractures increased from 40.8 per 100,000 (95 % CI, 29.2–55.3) in 1984–1995 to 76.1 per 100,000 (95 % CI, 61.7–93.0) in 1996–2007 ($p = 0.001$)

epidemiology of classic osteoporosis-related hip fractures in terms of increasing incidence with age and higher rates in females than males [8, 14].

Danish administrative data [15] were queried to investigate the relationship between bisphosphonate use and subtrochanteric or femoral shaft fractures among a large number of alendronate users ($n = 39,567$) and nonusers ($n = 158,268$). Alendronate users were more likely to have hip fractures than nonusers (HR, 1.5; 95 % CI, 1.4–1.5). In addition, alendronate users were more likely to have subtrochanteric or femoral shaft fractures (HR, 2.0; CI, 1.8–2.3); however, the risk did not vary with length of bisphosphonate use. Of note, these were not AFF since there was no radiographic review. A similar lack of association between BP use and ST/FS fractures was found in another Danish study using untreated controls and in both a US study and one based on data from Taiwan both of which used other osteoporosis drug users as controls [16–18]. A nested case -control study in Canada did find that BP use for more than 5 years as compared to transient use was associated with ST/FS fracture (OR = 2.7, 95 % CI 1.25, 6.02), although as expected there was a concomitant reduced odds of classic hip fractures [19]. Again, there was no radiographic review, so these were not AFFs.

Risk Factors from Case Reports and Other Studies

Several clinical and radiographic features were identified from numerous case reports and series [20–29] which have helped to differentiate atypical fractures as being distinct from osteoporosis-related, prosthesis-related, or major trauma-related fractures. Asian women appear to represent a greater proportion of persons with AFF as compared to the population proportion [30, 31]. One of these features is now included in the minor features of AFF prodromal pain in the thigh or leg for weeks or months prior to the fracture [20, 24, 25, 32, 33], lack of trauma precipitating a fracture [20, 21, 24, 25], bilaterality in approximately 30 % (either simultaneous or sequential) [21, 25, 27, 28] and typically at the same location in the

contralateral leg [34], transverse fractures [24], cortical hypertrophy or thickness [25], stress reaction on the affected and/or unaffected side [20, 22, 24, 25, 27], and poor fracture healing [25, 26]. Other features identified with AFF include use of proton pump inhibitors, steroid therapy, in addition to the bisphosphonate [22, 25, 28, 35–38], and adherence to bisphosphonates [39] and other antiresorptive agents [38, 40–42], although in some cases there was prior bisphosphonate use. Normal or low bone mass but not osteoporosis in the hip region [28, 43–45] has also been reported. Comorbid conditions (e.g., vitamin D deficiency, rheumatoid arthritis, hypophosphatasia) have also been related to AFF [45, 46]. A recent study of 11 AFFs compared to those with typical femoral fractures ($n = 58$) identified hypocalcemia due to latent hypoparathyroidism as primary risk factor for AFF; younger age, higher BMI, early menopause, and less compromised BMD may also influence the development of AFF [47]. Structural features and hip geometry [34, 48] may also be important, and in fact 12 elderly women had AFF associated with bowing deformity, and only 6 of 12 had prior bisphosphonate use [49]. This is further described in Chap. 7. Although cortical thickening was thought to relate to long-term BP use, this is not true, and increased subtrochanteric femoral cortical thickening may instead be a risk factor. In fact, many AFFs occur at the point of greatest cortical thickening [50, 51]. A registry for AFF would help to identify more commonly underlying features since additional case series are unlikely to continue to be published.

Studies of Atypical Subtrochanteric and Femoral Shaft Fractures with Radiographic Review

The ASBMR Task Force [1] had extensively reviewed the epidemiologic studies concerning AFF, and these studies are found in Table 6.2 [30, 33, 52–61]. Many of these studies found an association between bisphosphonate use and AFF [30, 33, 52–58]. The benefits of bisphosphonates have been estimated to be 100-fold greater than the risk of AFF [38].

Table 6.2 Studies of atypical subtrochanteric and femoral shaft fractures with radiograph review

Author/date country	Design/time frame	Population	ST/FS N	AFF criteria	AFFs N (%)	AFFs on BPs N (%)	Incidence rate	Relative risk for BP use OR (95 % CI)	Absolute risk for BP use OR (95 % CI)	Comments
Lenart, 2009, USA [52]	Retrospective case-control 2000–2007	PM women admitted to level 1 trauma center in NY with ST/FS # matched by age, race, BMI to 1 IT and 1 FN # excluded GCs and low D levels	41	Transverse or oblique orientation. Cortical thickening. "Beaking" of lateral cortex. No kappa: all 3 had to agree	10 (24)	Hard to calculate	NA	15.33 (3.1–76.9)	NA	FN/IT# decreased with longer duration of BP use. AFFs associated with longer duration of BP use. Patients with AFFs on BPs were younger (70.4 vs. 82.5)
Girgis, 2010, Australia [53]	Retrospective case-control 2003–2008	152 M + W of any age admitted with ST/FS #	152	Lateral transverse or <30° oblique. Fracture line in area of cortical thickening. Medial unicortical beak. Kappa 0.8	20 (13)	17 (85)	NA	37.4 (12.9–113.3)	NA	Specificity of atypical pattern for BP use 96.7 %. No clear association with duration of BP use. Associated with GC exposure (OR 5.2; 95 % CI, 1.3–31)
Giusti, 2011, Netherlands [54]	Retrospective cohort case-control 1997–2007	906 M + W ≥ 50 admitted with new femur # each ST/FS # matched 1:2 to hip # matched for age, gender	63 (low energy)	Transverse or short oblique Non-comminuted in an area of thickened cortices Unicortical beaking. Kappa 0.83	10 (16)	5 (50)	NA	17.0 (2.6–113.3)	NA	No change in frequency of IT/FN or ST/FS fractures over 11 years. No difference in duration of BP between AFFs and ST/FS. AFFs associated with GC exposure, but not significant
Schilcher, 2011, Sweden [55]	Retrospective cohort case-control 2008	12,777 women ≥ 55 of whom 3515 admitted with proximal femur # in 2008 59 women with AFFs matched to 263 women with # at similar site representative of women vulnerable to #	1234	Transverse. Initiated on lateral side. Non-comminuted. Thickened lateral cortex at fracture site. No kappa	59 (5)	46 (78)	Ever use of BP 5.5/10,000 patient-year 1.9/10,000 for <1–1.9 years of use 8.4/10,000 for ≥2.0 years	Cohort: age-adjusted 47.3 (25.6, 87.3). Case-control: multivariate-adjusted 33.3 (14.3–77.8)	5 per 10,000 patient-years (4–7)	AFFs associated with longer duration of BP use. Risk diminished by 70 % per year after last use. No association with GC or PPI exposure. Drug use only captured from 2005 onward; uncaptured prior BP exposure may have inflated rates
Thompson, 2012, UK [56]	Retrospective case series no controls 2008–2010	3515 M + W admitted with proximal femur fracture	407	Simple transverse fracture line in a region of cortical hypertrophy. No kappa	27 (7)	22 (81)	NA	N/A	NA	30 % of patients with AFFs were on GCs. Mean duration of BP use 4.6 years (0.4–12.1)

(continued)

Table 6.2 (continued)

Author/date country	Design/time frame	Population	ST/FS N	AFF criteria	AFFs N (%)	AFFs on BPs N (%)	Incidence rate	Relative risk for BP use OR (95 % CI)	Absolute risk for BP use OR (95 % CI)	Comments
Feldstein, 2012, USA [57]	Retrospective cohort case-control 1996–2009	W ≥ 50; M ≥ 65 KPNW members 5034 new femur # All qualifying # matched to 300 FN and 300 IT #	197 femoral shaft # (FSF) with X rays	**ASBMR major:** ST/FS location. Low trauma. Transverse or short oblique fracture (see comments). Non-comminuted. Kappa 0.62	AFFM 53 (27) AFF major + minor 22 (11)	Any BP dispenses past 6M AFFM 6 (12)	AFFM: 5.9 per 100,000 person-years (4.6–7.4)	Unadjusted 2.29[a] (1.12–4.67). Age-adjusted 2.11[a] (0.99–4.49)	AFFM: 5.9 per 100,000 person-years (4.6–7.4)	Incidence of AFFs with ASBMR major + minor criteria increased by 10.7 % annually and was more strongly associated with BP use and with duration of BP and GC use than AFFs with only AFF Major criteria. These authors designated 35 fractures with angles of <30° as transverse, 43 fractures with angles of 30–60° as short oblique, and also included 3 fractures > 60°. Many would not agree that fractures with angles >30° are atypical
	Incidence based on 1,271,575 person-years of observation with 98,580 people/year			**ASBMR minor:** Localized periosteal reaction of the lateral cortex (beaking). Thick cortices. Unicortical stress fracture. Kappa 0.84		AFF major + minor 11 (52)			NA	
Lo, 2012, USA [30]	Retrospective case-control 2007–2008	3078 W ≥ 60 from KPNW with a hip/ femur # in 07-8	79	Transverse or short oblique pattern (with a medial spike). Non-comminuted. Lateral cortical thickening at fracture site. No kappa	38 (48)	37 (97)	NA	N/A	NA	No definition of short oblique. Bisphosphonate duration longer in AFFs than controls (5.1 vs. 2.3 years). No difference in GC exposure. Patients with AFFs more likely to be Asian

Dell, 2012, USA [62]	Prospective cohort incidence 2007–2011	All femur # over 5-year period in 1,835,116 M+W≥45 enrolled in Healthy Bones Program in KPSW 11,466 # reviewed	4036	ST/FS location. Transverse or with short oblique extension. Thickening of lateral cortex at fracture site	142 (4)	128 (90) Duration of use 1 M–13 Y mean 5.5±3.4 Y	Age-adjusted IR of AFFs with BP use 1.78/100,000 (1.5–2.0) with 0.1–1.9 Y 113.1/100,000 (69.3–156.8) with 8-8.9 Y	N/A	NA	For comparison, IR of all hip fractures in BP-exposed pts at KPSW was 463/100,000 patient-years in those on BPs for 0–1 Y. IR of all hip fractures decreased on BPs out to 5 years (384, 367–400), then stabilized, and was slightly increased after 8–9 years (544/100,000 (522–565). Incidence of AFFs increased markedly with increasing duration of BP use. 49 % of patients with AFFs were Asian. 12 % of patients with AFFs were on GCs
Meier, 2012, Switzerland [58]	Retrospective case-control cases were 39 AFFs, and 438 controls were patients with "classic" # in same region 1999–2010	477 M+W≥50 hospitalized with ST or FS # denominator for IR state population >50	477	Transverse or short oblique. Originating at lateral femoral cortex. Kappa 0.96	39 (8)	32 (82)	Over 12 Y, IR for classic # was 357/1,000,000 p-y and was stable. For AFFs IR was 32/1,000,000 and increased by 10.7 % (+1.2 to +20.3 %; $p=0.03$)	Crude OR 66.9 (627.1–165.1). Adjusted OR (Vit D, GCs, PPIs, sex, age) 69.1 (22.8–209.5)	For AFFs IR was 32/1,000,000 and increased by 10.7 % (+1.2 to +20.3 %; $p=0.03$)	OR for recurrence in patients with AFF was 42.6 (12.8–142.4) compared to classic #. OR for AFF vs. classic fractures increased with increasing BP duration from 35.1 (10.1–123.6) for <2 years, 46.9 (14.2–154.4) for 2–5 Y, 117.1 (34.2–401.7) for 5–9 Y, 175.7 (30.0–1027.6) for ≥9 Y, compared with no BP use. Mean duration of use 5.1±3.1 Y for AFF vs. 3.3±2.6 Y for classic ($p=0.02$)
Warren, 2012, New Zealand [59]	Retrospective case-control cases were 6 AFFs, and 65 controls were patients with fractures in same region 2003–2008	528 M+W≥20 hospitalized with ST or FS #, excluding those associated with coding errors, high trauma, tumors, or other pathology, prostheses, minor comminution	528	Thickened cortices. Transverse orientation. Medial spike. Single observer. No kappa	6 (1)	3 (50)	NA	Crude OR 5.5 (0.97–31)	NA	AFFs and ordinary fractures did not differ by age. 2/6 AFFS on GCs compared to 6/65 ordinary # (OR 4.9; 95 % CI 0.74–32.7). Relationship to BPs and GCs was not significant

(continued)

Table 6.2 (continued)

Author/date country	Design/time frame	Population	ST/FS N	AFF criteria	AFFs N (%)	AFFs on BPs N (%)	Incidence rate	Relative risk for BP use OR (95 % CI)	Absolute risk for BP use OR (95 % CI)	Comments
Shkolikova, 2012, Australia [60]	Retrospective case-control cases were 16 M+W with 20 AFFs and 46 patients with 46 ordinary fractures in same region 2007–2012	62 M+W with 66 ST/FS fractures, no age exclusion, admitted to a single hospital	66	ST/FS location. Cortical thickening. Cortical beaking. Lateral transverse fracture with or without medial oblique portion. Two observers, kappa 1.0, no information provided on blinding to clinical information	20 (30)	18 (90)	NA	Crude OR 128 (18–838)	NA	4 patients had bilateral AFFs. Patients with AFFs were younger (70.7 vs. 79.9, $p=0.01$) and more physically active before the fracture than those with typical ST/FS fractures
Beaudouin-Bazire, 2012, France [61]	Retrospective frequency study 2005–2010	4080 M+W >age 50 admitted for any femoral fracture	300 of 780 fractures with ST/FS codes, 206 had unavailable data, and 274 had erroneous codes. After exclusion of prostheses, pathological fractures and high-trauma fractures, 92 ST/FS fragility fractures remained	ASBMR major criteria: ST/FS location, no or minimal trauma. Transverse or short oblique (fracture line <30°) orientation. Non-comminuted. Complete +/− medial spike or incomplete. No kappa	12 (4 % of all ST/FS fractures and 13 % of low trauma ST/FS fractures, not associated with prostheses or pathological fractures)	5 (41.6)	NA	NA	NA	Patients with AFFs were predominantly women (10/12) with a mean age of 71.5. Information on BP therapy unknown in 2/12 AFF patients. 6/12 AFF patients also had "cortical hypertrophy"; 3 of these patients (50 %) were on BPs, and in one, BP status was unknown. There was a very high rate of erroneous coding, but with respect to fracture site and diagnosis of atypia; of 29 patients with radiographic features of atypia, 6 were excluded because of osteolytic lesions and 11 were excluded by chart review that revealed evidence of high-trauma or pathological fracture

All studies excluded peri-prosthetic and high-trauma fractures and fractures associated with malignancy

OR odds ratio, *IR* incidence rate, *#* fracture, *ST/FS* subtrochanteric/femoral shaft, *AFF* atypical femoral fracture, *BP* bisphosphonate, *GC* glucocorticoid, *ASBMR* American Society for Bone and Mineral Research, *PPI* proton pump inhibitors, *Y* years, *M* men, *W* women, *KPSW* Kaiser Permanente Southwest, *KPNW* Kaiser Permanente Northwest

From Shane E, et al. Atypical subtrochanteric and diaphyseal femoral fractures: Second report of a task force of the American Society for Bone and Mineral Research. J Bone Miner Res. May 28 2013. Reprinted with permission from John Wiley and Sons

[a]OR for atypical fractures with ASBMR major + minor criteria

One of the important papers in this selection was the paper by Feldstein et al. [57] that used data from patients registered in Kaiser Permanente Northwest and concluded that patients with atypical fractures and one or more of the ASBMR minor *radiographic* criteria (beaking, cortical thickening, and stress fracture) appear to differ in several ways from those with only major radiographic criteria (low force, location at ST/FS, transverse, non-comminuted). Some of the differences they noted were that patients with both major and minor radiographic criteria were younger, were more likely to use glucocorticoids, were more likely to report long-term bisphosphonate use, and were more likely to report prodromal pain as compared to patients with only major criteria. As noted in the commentary by Abrahamsen [7], future studies should separate our AFF based on if they only display ASBMR major radiographic criteria from those that also have one or more minor criteria. These radiographic features used for the minor criteria may also help to elucidate the mechanism by which AFF occur.

Lo [30] from Kaiser Permanente Northwest studied women aged ≥60 hospitalized with a hip or femur fracture ($n=3078$), and of these fractures, 38 were determined to be AFF with the minor feature of lateral cortical thickening. One striking finding was the preponderance of Asian women in the AFF group.

In another Kaiser Permanente study [62], the age-adjusted incidence of AFF was found to increase with duration of bisphosphonate use from 1.8/100,000 cases per year <2 years of use to 113.1/100,000 cases per year for >8.0 years of use, while hip fracture rates decreased with bisphosphonate use. Similar results of increasing risk with increasing bisphosphonate use were found in a case-control study in a Swiss hospital [58] where they identified several risk factors for AFF including use of glucocorticoids, vitamin D supplements, and proton pump inhibitors and also estimated that 28 % of AFF had a fracture in the contralateral leg.

Another important contribution was the paper by Schilcher [55] in which 1234 radiographs of subtrochanteric or femoral shaft fractures in women over age 55 were reviewed and 59 cases with atypical features were identified and compared to 263 controls with subtrochanteric or femoral shaft fractures that were not transverse. In a cohort of 1.5 million women 55 years or older residing in Sweden in 2008, 83,311 received bisphosphonates during the 3 years preceding the fracture (only prior 3 years' drug use was available in database), and 59 had atypical fractures, with an absolute risk of five cases per 10,000 patient-years (95 % CI, 4–7) and longer duration of use was associated with 30 % increased risk per 100 daily doses (1.3; 95 % CI, 1.1–1.6). Importantly, after bisphosphonates were stopped, the risk of AFF was reduced by 70 % per year (OR, 0.28; 95 % CI, 0.21, 0.38).

Several papers have been published subsequent to the ASBMR publication and will be summarized here. Wang et al. [39] found that the rate of subtrochanteric/femoral shaft fractures, but not intertrochanteric/femoral neck fractures, was positively associated with higher adherence to long-term (≥3 years) oral bisphosphonates in the elderly female Medicare population. This study could not evaluate X-rays, so the study did not specifically look at AFF.

A retrospective blinded review of 2238 radiographs in Japan by orthopedic surgeons were used to identify AFF based on meeting all of ASBMR established major criteria (including beaking of the lateral cortex), and these AFFs were further confirmed by other orthopedists. In a case-control analysis of the 10 identified AFF subjects compared to 30 typical ST/FS fractures, it was found that a higher percentage of patients with AFFs used bisphosphonates and glucocorticoids and were suffering from collagen disease than those with typical femoral fractures [63]. In Korea, a total of 108 consecutive patients with displaced atypical femoral fracture after minimal trauma that occurred between January 2005 and June 2011 were reviewed, and 76 patients were found to have AFF based on ASBMR 2013 criteria [37]. They noted that bisphosphonate use was more than 3 years in 75 % of cases and that in these individuals there was more nonunion and more bilateral fractures than in shorter bisphosphonate use. A recent nested case-control study in Spain used a general practice research database and matched five controls (no history of AFF or hip fracture) for each AFF case and reported that there was an increase of atypical fracture risk among ever users of bisphosphonates versus never users, and that risk was greater in those with longer duration of use [64].

Conclusion

Atypical femur fractures are uncommon but appear to be more frequent among individuals who are being treated with oral and intravenous bisphosphonates and longer duration of use further increases the risk. Additional studies of atypical fractures are needed to clarify the mechanism by which they occur (however, the benefits of bisphosphonates have been estimated to be 100-fold greater than the risk of AFF) [38] and to identify other key risk factors as well as to confirm that discontinuation of treatment after long-term use substantially lowers the risk. A better understanding of the mechanisms that may lead to AFF and their risk factors using clinical models, genetics, and imaging may help to target those individuals who are at high risk and should avoid the use of bisphosphonates.

References[1]

1. *Shane E, Burr D, Abrahamsen B, et al. Atypical subtrochanteric and diaphyseal femoral fractures: second report of a task force of the American Society for Bone and Mineral Research. J Bone Miner Res. 2014;29(1):1–23. *This provides an excellent overview of knowledge to date on AFFs.
2. Salminen S, Pihlajamaki H, Avikainen V, Kyro A, Bostman O. Specific features associated with femoral shaft fractures caused by low-energy trauma. J Trauma. 1997;43(1):117–22.
3. Butler JE, Brown SL, McConnell BG. Subtrochanteric stress fractures in runners. Am J Sports Med. 1982; 10(4):228–32.
4. Mullaji AB, Thomas TL. Low-energy subtrochanteric fractures in elderly patients: results of fixation with the sliding screw plate. J Trauma. 1993;34(1):56–61.
5. Salminen ST, Pihlajamaki HK, Avikainen VJ, Bostman OM. Population based epidemiologic and morphologic study of femoral shaft fractures. Clin Orthop Relat Res. 2000;372:241–9.
6. Koeppen VA, Schilcher J, Aspenberg P. Dichotomous location of 160 atypical femoral fractures. Acta Orthop. 2013;84(6):561–4.
7. Abrahamsen B. Atypical femur fractures: refining the clinical picture. J Bone Miner Res. 2012;27(5): 975–6.
8. Nieves JW, Bilezikian JP, Lane JM, et al. Fragility fractures of the hip and femur: incidence and patient characteristics. Osteoporos Int. 2010;21(3):399–408.
9. Wang Z, Bhattacharyya T. Trends in incidence of subtrochanteric fragility fractures and bisphosphonate use among the US elderly, 1996-2007. J Bone Miner Res. 2011;26(3):553–60.
10. Ng AC, Drake MT, Clarke BL, et al. Trends in subtrochanteric, diaphyseal, and distal femur fractures, 1984-2007. Osteoporos Int. 2012;23(6):1721–6.
11. Spangler L, Ott SM, Scholes D. Utility of automated data in identifying femoral shaft and subtrochanteric (diaphyseal) fractures. Osteoporos Int. 2011;22(9): 2523–7.
12. Maravic M, Ostertag A, Cohen-Solal M. Subtrochanteric/femoral shaft versus hip fractures: incidences and identification of risk factors. J Bone Miner Res. 2012; 27(1):130–7.
13. Lee YK, Ha YC, Park C, Yoo JJ, Shin CS, Koo KH. Bisphosphonate use and increased incidence of subtrochanteric fracture in South Korea: results from the National Claim Registry. Osteoporos Int. 2013;24(2): 707–11.
14. Abrahamsen B, Eiken P, Eastell R. Subtrochanteric and diaphyseal femur fractures in patients treated with alendronate: a register-based national cohort study. J Bone Miner Res. 2009;24(6):1095–102.
15. Abrahamsen B, Eiken P, Eastell R. Cumulative alendronate dose and the long-term absolute risk of subtrochanteric and diaphyseal femur fractures: a register-based national cohort analysis. J Clin Endocrinol Metab. 2010;95(12):5258–65.
16. Vestergaard P, Schwartz F, Rejnmark L, Mosekilde L. Risk of femoral shaft and subtrochanteric fractures among users of bisphosphonates and raloxifene. Osteoporos Int. 2011;22(3):993–1001.
17. Kim SY, Schneeweiss S, Katz JN, Levin R, Solomon DH. Oral bisphosphonates and risk of subtrochanteric or diaphyseal femur fractures in a population-based cohort. J Bone Miner Res. 2011;26(5):993–1001.
18. Hsiao FY, Huang WF, Chen YM, et al. Hip and subtrochanteric or diaphyseal femoral fractures in alendronate users: a 10-year, nationwide retrospective cohort study in Taiwanese women. Clin Ther. 2011; 33(11):1659–67.
19. Park-Wyllie LY, Mamdani MM, Juurlink DN, et al. Bisphosphonate use and the risk of subtrochanteric or femoral shaft fractures in older women. JAMA. 2011;305(8):783–9.

[1] *Important References

20. Lee P, van der Wall H, Seibel MJ. Looking beyond low bone mineral density: multiple insufficiency fractures in a woman with post-menopausal osteoporosis on alendronate therapy. J Endocrinol Invest. 2007; 30(7):590–7.

21. Cheung RK, Leung KK, Lee KC, Chow TC. Sequential non-traumatic femoral shaft fractures in a patient on long-term alendronate. Hong Kong Med J. 2007;13(6): 485–9.

22. Demiralp B, Ilgan S, Ozgur Karacalioglu A, Cicek EI, Yildrim D, Erler K. Bilateral femoral insufficiency fractures treated with inflatable intramedullary nails: a case report. Arch Orthop Trauma Surg. 2007;127(7): 597–601.

23. Armamento-Villareal R, Napoli N, Panwar V, Novack D. Suppressed bone turnover during alendronate therapy for high-turnover osteoporosis. N Engl J Med. 2006;355(19):2048–50.

24. Kumm DA, Rack C, Rutt J. Subtrochanteric stress fracture of the femur following total knee arthroplasty. J Arthroplasty. 1997;12(5):580–3.

25. Schneider JP. Should bisphosphonates be continued indefinitely? An unusual fracture in a healthy woman on long-term alendronate. Geriatrics. 2006;61(1):31–3.

26. Sayed-Noor AS, Sjoden GO. Case reports: two femoral insufficiency fractures after long-term alendronate therapy. Clin Orthop Relat Res. 2009;467(7):1921–6.

27. Husada G, Libbeerecht K, Peeters T, Populaire J. Bilateral mid-diaphyseal femoral stress fractures in the elderly. Eur J Trauma. 2005;1:68–71.

28. Somford MP, Draijer FW, Thomassen BJ, Chavassieux PM, Boivin G, Papapoulos SE. Bilateral fractures of the femur diaphysis in a patient with rheumatoid arthritis on long-term treatment with alendronate: clues to the mechanism of increased bone fragility. J Bone Miner Res. 2009;24(10):1736–40.

29. Nieves JW, Cosman F. Atypical subtrochanteric and femoral shaft fractures and possible association with bisphosphonates. Curr Osteoporos Rep. 2010;8(1): 34–9.

30. Lo JC, Huang SY, Lee GA, et al. Clinical correlates of atypical femoral fracture. Bone. 2012;51(1):181–4.

31. Marcano A, Taormina D, Egol KA, Peck V, Tejwani NC. Are race and sex associated with the occurrence of atypical femoral fractures? Clin Orthop Relat Res. 2014;472(3):1020–7.

32. Neviaser AS, Lane JM, Lenart BA, Edobor-Osula F, Lorich DG. Low-energy femoral shaft fractures associated with alendronate use. J Orthop Trauma. 2008; 22(5):346–50.

33. Dell RM, Adams AL, Greene DF, et al. Incidence of atypical nontraumatic diaphyseal fractures of the femur. J Bone Miner Res. 2012;27(12):2544–50.

34. Saita Y, Ishijima M, Mogami A, et al. The fracture sites of atypical femoral fractures are associated with the weight-bearing lower limb alignment. Bone. 2014;66C:105–10.

35. Odvina CV, Levy S, Rao S, Zerwekh JE, Rao DS. Unusual mid-shaft fractures during long-term bisphosphonate therapy. Clin Endocrinol (Oxf). 2010;72(2):161–8.

36. Giusti A, Hamdy NA, Papapoulos SE. Atypical fractures of the femur and bisphosphonate therapy: a systematic review of case/case series studies. Bone. 2010;47(2):169–80.

37. Kang JS, Won YY, Kim JO, et al. Atypical femoral fractures after anti-osteoporotic medication: a Korean multicenter study. Int Orthop. 2014;38(6):1247–53.

38. Edwards BJ, Bunta AD, Lane J, et al. Bisphosphonates and nonhealing femoral fractures: analysis of the FDA Adverse Event Reporting System (FAERS) and international safety efforts: a systematic review from the Research on Adverse Drug Events And Reports (RADAR) project. J Bone Joint Surg Am. 2013; 95(4):297–307.

39. Wang Z, Ward MM, Chan L, Bhattacharyya T. Adherence to oral bisphosphonates and the risk of subtrochanteric and femoral shaft fractures among female medicare beneficiaries. Osteoporos Int. 2014; 25(8):2109–16.

40. Thompson RN, Armstrong CL, Heyburn G. Bilateral atypical femoral fractures in a patient prescribed denosumab—a case report. Bone. 2014;61:44–7.

41. Khow KS, Yong TY. Atypical femoral fracture in a patient treated with denosumab. J Bone Miner Metab. 2015;33(3):355–8.

42. Bone HG, Chapurlat R, Brandi ML, et al. The effect of three or six years of denosumab exposure in women with postmenopausal osteoporosis: results from the FREEDOM extension. J Clin Endocrinol Metab. 2013;98(11):4483–92.

43. Odvina CV, Levy S, Rao S, Zerwekh JE, Sudhaker RD. Unusual mid-shaft fractures during long term bisphosphonate therapy. Clin Endocrinol (Oxf). 2010;72(2):161–8.

44. Visekruna M, Wilson D, McKiernan FE. Severely suppressed bone turnover and atypical skeletal fragility. J Clin Endocrinol Metab. 2008;93(8):2948–52.

45. Markman LH, Allison MB, Rosenberg ZS, et al. A retrospective review of patients with atypical femoral fractures while on long-term bisphosphonates: including pertinent biochemical and imaging studies. Endocr Pract. 2013;19(3):456–61.

46. Shane E, Burr D, Ebeling PR, et al. Atypical subtrochanteric and diaphyseal femoral fractures: report of a task force of the American Society for Bone and Mineral Research. J Bone Miner Res. 2010;25(11): 2267–94.

47. Franceschetti P, Bondanelli M, Caruso G, et al. Risk factors for development of atypical femoral fractures in patients on long-term oral bisphosphonate therapy. Bone. 2013;56(2):426–31.

48. Taormina DP, Marcano AI, Karia R, Egol KA, Tejwani NC. Symptomatic atypical femoral fractures are related to underlying hip geometry. Bone. 2014;63:1–6.

49. Oh Y, Wakabayashi Y, Kurosa Y, Ishizuki M, Okawa A. Stress fracture of the bowed femoral shaft is another cause of atypical femoral fracture in elderly Japanese: a case series. J Orthop Sci. 2014;19(4):579–86.

50. Chen F, Wang Z, Bhattacharyya T. Absence of femoral cortical thickening in long-term bisphosphonate

users: implications for atypical femur fractures. Bone. 2014;62:64–6.

51. Unnanuntana A, Ashfaq K, Ton QV, Kleimeyer JP, Lane JM. The effect of long-term alendronate treatment on cortical thickness of the proximal femur. Clin Orthop Relat Res. 2012;470(1):291–8.

52. Lenart BA, Neviaser AS, Lyman S, et al. Association of low-energy femoral fractures with prolonged bisphosphonate use: a case control study. Osteoporos Int. 2009;20(8):1353–62.

53. Girgis CM, Seibel MJ. Atypical femur fractures: a complication of prolonged bisphosphonate therapy? Med J Aust. 2010;193(4):196–8.

54. Giusti A, Hamdy NA, Dekkers OM, Ramautar SR, Dijkstra S, Papapoulos SE. Atypical fractures and bisphosphonate therapy: a cohort study of patients with femoral fracture with radiographic adjudication of fracture site and features. Bone. 2011;48(5):966–71.

55. *Schilcher J, Michaelsson K, Aspenberg P. Bisphosphonate use and atypical fractures of the femoral shaft. N Engl J Med. 2011;364(18):1728–37. *This paper highlights the risk of fractures, association with bisphosphonate and reduction in risk when bisphosphonates are stopped.

56. Thompson RN, Phillips JR, McCauley SH, Elliott JR, Moran CG. Atypical femoral fractures and bisphosphonate treatment: experience in two large United Kingdom teaching hospitals. J Bone Joint Surg Br. 2012;94(3):385–90.

57. *Feldstein AC, Black D, Perrin N, et al. Incidence and demography of femur fractures with and without atypical features. J Bone Miner Res. 2012;27(5):977–86. *Helps to clarify that there may be a subset of AFF that are more likely associated with bisphosphonates based on the presence of major and minor criteria.

58. Meier RP, Perneger TV, Stern R, Rizzoli R, Peter RE. Increasing occurrence of atypical femoral fractures associated with bisphosphonate use. Arch Intern Med. 2012;172(12):930–6.

59. Warren C, Gilchrist N, Coates M, et al. Atypical subtrochanteric fractures, bisphosphonates, blinded radiological review. ANZ J Surg. 2012;82(12):908–12.

60. Shkolnikova J, Flynn J, Choong P. Burden of bisphosphonate-associated femoral fractures. ANZ J Surg. 2013;83(3):175–81.

61. Beaudouin-Bazire C, Dalmas N, Bourgeois J, et al. Real frequency of ordinary and atypical subtrochanteric and diaphyseal fractures in France based on X-rays and medical file analysis. Joint Bone Spine. 2013;80(2):201–5.

62. Dell R. Fracture prevention in Kaiser Permanente Southern California. Osteoporos Int. 2011;22 Suppl 3:457–60.

63. Saita Y, Ishijima M, Mogami A, et al. The incidence of and risk factors for developing atypical femoral fractures in Japan. J Bone Miner Metab. 2015;33(3):311–8.

64. Erviti J, Alonso A, Oliva B, et al. Oral bisphosphonates are associated with increased risk of subtrochanteric and diaphyseal fractures in elderly women: a nested case-control study. BMJ Open. 2013 Jan 30;3(1).

Bisphosphonate-Related Atypical Femur Fractures and Their Radiographic Features

Joseph C. Giaconi and C. Travis Watterson

Summary

- Defining features of Atypical femur fractures include subtrochanteric lateral cortical thickening ("beaking"), a transverse fracture line (within 15° of 90°), and lateral to medial progression of the fracture line.
- Typically occur within 5 cm of the lesser trochanter.
- Best evaluated on MRI; however, X-ray and DXA may be appropriate for screening.
- Typically progress to full fracture over 2–6 months.
- Resolution of incomplete fractures is confirmed by resolution of findings on MRI.
- Conservative therapy is typically considered to have failed if there is no resolution of MRI findings over 2–3 months.

As a response to the particularly devastating nature of femoral fractures, the last decade has seen an explosion of drugs to promote bone health. Foremost among these are the bisphosphonates, osteoclast inhibitors, that help improve bone density by decreasing mineral resorption.

As with all medications, they are not without undesired side effects. In particular, the atypical femoral fracture is one side effect that has come to recent attention. This type of fracture, as the name implies, is unusual for a number of reasons including its characteristic location inferior to the lesser trochanter and its progression from the lateral to the medial cortex. The most concerning feature, however, is that a patient may suffer a complete transverse fracture from low-energy trauma, such as tripping over a rug or stepping off a curb. Because of such dramatic consequences with little-to-no warning, a tremendous effort has been summoned to better understand bisphosphonate-related fractures and to better inform therapy.

History and Mechanism of Action

The effect of phosphate exposure on bone health dates to the 1840s when British matchstick makers began to develop what would eventually be recognized as a precursor syndrome to long-term bisphosphonate toxicity. "Phossy jaw" caused by exposure to the phosphate used in matchstick heads was characterized by osteonecrosis of the jaw and phospholuminescence that would later progress to brain damage and diffuse organ failure [1, 2]. It would not be until the 1970s that medicines were developed to inhibit resorption without inhibiting growth.

J.C. Giaconi, MD (✉) • C.T. Watterson, MD
Musculoskeletal Radiology, S. Mark Taper
Foundation Imaging Center, Cedars Sinai Medical
Center, 8700 Beverly Blvd, Suite M-335,
Los Angeles, CA, 90048, USA
e-mail: joseph.giaconi@cshs.org

© Springer International Publishing Switzerland 2016
S.L. Silverman, B. Abrahamsen (eds.), *The Duration and Safety of Osteoporosis Treatment*, DOI 10.1007/978-3-319-23639-1_7

Originally derived from pyrophosphate, these medicines actively inhibit and even induce apoptosis of osteoclasts [3–5]. In doing so, the balance of continual bone turnover shifts to favor growth. This principle has been successfully exploited to prevent refracture of the vertebral bodies and femora of patients with a variety of diseases. The most commonly treated diseases include osteoporosis, Paget's disease, osteogenesis imperfecta, multiple myeloma, and osteolytic metastatic disease.

As pyrophosphate derivatives preferentially target active osteoclasts, there has always been a theoretical risk that bone turnover may be more severely suppressed in more stressed areas of bone. Sure enough, studies began to present cases of low-impact fracture, with the most apparent explanation being a disorganized bony remodeling secondary to disrupted turnover, similar to that found in osteopetrosis.

It has been widely reported that bisphosphonates work to decrease the rate of classical femoral fractures [6]. Multinational registry studies have shown a dramatic decrease in femoral fractures coinciding with increased bisphosphonate use over the last decade [7–9]. What's more, patients placed on a bisphosphonate following an initial osteoporotic, classic fracture are less likely to be rehospitalized for subsequent fracture [10]. Despite this, there has been as much as a 10 % increase in the number of subtrochanteric femoral fractures [8]. The incidence of subtrochanteric fractures among bisphosphonate users ranges from 3.2 to 50/100,000 [7, 8, 11].

Epidemiology

Conflicting information has been presented regarding the epidemiology of atypical fractures. While some studies have demonstrated that the patients at the highest risk for fracture are those who have taken these medicines for less than 3 years [12, 13], the majority of research favors increased risk with longer duration of therapy [8, 14–17]. On the other hand, there has been some suggestion that those suffering AFFs may have a lower baseline level of health than those who have taken a bisphosphonate for years without issue. Even more enshrouded is the efficacy of drug holidays. Still under active investigation are the length of time a patient remains at risk for atypical fracture after suspending specific bisphosphonates [8, 18] and whether risk is dose-related [13].

A variety of risk factors are being evaluated. Evidence exists for increased risk in patients with concomitant long-term steroid use, active rheumatoid arthritis, low vitamin D levels [19], and Asian ethnic background [20, 21]. Patients suffering fracture are typically younger, averaging 71 years old in contrast to the average age of bisphosphonate users in general, 80 years old [11]. They also tend to be more ambulatory prior to fracture. Conflicting information exists regarding whether diabetes or proton-pump inhibitors play any role.

Histology

Under the microscope, a minority of patients show a decreased numbers of osteoclasts with a high proportion of osteoclasts with abnormal, pyknotic nuclei [22, 23]. There is also an increased prevalence of nonfunctioning "atypical giant osteoclasts." In the majority, however, there is normal histology with the only finding being an up to 90 % reduction in bone remodeling [4]. These findings are similar to those in osteopetrosis and help to support the theory that disorganized remodeling progresses to bone weakness despite normal or increased mineralization.

Imaging

For the radiologist, there are several important considerations. As many as 50 % of patients may be asymptomatic [24]. Given this, radiology has a strong role in early screening. In addition, it is important to remember that Atypical femur fractures make up a minority of subtrochanteric femoral fractures, and there are several imaging features that must be kept in mind when suggesting this diagnosis.

In 2013, the Society for Bone and Mineral Research published an updated set of criteria for making the diagnosis of atypical femoral fracture [25]:

Major features

1. The fracture is associated with minimal or no trauma, as in a fall from a standing height or less.
2. The fracture line originates at the lateral cortex and is substantially transverse in its orientation [90° ± 15], although it may become oblique as it progresses medially across the femur.
3. Complete fractures extend through both cortices and may be associated with a medial spike; incomplete fractures involve only the lateral cortex.
4. The fracture is non-comminuted or minimally comminuted.
5. Localized periosteal or endosteal thickening of the lateral cortex is present at the fracture site ("beaking" or "flaring").

Minor features

1. Generalized increase in cortical thickness of the femoral diaphysis
2. Unilateral or bilateral prodromal symptoms such as dull or aching in the groin or thigh
3. Bilateral incomplete or complete femoral diaphysis fractures
4. Delayed fracture healing

At least four of the five major features must be present to diagnose an atypical femoral fracture. No minor criteria are required. Figures 7.1, 7.2, 7.3, 7.4, 7.5, 7.6, 7.7, 7.8, 7.9, and 7.10 demonstrate a classic appearance of an AFF over several modalities in a 58-year-old male on bisphosphonates.

Conventional Radiography

Atypical femur fractures are defined by their radiographic appearance. Currently, they are defined as transverse fractures arising from the lateral cortex of

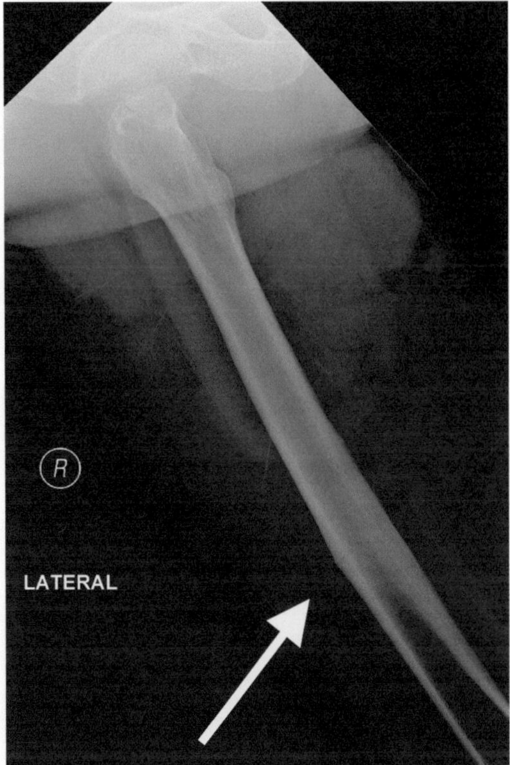

Fig. 7.1 This lateral radiograph of the right femur shows lateral, mid-diaphyseal cortical thickening

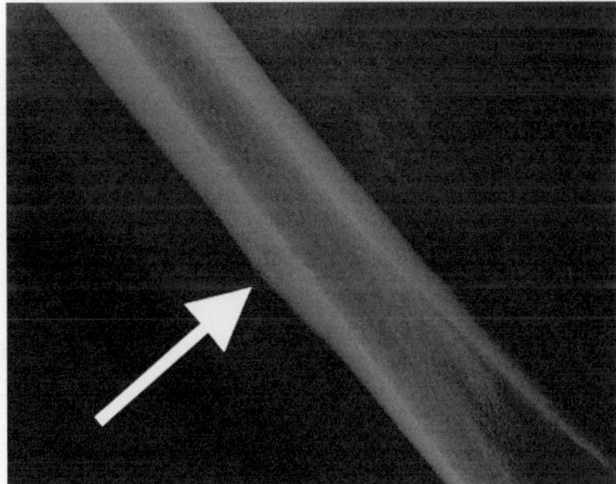

Fig. 7.2 Frontal radiograph better demonstrates some intracortical lucency, possibly an early fracture line

the femur, inferior to the lesser trochanter. Seventy-nine percent of all atypical fractures occur within 5 cm of the lesser trochanter and, by definition, lie above the supracondylar flare [26]. Early on, there will be thickening ("beaking") of the medial or lateral aspect of the lateral cortex.

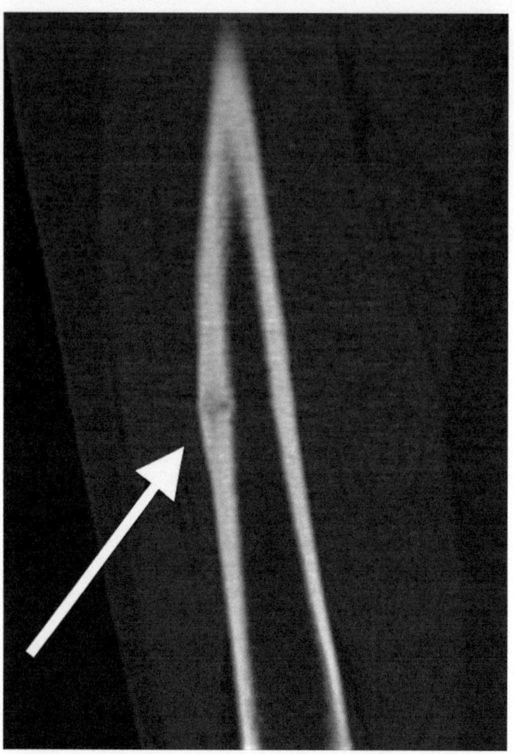

Fig. 7.3 Coronal CT reformation shows lateral cortical thickening with a linear lucency developing. The medial cortex is uninvolved

With progression, a fracture line will develop and extend medially. There have been several examples of multiple foci developing simultaneously; however, these fractures are rarely comminuted [27–29].

The angle made by the fracture and lateral femoral cortex is important in elucidating the etiology. Atypical femur fractures comprise only about 1/3 of all subtrochanteric fractures, and, in cases where the fracture angle is shallow, it can be difficult to differentiate bisphosphonate-related fractures from other diagnoses [16]. A fracture angle of $90° \pm 15$ with associated periosteal beaking has a 90 % specificity for bisphosphonate use [30]. Fatigue fractures will typically be more oblique, in addition to propagating from the medial to lateral cortex [31, 32]. Additional considerations for differential diagnoses are described in conjunction with the figures found at the end of this chapter. Distinguishing bisphosphonate-related injury from classic fractures may become increasingly important in determining prognosis and guiding specific therapy.

Progression to the middle and late stages of the fracture are marked by involvement of the medial cortex and complete displacement of

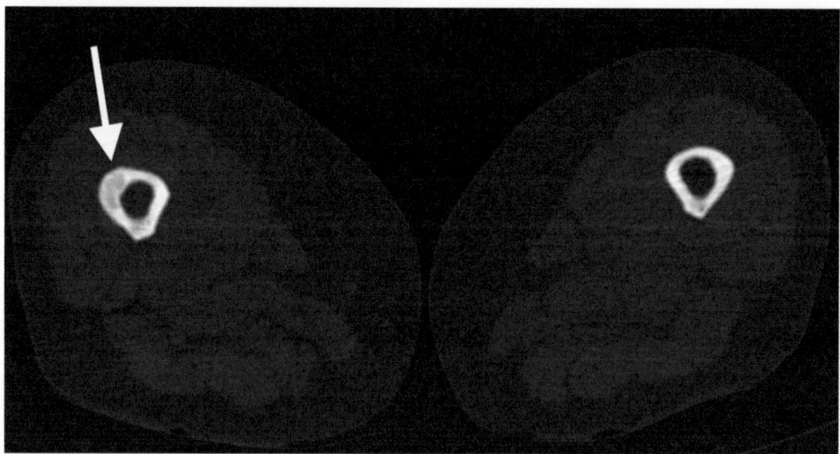

Fig. 7.4 Transverse CT shows thickening and lucency of the right femoral lateral cortex

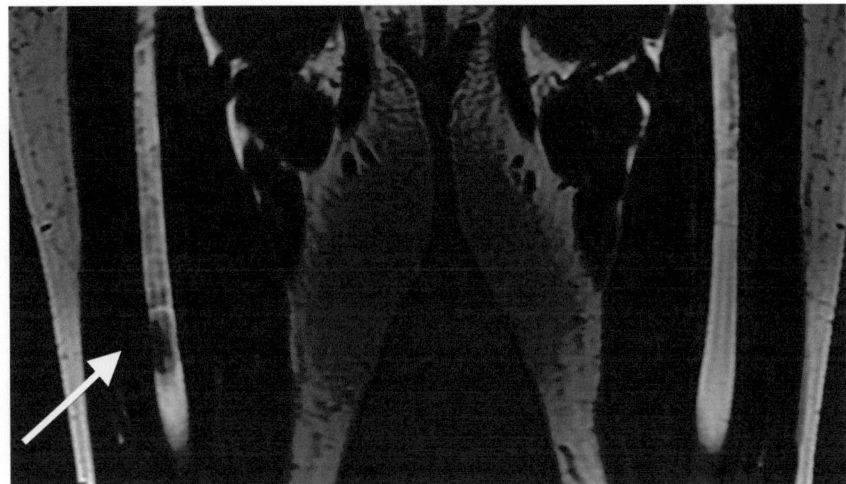

Fig. 7.5 Coronal T1-weighted 1.5 T MRI shows lateral cortical thickening of the right femur with a confluent, decreased marrow signal. The left femur is unremarkable

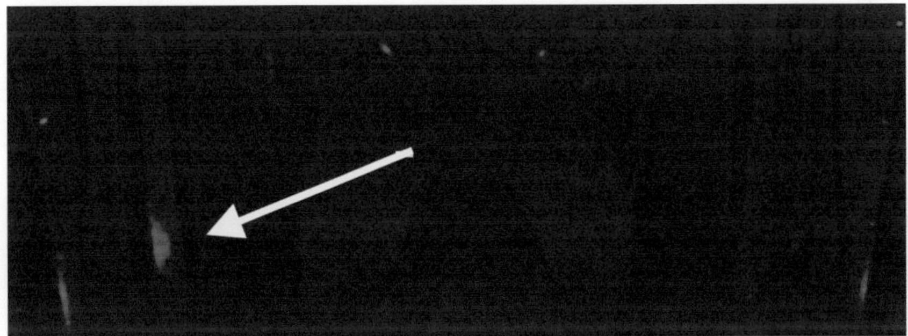

Fig. 7.6 Coronal T2-weighted, fat-saturated 1.5 T MRI shows increased signal intensity of the bone marrow at the non-displaced atypical femoral fracture site

Fig. 7.7 Transverse T2 1.5 T MRI with fat saturation shows increased bone marrow signal

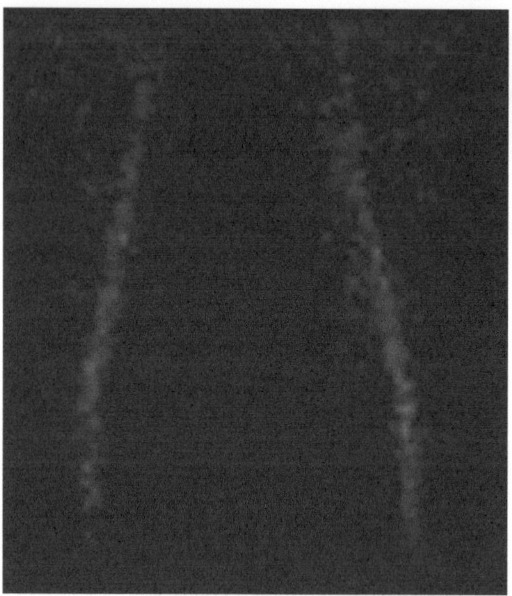

Fig. 7.8 Flow (early) phase of a bone scan. No abnormality is identified

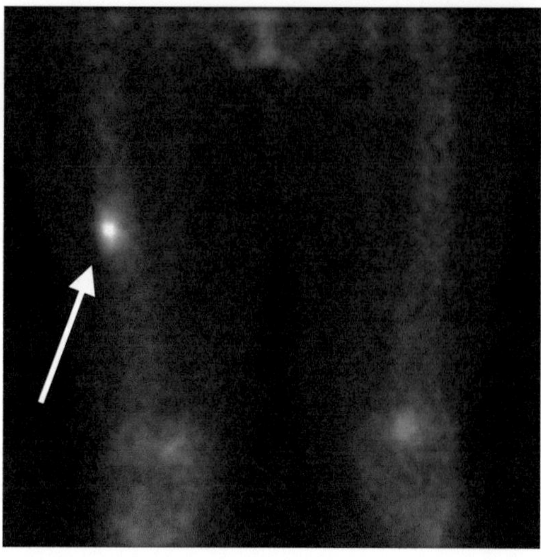

Fig. 7.10 Delayed phase on bone scan shows significantly increased radiotracer uptake. This appearance can be seen in conditions of increased bone turnover, such as osteoblastic metastases and stress fractures, and in this case of non-displaced atypical femoral fracture (AFF)

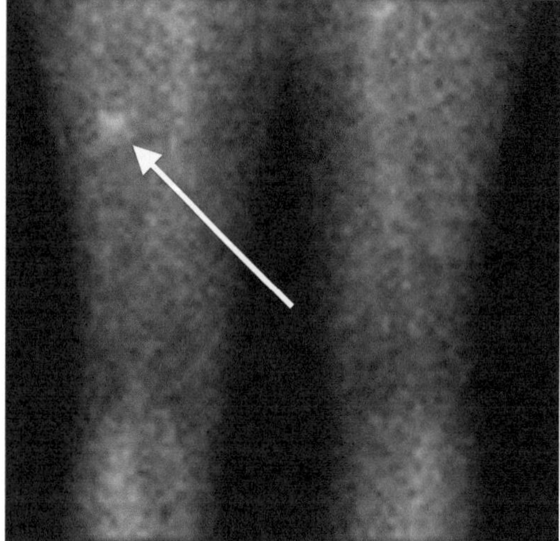

Fig. 7.9 Blood pool phase on bone scan. Increased radiotracer uptake is noted within the right mid-diaphysis

the distal femoral fragment. There is invariably varus angulation, which can help distinguish AFFs from other fracture etiologies.

X-ray evaluation of patients with hip, thigh, or groin pain on long-term bisphosphonates should include a frontal view of the pelvis and two views of the full length of each femur.

MRI

The MRI characteristics of an atypical femoral fracture are much like any other stress fracture, save for the lateral to medial transverse pattern, as described above. The earliest findings include high-signal periosteal reaction about the lateral cortex with normal marrow signal [33]. MRI is presumed to be the most sensitive modality prior to fracture [33]. Progression is marked by linear low T1 and high STIR or T2 signal within the marrow as the fracture extends medially. Conversely, non-progression or reversal of marrow signal changes on MRI may be a guide for therapeutic efficacy.

MRI may also be of particular benefit in patients with known atypical fracture as a screening technique for the contralateral leg. Risk of contralateral fracture appears to be between 22 and 64 %, and increasing attention is being devoted to prevention of these fractures [20, 21, 24].

A pelvis MRI without contrast protocolled for musculoskeletal purposes will evaluate both hips, the pubic symphysis and sacroiliac joints, and the musculature and tendons of both hips and thus can provide an explanation for pain other than atypical femur fracture. MRI of the entire length of both femora without contrast is also recommended as the next step, as cortical thickening can be subtle, and having the other side for comparison can improve the diagnostic capability of the scan. Furthermore, the marrow lesions can be far down the shaft of the femur, which would be missed if only the hips were imaged. By scanning both femora, asymptomatic lesions can be picked up on the opposite side. Both femora should be scanned simultaneously, thereby not resulting in any increased scanner time, patient discomfort, or cost. And since MRI does not result in any deleterious effects to human tissue, no collateral damage is incurred by scanning both femora. Contrast-enhanced MRI is not needed, as the findings are present on the non-contrast MRI scans.

Nuclear Medicine (DXA and Bone Scan)

Two studies under the domain of nuclear medicine have been found to be helpful: dual-energy X-ray absorptiometry (DXA) and bone scintigraphy (or more commonly referred to as a "bone scan"). DXA describes a technique in which X-rays of two different energy levels are used to acquire images of the lumbar spine and hips. The difference in through-transmission of X-rays through these bones can be used to calculate the density of the bones to a high degree of certainty. This is currently the gold standard in the clinical evaluation of bone density and is commonly performed annually to biennially in patients at risk for the development of osteoporosis. For obvious reasons, a large number of patients receiving bisphosphonates likely undergo regular DXA scans. The findings of Atypical femur fractures on DXA appear much like those on conventional radiography, with the exception being that DXA demonstrates a lower degree of spatial resolution. It should also be highlighted that conventional DXA studies include only 1–2 cm below the lesser trochanter. Given that AFFs typically occur within 5 cm of the lesser trochanter, conventional

DXA may miss a large percentage of developing lesions. Many advocate extending the length of the DXA scan in patients on bisphosphonates.

Bone scintigraphy, on the other hand, uses a radioisotope (most commonly technetium-99m-labeled methylene diphosphonate) that shows active bone turnover when imaged with a gamma camera. The basic principle is that labeled methylene diphosphonate (MDP) will attach to phosphate binding sites and radioactivity will accumulate in areas of high turnover. Devices called gamma cameras can then detect this radiation. A subset of bone scans, the "triple-phase" bone scans, are imaged at three times: in the first several moments to show perfusion; several minutes later to show "blood pooling," i.e., inflammation or autonomic dysfunction; and after several hours, at which point any tracer not bound to the bone should have been cleared by the patient's kidneys. It is during this third, "delayed," phase that stress fractures and AFFs are most easily identified. As the compound actively seeks out sites of bone turnover, bone scintigraphy can be highly sensitive for developing stress fractures; however, its specificity is extremely limited by a lack of spatial resolution. Atypical femur fractures appear as increased activity in the subtrochanteric region, again, with a predilection for the lateral cortex.

Differential Diagnosis

While AFFs demonstrate a specific and recognizable pattern, several other conditions may simulate this appearance. Stress fractures of the femur may occur in a subtrochanteric location; however, they most typically begin along the medial cortex and propagate laterally. Pathologic fractures related to underlying osseous lesions may simulate the cortical "beaking" that classically defines a developing bisphosphonate-related fracture. A sinus tract along a region of chronic osteomyelitis may appear similar to a fracture like, with adjacent osseous irregularity. Figures 7.11, 7.12, 7.13, 7.14, 7.15, 7.16, 7.17, 7.18, and 7.19 demonstrate several such mimics.

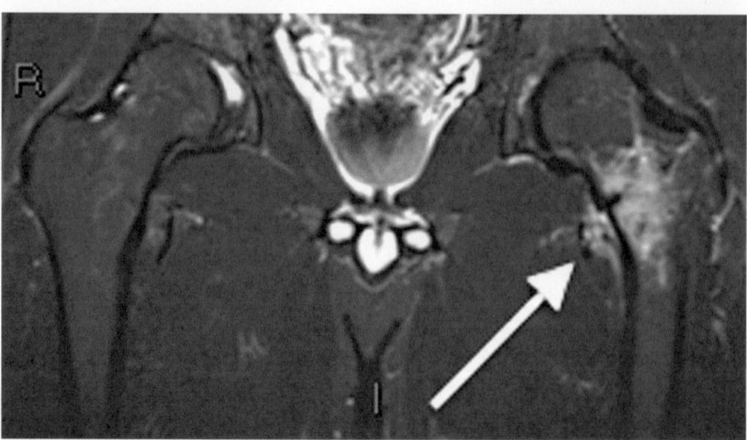

Fig. 7.11 Coronal STIR 1.5 T MRI of a 36-year-old shows a stress fracture of the left femoral neck. A dark fracture line is progressing from medial to lateral and is surrounded by extensive edema signal. Note the predilection for the medial cortex of the femoral neck in contrast to Atypical femur fractures, which begin on the lateral cortex of the subtrochanteric region

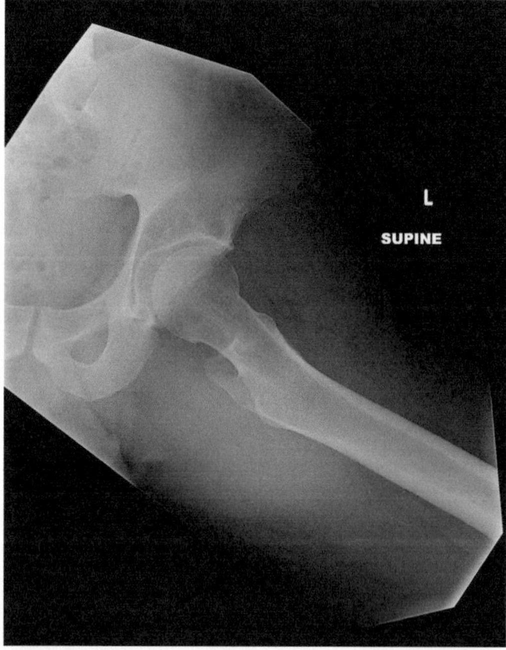

Fig. 7.12 Frog-leg lateral radiograph of the same patient in Fig 7.11. Slight medial cortical thickening with sclerotic, non-displaced fracture line oriented perpendicular to the trabecular lines of the femoral neck is characteristic of a stress fracture

Screening Considerations

A prodromal pain syndrome only exists in 50–76 % of patients who demonstrate incomplete or developing fractures [24]. Progression from the earliest findings to complete fracture typically takes between 2 and 6 months [34]. Lastly, quantitative risk stratification based on risk factors or by a general tool such as the fracture risk assessment tool (FRAX) has yet to be fully elaborated. This being said, there is a growing emphasis on finding the best screening test for early fractures. MRI may be an excellent choice for those with the classic prodrome of unrelenting groin pain. For those who are asymptomatic, however, other modalities may prove to be more cost-effective initial screens. One promising suggestion has been to increase the length of femur included in DXA scans, which most bisphosphonate patients undergo routinely [35]. It is unlikely, however, that the routine DXA scan interval is appropriate for the prevention of complete fractures. Nuclear scintigraphy is another possibility with areas of developing fracture appearing

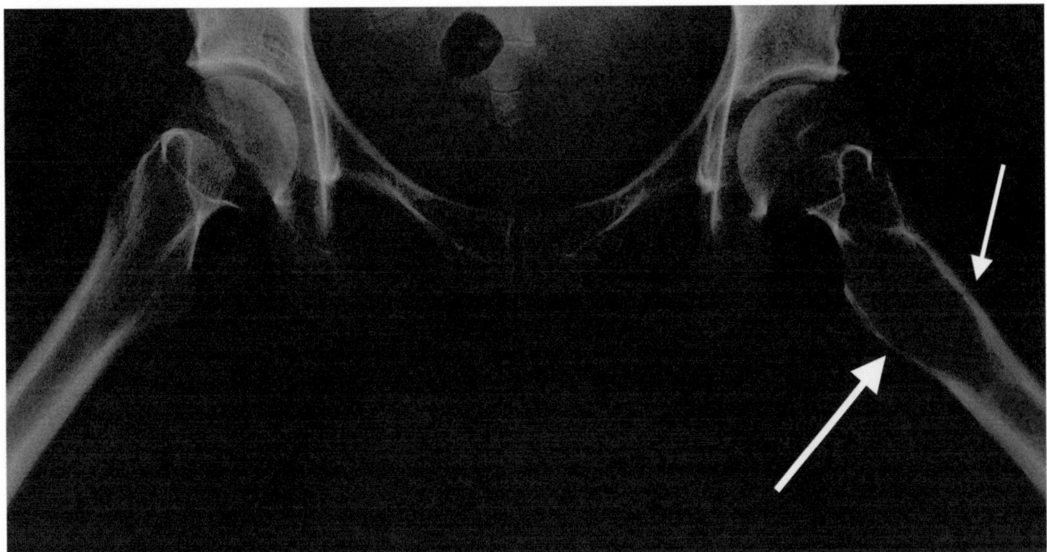

Fig. 7.13 AP radiograph of the hips in frog-leg position of a 38-year-old. There is a nearly transverse fracture line progressing from lateral to medial cortex of the left subtrochanteric femur through a lytic lesion in the intertro-chanteric and subtrochanteric femur. In this case, the etiology is a pathologic fracture through bone that has been weakened by fibrous dysplasia

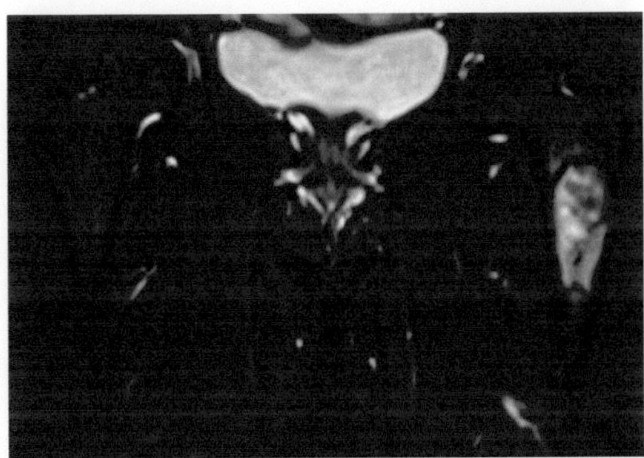

Fig. 7.14 Coronal STIR 1.5 T MRI of the same patient as in Fig 7.13 shows a region of increased signal that could mimic marrow edema on first glance. In contrast, this is well-marginated lesion with a narrow zone of transition, with a low signal sclerotic rim, representing fibrous dysplasia. While there is a beaking of the lateral cortex, the cortex is not thickened as one would see in a developing AFF

similar to a lateral cortical stress fracture. This, however, tends to be positive only in symptomatic patients and may prove to be too insensitive for screening [26]. At our institution, it has become common practice to include the most commonly involved part of the femur in all routine emergency department and outpatient pelvic X-rays as well as all DXA scans. Anecdotally, this has led to a sharp increase in the number of incidentally discovered early AFFs. Regardless of whether initial findings are discovered on conventional radiography or DXA, it is recommended that MRI or CT confirmation should be pursued [25].

Another area that has yet to be addressed is whether there is any benefit to whole-body or targeted non-femoral screening. Bisphosphonate-related low-impact fractures have also been described of the tibia and forearm [36, 37]. It remains uncertain whether these are simply too rare to warrant non-femoral screening in populations at higher risk, such as those using walkers for partial weight-bearing.

Follow-Up

The primary goals of imaging atypical fractures are primary and secondary prevention. Many now recommend imaging of the contralateral leg as soon as an AFF is identified [38, 39]. The recommended modalities are combined X-rays and MRI or DXA and MRI. Radionuclide scans are currently recommended against, given a lack of specificity.

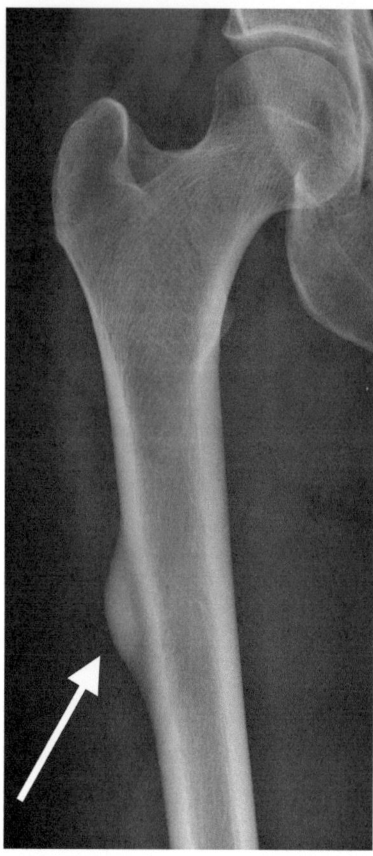

Fig. 7.15 Apparent lateral cortical thickening in a 41-year-old. This shows an underlying linear lucency and lacks the medial beaking seen in AFFs. This is an osteochondroma, with characteristic continuity of the cortex and medullary space

Fig. 7.16 AP radiograph of the distal femur and knee in a 45-year-old with thigh pain. Large expansile mass with osteoid matrix and cortical bone destruction suggest osteosarcoma, which was proven on biopsy

Summarization of Diagnosis and Management

While there have been relatively few randomized-controlled trials to definitively demonstrate the relative efficacy of different management algorithms, a task force assembled by the American Society for Bone and Mineral Research has proposed an algorithm based on the current available data [25]. Patients at risk for complete fracture will present in one of two ways: asymptomatically, with incidentally discovered fractures, or as part of a workup for vague hip or groin pain. If not already acquired, conventional radiographs should be part of the initial workup, with any concerning findings

followed by advanced imaging. X-rays should consist of a frontal view of the pelvis, which includes both hips, and bilateral femora. Strong evidence on what should be the next test in the workup of a patient with groin or hip pain with negative X-rays who are on long-term bisphosphonates is lacking, but based on its superior anatomic detail, MRI of the musculoskeletal pelvis and bilateral femora without contrast is recommended as the next test. MRI is the preferred advanced modality for its ability to delineate subtle marrow signal abnormality and to assess cortical abnormality [25]. CT is insensitive to early stress reaction and, given its radiation, is not recommended in the workup of atypical fracture. Nuclear bone scan is relatively sensitive to early change in

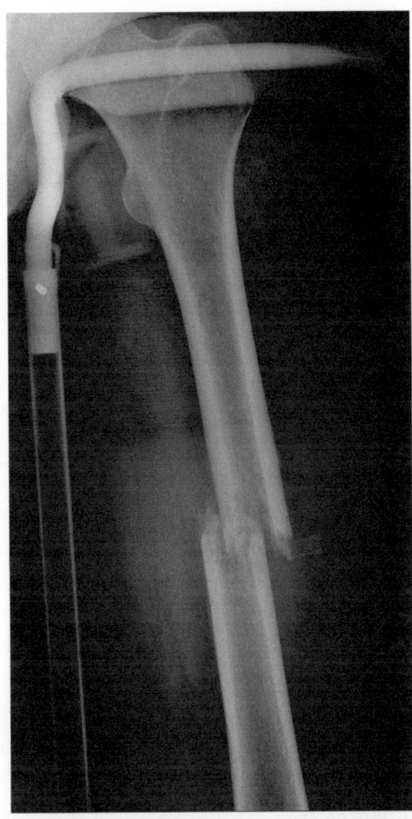

Fig. 7.17 Radiograph of the femur demonstrates a transverse subtrochanteric fracture in a previously asymptomatic 54-year-old patient. Faintly moth-eaten cortex and intramedullary cavity hints at the patient's underlying lymphoma which resulted in this pathologic fracture. Note that there is no cortical thickening and the jaggedness of the fracture line

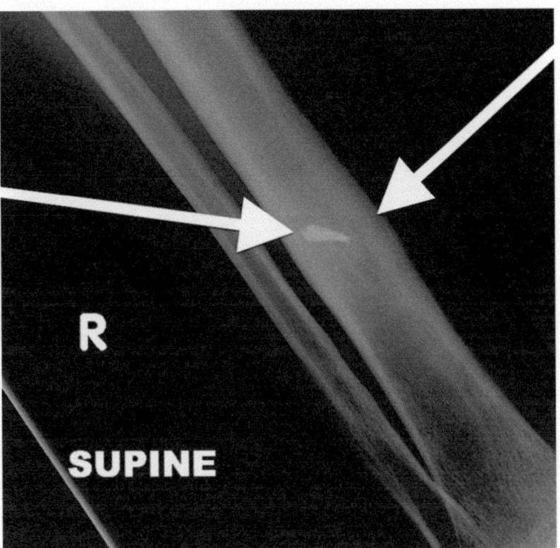

Fig. 7.18 Frontal radiograph of the right tibia demonstrates healed tibia fracture complicated by chronic osteomyelitis. Note the fusiform medial and lateral distal cortical thickening. Can mimic a developing AFF when it occurs in the femur. The presence of a retained drill bit indicates prior surgical intervention (white arrows). Also note a healed distal fibula fracture

symptomatic patients, but is nonspecific. Nuclear medicine bone scan is recommended if MRI is inconclusive, unavailable, or contraindicated. Triple-phase bone scan is unnecessary, as the stress reaction is found on the delayed phase. A whole-body delayed phase bone scan is recommended if X-ray and MRI are negative, as the whole-body bone scan may pick up other abnormal sites of disease other than both femora.

Following an initial workup, patients can be classified in one of three proposed prognostic categories: stress reaction/stress fracture without cortical lucency, incomplete cortical fracture, and complete cortical fracture. For those with painful, incomplete cortical fractures, intra-

medullary nail fixation is currently advised [25]. Asymptomatic patients with an incomplete cortical fracture, as well as those with stress reaction or fracture without cortical lucency, can be managed medically [25]. Recommendations for medical management involve suspending all anti-resorptive therapy and optimizing vitamin D and calcium. There is no definitive recommendation regarding additional medication, such as teriparatide, though this is sometimes considered in the treatment regimen. Painless incomplete cortical fractures should be on a strict regimen of non-weight-bearing, while those without cortical involvement (stress reaction and some stress fracture patients) are advised to limit weight-bearing and reduce high-impact activity [25]. All patients being treated conservatively should be followed with MRI or bone scans until there is no evidence of marrow signal change or increased metabolic activity [25]. The frequency of follow-up imaging remains uncertain; however, repeat MRI at 4–6 months is recommended. Early surgical fixation is controversial. Figures 7.20, 7.21, 7.22, 7.23, 7.24, 7.25, 7.26, 7.27, 7.28, and 7.29 demonstrate two severely osteoporotic patients who had suf-

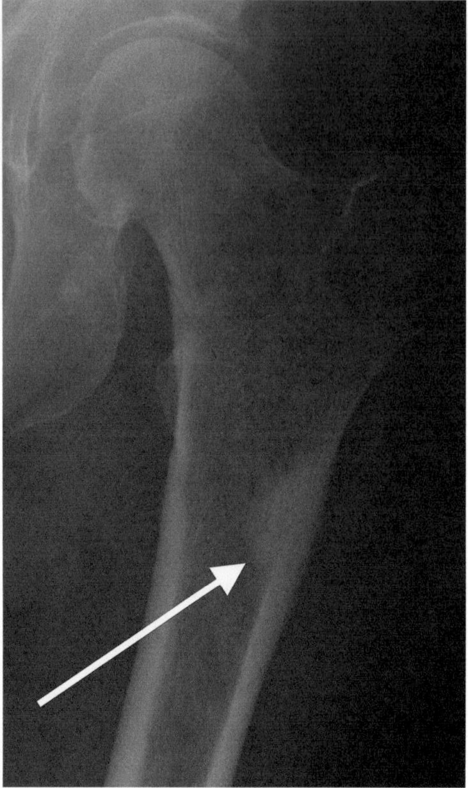

Fig. 7.19 Sclerotic non-ossifying fibroma masquerading as lateral cortical thickening. In contrast to the smooth contour of a developing AFF endosteal "beak," this lesion demonstrates a more acute shoulder at its interface with the cortex as well as an indistinct "brush border"

fered complete fractures and showed signals of multiple developing contralateral fractures. Both cases went on to prophylactic surgical fixation.

Conclusion

Bisphosphonates are a widespread class of medications used to decrease fractures of the hips and lumbar spine, with a primary goal of preventing morbidity. The medical community is increasingly aware that, while these medicines decrease the rate of both femoral and lumbar fractures, there has been an increase in the proportion of severely debilitating, low-impact subtrochanteric fractures. The goals of imaging are to effectively screen for these fractures during the 2–6 months in which they develop, to provide evidence of the efficacy of conservative therapy, to help decide when surgery would be warranted, and to screen for associated fractures that may develop. Debate about the best screening method is ongoing, but MRI appears to be the most sensitive modality; DXA provides a low-cost alternative; and X-rays show classic findings. Nuclear medicine techniques are less favored given a lack of specificity. Subtrochanteric fractures, as a class, are especially debilitating, and diagnostic imaging plays a strong role in preventing their progression.

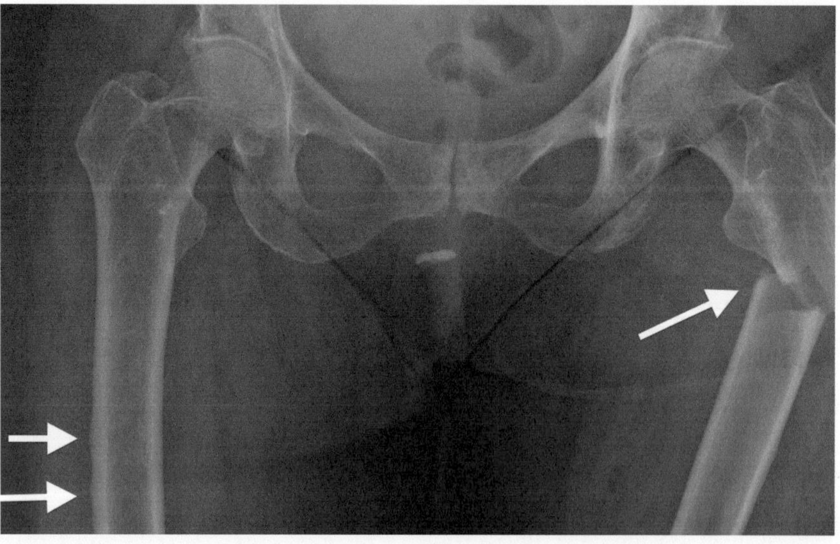

Fig. 7.20 This frontal pelvic radiograph shows a complete AFF of the proximal left femur. Two areas of lateral cortical beaking are also seen in the mid-diaphyseal right femoral cortex

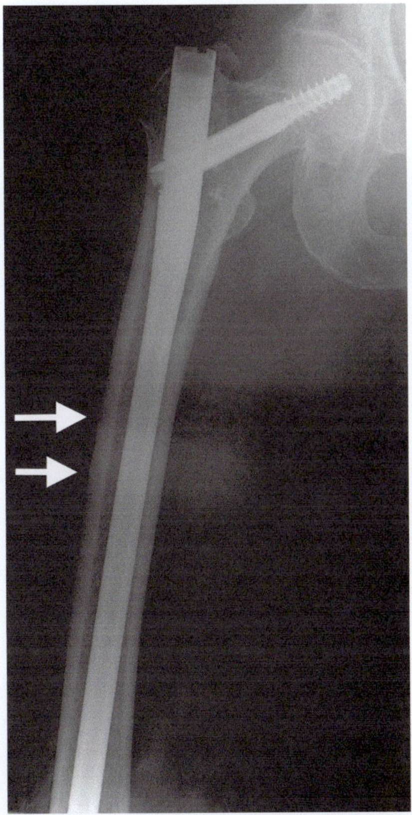

Fig. 7.21 Frontal radiograph of the right hip following prophylactic intramedullary nail fixation. Again seen are two areas of lateral cortical beaking

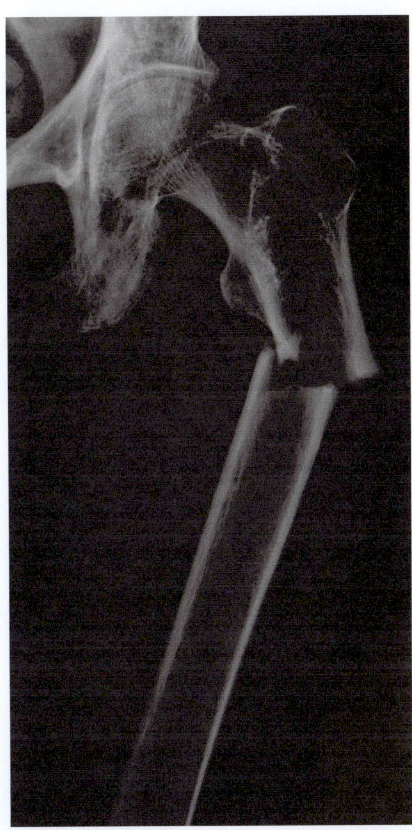

Fig. 7.22 Frontal radiograph of the same patient as in Fig 7.20 better demonstrates the complete fracture of the patient's left femur. Note the varus angulation of the distal fragment

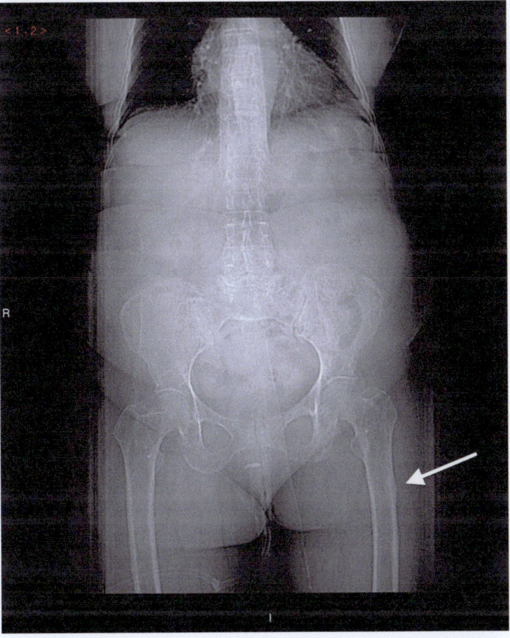

Fig. 7.23 Scout image from an abdominal-pelvic CT obtained of the same patient as in Fig 7.20 7 months prior for abdominal pain shows beaking of the left femoral cortex

Fig. 7.24 Transverse CT image from the same scan as in Fig 7.23 shows lateral cortical thickening of the left femur

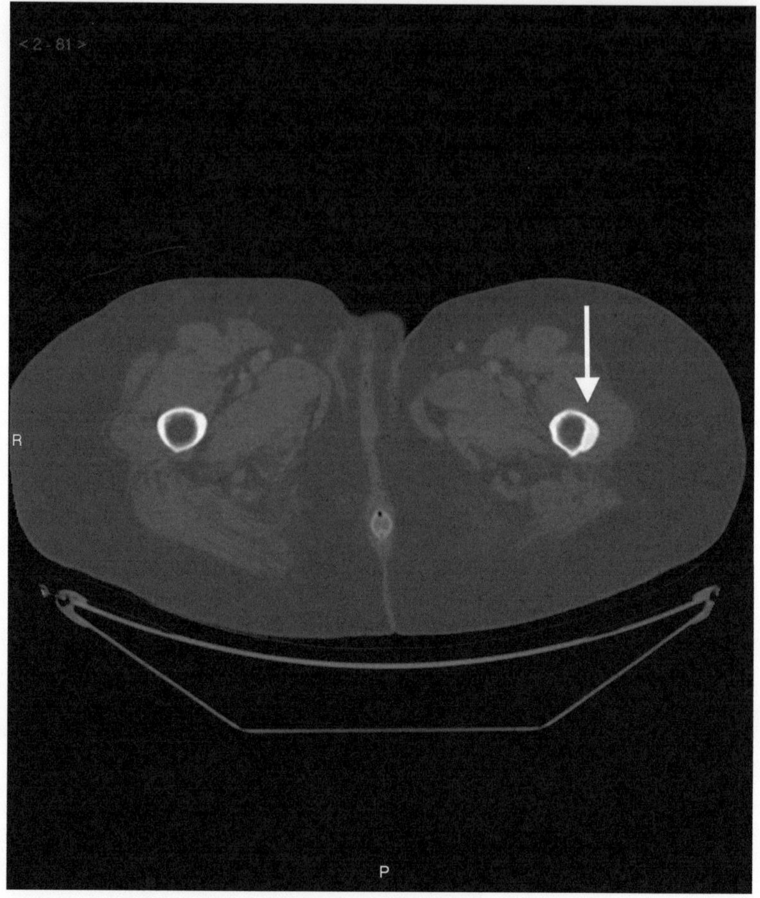

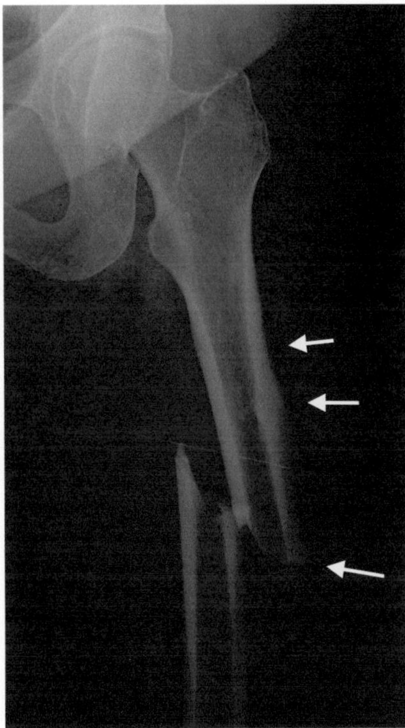

Fig. 7.25 AP radiograph of the left hip shows a complete AFF. Note the lateral cortical beaking and the presence of a developing AFF superior to the fracture. Note the varus angulation, another classic finding

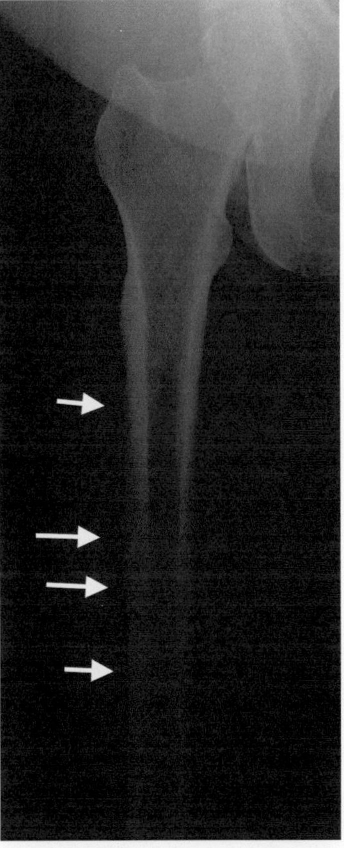

Fig. 7.26 X-ray of the contralateral femur was performed to rule out developing AFFs. Multiple areas of lateral cortical thickening are present

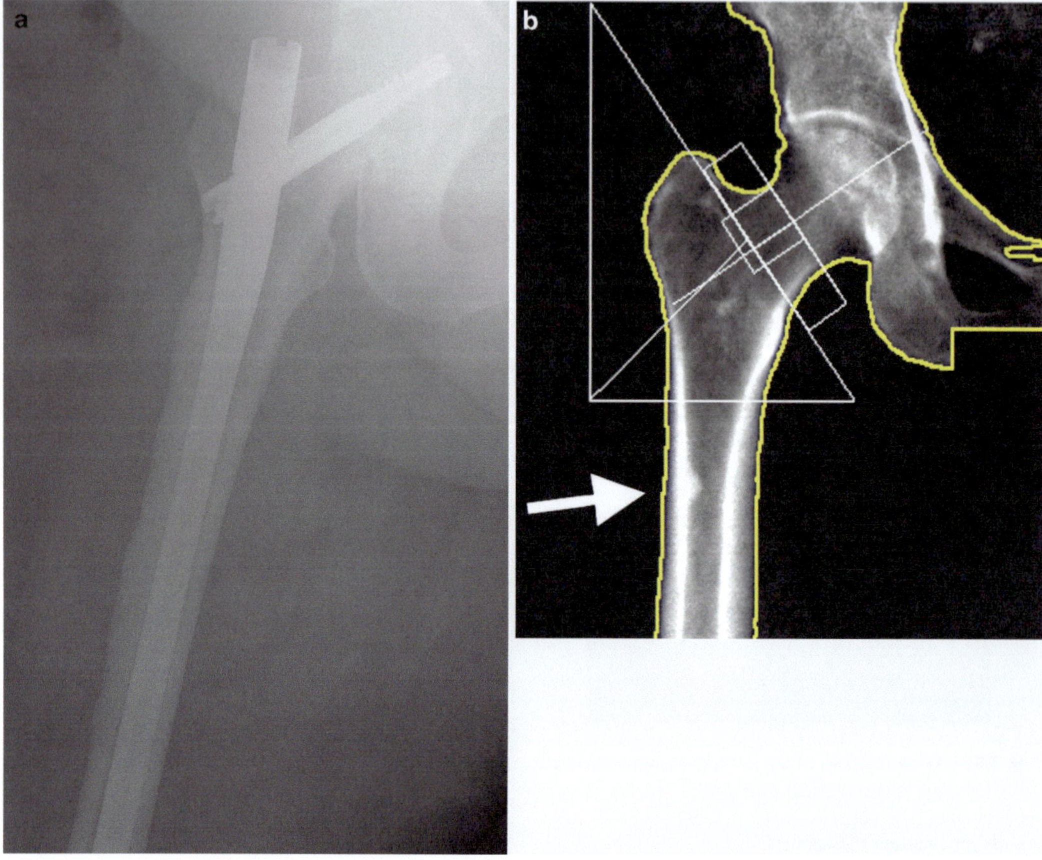

Fig. 7.27 (**a**) Radiograph after prophylactic femur fixation with a long intramedullary gamma nail (patient C). (**b**) Dual-energy X-ray absorptiometry (DXA) of a 59-year-old (patient D) on current bisphosphonate therapy. There is beaking of the medullary aspect of the lateral femoral cortex

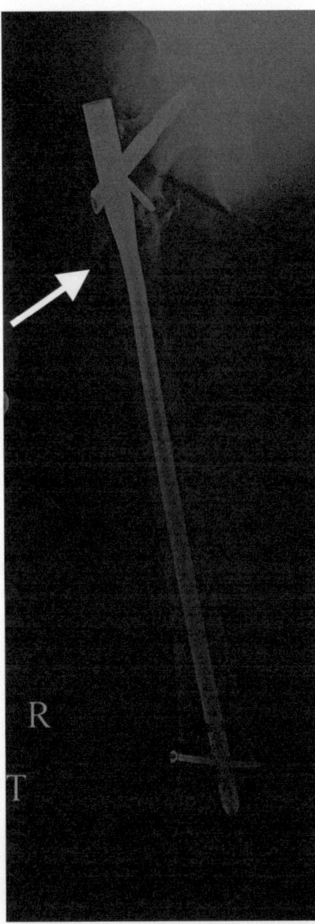

Fig. 7.28 Frontal radiograph of the right femur in a patient (patient E) who suffered a complete AFF 2-and-a-half years prior. The fracture shows nonunion despite conventional fixation with a long cephalomedullary nail. Note that subtle cortical buttressing (thickening) of the lateral and medial cortex is still present

Fig. 7.29 The same patient E, following removal of the cephalomedullary nail and revision fixation with a blade plate. There is now increased bridging osseous callus at the site of the fracture, demonstrating improved bone healing

References[1]

1. Jacobsen C, et al. The phosphorous necrosis of the jaws and what can we learn from the past: a comparison of "phossy" and "bisphossy" jaw. Oral Maxillofac Surg. 2014;18(1):31–7.
2. Marx RE. Uncovering the cause of "phossy jaw" Circa 1858 to 1906: oral and maxillofacial surgery closed case files-case closed. J Oral Maxillofac Surg. 2008;66(11):2356–63.
3. Ahn JK, et al. Non-traumatic fracture of the femoral shaft in a patient taking long-term bisphosphonate therapy. Rheumatol Int. 2011;31(7):973–5.
4. Visekruna M, Wilson D, McKiernan FE. Severely suppressed bone turnover and atypical skeletal fragility. J Clin Endocrinol Metab. 2008;93(8):2948–52.
5. Luckman SP, et al. JBMR anniversary classic. Nitrogen-containing bisphosphonates inhibit the mevalonate pathway and prevent post-translational prenylation of GTP-binding proteins, including Ras. Originally published in Volume 7, number 4, pp 581-9 (1998). J Bone Miner Res. 1998;20(7):1265–74.
6. Abrahamsen B, Eiken P, Eastell R. Subtrochanteric and diaphyseal femur fractures in patients treated with alendronate: a register-based national cohort study. J Bone Miner Res. 2009;24(6):1095–102.
7. Schilcher J, Aspenberg P. Incidence of stress fractures of the femoral shaft in women treated with bisphosphonate. Acta Orthop. 2009;80(4):413–5.
8. Meier RP, et al. Increasing occurrence of Atypical femur fractures associated with bisphosphonate use. Arch Intern Med. 2012;172(12):930–6.
9. Wang Z, Bhattacharyya T. Trends in incidence of subtrochanteric fragility fractures and bisphosphonate use among the US elderly, 1996-2007. J Bone Miner Res. 2011;26(3):553–60.

[1]*Important References

10. Hsiao FY, et al. Hip and subtrochanteric or diaphyseal femoral fractures in alendronate users: a 10-year, nationwide retrospective cohort study in Taiwanese women. Clin Ther. 2011;33(11):1659–67.

11. Feldstein AC, et al. Incidence and demography of femur fractures with and without atypical features. J Bone Miner Res. 2012;27(5):977–86.

12. Park-Wyllie LY, et al. Bisphosphonate use and the risk of subtrochanteric or femoral shaft fractures in. JAMA. 2011;305(8):783–9.

13. Abrahamsen B, Eiken P, Eastell R. Cumulative alendronate dose and the long-term absolute risk of subtrochanteric. J Clin Endocrinol Metab. 2010;95(12):5258–65.

14. Erviti J, et al. Oral bisphosphonates are associated with increased risk of subtrochanteric and diaphyseal fractures in elderly women: a nested case-control study. BMJ Open. 2013;3(1):e002091.

15. Isaacs JD, et al. Femoral insufficiency fractures associated with prolonged bisphosphonate therapy. Clin Orthop Relat Res. 2010;468(12):3384–92.

16. Neviaser AS, et al. Low-energy femoral shaft fractures associated with alendronate use. J Orthop Trauma. 2008;22(5):346–50.

17. Gedmintas L, Solomon DH, Kim SC. Bisphosphonates and risk of subtrochanteric, femoral shaft, and atypical femur fracture: a systematic review and meta-analysis. J Bone Miner Res. 2013;28(8):1729–37.

18. Abrahamsen B. Adverse effects of bisphosphonates. Calcif Tissue Int. 2010;86(6):421–35.

19. Girgis CM, Sher D, Seibel MJ. Atypical femur fractures and bisphosphonate use. N Engl J Med. 2010;362(19):1848–9.

20. Lo JC, et al. Clinical correlates of atypical femoral fracture. Bone. 2012;51(1):181–4.

21. Dell RM, et al. Incidence of atypical nontraumatic diaphyseal fractures of the femur. J Bone Miner Res. 2012;27(12):2544–50.

22. Jamal SA, Dion N, Ste-Marie LG. Atypical femur fractures and bone turnover. N Engl J Med. 2011;365(13):1261–2.

23. Weinstein RS, Roberson PK, Manolagas SC. Giant osteoclast formation and long-term oral bisphosphonate therapy. N Engl J Med. 2009;360(1):53–62.

24. Kwek EB, Koh JS, Howe TS. More on atypical fractures of the femoral diaphysis. N Engl J Med. 2008;359(3):316–7. Author reply 317–8.

25. Shane E, et al. Atypical subtrochanteric and diaphyseal femoral fractures: second report of a task force of the American Society for Bone and Mineral Research. J Bone Miner Res. 2014;29(1):1–23.

26. Chan SS, et al. Subtrochanteric femoral fractures in patients receiving long-term alendronate therapy: imaging features. AJR Am J Roentgenol. 2010;194(6):1581–6.

27. Cheung RK, et al. Sequential non-traumatic femoral shaft fractures in a patient on long-term. Hong Kong Med J. 2007;13(6):485–9.

28. *Mohan PC, et al. Radiographic features of multifocal endosteal thickening of the femur in patients. Eur Radiol. 2013;23(1):222–7. *A case series showing the multifocal nature of bisphosphonate-related injury.

29. Probst S, Rakheja R, Stern J. Atypical bisphosphonate-associated subtrochanteric and femoral shaft stress. Clin Nucl Med. 2013;38(5):397–9.

30. Schilcher J, et al. Atypical femur fractures are a separate entity, characterized by highly specific radiographic features. A comparison of 59 cases and 218 controls. Bone. 2013;52(1):389–92.

31. Deutsch AL, Coel MN, Mink JH. Imaging of stress injuries to bone. Radiography, scintigraphy, and MR imaging. Clin Sports Med. 1997;16(2):275–90.

32. Spitz DJ, Newberg AH. Imaging of stress fractures in the athlete. Radiol Clin North Am. 2002;40(2):313–31.

33. Haworth AE, Webb J. Skeletal complications of bisphosphonate use: what the radiologist should know. Br J Radiol. 2012;85(1018):1333–42.

34. Goh SK, et al. Subtrochanteric insufficiency fractures in patients on alendronate therapy: a caution. J Bone Joint Surg Br. 2007;89(3):349–53.

35. Ahlman MA, Rissing MS, Gordon L. Evolution of bisphosphonate-related atypical fracture retrospectively observed with DXA scanning. J Bone Miner Res. 2012;27(2):496–8.

36. Bissonnette L, et al. Atypical fracture of the tibial diaphysis associated with bisphosphonate therapy: a case report. Bone. 2013;56(2):406–9.

37. Moon J, Bither N, Lee T. Atypical forearm fractures associated with long-term use of bisphosphonate. Arch Orthop Trauma Surg. 2013;133(7):889–92.

38. Das De S, Setiobudi T, Shen L. A rational approach to management of alendronate-related subtrochanteric fractures. J Bone Joint Surg Br. 2010;92(5):679–86.

39. Hsu JH, et al. Bisphosphonate-related atypical femoral fracture. Kaohsiung J Med Sci. 2013;29(6):345–6.

Factors Contributing to Atypical Femoral Fractures

8

Adele L. Boskey and
Marjolein C.H. van der Meulen

List of Abbreviations

AFF	Atypical femoral fracture
ASBMR	American Society for Bone and Mineral Research
BMI	Body mass index
BMU	Basic multicellular unit
BP	Bisphosphonate
GC	Glucocorticoid
PTH	Parathyroid hormone
RPI	Reference point indentation

Summary

- Atypical fractures are stress fracture-like breaks that occur during normal activity at unusual, i.e., atypical sites, in the bone; the most common site is the femur.
- The incidence of AFFs is very low compared to the number of osteoporotic fractures prevented by bisphosphonates and other antiresorptive therapies.
- Common characteristics of these fractures include a beak-like appearance on the lateral cortex, thickened cortices, and bilateral occurrence; they often are preceded by prodermal pain.
- Atypical femoral fractures (AFFs) occur most frequently in patients given antiresorptive drugs, including bisphosphonates.
- Several features of AFFs suggest that these failures result from repetitive loading.
- These rare occurrences do not have a well-defined etiology, but likely contributing factors include use of bisphosphonates and other antiresorptives, variations in skeletal morphology, and the presence of metabolic disorders.
- Antiresorptive agents can affect bone material properties by retarding turnover, increasing bone mineral content, reducing bone tissue heterogeneity, increasing collagen cross-linking, increasing microdamage, and decreasing toughness.
- Changes in lower limb skeletal geometry, such as femoral neck-shaft angle and femoral curvature, alter the stresses and strains experienced in the femoral diaphysis with loading.
- Patients with complete or partial AFFs are generally treated by surgical intervention, withdrawal of bisphosphonate treatment, and either a "drug" holiday or treatment with an anabolic agent.

A.L. Boskey, PhD (✉)
Mineralized Tissue Research, Musculoskeletal
Integrity Program, Hospital for Special Surgery,
535 E. 70th St., New York, NY 10021, USA
e-mail: boskeya@hss.edu

M.C.H. van der Meulen, PhD
Biomedical Engineering and Mechanical &
Aerospace Engineering, Cornell University,
Ithaca, NY, USA

© Springer International Publishing Switzerland 2016
S.L. Silverman, B. Abrahamsen (eds.), *The Duration and Safety
of Osteoporosis Treatment*, DOI 10.1007/978-3-319-23639-1_8

Atypical Femoral Fractures: Definition

Atypical femoral fractures (AFFs) and perhaps, by analogy, "atypical" fractures in other long bones that match the case description (see below) for AFFs [1, 2], are stress fracture-like breaks that occur during normal activity at unusual, i.e., atypical, sites in the bone. A task force of the American Society for Bone and Mineral Research (ASBMR) defined AFFs as "atraumatic or low-trauma fractures located in the subtrochanteric region or femoral shaft" [3]. Radiographically, these fractures are characterized by a "beaking" appearance on the lateral cortex with cortical thickening and a medial spike in the fracture (Fig. 8.1) (see also Chap. 12). A transverse fracture line is present at the point of origin in the lateral cortex. Focal or diffuse periosteal, and sometimes endosteal, reactions of the lateral cortex may surround the origin of the fracture. Patients with AFFs often complained of "prodermal" pain before the fracture(s) were noted, and fractures often occur bilaterally. AFFs occur most frequently in patients given antiresorptive drugs, including bisphosphonates, which were associated with the first case reports [4–6]. To date, one case has been reported with denosumab [7]. The ASBMR Task Force initial report provided the case definition of "atypical femoral fractures" [3]. The second ASBMR report refined the initial definition [8].

The incidence of AFFs is very low [8], especially when compared to the number of osteoporotic fractures prevented by bisphosphonates and other antiresorptive therapies [9, 10]. The relative risk (or odds ratio) of AFFs is more variable and has been reported as ranging from 2 to 47 [11]. Factors contributing to the variability of the relative risk are important to consider: does the variability just reflect regional variation, specifically the relative length of time patients in different geographic areas have been on antiresorptive drugs or, as recently suggested [12], variations in the authors' definitions of an atypical fracture? Since the calculation of relative risk depends on the types of patients in the case and control groups, the latter is likely the case. In a letter to the editor of *Journal of Bone and Mineral Research* that was published in *Acta Orthopaedica* [12] explaining the variation in observed AFF rate in different studies, the authors of the letter

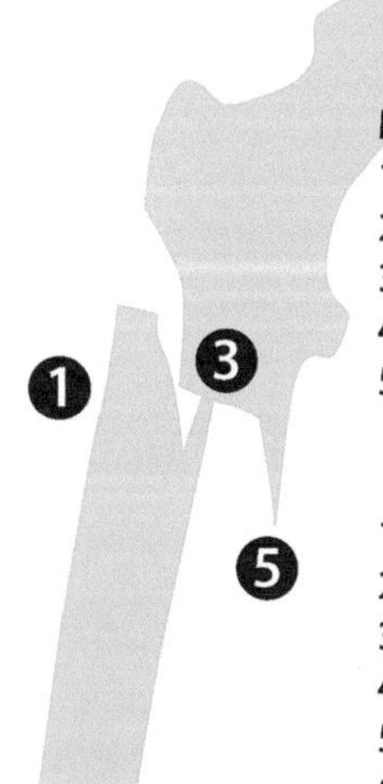

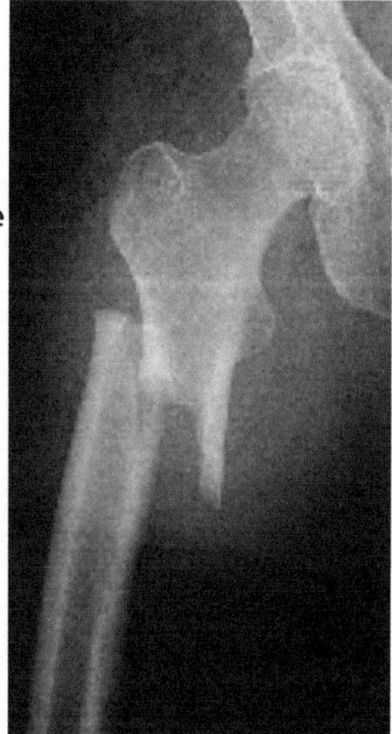

Fig. 8.1 ASBMR-established AFF criteria and schematic with radiograph illustrating the major features of AFFs

pointed out that the "fatigue-type" fracture noted in elderly populations and associated with material failure was referred to as atypical whether or not the fracture occurred in the femoral shaft or in the subtrochanteric region. Hence, AFFs reported in some studies did not meet the ASBMR definition. Factors contributing to the discrepancy in odds ratio could include the absence of radiographic data, a broad definition of shaft fractures, and the absence of a fracture line perpendicular to the cortex [13].

Conditions and Treatments Associated with AFFs

Independent of the relative risk of AFF, the majority of existing studies that based their evaluation of AFFs on the ASBMR criteria found an association between duration of use of bisphosphonates and incidence of AFF [8, 14–16], with incidence increasing with prolonged use of antiresorptive drugs. Association of bisphosphonates with AFF, however, remains debatable as AFFs continue to be reported in bisphosphonate-free patients [17]. Large population-based studies of older women, with validated fracture codes, support the association of long-term bisphosphonate (BP) use and AFFs [18]. In contrast, based on propensity data, AFFs were equally common to people using bisphosphonates and to those using raloxifene (a selective estrogen receptor modulator) or calcitonin [19]. Notably, reports of subtrochanteric (atypical) fractures began after the introduction of bisphosphonates [20]. This observation, and the radiographic findings indicating the association of AFF with long-term (>5 years) bisphosphonate use [21, 22], lends support to the association between AFFs and antiresorptive drugs, but the data to date have not been conclusive. Readers are again reminded that today, bisphosphonates and other antiresorptive drugs have been remarkably effective in reducing osteoporotic fracture incidence [3, 8–10].

The question to be addressed in this review is why the use of antiresorptive medication results in AFFs. Although this fracture is a rare occurrence, the etiology is important. Possible answers to the association between bisphosphonate treatment and AFF include (1) patients who get AFFs did not need bisphosphonates or related drugs but were treated, resulting in a situation in which bone remodeling is oversuppressed; (2) oversuppression alters the material properties of bone to such an extent that the tissue becomes more brittle; (3) alterations in bone morphology increase the stresses on the femur and put specific sets of patients at risk; and (4) the patients were receiving other medications, such as glucocorticoids (GC), that also affect the bone tissue properties, and the combined treatment is adverse. Each of these possibilities is supported by existing data as discussed below, and finally, some component of each of these factors likely contributes to the development of AFFs. One key issue in looking at both etiology and mechanism is the variability in the profiles of the small number of AFF patients.

Serum and Other Noninvasive Clinical Markers of AFFs

Serum or other noninvasive clinical markers would be desirable to detect early signs of AFFs or to recognize individuals at risk for AFFs who should not be treated with antiresorptive drugs associated with AFFs. To date, unfortunately, no definitive associations have been identified between AFF and serum markers. However, through these studies, other metabolic contributors to AFFs have been identified (see section "Contribution of Metabolic Disease to Development of AFF") [23, 24].

Histological Markers of AFF

Studies examining bone tissue next to the fracture site generally found decreased bone formation but normal bone remodeling and no evidence of a mineralization defect in patients with AFFs. Because these tissues were collected at variable times after the fracture occurred and did not always include double labeling to measure bone formation rate, the meaning of the overall histomorphometric data is difficult to interpret.

The presence of a fracture callus and radiolucency on the lateral cortex where these fractures initiate suggests that bone tissue is still actively formed and resorbed. However, a limited number of case reports of AFFs show no or very few double labels indicating that mineralization is not occurring [25].

Are AFFs "Stress" Fractures Rather than "Insufficiency" Fractures?

Insufficiency fracture

Insufficiency fracture is a fracture that occurs at a load that would normally not cause failure, because the mechanical strength of the bone is compromised. The same load applied to the skeleton of a healthy individual would not result in a fracture.

Stress fractures are fractures which occur as a result of repetitive loading at subfailure loads in the skeleton of a healthy individual.

Several features of AFFs suggest that these failures result from repetitive loading (fatigue-type fractures). AFFs occur with minimal or low loads. Fracture occurs when the applied loads exceed the load-bearing capacity of a structure such as a long bone. This process can result either due to a single high overload (traumatic failure) or as a result of repeated subfailure loads (fatigue failure). Fatigue failure results from cyclic loading over time at loads that are below the single fracture load, which appears to correspond to the AFF mechanism. Repetitive loading in fatigue initiates damage in the form of cracks or microcracks, damage accumulates with continued loading until these cracks propagate and coalesce to produce catastrophic structural failure. This process of damage development and propagation depends on cortical geometry and tissue mechanical properties. Therefore, AFFs likely result from a fatigue-based mechanism.

A further indication that AFFs are stress fractures is the presence of a localized periosteal response and the prodromal symptoms. The periosteal response includes not only a general thickening of the cortex but also the "beaking" seen on the lateral cortex and is often accompanied by a radiolucent line that is presumably a localized healing or remodeling response. Similar local tissue responses are present in stress fractures induced through strenuous athletic activity. The cortices of bones of patients with AFFs appear thicker, but whether this reflects bisphosphonate treatment or AFF development or a combination of the two is not known.

If AFFs are indeed stress fractures, then two bone tissue properties are critical to characterizing the tissue-level changes: fatigue behavior for understanding the performance under repetitive, non-failure loading, and fracture toughness for understanding crack propagation. While these properties have been reported for healthy human cortical bone tissue, our knowledge of the effects with bisphosphonate treatment and remodeling suppression is limited.

Factors Contributing to AFFs

As mentioned above, a variety of causes may contribute to the development of AFFs. Conceptually, these factors that may underlie AFF can be considered in three broad categories. First, the use of antiresorptive drugs, particularly bisphosphonates, can lead to oversuppression of remodeling and result in alterations in bone material properties that adversely affect the mechanical behavior of the femur and the properties of cortical bone tissue (Fig. 8.2). Alterations in cancellous bone with bisphosphonate treatment that contribute to reductions in typical osteoporotic fractures will not be addressed here. Second, individual variations in skeletal morphology could contribute to the presence of high stresses in femoral cortex, a location that bears high loads and normally does not fracture. Finally, as introduced above, the presence of underlying metabolic disease likely also contributes. Here, we

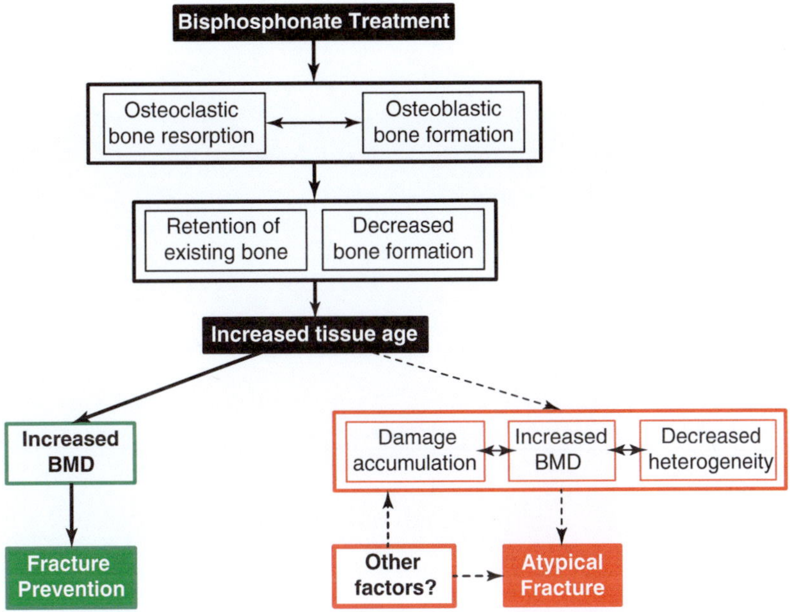

Fig. 8.2 Illustration of the possible actions of bisphosphonates leading to either reduced typical fracture rates (primary pathway leading to *green box*) or to altered material properties in patients with AFFs (secondary pathway leading to *red box*). Bisphosphonate treatment inhibits the activity of osteoclasts, disrupts the coupling between osteoblasts and osteoclasts, and, to a lesser extent, inhibits osteoblastic action

review the data supporting each of these mechanisms and the impact on the ability of the femur to bear functional loads.

BP-Induced Remodeling Suppression Leads to Adverse Tissue Material Changes

Bisphosphonates are administered to reduce bone turnover in individuals with osteoporosis. Therefore, impaired bone turnover is a likely suspect as a cause underlying AFFs. However, the histological evidence is limited and mixed, based on double labeling of tissue to indicated active bone remodeling. AFF patients given dual tetracycline labels prior to biopsy have been reported to show only single or no labels [25, 26], while well-defined double labels have been reported in a patient on long-term bisphosphonate treatment (>9 years) [27]. Thus, oversuppression of bone remodeling may not be the sole cause of AFFs. This suppression of bone turnover may contribute to multiple material changes including increased bone mineral content of the tissue, reduced tissue heterogeneity, and increased microdamage formation (Fig. 8.3). These individual material changes can combine to lead to brittle failure of the tissue and whole bone.

Increased Bone Mineral Content

Increased bone mineral content of bone tissue is a positive outcome of reduced turnover rates and the primary reason osteoporotic individuals are treated with bisphosphonates. However, this positive effect has limitations that may contribute to AFF development in the small cohort of individuals who develop these fractures. In particular, this increase in mineral content is accompanied by an increase in the mean age of the tissue. The absence of remodeling produces not only a greater volume of mineralized tissue but also a reduced volume of newer younger tissue, resulting a more homogeneous tissue with an increased degree of mineralization.

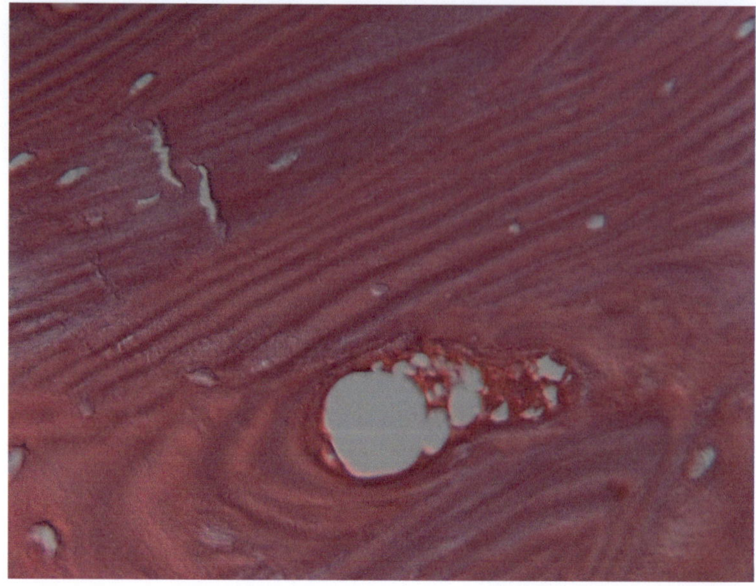

Fig. 8.3 Photomicrograph showing multiple cracks in a hematoxylin- and eosin-stained biopsy of a female patient with osteoporosis treated for 6 years with alendronate who sustained an atypical femoral fracture. Courtesy of Dr. M. Klein, Department of Pathology, HSS

Reduced Tissue Heterogeneity

BP treatment has multiple effects on tissue composition and ultimately results in a more homogenous tissue without the heterogeneity in composition that is normally a hallmark of bone tissue. Changes in bone composition have also been reported both in short-term iliac crest biopsies from alendronate-treated women [28], iliac crest biopsies from individuals with AFF on bisphosphonates [25], and in biopsies obtained adjacent to the fracture site in bisphosphonate-treated women [25, 29]. Compositional variability was reduced in biopsies from individuals with AFFs [25, 29]. When mineral composition was examined as a function of typical or atypical fracture morphology in patients on bisphosphonates, the compositional properties of tissue from patients with AFFs ($n=6$) fell within the range of values from patients with typical fractures ($n=14$), except the mean cortical degree of mineralization was 8 % greater in AFF tissue (atypical 5.6±0.3 versus typical 5.2±0.5) than in bisphosphonate-treated patients with typical osteoporotic fractures [29]. Biopsies were also included from bisphosphonate-naïve individuals with fragility fractures, none of whom experienced AFFs. Although the mean values of most compositional properties

were similar in both fracture groups, the tissue in bisphosphonate-treated patients had a more uniform composition than that of bisphosphonate-naïve patients with typical fractures. A study of iliac crest biopsies from AFF and control patients focused on trabecular tissue and examined similar compositional outcome measures [25]. While AFFs were not only present with bisphosphonate treatment, the biopsies were obtained from four patients on long-term bisphosphonate therapy. Trabecular tissue from the iliac crest of individuals with AFF had increased degree of mineralization, increased collagen maturity, and decreased mineralization heterogeneity. These compositional and morphological features could explain the higher incidence of fracture in these patients. Similar decreases in bone material heterogeneity were reported with treatment by different bisphosphonates including alendronate [28–32], risedronate [33], and zoledronic acid [34]. Oversuppression of remodeling by long-term treatment with bisphosphonates allows the proliferation of microcracks that weaken the bone tissue. Thus, loss of heterogeneity may reflect suppressed bone remodeling and inability to repair microcracks while also resulting in less resistance to crack formation and propagation.

Increased Collagen Cross-Linking

A further material change with bisphosphonate treatment is increased nonenzymatic collagen cross-links [28, 29]. At the tissue level, reductions in post-yield toughness were associated with increased nonenzymatic collagen glycation in cortical tissue of the tibia from dogs treated with high doses of alendronate, but not when clinically equivalent doses were administered [35]. While limited data exist for the composition of bone in individuals with AFF, changes in the collagen maturity, a measure of the ratio of non-reducible to reducible collagen cross-links, were reported in both cortical and cancellous tissue [25, 29] and suggest that they may arise from prolonged bisphosphonate treatment.

Increased Microdamage Formation

Suppression of remodeling by bisphosphonates increases microdamage in cortical bone tissue. Bone microdamage increases due to diminished repair [36–39] and increased crack burden, possibly due to a less heterogeneous tissue, leading to failure at lower energy and in a more "brittle" mode. Reduced post-yield toughness of bone tissue was associated with increased crack lengths and density in dogs treated with high doses of either alendronate or risedronate [40, 41]; however, increased microdamage was not present in animals treated with etidronate [42]. As described above, remodeling suppression reduces or eliminates "normal" bone tissue microstructural heterogeneity that results from having osteons and cement lines of different ages. In healthy tissue, the local differences in material properties produced by microstructural features are essential in dissipating energy and blunting crack propagation. Loss of these natural interfaces and crack-blunting processes can result in brittle-mode-type fractures [36, 37, 42, 43]. In addition, the lack of remodeling limits the repair of this damage.

Both brittleness and loss of heterogeneity allow greater progression of microscopic cracks (Fig. 8.2) that can occur with usual physical activity. Material heterogeneity is a mechanism that normally dissipates crack tip growth energy, thereby limiting crack growth. In a more homogeneous tissue, the energy to grow a crack is reduced and crack progression is less impeded. Targeted repair of cracks by newly activated BMUs appears to be preferentially suppressed by BPs [38]. In classical fracture mechanics, loss of material heterogeneity is associated with increased crack initiation and less resistance to crack propagation, leading to a greater risk of fracture [44, 45]. In cortical bone, transverse cracks are normally deflected longitudinally, limiting the effects of damage when the tissue is loaded. The remarkable straight transverse fracture line seen with AFF is an indicator of the dramatically altered tissue material properties and the failure of usual mechanisms to bridge or deflect the crack.

Decreased Toughness of Cortical Bone

In cortical bone, the functional outcome of these multiple effects of BP treatment can be to alter the mechanical behavior of bulk samples as in the case of AFF, presumably reflecting the combined effects of the increased bone mineral content, reduced heterogeneity, and increased microdamage associated with suppressed bone turnover. In general, bone material strength and stiffness were not altered in cortical bone, but post-yield toughness decreased at high doses [40, 46]. Preclinical studies examining bone properties primarily have been performed in estrogen-replete dog models using supraphysiological BP doses [37]. The majority of these studies have examined alendronate treatment, but these changes are also reported with risedronate and etidronate. The reduced post-yield deformation likely reflects increased damage formation, contributing to the brittle failure evident in AFF. Excessively reduced post-yield toughness produces brittle behavior, which is defined as the absence of post-yield deformation.

Nanomechanical Behavior

When the mechanical behavior is examined in small volumes of cortical bone tissue, the elastic behavior has been reported to be both reduced and unaffected. The reported differences may reflect levels of scale. Reference point indentation (RPI) has previously shown differences in the in vivo bone microindentation properties at the anterior tibial cortex of patients with hip fractures compared to age-matched controls [47]. Using RPI, no differences were present among typical and atypical fracture cases at the mid-tibia for microindentation properties nor were these cases different from patients on long-term bisphosphonate treatment, whose values were intermediate between controls and those who sustained fractures [48]. The similarity of properties among fracture cases suggests that the alterations in tissue-level material properties in individuals with AFF are similar to those of individuals who sustain osteoporotic fractures. Micromechanical properties were reduced in patients using alendronate for 6–10 years, corresponding with decreased mineral crystallinity, elastic modulus, and contact microhardness [49]. Tissue from patients with AFF was not examined. These relatively larger sampled volumes may include damage and other effects, but these effects would also be present with RPI, so in vivo measurement may be a critical difference. Nanomechanical analysis of iliac crest biopsies of individuals with severely suppressed bone turnover and atypical fractures (SSBT) showed no differences in cortical modulus or hardness of cortical tissue from AFF patients relative to age-matched and young female controls and osteoporotic individuals who had experienced vertebral fractures [50]. Plastic deformation resistance was greater in tissue from individuals with SSBT. Nanomechanical differences were present in their cancellous tissue. Tissue-level heterogeneity of the elastic modulus and plastic deformation resistance was reduced in the cortical bone of the biopsies from patients with suppressed bone turnover. While hardness and plastic deformation resistance are inelastic measures, their relationship to the tissue-level toughness has not been established.

Finally, if AFFs are due to impaired remodeling and associated mechanisms, as described, a similar fracture pattern might be expected in individuals with pycnodysostosis, a rare disorder with mutations in cathepsin K, the enzyme that digests the organic matrix of bone during the remodeling process [51]. In fact, AFFs have been reported in some patients with pycnodysostosis [52]. However, AFFs have not been reported in other cases of pycnodysostosis or in patients with other defects in remodeling, such as osteopetrosis.

Lower Limb Morphology Alters Stresses in the Femur

The frequent bilateral incidence of AFF suggests a mechanical etiology associated with individual anatomy, in addition to any remodeling-induced changes. Changes in lower limb skeletal geometry, such as femoral neck-shaft angle and femoral curvature [53], will alter the stresses and strains experienced in the femoral diaphysis with loading. Skeletal structure and kinematics have been correlated with the risk of stress fracture in young active individuals [54–56]. The incidence of typical osteoporotic hip fractures is lower in Asian women [57], yet the incidence of AFF is higher [22, 58]. Femoral geometry differs between Asian and Caucasian women, including shorter hip axis lengths and smaller femoral neck-shaft angles in Asian women [59]. If such geometric variations contribute to typical fracture rate differences, similar factors may also explain AFF incidence rates. The exact contribution of lower limb skeletal morphology to AFFs is yet to be determined, but the evidence shows morphology is likely a contributing factor [60].

Contribution of Metabolic Disease to Development of AFF

In addition to osteoporosis, other metabolic abnormalities may be present in AFF patients. Comorbidities of AFFs such as bisphosphonate therapy, use of GCs, and other complications likely contribute to the alterations in tissue properties that result in AFFs. In a review of 31 published cases and one unpublished case, proton pump inhibitor and GC use were found in a majority of the AFF patients [24]. Moreover, ~76 % of the AFF patients had at least one major chronic disorder. AFFs occurred in patients with hypophosphatemia, indicating that some underlying disorder in metabolic status was a contributing factor to AFFs. A recent study using ASBMR criteria to identify AFFs examined serum markers in an Italian population comparing women with AFF ($n=11$) to women with typical fractures ($n=58$) admitted to a single hospital over a period of 3 years [23]. Younger age, use of bisphosphonates, and hypercalcemia were features of the AFF patients, while elevated PTH was reported to be protective. The younger age of the patients is supported by other studies [24, 61]; however, hypercalcemia, earlier menopause, and higher BMI associated with AFFs have not been confirmed.

Treatment and Prevention of AFFs

In general, most patients with complete or partial AFFs are treated by surgical intervention (rodding or pinning), withdrawal of bisphosphonate treatment, and either a "drug" holiday or treatment with an anabolic agent [62].

Drug Holiday

Cessation of bisphosphonate treatment for what is termed a "drug holiday" is a common treatment for AFF and prophylaxis for individuals on long-term bisphosphonate treatment. However, the duration and effectiveness have not been established. Yet the literature contains numerous recommendations of a "drug holiday" for users of bisphosphonates [63–67]. The suggested length of such a holiday ranges from 1 year to longer indeterminate times [68, 69]. When the drug holiday should start is also unresolved, although suggested times range from 2 to 5 years or longer [70, 71]. The use of denosumab, which has been shown to have fully reversible effects on bone turnover [72], might also be considered, although AFF has been associated with denosumab use [7]. Generally, the initiation and length of the holiday should be based on clinical judgment.

Use of Anabolic Agents

A recent alternative approach to treating AFFs rather than starting a "drug holiday" is to switch the patient to an anti-catabolic or anabolic therapy such as parathyroid hormone [73] or newer modalities such as sclerostin antibody [74]. Until the mechanism through which AFFs develop is established, selecting the appropriate therapy will be difficult. Both positive and negative results have been reported using these treatment modalities. However, the effectiveness of these therapies assumes that antiresorptives are the causative factor of AFF [8].

Conclusion

AFFs or, as the definition is widened, atypical fractures (AFs) are stress fracture-like fractures that occur at unexpected locations in weight-bearing bones. Characterized by a beak-like appearance on the lateral cortex, thickened cortices, bilateral occurrence, and often preceded by prodermal pain, these rare occurrences do not have a well-defined etiology. Often associated with long-term bisphosphonate use, having bone tissue of reduced heterogeneity and increased numbers of microcracks, their material properties generally do not appear different from typical fractures in age-matched patients. To date, no evidence exists for other causes beyond increased remodeling suppression, yet most individuals taking antiresorptive agents long-term do not have this adverse reaction. Thus, further clues must be sought to the etiology, while at the same time attempting to minimize risk in those patients taking bisphosphonates long-term.

Acknowledgments The authors work reported in this manuscript was supported by NIH grants R01-AR041325 and R01-AR053571.

References[1]

1. Imbuldeniya AM, Jiwa N, Murphy JP. Bilateral atypical insufficiency fractures of the proximal tibia and a unilateral distal femoral fracture associated with long-term intravenous bisphosphonate therapy: a case report. J Med Case Reports. 2012;6(1):50.
2. Breglia MD, Carter JD. Atypical insufficiency fracture of the tibia associated with long-term bisphosphonate therapy. J Clin Rheumatol. 2010;16(2):76–8.
3. *Shane E, Burr D, Ebeling PR, Abrahamsen B, Adler RA, Brown TD, et al. Atypical subtrochanteric and diaphyseal femoral fractures: report of a task force of the American Society for Bone and Mineral Research. J Bone Miner Res. 2010;25(11):2267–94. *This paper summarizes the initial recommendation of the ASBMR Taskforce on the definition of AFFs.
4. Alfahad A, Thet EM, Radwan F, Sudhakar J, Nini K, Tachtatzis P. Spontaneous incomplete transverse subtrochanteric femoral fracture with cortical thickening possibly secondary to risedronate use: a case report. J Med Case Reports. 2012;6(1):272.
5. Kim YS, Park WC. Atypical subtrochanteric femur fracture in patient with metastatic breast cancer treated with zoledronic acid. J Breast Cancer. 2012;15(2):261–4.
6. *Odvina CV, Zerwekh JE, Rao DS, Maalouf N, Gottschalk FA, Pak CY. Severely suppressed bone turnover: a potential complication of alendronate therapy. J Clin Endocrinol Metab. 2005;90(3):1294–301. *This report was the first regarding unusual fractures associated with long-term bisphosphonate use.
7. Paparodis R, Buehring B, Pelley EM, Binkley N. A case of an unusual subtrochanteric fracture in a patient receiving denosumab. Endocr Pract. 2013;19(3):e64–8.
8. *Shane E, Burr D, Abrahamsen B, Adler RA, Brown TD, Cheung AM, et al. Atypical subtrochanteric and diaphyseal femoral fractures: second report of a task force of the American Society for Bone and Mineral Research. J Bone Miner Res. 2014;29(1):1–23. *This paper is a refinement of the initial ASBMR taskforce on AFFs, including a revised definition and more definitive recommendations for diagnosis and treatment.
9. Eriksen EF, Halse J, Moen MH. New developments in the treatment of osteoporosis. Acta Obstet Gynecol Scand. 2013;92(6):620–36.
10. Epstein S. Update of current therapeutic options for the treatment of postmenopausal osteoporosis. Clin Ther. 2006;28(2):151–73.
11. Schilcher J, Michaelsson K, Aspenberg P. Bisphosphonate use and atypical fractures of the femoral shaft. N Engl J Med. 2011;364(18):1728–37.
12. Rydholm A. Highly different risk estimates for atypical femoral fracture with use of bisphosphonates—debate must be allowed! Acta Orthop. 2012;83(4):319–20.
13. Feldstein AC, Black D, Perrin N, Rosales AG, Friess D, Boardman D, et al. Incidence and demography of femur fractures with and without atypical features. J Bone Miner Res. 2012;27(5):977–86.
14. Cakmak S, Mahirogullari M, Keklikci K, Sari E, Erdik B, Rodop O. Bilateral low-energy sequential femoral shaft fractures in patients on long-term bisphosphonate therapy. Acta Orthop Traumatol Turc. 2013;47(3):162–72.
15. Donnelly E, Saleh A, Unnanuntana A, Lane JM. Atypical femoral fractures: epidemiology, etiology, and patient management. Curr Opin Support Palliat Care. 2012;6(3):348–54.
16. Gedmintas L, Solomon DH, Kim SC. Bisphosphonates and risk of subtrochanteric, femoral shaft, and atypical femur fracture: a systematic review and meta-analysis. J Bone Miner Res. 2013;28(8):1729–37.
17. *Tan SC, Koh SB, Goh SK, Howe TS. Atypical femoral stress fractures in bisphosphonate-free patients. Osteoporos Int. 2011;22(7):2211–2. *Four patients who were bisphosphonate-free presented with fractures fitting the "AFF- characteristics," casting doubt on the association of bisphosphonates and atypical fractures.
18. Park-Wyllie LY, Mamdani MM, Juurlink DN, Hawker GA, Gunraj N, Austin PC, et al. Bisphosphonate use and the risk of subtrochanteric or femoral shaft fractures in older women. JAMA. 2011;305(8):783–9.
19. Kim SY, Schneeweiss S, Katz JN, Levin R, Solomon DH. Oral bisphosphonates and risk of subtrochanteric or diaphyseal femur fractures in a population-based cohort. J Bone Miner Res. 2011;26(5):993–1001.
20. Isaacs JD, Shidiak L, Harris IA, Szomor ZL. Femoral insufficiency fractures associated with prolonged bisphosphonate therapy. Clin Orthop Relat Res. 2010;468(12):3384–92.
21. La Rocca Vieira R, Rosenberg ZS, Allison MB, Im SA, Babb J, Peck V. Frequency of incomplete atypical femoral fractures in asymptomatic patients on long-term bisphosphonate therapy. AJR Am J Roentgenol. 2012;198(5):1144–51.
22. Lo JC, Huang SY, Lee GA, Khandelwal S, Provus J, Ettinger B, et al. Clinical correlates of atypical femoral fracture. Bone. 2012;51(1):181–4.
23. Franceschetti P, Bondanelli M, Caruso G, Ambrosio MR, Lorusso V, Zatelli MC, et al. Risk factors for development of atypical femoral fractures in patients on long-term oral bisphosphonate therapy. Bone. 2013;56(2):426–31.
24. Giusti A, Hamdy NA, Dekkers OM, Ramautar SR, Dijkstra S, Papapoulos SE. Atypical fractures and bisphosphonate therapy: a cohort study of patients with femoral fracture with radiographic adjudication of fracture site and features. Bone. 2011;48(5):966–71.
25. Tamminen IS, Yli-Kyyny T, Isaksson H, Turunen MJ, Tong X, Jurvelin JS, et al. Incidence and bone biopsy findings of atypical femoral fractures. J Bone Miner Metab. 2013;31(5):585–94.
26. Odvina CV, Levy S, Rao S, Zerwekh JE, Rao DS. Unusual mid-shaft fractures during long-term

---

[1] *Important References

bisphosphonate therapy. Clin Endocrinol (Oxf). 2010;72(2):161–8.

27. Jamal SA, Dion N, Ste-Marie LG. Atypical femoral fractures and bone turnover. N Engl J Med. 2011;365(13):1261–2.

28. Boskey AL, Spevak L, Weinstein RS. Spectroscopic markers of bone quality in alendronate-treated postmenopausal women. Osteoporos Int. 2009;20(5): 793–800.

29. Donnelly E, Meredith DS, Nguyen JT, Gladnick BP, Rebolledo BJ, Shaffer AD, et al. Reduced cortical bone compositional heterogeneity with bisphosphonate treatment in postmenopausal women with intertrochanteric and subtrochanteric fractures. J Bone Miner Res. 2012;27(3):672–8.

30. Boivin GY, Chavassieux PM, Santora AC, Yates J, Meunier PJ. Alendronate increases bone strength by increasing the mean degree of mineralization of bone tissue in osteoporotic women. Bone. 2000;27(5): 687–94.

31. Gourion-Arsiquaud S, Allen MR, Burr DB, Vashishth D, Tang SY, Boskey AL. Bisphosphonate treatment modifies canine bone mineral and matrix properties and their heterogeneity. Bone. 2010;46(3):666–72.

32. Gourion-Arsiquaud S, Lukashova L, Power J, Loveridge N, Reeve J, Boskey AL. Fourier transform infrared imaging of femoral neck bone: reduced heterogeneity of mineral-to-matrix and carbonate-to-phosphate and more variable crystallinity in treatment-naive fracture cases compared with fracture-free controls. J Bone Miner Res. 2013;28(1):150–61.

33. Zoehrer R, Roschger P, Paschalis EP, Hofstaetter JG, Durchschlag E, Fratzl P, et al. Effects of 3- and 5-year treatment with risedronate on bone mineralization density distribution in triple biopsies of the iliac crest in postmenopausal women. J Bone Miner Res. 2006;21(7):1106–12.

34. Misof BM, Roschger P, Gabriel D, Paschalis EP, Eriksen EF, Recker RR, et al. Annual intravenous zoledronic acid for three years increased cancellous bone matrix mineralization beyond normal values in the HORIZON biopsy cohort. J Bone Miner Res. 2013;28(3):442–8.

35. *Tang SY, Allen MR, Phipps R, Burr DB, Vashishth D. Changes in non-enzymatic glycation and its association with altered mechanical properties following 1-year treatment with risedronate or alendronate. Osteoporos Int. 2009;20(6):887–94. *This paper correlates accumulation of advanced glycation endproducts (AGEs) in bone with loss of whole bone mechanical strength.

36. Allen MR, Iwata K, Phipps R, Burr DB. Alterations in canine vertebral bone turnover, microdamage accumulation, and biomechanical properties following 1-year treatment with clinical treatment doses of risedronate or alendronate. Bone. 2006;39(4):872–9.

37. *Allen MR, Burr DB. Bisphosphonate effects on bone turnover, microdamage, and mechanical properties: what we think we know and what we know that we don't know. Bone. 2011;49(1):56–65. *This review summarizes the state of knowledge on AFFs in 2011 and indicates the key questions that remain to be addressed.

38. Li J, Mashiba T, Burr DB. Bisphosphonate treatment suppresses not only stochastic remodeling but also the targeted repair of microdamage. Calcif Tissue Int. 2001;69(5):281–6.

39. Wang X, Zauel RR, Rao DS, Fyhrie DP. Cancellous bone lamellae strongly affect microcrack propagation and apparent mechanical properties: separation of patients with osteoporotic fracture from normal controls using a 2D nonlinear finite element method (biomechanical stereology). Bone. 2008;42(6):1184–92.

40. Allen MR, Reinwald S, Burr DB. Alendronate reduces bone toughness of ribs without significantly increasing microdamage accumulation in dogs following 3 years of daily treatment. Calcif Tissue Int. 2008;82(5): 354–60.

41. Mashiba T, Hirano T, Turner CH, Forwood MR, Johnston CC, Burr DB. Suppressed bone turnover by bisphosphonates increases microdamage accumulation and reduces some biomechanical properties in dog rib. J Bone Miner Res. 2000;15(4):613–20.

42. Hirano T, Turner CH, Forwood MR, Johnston CC, Burr DB. Does suppression of bone turnover impair mechanical properties by allowing microdamage accumulation? Bone. 2000;27(1):13–20.

43. Tarnowski CP, Ignelzi Jr MA, Wang W, Taboas JM, Goldstein SA, Morris MD. Earliest mineral and matrix changes in force-induced musculoskeletal disease as revealed by Raman microspectroscopic imaging. J Bone Miner Res. 2004;19(1):64–71.

44. Zioupos P, Gresle M, Winwood K. Fatigue strength of human cortical bone: age, physical, and material heterogeneity effects. J Biomed Mater Res A. 2008;86(3): 627–36.

45. Ettinger B, Burr DB, Ritchie RO. Proposed pathogenesis for atypical femoral fractures: lessons from materials research. Bone. 2013;55(2):495–500.

46. Allen MR, Follet H, Khurana M, Sato M, Burr DB. Antiremodeling agents influence osteoblast activity differently in modeling and remodeling sites of canine rib. Calcif Tissue Int. 2006;79(4):255–61.

47. Diez-Perez A, Guerri R, Nogues X, Caceres E, Pena MJ, Mellibovsky L, et al. Microindentation for in vivo measurement of bone tissue mechanical properties in humans. J Bone Miner Res. 2010;25(8):1877–85.

48. Guerri-Fernandez RC, Nogues X, Quesada Gomez JM, Torres Del Pliego E, Puig L, Garcia-Giralt N, et al. Microindentation for in vivo measurement of bone tissue material properties in atypical femoral fracture patients and controls. J Bone Miner Res. 2013;28(1):162–8.

49. Bala Y, Depalle B, Farlay D, Douillard T, Meille S, Follet H, et al. Bone micromechanical properties are compromised during long-term alendronate therapy independently of mineralization. J Bone Miner Res. 2012;27(4):825–34.

50. Tjhia CK, Odvina CV, Rao DS, Stover SM, Wang X, Fyhrie DP. Mechanical property and tissue mineral

density differences among severely suppressed bone turnover (SSBT) patients, osteoporotic patients, and normal subjects. Bone. 2011;49(6):1279–89.

51. Xue Y, Cai T, Shi S, Wang W, Zhang Y, Mao T, et al. Clinical and animal research findings in pycnodysostosis and gene mutations of cathepsin K from 1996 to 2011. Orphanet J Rare Dis. 2011;6:20.

52. Yates CJ, Bartlett MJ, Ebeling PR. An atypical subtrochanteric femoral fracture from pycnodysostosis: a lesson from nature. J Bone Miner Res. 2011;26(6):1377–9.

53. Wang Q, Teo JW, Ghasem-Zadeh A, Seeman E. Women and men with hip fractures have a longer femoral neck moment arm and greater impact load in a sideways fall. Osteoporos Int. 2009;20(7):1151–6.

54. Crossley K, Bennell KL, Wrigley T, Oakes BW. Ground reaction forces, bone characteristics, and tibial stress fracture in male runners. Med Sci Sports Exerc. 1999;31(8):1088–93.

55. Milner CE, Hamill J, Davis IS. Distinct hip and rearfoot kinematics in female runners with a history of tibial stress fracture. J Orthop Sports Phys Ther. 2010;40(2):59–66.

56. Pohl MB, Mullineaux DR, Milner CE, Hamill J, Davis IS. Biomechanical predictors of retrospective tibial stress fractures in runners. J Biomech. 2008;41(6):1160–5.

57. Nakamura T, Turner CH, Yoshikawa T, Slemenda CW, Peacock M, Burr DB, et al. Do variations in hip geometry explain differences in hip fracture risk between Japanese and white Americans? J Bone Miner Res. 1994;9(7):1071–6.

58. Marcano A, Taormina D, Egol KA, Peck V, Tejwani NC. Are race and sex associated with the occurrence of atypical femoral fractures? Clin Orthop Relat Res. 2014;472(3):1020–7.

59. Cummings SR, Cauley JA, Palermo L, Ross PD, Wasnich RD, Black D, et al. Racial differences in hip axis lengths might explain racial differences in rates of hip fracture. Study of Osteoporotic Fractures Research Group. Osteoporos Int. 1994;4(4):226–9.

60. Taormina DP, Marcano AI, Karia R, Egol KA, Tejwani NC. Symptomatic atypical femoral fractures are related to underlying hip geometry. Bone. 2014;63(1):1–6.

61. Allison MB, Markman L, Rosenberg Z, Vieira RL, Babb J, Tejwani N, et al. Atypical incomplete femoral

fractures in asymptomatic patients on long term bisphosphonate therapy. Bone. 2013;55(1):113–8.

62. Lee YK, Ha YC, Kang BJ, Chang JS, Koo KH. Predicting need for fixation of atypical femoral fracture. J Clin Endocrinol Metab. 2013;98(7):2742–5.

63. Abrahamsen B, Clark EM. Disentangling the emerging evidence around atypical fractures. Curr Rheumatol Rep. 2012;14(3):212–6.

64. Diab DL, Watts NB. Bisphosphonates in the treatment of osteoporosis. Endocrinol Metab Clin North Am. 2012;41(3):487–506.

65. Dunn RL, Bird ML, Conway SE, Stratton MA. Use of bisphosphonates in older adults: how long is long enough? Consult Pharm. 2013;28(1):39–57.

66. Rebolledo BJ, Unnanuntana A, Lane JM. A comprehensive approach to fragility fractures. J Orthop Trauma. 2011;25(9):566–73.

67. Ro C, Cooper O. Bisphosphonate drug holiday: choosing appropriate candidates. Curr Osteoporos Rep. 2013;11(1):45–51.

68. Sellmeyer DE. Atypical fractures as a potential complication of long-term bisphosphonate therapy. JAMA. 2010;304(13):1480–4.

69. Kong SY, Kim DY, Han EJ, Park SY, Yim CH, Kim SH, et al. Effects of a 'drug holiday' on bone mineral density and bone turnover marker during bisphosphonate therapy. J Bone Metab. 2013;20(1):31–5.

70. Ott SM. What is the optimal duration of bisphosphonate therapy? Cleve Clin J Med. 2011;78(9):619–30.

71. McClung M, Harris ST, Miller PD, Bauer DC, Davison KS, Dian L, et al. Bisphosphonate therapy for osteoporosis: benefits, risks, and drug holiday. Am J Med. 2013;126(1):13–20.

72. Brown JP, Dempster DW, Ding B, Dent-Acosta R, San Martin J, Grauer A, et al. Bone remodeling in postmenopausal women who discontinued denosumab treatment: off-treatment biopsy study. J Bone Miner Res. 2011;26(11):2737–44.

73. Chiang CY, Zebaze RM, Ghasem-Zadeh A, Iuliano-Burns S, Hardidge A, Seeman E. Teriparatide improves bone quality and healing of atypical femoral fractures associated with bisphosphonate therapy. Bone. 2013;52(1):360–5.

74. Das S, Sakthiswary R. Bone metabolism and histomorphometric changes in murine models treated with sclerostin antibody: a systematic review. Curr Drug Targets. 2013;14(14):1667–74.

Clinical Presentation of Atypical Femur Fractures

Yelena Bogdan and Thomas A. Einhorn

Summary

- Atypical femur fractures (AFFs) have a specific clinical presentation discussed in the American Society of Bone and Mineral Research (ASBMR) task force document.
- These fractures are associated with very minimal to no trauma, the presence of prodromal pain, and the presence of contralateral symptoms or fractures.
- Certain patients may be more at risk for AFFs, including those with rheumatoid arthritis, breast cancer, and hypophosphatasia or those taking medications such as bisphosphonates, glucocorticoids, and proton pump inhibitors.
- Careful evaluation of the contralateral side in a patient with an AFF is paramount.

Introduction

The clinical presentation of AFFs exhibits specific characteristics not seen in traumatic injuries and typical hip fractures occurring in the elderly.

Y. Bogdan, MD (✉) • T.A. Einhorn, MD
Department of Orthopaedic Surgery, Boston
University Medical Center, 850 Harrison Ave,
Dowling 2 North, Boston, MA 02118, USA
e-mail: ybogdan@gmail.com

The 2013 ASBMR task force document [1] presents the most current definition of AFFs (Table 9.1). This definition includes both radiologic and clinical criteria, and it is the latter that comprises the focus of this chapter.

Patient Characteristics

The vast majority of subtrochanteric and diaphyseal femur fractures are caused by major trauma such as motor vehicle accidents, particularly in men. However, with increased age, the incidence of lower-energy trauma as a cause of these fractures rises until the incidence in women overtakes that of men [2]. This parallels the rise in hip fractures in elderly women [3]. AFFs, like hip and other fragility fractures, also predominantly affect the older female patient population.

There is some evidence that patients affected by AFFs differ from "typical" hip fracture patients with regard to level of functioning, particularly after surgery. A study of 191 operatively treated AFF patients recently presented at the Orthopaedic Trauma Association meeting [4] noted that 93 % were living in their homes at the time of final follow-up, with a mortality rate of 2 %. In contrast, a study of 87 subtrochanteric fracture patients showed a mortality rate of 25 % at 1 year, and 71 % of patients were unable to return to their previous living arrangement [5]. This suggests that there may be a difference in the two

© Springer International Publishing Switzerland 2016
S.L. Silverman, B. Abrahamsen (eds.), *The Duration and Safety of Osteoporosis Treatment*, DOI 10.1007/978-3-319-23639-1_9

Table 9.1 Updated criteria to the definition of atypical femur fractures, as listed in the 2013 ASBMR task force document [1]

All fractures are located along the femur from distal to lesser trochanter to proximal to supracondylar flare
PLUS

Major features: (four of five are required)
- **No trauma or minimal trauma**
- Fracture originates in lateral cortex and is substantially transverse but may become oblique as progresses medially
- Fracture is noncomminuted or minimally comminuted
- Complete fractures extend through both cortices and may be associated with medial spike; incomplete fractures involve only lateral cortex
- Localized periosteal or endosteal thickening of lateral cortex is present at fracture site (beaking or flaring)

Minor features: (none are required)
- Generalized increase in cortical thickness of femoral diaphysis
- **Unilateral or bilateral prodromal symptoms**
- **Bilateral incomplete or complete femoral diaphysis fractures**
- Delayed fracture healing

Definitions specifically discussed are in **bold**

Data from Shane E, et al. Atypical subtrochanteric and diaphyseal femoral fractures: Second report of a task force of the American Society for Bone and Mineral Research. J Bone Miner Res 2013. Epub May 28

populations at baseline, as well as in their response to the same operative treatment (cephalomedullary nailing).

Task Force Document: Major Features

The ASBMR task force definition lists "minimal to no trauma" as a major feature of AFFs that must be present in order for a fracture to be classified as such. While low-energy trauma that causes hip (femoral neck and intertrochanteric) fractures is common among the elderly, the vast majority of subtrochanteric and femoral shaft fractures in the general population are caused by major trauma such as motor vehicle accidents. Even in cases where low-energy trauma results in femoral shaft fractures in older patients, however, the fracture configurations are different than those seen in AFFs [6].

The most common mechanism of injury for AFFs appears to be either a ground-level fall or nontraumatic activities such as walking or stepping off a curb. In an early study [7], five of nine patients with AFFs had femoral shaft fractures, and all occurred during walking or turning. Another study of 25 patients [8] with AFFs who were matched with a cohort of similar age showed a ground-level fall to be the cause of 96 % of the AFFs.

Task Force Document: Minor Features

The presence of prodromal symptoms in the affected extremity is very common in AFFs, occurring at a rate of approximately 70 % [1]. This figure is based on data accumulated from case series reviewed by the ASBMR task force, but the number in individual studies varies, and a recent large series noted a 32 % rate of prodromal symptoms [4]. Smaller series vary, with 41 % [9], 63 % [10], 67 % [11], and 76 % [12] rates of prodromal pain, although those series involved low patient numbers (maximum $n = 22$).

Prodromal pain first occurs any time from 2 weeks to several years prior to the fracture [9, 12]. It commonly presents as pain in the anterior or lateral thigh and often in the groin as well [12]. The presence of prodromal pain may be the first sign necessitating a radiograph in these patients, which may then show a stress lesion in the cortex (discussed elsewhere in this book). Both stress lesions and the presence of prodromal pain have been shown to increase the risk of subsequent fracture [13]. The presence of prodromal pain, particularly in a patient on bisphosphonates, should be a concerning signal that warrants clinical and radiologic investigation.

Another major clinical characteristic of AFFs is the presence of contralateral symptoms and/or fractures. These fractures can occur both sequentially and simultaneously and are often associated with prodromal pain. Initial small studies [12, 14] showed an approximately 20 % rate of contralateral fractures, and in one study, two out of the three patients with bilateral fractures had sustained them simultaneously [14]. Another study of seven patients with AFFs identified four with a stress reaction on the contralateral side, with all four patients presenting with prodromal pain [15]. One of the four eventually fractured through the site of stress reaction after a fall, while the other three patients received a prophylactic cephalomedullary nail.

One recent series of 191 operatively treated AFFs confirmed the contralateral fracture rate reported in a smaller series [12], noting a 19 % rate of contralateral fractures, 20 months on average after their index procedure [4]. Notably, 50 % of those patients had discontinued bisphosphonate treatment at the time of their first procedure. Also in that study, 32 % of the patients with contralateral fractures who had information available had prodromal pain, and 59 % (10/17 with available data) had a stress reaction on X-ray prior to their contralateral fracture [4]. These data underscore the need to carefully evaluate the contralateral femur in AFF patients, even if prodromal symptoms are not present.

Another clinical feature of AFFs that may be found in the patient history is an association with several comorbid conditions. One is hypophosphatasia, an error of metabolism in which a loss-of-function mutation occurs in the gene encoding alkaline phosphatase. This results in pyrophosphate accumulation and causes osteomalacia due to impaired mineralization. This, in turn, can result in femoral pseudofractures that are often bilateral and occur in the subtrochanteric region [16]. This further supports the hypothesis that bisphosphonate treatment is related to AFFs, because bisphosphonates are analogs of inorganic pyrophosphate. Other conditions that may be found on presentation of AFFs are rheumatoid arthritis and breast cancer. An analysis of the FDA Adverse Effect Reporting System (FAERS) showed a 7 % rate of rheumatoid arthritis and a 2 % rate of breast cancer in suspected AFF patients. In the case of breast cancer, it is unclear whether concomitant administration of bisphosphonates is the cause of the association between this malignancy and AFFs, and several studies [17, 18] have examined this question.

The last aspect of AFF presentation mentioned in the task force document is the association with medication use in the patient's history. In a 2011 study, Park et al. [19] showed that although the absolute risk of AFFs was very low, the odds ratio was 2.74 in the case of older women taking bisphosphonates for greater than 5 years. Another cohort analysis of 12,777 women greater than age 55 isolated 59 patients with AFFs, with an adjusted odds ratio of 33.3 for bisphosphonate use (i.e., 78 % of the AFFs vs. 10 % who did not have AFFs used bisphosphonates) [20]. The popularity of bisphosphonates has come hand in hand with a rise in subtrochanteric fractures and a decline of "typical" hip fractures, particularly in females [21]. Glucocorticoids are also implicated in AFFs [22, 23], as well as in general osteoporotic fractures [24]; one study of 20 AFF patients gave a 5.2 odds ratio for developing an AFF if a patient used glucocorticoids for more than 6 months [23]. Lastly, proton pump inhibitors such as omeprazole have been found in the medication history of approximately 34–39 % of AFF patients [1]. Like glucocorticoids, proton pump inhibitors are also noted to be associated with osteoporotic hip and wrist fractures if they are used long-term [25].

Conclusion

The clinical presentation of AFFs is noted in the ASBMR task force document. The physician should be aware of warning signs such as prodromal pain, which may signal an impending fracture, as well as bilateral symptoms. The presence of these symptoms, particularly in a patient with risk factors such as rheumatoid arthritis, breast cancer, or use of bisphosphonates, is concerning and should be evaluated thoroughly. Radiologic findings and current treatment recommendations are discussed elsewhere in this book.

References[1]

1. *Shane E, Burr D, Abrahamsen B, et al. Atypical subtrochanteric and diaphyseal femoral fractures: second report of a task force of the American society for bone and mineral research. J Bone Miner Res. 2013. Epub May 28. *Description: 2013 ASBMR Task Force Document, second update. Details the latest research

---

[1] *Important References

into atypical femur fractures and presents an updated definition, both clinical and radiologic. Much of this chapter is based on this definition.

2. Hedlund R, Lindgren U. Epidemiology of diaphyseal femoral fracture. Acta Orthop Scand. 1986;57(5): 423–7.

3. Nieves JW, Bilezikian JP, Lane JM, et al. Fragility fractures of the hip and femur: incidence and patient characteristics. Osteoporos Int. 2010;21(3):399–408.

4. *Bogdan Y, Tornetta P III, Einhorn TA, et al. Healing time and complications in operatively treated atypical femur fractures associated with bisphosphonate use: a multicenter retrospective cohort. In: OTA annual meeting podium presentation. p. 4. http://ota.org/media/77960/Geriatric-Papers.pdf. *Author Note/Disclosure: Large retrospective study of operatively treated fractures by same author as author of this chapter (Dr. Bogdan). At time of chapter writing, the above study has been submitted for publication; the findings noted in the chapter are from the most recent data analysis and are thus more current than the data presented in the reference.

5. Ekstrom W, Nemeth G, Samnegard E, et al. Quality of life after a subtrochanteric fracture: a prospective cohort study on 87 elderly patients. Injury. 2009;40: 371–6.

6. Salminen S, Pihlajamaki H, Avikainen V, et al. Specific features associated with femoral shaft fractures caused by low energy trauma. J Trauma. 1997;43:117–22.

7. Odvina CV, Zerwekh JE, Rao DS, et al. Severely suppressed bone turnover: a potential complication of alendronate therapy. J Clin Endocrinol Metab. 2005;90(3):1294–301.

8. Prasarn ML, Ahn J, Helfet DL, et al. Bisphosphonate-associated femur fractures have high complication rates with operative fixation. Clin Orthop Relat Res. 2012;470(8):2295–301.

9. Thompson RN, Phillips JR, McCauley SH, et al. Atypical femoral fractures and bisphosphonate treatment: experience in two large United Kingdom teaching hospitals. Bone Joint J. 2012;94(3):385–90.

10. Wang K, Moaveni A, Dowrick A. Alendronate-associated femoral insufficiency fractures and femoral stress reaction. J Orthop Surg. 2011;19(1):89–92.

11. Visekruna N, Wilson D, McKiernan FE. Severely suppressed bone turnover and atypical skeletal fragility. J Clin Endocrinol Metab. 2008;93(8):2948–52.

12. Kwek EB, Goh SK, Koh JS, et al. An emerging pattern of subtrochanteric stress fractures: a long-term complication of alendronate therapy? Injury. 2008;39(2):224–31.

13. Koh JS, Goh SK, Png MA, et al. Femoral cortical stress lesions in long-term bisphosphonate therapy: a herald of impending fracture? J Orthop Trauma. 2010;24(2):75–81.

14. Weil YA, Rivkin G, Safran O, et al. The outcome of surgically treated femur fractures associated with long-term bisphosphonate use. J Trauma. 2011;71(1): 186–90.

15. Capeci CM, Tejwani NC. Bilateral low-energy simultaneous or sequential femoral fractures in patients on long-term alendronate therapy. J Bone Joint Surg Am. 2009;91(11):2556–61.

16. Whyte MP. Atypical femoral fractures, bisphosphonates, and adult hypophosphatasia. J Bone Miner Res. 2009;24(6):1132–4.

17. Chang ST, Tenforde AS, Grimsrud CD, et al. Atypical femur fractures among breast cancer and multiple myeloma patients receiving intravenous bisphosphonate therapy. Bone. 2012;51(3):524–7.

18. Puhaindran ME, Farooki A, Steensma MR, et al. Atypical subtrochanteric femoral fractures in patients with skeletal malignant involvement treated with intravenous bisphosphonates. J Bone Joint Surg Am. 2011;93(13):1235–42.

19. Park-Wyllie LY, Mamdani MM, Juurlink DL, et al. Bisphosphonate use and the risk of subtrochanteric or femoral shaft fractures in older women. JAMA. 2011; 305(8):783–9.

20. Schilcher J, Michaëlsson K, Aspenberg P. Bisphosphonate use and atypical fractures of the femoral shaft. N Engl J Med. 2011;364(18):1728–37.

21. Wang Z, Bhattachariyya T. Trends in incidence of subtrochanteric fragility fractures and bisphosphonate use among the US elderly, 1996–2007. J Bone Miner Res. 2011;26(3):553–60.

22. *Edwards BJ, Bunta AD, Lane J. Bisphosphonates and nonhealing femoral fractures: analysis of the FDA adverse event reporting system (FAERS) and international safety efforts: a systematic review from the research on adverse drug events and reports (RADAR) project. J Bone Joint Surg Am. 2013;95(4):297–307. *Description: Review of 317 atypical femoral fractures associated with alendronate use from a large database demonstrating that many of these fractures show a delayed healing response. Also includes a literature review.

23. Girgis CM, Sher D, Seibel MJ. Atypical femoral fractures and bisphosphonate use. N Engl J Med. 2010;362(19):1848–9.

24. Kanis JA, Johansson H, Oden A. A meta-analysis of prior corticosteroid use and fracture risk. J Bone Miner Res. 2004;19(6):893–9.

25. Targownik LE, Lix LM, Metge CJ. Use of proton pump inhibitors and risk of osteoporosis-related fractures. CMAJ. 2008;179(4):319–26.

Effects of Antiresorptive Therapy on Bone Microarchitecture

Joy N. Tsai and Mary L. Bouxsein

List of Abbreviations

DXA	Dual-energy X-ray absorptiometry
HR-pQCT	High-resolution peripheral quantitative CT
BMD	Bone mineral density
2-D	Two-dimensional
BV/TV	Trabecular bone volume fraction
3-D	Three-dimensional
vBMD	Volumetric bone mineral density
ITS	Individual trabecula segmentation

Summary

- Bone mineral density (BMD) is only one determinant of bone strength. Another major contributor is change in bone microarchitecture.
- Trabecular and cortical microarchitectures are generally preserved or improved with antiresorptive therapy.

J.N. Tsai, MD (✉)
Endocrine Unit, Massachusetts General Hospital, 50 Blossom Street, Thier 1051, Boston, MA 02114, USA
e-mail: jntsai@mgh.harvard.edu

M.L. Bouxsein, PhD
Department of Orthopedic Surgery, Beth Israel Deaconess Medical Center, Boston, MA, USA

- In vivo approaches for assessment of bone microarchitecture are useful research tools, but their utility in clinical management of patients remains to be established.

Introduction

Measurement of BMD by dual-energy X-ray absorptiometry (DXA) is widely accepted for both clinical and research use. Although the measurement of BMD measurement by DXA is a validated predictor of fracture, most fracture victims have only modestly reduced BMD, and the changes in BMD with osteoporosis therapy do not fully explain the degree of fracture reduction [1–5]. For example, in postmenopausal women with low femoral neck bone density and at least one vertebral fracture, alendronate increased spine and femoral neck BMD by 6.2 % and 4.1 %, respectively, which was sufficient to reduce the risk of vertebral fracture by approximately 50 % and nonvertebral fractures by approximately 30 %, reductions that are significantly greater than would be predicted based on BMD changes alone [6].

One possible reason that changes in BMD following treatment underestimate the observed reductions in fracture risk is that BMD is only one determinant of bone strength. Other potential contributors to fracture risk reduction following osteoporosis therapies include changes in bone

© Springer International Publishing Switzerland 2016
S.L. Silverman, B. Abrahamsen (eds.), *The Duration and Safety of Osteoporosis Treatment*, DOI 10.1007/978-3-319-23639-1_10

morphology, bone microarchitecture, and/or the intrinsic properties of bone tissue (such as degree of mineralization or collagen cross-linking). DXA is a two-dimensional imaging method that assesses areal BMD and thus cannot separately delineate changes in the trabecular and cortical compartments or bone microarchitecture. Trabecular and cortical bone have unique responses to treatment and possibly distinct contributions to overall bone strength. The development of high-resolution imaging with ex vivo micro-CT and in vivo high-resolution peripheral quantitative computed tomography (HR-pQCT) allows for the assessment of compartment-specific bone densities, as well as parameters of bone microarchitecture [7–10].

This chapter focuses on change in bone microarchitecture in response to antiresorptive therapy as evaluated by histomorphometry and ex vivo micro-CT analyses of iliac crest biopsies and noninvasive high-resolution imaging.

Effect of Antiresorptive Therapy on Bone Microarchitecture as Assessed by Histomorphometry and Ex Vivo Micro-CT

Trabecular and cortical microarchitecture can be assessed using two-dimensional (2-D) histomorphometry of iliac crest bone biopsies. Trabecular bone volume fraction (BV/TV), trabecular thickness, trabecular separation, trabecular number, cortical thickness, and cortical porosity may be evaluated [11]. The addition of micro-CT allows for nondestructive imaging of ex vivo human samples and provides for three-dimensional (3-D) assessment of many of the same morphologic parameters assessed by histomorphometry [7, 8]. The potential advantage of micro-CT is that the evaluation is done in 3-D and, perhaps more importantly, incorporates a much larger volume of bone than is evaluated in a few thin histologic sections. This larger volume of bone may provide a more robust indication of the skeletal response to treatment. However, it is unclear how closely changes in bone structure at the iliac crest reflect changes in bone structure elsewhere in the body.

Effect of Antiresorptive Therapy on Trabecular Microarchitecture

Numerous studies have reported antiresorptive treatment-induced changes in trabecular microarchitecture as assessed by 2-D histomorphometry and 3-D micro-CT of iliac crest biopsies [12–28]. Most of these studies are cross-sectional, with comparisons made between a treated and placebo group at the end of the study [12–20]. A few studies are longitudinal, with baseline and follow-up iliac crest biopsies in the treated and placebo groups [21–28].

Treatment with raloxifene for 6 months showed no significant change in trabecular BV/TV, thickness, or number as assessed by 2-D histomorphometry of paired baseline and end-of-study biopsies [22]. Similarly, Bravenboer et al. assessed 12 paired iliac biopsies and reported no change in trabecular bone volume or thickness after 2 years of pamidronate [21]. In contrast, trabecular BV/TV and thickness were higher, while trabecular spacing was lower after 2 or 3 years of alendronate ($n=29$) compared to the placebo group ($n=59$) in a cross-sectional study [16]. Results from 3-D micro-CT were also consistent with these favorable trabecular histomorphometric findings. Evaluated using baseline and follow-up biopsies, risedronate treatment showed preservation of trabecular BV/TV and microarchitecture after 1 and 5 years of treatment [25, 29]. In the HORIZON trial, micro-CT analyses of end-of-study iliac biopsies revealed that trabecular BV/TV and number were higher, whereas trabecular separation was lower in postmenopausal women who received 3 years of zoledronic acid ($n=79$) compared to those who received placebo ($n=68$) [17]. In contrast, micro-CT analyses of end-of-study biopsies revealed no difference in trabecular architecture between postmenopausal women treated for 2 ($n=31$) or 3 ($n=22$) years with denosumab compared to placebo-treated controls ($n=37$ at 2 years, $n=25$ at 3 years) [20]. Data from iliac biopsies following treatment with the cathepsin K inhibitor odanacatib (a novel agent that reduces bone resorption while maintaining bone formation) are limited. Though no statistical analyses were reported after 2 years of treatment, trabecular thickness and number were similar or higher in odanacatib-treated subjects ($n=6$) than placebo-treated controls ($n=5$) as measured by 3-D micro-CT [19]. Clearly, more data are needed to draw conclusions about the effects of odanacatib on trabecular bone microarchitecture in iliac biopsies. Altogether, these studies show that trabecular microarchitecture parameters are generally preserved or improved with antiresorptive therapy.

Effect of Antiresorptive Therapy on Cortical Microarchitecture

The effect of antiresorptive therapy on cortical bone microarchitecture as assessed by bone histomorphometry and ex vivo micro-CT is less well studied. Two years of pamidronate showed no change in cortical thickness [21]. One to three years of risedronate treatment showed no change in cortical thickness compared to baseline [25, 26]. In comparison, 2–3 years of alendronate, risedronate, or denosumab treatment lead to lower cortical porosity in iliac crest biopsy specimens [13, 20, 26]. Cortical porosity values were not reported in the assessment of iliac crest biopsies after zoledronic acid treatment, though in one stratum, cortical thickness was reported to be higher in women treated with zoledronic acid when compared to placebo-treated controls [17]. Altogether, antiresorptive treatment is reported to have either no effect on iliac crest cortical bone microstructure or to slightly reduce cortical porosity and increase cortical thickness. The variability in outcomes likely depends on the cross-sectional study designs, small sample sizes, and high variability of cortical thickness as assessed from iliac crest biopsies.

Effect of Antiresorptive Therapy on Bone Microarchitecture as Assessed by Noninvasive High-Resolution Imaging

Until recently, treatment-induced microarchitectural changes could only be assessed by histomorphometric analyses of iliac crest bone biopsies.

The development of high-resolution peripheral quantitative computed tomography (HR-pQCT) (XtremeCT, SCANCO Medical AG, Switzerland) allows for assessment of bone microarchitecture at the distal radius and distal tibia in vivo. In particular, with the standard analysis, 110 slices within a 9.02 mm long region of interest are obtained. Advantages of HR-pQCT include a short scan time of approximately 3 min and minimal radiation exposure (<3 μSv). The small voxel size (82 μm) enables measurement of not only cortical and trabecular volumetric bone mineral density (vBMD) but also geometry (cortical area, trabecular area) and structure (cortical thickness, trabecular thickness, trabecular number, and trabecular separation) [30]. However, a limitation in current methodology is that the trabecular BV/TV and thickness are not directly measured, but rather are derived [31]. Nonetheless, the potential value of bone architecture assessed by HR-pQCT is demonstrated by studies reporting that HR-pQCT variables were better able to discriminate between women with and without a history of fractures than standard DXA, including a prospective study showing predictive value of altered cortical and trabecular microarchitectural parameters [9, 32–42]. Furthermore, many of these HR-pQCT measures associated with fracture are independent of those assessed by DXA [38–40].

Adding to standard analysis of HR-pQCT images as described above, extended cortical analysis enables detailed imaging of cortical microarchitecture. Cortical vBMD, porosity, and thickness are assessed by direct 3-D measurements [43, 44]. This technique consists of segmentation of cortical bone compartment by an autocontouring process, generating periosteal and endosteal contours, and cortical porosity segmentation by identifying resolved Haversian canals within the cortical compartment. Using this algorithm, cortical bone volume, pore volume, porosity, and pore diameter can be assessed. Of note, with this approach, HR-pQCT measurements only capture cortical pores with a diameter larger than approximately 100 μm. Smaller pores are difficult to resolve given the 82 μm voxel size. Nonetheless, cortical vBMD measurements have high precision and reflect both the larger and smaller pores and may be a reasonable surrogate of cortical porosity. Alternate methods for assessing cortical porosity have also been introduced, but to date have been used less frequently than the extended cortical analysis method to assess the effects of antiresorptive therapies [45, 46]. The approach proposed by Zebaze and colleagues defines porosity via a "segmentation-free" algorithm that depends on knowledge and constancy of the tissue density of fully mineralized bone and computes porosity in inner and outer "transitional zones," as well as the "compact-appearing cortex." The potential value of cortical microarchitecture measurements is demonstrated in studies reporting that cortical porosity discriminates fracture cases from controls [37, 47].

A summary of effects of antiresorptive therapy on trabecular and cortical microarchitecture as assessed by HR-pQCT is outlined below and summarized in Tables 10.1 and 10.2. Given that the measurements are made in vivo, these are all longitudinal studies.

Effect of Antiresorptive Therapy on Trabecular Microarchitecture

Overall, the effect of antiresorptive therapy on trabecular vBMD and microarchitecture varies by treatment, skeletal site, and study. Two years of ibandronate treatment in postmenopausal women with osteopenia did not lead to significant improvement in trabecular vBMD in comparison to the placebo control group at either the distal radius or distal tibia [48]. Similarly, in a placebo-controlled study of postmenopausal women with low bone density, Burghardt et al. reported that 2 years of alendronate therapy also did not change trabecular vBMD at the distal radius [49]. This finding was also observed at the distal radius in two other studies of postmenopausal women treated with alendronate [50, 51]. However, Seeman et al. and Burghardt et al. reported an increase in trabecular vBMD at the distal tibia after 12 and 24 months of alendronate, respectively [49, 51]. Treatments with 12 months of denosumab, 18 months of zoledronic acid, and 24 months of odanacatib in postmenopausal women were all reported to increase trabecular vBMD at both skeletal sites [51–53].

Despite advancements in high-resolution imaging, changes in trabecular microarchitectural parameters in response to antiresorptive therapy have generally not been detected by HR-pQCT [48–54]. The lack of significant findings may be due to limited resolution and/or poor measurement precision relative to the expected change induced by the treatment. Although the reconstructed voxel size is 82 µm for the standard patient HR-pQCT protocol, the actual spatial resolution of the image is approximately 130–140 µm, which is about equal to the width of human trabeculae [55]. Moreover, subtle motion during the scan, more common at the radius than the tibia, can negatively affect the precision of HR-pQCT measurements thereby adding to the challenge of detecting small changes. Indeed, whereas the short-term precision of trabecular density measurements by HR-pQCT is excellent (<1 %), the short-term precision of trabecular microarchitecture measurements is substantially worse (1.8–4.4 %) [9, 10]. Though not routinely used, 3-D registration of follow-up images to the baseline image may improve the ability to detect changes in bone microstructure [56, 57].

A recently developed technique called individual trabecula segmentation (ITS) enables detailed quantification of trabecular morphology (plates or rods) and direct measurements of each individual trabecula [58]. The effect of anabolic therapy on HR-pQCT-based ITS parameters has been reported and thus may be a useful method to characterize other treatment-induced changes in trabecular microarchitecture in the future [59].

Effect of Antiresorptive Therapy on Cortical Microarchitecture

Several studies have reported no effect or positive effects on cortical microarchitecture in response to oral and intravenous bisphosphonate treatments, denosumab, and odanacatib.

Reports of changes in cortical microarchitecture following bisphosphonate treatment have been inconsistent (Tables 10.1 and 10.2). Rizzoli and colleagues reported that 2 years of alendronate treatment in postmenopausal osteoporotic women had no influence on cortical vBMD,

Table 10.1 Effect of antiresorptive therapy on trabecular and cortical density and cortical thickness at the distal radius, as assessed in vivo by HR-pQCT

Study	Drug	Duration (months)	N	Age (years)	Distal radius Tb.vBMD or BV/TV	Distal radius Ct.vBMD	Distal radius Ct.Th
Burghardt et al. (2010)	Alendronate	24	13	56±4	NS	NS	NS
	Placebo	24	20	56±2	NS	NS	NS
Rizzoli et al. (2012)	Alendronate	24	42	64±8	NS	NS	NS
	Strontium	24	41	64±8	NS	NS	NS
Seeman et al. (2010)	Alendronate	12	82	61±5	NS	NS	~+2 to 3 %[a]
	Denosumab	12	83	60±6	~0 to +1 %[a]	~0 to +0.5 %[a]	~+3 to 4 %[a]
	Placebo	12	82	61±5	~ −2 %[a]	~ −1.5 %[a]	~0 to −1 %[a]
Chapurlat et al. (2013)[b]	Ibandronate	24	72	63±5	No difference between groups	No difference between groups	No difference between groups
	Placebo	24	76	63±5			
Bala et al. (2014)	Risedronate (<55 year)	12	112	53±2	−1.60±4.49	NS	Not reported
	Placebo (<55 year)	12	49	53±2	−3.61±8.21	NS	Not reported
	Risedronate (>55 year)	12	109	62±6	NS	NS	Not reported
	Risedronate (>55 year)	12	54	61±4	NS	NS	Not reported
Hansen et al. (2013)	Zoledronic acid	18	33	70 (54–86)	+2.5±5.1 %	NS	NS
	PTH(1-34)	18	18	72 (59–80)	NS	−2.4±4.5 %	+2.0±3.8 %
	PTH(1-84)	18	20	70 (61–86)	NS	−3.5±3.3 %	NS
Cheung et al. (2014)	Odanacatib	24	109	64±7	+2.57 %[a]	+0.78 %[a]	+1.57 %[a]
	Placebo	24	105	64±6	NS	−1.65 %[a]	−5.28 %[a]
Schafer et al. (2012)	Ibandronate and PTH(1-84)[c]	24	43	62±4	+2.26 % (1.37, 3.14)[a]	−0.76 (−1.33, −0.20)[a]	−1.90 (−2.61, −1.18)[a]
Tsai et al. (2014)	PTH(1-34)	12	31	66±8	NS	−1.9±2.8 %	NS
	Denosumab	12	33	66±8	+1.3±2.8 %	+0.7±1.4 %	+2.3±4.8
	Denosumab and PTH(1-34)	12	30	66±9	+3.1±3.3 %	+1.0±1.6 %	+2.3±4.8

NS not significant

Values are means±SD unless otherwise noted as [a]Least squares means, and if values reported, with 95 % CIs

[b]For the Chapurlat et al. (2013) study, significance of within-group changes was not reported

[c]For the Schafer et al. (2012) study, subjects were treated with 6 months of PTH(1-84), either as one 6- or two 3-month courses, in combination with ibandronate over 2 years

Summary of within-group changes from baseline of trabecular density (trabecular vBMD or calculated BV/TV), cortical vBMD, and cortical thickness (Ct.Th) at the distal radius in HR-pQCT studies evaluating antiresorptive treatment

Table 10.2 Effect of antiresorptive therapy on trabecular and cortical density and cortical thickness at the distal tibia, as assessed in vivo by HR-pQCT

Study	Drug	Duration (months)	N	Age (years)	Distal tibia Tb.vBMD or BV/TV	Distal tibia Ct.vBMD	Distal tibia Ct.Th
Burghardt et al. (2010)	Alendronate	24	13	56±4	~ +1 to 2 %	NS	~ +3 to 4 %
	Placebo	24	20	56±2	NS	NS	NS
Rizzoli et al. (2012)	Alendronate	24	42	64±8	NS	NS	NS
	Strontium	24	41	64±8	+2.5±5.1 %	+1.4±2.8 %	+6.3±9.5 %
Seeman et al. (2010)	Alendronate	12	82	61±5	+0.5 to 1 %[a]	NS	+4 to 5 %[a]
	Denosumab	12	83	60±6	+1 to 1.5 %[a]	+0.5 to 1 %[a]	+5 to 6 %[a]
	Placebo	12	82	61±5	−0.5 to −1 %[a]	−0.5 to −1 %[a]	+1 to 2 %[a]
Chapurlat et al. (2013)[b]	Ibandronate	24	72	63±5	No difference between groups	Greater increase in ibandronate group	Greater increase in ibandronate
	Placebo	24	76	63±5			
Bala et al. (2014)	Risedronate (<55 year)	12	112	53±2	NS	−1.09±2.41	Not reported
	Placebo (<55 year)	12	49	53±2	NS	NS	Not reported
	Risedronate (>55 year)	12	109	62±6	NS	NS	Not reported
	Risedronate (>55 year)	12	54	61±4	+0.40±1.51	+0.50±1.68	Not reported
Hansen et al. (2013)	Zoledronic acid	18	33	70 (54–86)	+2.2 %±2.2 %	+1.5 %±2.0	+3.0±3.5 %
	PTH(1-34)	18	18	72 (59–80)	+3.3 %±5.7 %	−1.6 %±4.4	+3.8±10.4 %
	PTH(1-84)	18	20	70 (61–86)	NS	−4.7 %±4.5	−2.8±4.7 %
Cheung et al. (2014)	Odanacatib	24	109	64±7	2.27 %[a]	NS	+2.15 %[a]
	Placebo	24	105	64±6	+0.84[a]	−1.05 %[a]	−3.03 %[a]
Schafer et al. (2012)	Ibandronate and PTH(1-84)[c]	24	43	62±4	+3.22 % (2.35, 4.10)[a]	NS	NS
Tsai et al. (2014)	PTH(1-34)	12	31	66±8	NS	−1.6 %±1.9	NS
	Denosumab	12	33	66±8	+2.1 %±3.0	+0.9 %±1.2	+3.3 %±3.3
	Denosumab and PTH(1-34)	12	30	66±9	+1.6 %±2.8	+1.5 %±1.5	+5.4 %±3.9

NS not significant

Values are means±SD unless otherwise noted as [a]Least squares means, and if values reported, with 95 % CIs

[b]For the Chapurlat et al. (2013) study, significance of within-group changes was not reported

[c]For the Schafer et al. (2012) study, subjects were treated with 6 months of PTH(1-84), either as one 6- or two 3-month courses, in combination with ibandronate over 2 years

Summary of within-group changes from baseline for trabecular density (trabecular vBMD or calculated BV/TV), cortical vBMD, and cortical thickness (Ct.Th) at the distal tibia in HR-pQCT studies evaluating antiresorptive treatment

thickness, or porosity at the distal radius or distal tibia [50]. In contrast, in another study of postmenopausal women with low bone density who received 2 years of alendronate, Burghardt et al. reported an increase in cortical thickness at the distal tibia and no change in cortical vBMD at the distal tibia or cortical vBMD and thickness at the distal radius [49]. A similar pattern with cortical changes primarily observed at the distal tibia rather than the distal radius was also observed with ibandronate [48]. Specifically, in comparison to placebo, 2 years of ibandronate increase cortical vBMD and cortical thickness at the distal tibia but not at the distal radius. However, Seeman et al. reported that 2 years of alendronate increase cortical thickness without an increase in cortical vBMD at both the distal tibia and the distal radius [51]. Treatment with zoledronic acid for 18 months increased cortical vBMD and cortical thickness but had no effect on cortical porosity at the distal tibia, as assessed using the standard Scanco algorithm [53]. Similar to other studies, at the distal radius, zoledronic acid had no effect on cortical vBMD, thickness, or porosity [53].

Using the "segmentation-free" approach to assess cortical porosity, Zebaze et al. reported that alendronate treatment reduces porosity in the inner cortical transitional zone at 1 year relative to baseline but not relative to controls [46]. Bala et al. assessed the effect of 1 year of risedronate treatment in women younger and older than age 55. Risedronate increased cortical vBMD at the distal tibia in women older than 55, but not in the younger cohort. Change in cortical thickness was not reported, however, using the "segmentation-free" approach, risedronate treatment prevented the increase in cortical porosity seen in the placebo group in the compact-appearing cortex at the distal radius in postmenopausal women under age 55 [47].

Like bisphosphonate treatment, denosumab and odanacatib have a similar overall positive effect on cortical microarchitecture. In the placebo-controlled study by Seeman et al., 2 years of denosumab increased cortical thickness and cortical vBMD at the distal tibia and distal radius as assessed by HR-pQCT [51]. In this same cohort, using the non-thresholding method

to assess cortical porosity, 12 months of denosumab treatment reduced radial cortical porosity more than alendronate [46]. Using a different technique of QCT-based cortical thickness mapping, 3 years of denosumab increased femoral cortical thickness, relative to placebo [60]. Lastly, Cheung et al. reported that 2 years of odanacatib increase cortical thickness at both the distal radius and distal tibia, with increases in cortical vBMD seen only at the distal radius [52].

Effect of Combined Anabolic and Antiresorptive Therapy on Microarchitecture

Most recently, data from the first HR-pQCT longitudinal trials with combination therapy of anabolic and antiresorptive agents were published. In the PTH and Ibandronate Combination Study (PICS) by Schafer et al., postmenopausal women with low bone mass were treated with 6 months of PTH(1-84), either as one 6- or two 3-month courses, in combination with ibandronate over 2 years [61]. As results were similar between the two treatment groups, data from the two treatment arms were pooled together for analyses. Schafer et al. reported an increase in trabecular vBMD at both the distal radius and distal tibia, but a decrease in cortical thickness and cortical vBMD at the distal radius, though not at the distal tibia. Furthermore, cortical porosity increased at the distal tibia but not the distal radius.

In the Denosumab and Teriparatide Administration (DATA) study, postmenopausal women with osteoporosis were treated with 1 year of denosumab, PTH(1-34), or both [54]. The DATA study demonstrated that 1 year of combined denosumab and teriparatide improves distal tibia and radius cortical microarchitecture more than either treatment alone (Fig. 10.1). For example, cortical thickness at the distal tibia did not change in the teriparatide monotherapy group, but increased in both other groups. The increase in cortical thickness at the distal tibia was greater in the combination group (5.4 ± 3.9 %) than both monotherapy groups (teriparatide, −0.6 ± 4.7 %; denosumab, 3.7 ± 3.3 %).

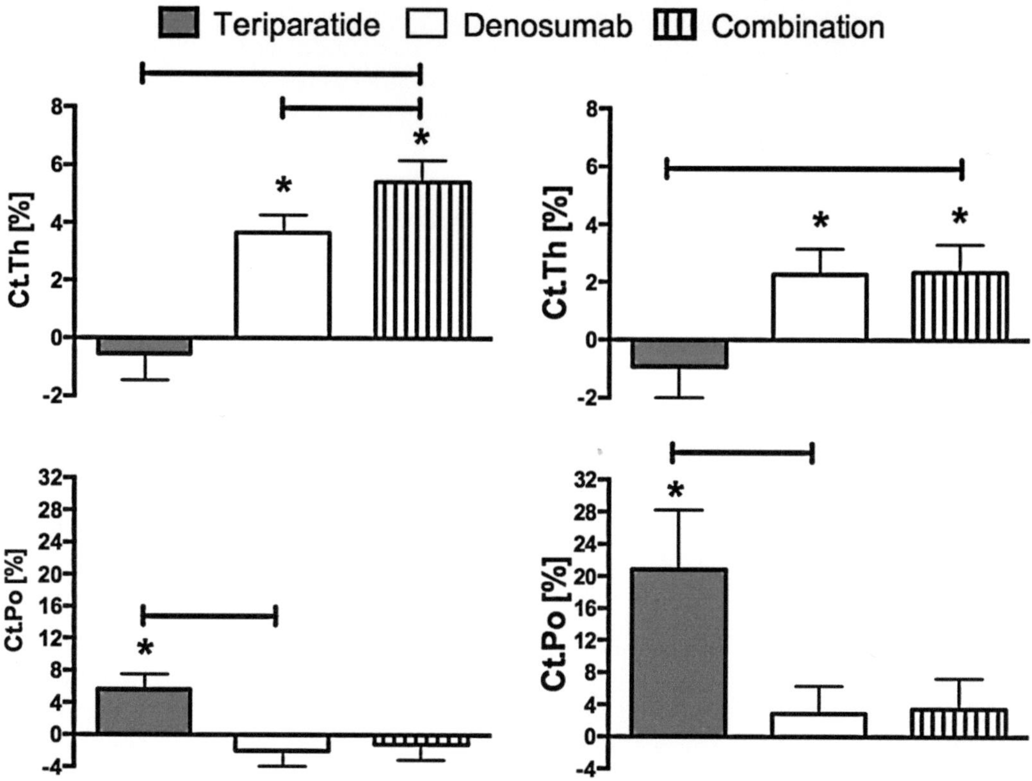

Fig. 10.1 Mean percent change (SEM) from baseline at distal tibia (*left*) and distal radius (*right*) in cortical thickness and cortical porosity at 12 months. $^*p$ value<0.05 versus baseline, bars represent p value<0.05 between groups. From Tsai JN, et al. Comparative Effects of Teriparatide, Denosumab, and Combination Therapy on Peripheral Compartmental Bone Density, Microarchitecture, and Estimated Strength: the DATA-HRpQCT Study. Journal of bone and mineral research : the official journal of the American Society for Bone and Mineral Research 2014;Epub 2014 Jul 7. Reprinted with permission from John Wiley and Sons

Additionally, cortical porosity did not change with combination therapy at either the distal tibia or distal radius. Consistent with Seeman et al. [51], the denosumab monotherapy group showed an increase in cortical thickness and cortical vBMD at both the distal tibia and distal radius in the DATA study.

Summary

Trabecular and cortical microarchitecture parameters are generally preserved or improved with antiresorptive therapy as evaluated by bone histomorphometry and ex vivo micro-CT of iliac crest biopsies and noninvasive methods with high-resolution imaging. Of note, a numerically greater effect and more consistent effect of antiresorptive therapy on microarchitecture as assessed by HR-pQCT are generally observed at the distal tibia in comparison to the distal radius. Beneficial effects that occur with weight bearing may, in part, explain this difference between skeletal sites, though differences in measurement precision between the two sites may also contribute to the reported differences.

There are several issues to consider when interpreting these findings. In particular, the cross-sectional design of several trials with bone histomorphometry severely limits interpretation of the effect of treatments on bone microarchitecture. Nonetheless, findings with histomorphometry were generally concordant with effects observed with longitudinal HR-pQCT trials.

Also, as previously discussed, detecting trabecular microarchitecture changes as assessed by HR-pQCT is limited by the image resolution available with current in vivo imaging methods. New imaging approaches with better resolution may be needed to determine whether trabecular microarchitecture changes following antiresorptive therapy. Lastly, motion artifact is a significant limitation of HR-pQCT, particularly at the distal radius. Thus, lack of significant changes detected at the distal radius may be reflective of this motion artifact limitation rather than a true lack of change in response to therapy.

Overall, the changes in trabecular and cortical microarchitecture parameters in response to the various antiresorptive treatments are favorable. In addition to demonstrating the differential effect of treatment on trabecular and cortical bone, these observed changes in microarchitecture in response to antiresorptive treatment may explain the anti-fracture benefit not captured by information obtained from standard DXA.

References[1]

1. Delmas PD. How does antiresorptive therapy decrease the risk of fracture in women with osteoporosis? Bone. 2000;27(1):1–3. PubMed.
2. Delmas PD, Seeman E. Changes in bone mineral density explain little of the reduction in vertebral or nonvertebral fracture risk with anti-resorptive therapy. Bone. 2004;34(4):599–604. PubMed.
3. Schuit SC, van der Klift M, Weel AE, de Laet CE, Burger H, Seeman E, et al. Fracture incidence and association with bone mineral density in elderly men and women: the Rotterdam study. Bone. 2004;34(1): 195–202. PubMed.
4. Siris ES, Miller PD, Barrett-Connor E, Faulkner KG, Wehren LE, Abbott TA, et al. Identification and fracture outcomes of undiagnosed low bone mineral density in postmenopausal women: results from the national osteoporosis risk assessment. JAMA. 2001;286(22):2815–22. PubMed.
5. Stone KL, Seeley DG, Lui LY, Cauley JA, Ensrud K, Browner WS, et al. BMD at multiple sites and risk of fracture of multiple types: long-term results from the study of osteoporotic fractures. J Bone Miner Res. 2003;18(11):1947–54. PubMed.
6. Black DM, Cummings SR, Karpf DB, Cauley JA, Thompson DE, Nevitt MC, et al. Randomised trial of effect of alendronate on risk of fracture in women with existing vertebral fractures. Fracture intervention trial research group. Lancet. 1996;348(9041):1535–41. PubMed.
7. Feldkamp LA, Goldstein SA, Parfitt AM, Jesion G, Kleerekoper M. The direct examination of three-dimensional bone architecture in vitro by computed tomography. J Bone Miner Res. 1989;4(1):3–11. PubMed.
8. Ruegsegger P, Koller B, Muller R. A microtomographic system for the nondestructive evaluation of bone architecture. Calcif Tissue Int. 1996;58(1):24–9. PubMed.
9. *Boutroy S, Bouxsein ML, Munoz F, Delmas PD. In vivo assessment of trabecular bone microarchitecture by high-resolution peripheral quantitative computed tomography. J Clin Endocrinol Metab. 2005;90(12): 6508–15. PubMed. *This cross-sectional study was the first to demonstrate that alterations of trabecular structure as measured by HR-pQCT discriminate between postmenopausal osteopenic women with and without a history of fragility fracture, whereas hip and spine areal BMD were no different between those with and without a history of fracture.*
10. *Khosla S, Riggs BL, Atkinson EJ, Oberg AL, McDaniel LJ, Holets M, et al. Effects of sex and age on bone microstructure at the ultradistal radius: a population-based noninvasive in vivo assessment. J Bone Miner Res. 2006;21(1):124–31. PubMed Pubmed Central PMCID: 1352156. *By examining differences in microarchitecture, this large population-based study proposes an explanation for the difference in age-related radial fracture risk between men and women.*
11. Parfitt AM, Drezner MK, Glorieux FH, Kanis JA, Malluche H, Meunier PJ, et al. Bone histomorphometry: standardization of nomenclature, symbols, and units. Report of the ASBMR histomorphometry nomenclature committee. J Bone Miner Res. 1987;2(6):595–610. PubMed.
12. Chavassieux PM, Arlot ME, Reda C, Wei L, Yates AJ, Meunier PJ. Histomorphometric assessment of the long-term effects of alendronate on bone quality and remodeling in patients with osteoporosis. J Clin Invest. 1997;100(6):1475–80. PubMed Pubmed Central PMCID: 508326.
13. Roschger P, Rinnerthaler S, Yates J, Rodan GA, Fratzl P, Klaushofer K. Alendronate increases degree and uniformity of mineralization in cancellous bone and decreases the porosity in cortical bone of osteoporotic women. Bone. 2001;29(2):185–91. PubMed.
14. Recker RR, Weinstein RS, Chesnut 3rd CH, Schimmer RC, Mahoney P, Hughes C, et al. Histomorphometric evaluation of daily and intermittent oral ibandronate in women with postmenopausal osteoporosis: results from the BONE study. Osteoporos Int. 2004;15(3): 231–7. PubMed.
15. Arlot M, Meunier PJ, Boivin G, Haddock L, Tamayo J, Correa-Rotter R, et al. Differential effects of

[1] *Important References
**Very important References

teriparatide and alendronate on bone remodeling in postmenopausal women assessed by histomorphometric parameters. J Bone Miner Res. 2005;20(7): 1244–53. PubMed.

16. Recker R, Masarachia P, Santora A, Howard T, Chavassieux P, Arlot M, et al. Trabecular bone microarchitecture after alendronate treatment of osteoporotic women. Curr Med Res Opin. 2005;21(2):185–94. PubMed.

17. Recker RR, Delmas PD, Halse J, Reid IR, Boonen S, Garcia-Hernandez PA, et al. Effects of intravenous zoledronic acid once yearly on bone remodeling and bone structure. J Bone Miner Res. 2008;23(1):6–16. PubMed.

18. Recker RR, Ste-Marie LG, Langdahl B, Masanauskaite D, Ethgen D, Delmas PD. Oral ibandronate preserves trabecular microarchitecture: micro-computed tomography findings from the oral iBandronate osteoporosis vertebral fracture trial in North America and Europe study. J Clin Densitom. 2009;12(1):71–6. PubMed.

19. Brixen K, Chapurlat R, Cheung AM, Keaveny TM, Fuerst T, Engelke K, et al. Bone density, turnover, and estimated strength in postmenopausal women treated with odanacatib: a randomized trial. J Clin Endocrinol Metab. 2013;98(2):571–80. PubMed.

20. Reid IR, Miller PD, Brown JP, Kendler DL, Fahrleitner-Pammer A, Valter I, et al. Effects of denosumab on bone histomorphometry: the FREEDOM and STAND studies. J Bone Miner Res. 2010;25(10):2256–65. PubMed Epub 2010/06/10. eng.

21. Bravenboer N, Papapoulos SE, Holzmann P, Hamdy NA, Netelenbos JC, Lips P. Bone histomorphometric evaluation of pamidronate treatment in clinically manifest osteoporosis. Osteoporos Int. 1999;9(6):489–93. PubMed.

22. Prestwood KM, Gunness M, Muchmore DB, Lu Y, Wong M, Raisz LG. A comparison of the effects of raloxifene and estrogen on bone in postmenopausal women. J Clin Endocrinol Metab. 2000;85(6):2197–202. PubMed.

23. Eriksen EF, Melsen F, Sod E, Barton I, Chines A. Effects of long-term risedronate on bone quality and bone turnover in women with postmenopausal osteoporosis. Bone. 2002;31(5):620–5. PubMed.

24. Ott SM, Oleksik A, Lu Y, Harper K, Lips P. Bone histomorphometric and biochemical marker results of a 2-year placebo-controlled trial of raloxifene in postmenopausal women. J Bone Miner Res. 2002;17(2):341–8. PubMed.

25. Dufresne TE, Chmielewski PA, Manhart MD, Johnson TD, Borah B. Risedronate preserves bone architecture in early postmenopausal women in 1 year as measured by three-dimensional microcomputed tomography. Calcif Tissue Int. 2003;73(5):423–32. PubMed.

26. Borah B, Dufresne TE, Chmielewski PA, Johnson TD, Chines A, Manhart MD. Risedronate preserves bone architecture in postmenopausal women with osteoporosis as measured by three-dimensional microcomputed tomography. Bone. 2004;34(4):736–46. PubMed.

27. Ste-Marie LG, Sod E, Johnson T, Chines A. Five years of treatment with risedronate and its effects on bone safety in women with postmenopausal osteoporosis. Calcif Tissue Int. 2004;75(6):469–76. PubMed.

28. Borah B, Dufresne T, Nurre J, Phipps R, Chmielewski P, Wagner L, et al. Risedronate reduces intracortical porosity in women with osteoporosis. J Bone Miner Res. 2010;25(1):41–7. PubMed.

29. Borah B, Dufresne TE, Ritman EL, Jorgensen SM, Liu S, Chmielewski PA, et al. Long-term risedronate treatment normalizes mineralization and continues to preserve trabecular architecture: sequential triple biopsy studies with micro-computed tomography. Bone. 2006;39(2):345–52. PubMed.

30. Ulrich D, Rietbergen B, Laib A, Ruegsegger P. Mechanical analysis of bone and its microarchitecture based on in vivo voxel images. Technol Health Care. 1998;6(5–6):421–7. PubMed.

31. *Cheung AM, Adachi JD, Hanley DA, Kendler DL, Davison KS, Josse R, et al. High-resolution peripheral quantitative computed tomography for the assessment of bone strength and structure: a review by the Canadian bone strength working group. Current Osteoporos Rep. 2013;11(2):136–46. PubMed Pubmed Central PMCID: 3641288. *This is an excellent review of HR-pQCT for assessment of bone microarchitecture in vivo.

32. Boutroy S, Van Rietbergen B, Sornay-Rendu E, Munoz F, Bouxsein ML, Delmas PD. Finite element analysis based on in vivo HR-pQCT images of the distal radius is associated with wrist fracture in postmenopausal women. J Bone Miner Res. 2008;23(3):392–9. PubMed.

33. *Liu XS, Stein EM, Zhou B, Zhang CA, Nickolas TL, Cohen A, et al. Individual trabecula segmentation (ITS)-based morphological analyses and microfinite element analysis of HR-pQCT images discriminate postmenopausal fragility fractures independent of DXA measurements. J Bone Miner Res. 2012;27(2):263–72. PubMed Pubmed Central PMCID: 3290758. *This case-control study demonstrates the utility of advanced individual trabecular segmentation (ITS), independent of DXA BMD measurements, to discriminate fracture subjects from controls..

34. Melton 3rd LJ, Christen D, Riggs BL, Achenbach SJ, Muller R, van Lenthe GH, et al. Assessing forearm fracture risk in postmenopausal women. Osteoporos Int. 2010;21(7):1161–9. PubMed Pubmed Central PMCID: 2889027.

35. Nishiyama KK, Macdonald HM, Hanley DA, Boyd SK. Women with previous fragility fractures can be classified based on bone microarchitecture and finite element analysis measured with HR-pQCT. Osteoporos Int. 2013;24(5):1733–40. PubMed.

36. Pialat JB, Vilayphiou N, Boutroy S, Gouttenoire PJ, Sornay-Rendu E, Chapurlat R, et al. Local topological analysis at the distal radius by HR-pQCT: application to in vivo bone microarchitecture and fracture assessment in the OFELY study. Bone. 2012;51(3): 362–8. PubMed.

37. **Sornay-Rendu E, Boutroy S, Chapurlat R. Bone Microarchitecture assessed by HR-pQCT as predictor of fracture risk in postmenopausal women: the OFELY study. J Bone Miner Metab Res. 2014;29 Suppl 1. ** *This recently presented abstract is the first study to prospectively show the utility of bone microarchitecture measurements by HR-pQCT for fracture risk assessment.*

38. Rozental TD, Deschamps LN, Taylor A, Earp B, Zurakowski D, Day CS, et al. Premenopausal women with a distal radial fracture have deteriorated trabecular bone density and morphology compared with controls without a fracture. J Bone Joint Surg Am. 2013;95(7):633–42. PubMed Pubmed Central PMCID: 3748976.

39. Sornay-Rendu E, Boutroy S, Munoz F, Delmas PD. Alterations of cortical and trabecular architecture are associated with fractures in postmenopausal women, partially independent of decreased BMD measured by DXA: the OFELY study. J Bone Miner Res. 2007;22(3):425–33. PubMed.

40. Sornay-Rendu E, Cabrera-Bravo JL, Boutroy S, Munoz F, Delmas PD. Severity of vertebral fractures is associated with alterations of cortical architecture in postmenopausal women. J Bone Miner Res. 2009;24(4):737–43. PubMed.

41. Stein EM, Liu XS, Nickolas TL, Cohen A, Thomas V, McMahon DJ, et al. Abnormal microarchitecture and stiffness in postmenopausal women with ankle fractures. J Clin Endocrinol Metab. 2011;96(7):2041–8. PubMed Pubmed Central PMCID: 3135193.

42. Vico L, Zouch M, Amirouche A, Frere D, Laroche N, Koller B, et al. High-resolution pQCT analysis at the distal radius and tibia discriminates patients with recent wrist and femoral neck fractures. J Bone Miner Res. 2008;23(11):1741–50. PubMed.

43. Burghardt AJ, Kazakia GJ, Ramachandran S, Link TM, Majumdar S. Age- and gender-related differences in the geometric properties and biomechanical significance of intracortical porosity in the distal radius and tibia. J Bone Miner Res. 2010;25(5):983–93. PubMed Pubmed Central PMCID: 3153365.

44. Nishiyama KK, Macdonald HM, Buie HR, Hanley DA, Boyd SK. Postmenopausal women with osteopenia have higher cortical porosity and thinner cortices at the distal radius and tibia than women with normal aBMD: an in vivo HR-pQCT study. J Bone Miner Res. 2010;25(4):882–90. PubMed.

45. *Zebaze R, Ghasem-Zadeh A, Mbala A, Seeman E. A new method of segmentation of compact-appearing, transitional and trabecular compartments and quantification of cortical porosity from high resolution peripheral quantitative computed tomographic images. Bone. 2013;54(1):8–20. PubMed. *This study introduces a new approach to assess intracortical porosity. Using a non-thresholding or "segmentation-free" method, this approach distinguishes cortical bone from trabecular bone and is unique in defining an inner and outer transitional zone.*

46. Zebaze RM, Libanati C, Austin M, Ghasem-Zadeh A, Hanley DA, Zanchetta JR, et al. Differing effects of denosumab and alendronate on cortical and trabecular bone. Bone. 2014;59:173–9. PubMed.

47. Bala Y, Chapurlat R, Cheung AM, Felsenberg D, LaRoche M, Morris E, et al. Risedronate slows or partly reverses cortical and trabecular microarchitectural deterioration in postmenopausal women. J Bone Miner Res. 2014;29(2):380–8. PubMed.

48. Chapurlat RD, Laroche M, Thomas T, Rouanet S, Delmas PD, de Vernejoul MC. Effect of oral monthly ibandronate on bone microarchitecture in women with osteopenia-a randomized placebo-controlled trial. Osteoporos Int. 2013;24(1):311–20. PubMed.

49. Burghardt AJ, Kazakia GJ, Sode M, de Papp AE, Link TM, Majumdar S. A longitudinal HR-pQCT study of alendronate treatment in postmenopausal women with low bone density: relations among density, cortical and trabecular microarchitecture, biomechanics, and bone turnover. J Bone Miner Res. 2010;25(12):2558–71. PubMed Pubmed Central PMCID: 3179276.

50. Rizzoli R, Chapurlat RD, Laroche JM, Krieg MA, Thomas T, Frieling I, et al. Effects of strontium ranelate and alendronate on bone microstructure in women with osteoporosis. Results of a 2-year study. Osteoporos Int. 2012;23(1):305–15. PubMed.

51. **Seeman E, Delmas PD, Hanley DA, Sellmeyer D, Cheung AM, Shane E, et al. Microarchitectural deterioration of cortical and trabecular bone: differing effects of denosumab and alendronate. J Bone Miner Res. 2010;25(8):1886–94. PubMed. ***This placebo-controlled trial is the first longitudinal study to describe effects of antiresorptive treatment on bone microarchitecture as assessed in vivo by HR-pQCT. This study is one of the first multi-center trials conducted with HR-pQCT..*

52. Cheung AM, Majumdar S, Brixen K, Chapurlat R, Fuerst T, Engelke K, et al. Effects of odanacatib on the radius and tibia of postmenopausal women: improvements in bone geometry, microarchitecture, and estimated bone strength. J Bone Miner Res. 2014;29(8):1786–94. PubMed.

53. Hansen S, Hauge EM, Beck Jensen JE, Brixen K. Differing effects of PTH 1-34, PTH 1-84, and zoledronic acid on bone microarchitecture and estimated strength in postmenopausal women with osteoporosis: an 18-month open-labeled observational study using HR-pQCT. J Bone Miner Res. 2013;28(4):736–45. PubMed.

54. *Tsai JN, Uihlein AV, Burnett-Bowie SA, Neer RM, Zhu Y, Derrico N, et al. Comparative effects of teriparatide, denosumab, and combination therapy on peripheral compartmental bone density, microarchitecture, and estimated strength: the DATA-HRpQCT study. J Bone Miner Res. 2014; Epub 2014 Jul 7. *This is the first clinical trial to assess the effects of combination therapy—denosumab plus PTH, compared to either therapy alone—on bone microarchitecture, assessed by HR-pQCT.*

55. Tjong W, Kazakia GJ, Burghardt AJ, Majumdar S. The effect of voxel size on high-resolution peripheral computed tomography measurements of trabecular and cortical bone microstructure. Med Phys. 2012;39(4):1893–903. PubMed Pubmed Central PMCID: 3316694.

56. Ellouz R, Chapurlat R, van Rietbergen B, Christen P, Pialat JB, Boutroy S. Challenges in longitudinal measurements with HR-pQCT: evaluation of a 3D registration method to improve bone microarchitecture and strength measurement reproducibility. Bone. 2014;63:147–57. PubMed.

57. Nishiyama KK, Pauchard Y, Nikkel LE, Iyer S, Zhang C, McMahon DJ, et al. Longitudinal HR-pQCT and image registration detects endocortical bone loss in kidney transplantation patients. J Bone Miner Res. 2014;11:554–61. PubMed.

58. *Liu XS, Sajda P, Saha PK, Wehrli FW, Bevill G, Keaveny TM, et al. Complete volumetric decomposition of individual trabecular plates and rods and its morphological correlations with anisotropic elastic moduli in human trabecular bone. J Bone Miner Res. 2008;23(2):223–35. PubMed Pubmed Central PMCID: 2665696. *This study utilizes an advanced method to assess trabecular morphology (plates or rods). This technique has the potential to improve non-invasive assessment of trabecular microarchitecture changes in response to treatment.

59. Nishiyama KK, Cohen A, Young P, Wang J, Lappe JM, Guo XE, et al. Teriparatide increases strength of the peripheral skeleton in premenopausal women with idiopathic osteoporosis: a pilot HR-pQCT study. J Clin Endocrinol Metab. 2014;99(7):2418–25. PubMed Pubmed Central PMCID: 4079304.

60. Poole, KE, Treece GM, Gee AH, Brown JP, McClung MR, Wang A, et al. Denosumab rapidly increases cortical bone in key locations of the femur: a 3D bone mapping study in women with osteoporosis. J Bone Miner Res. 2015;30(1):46–54.

61. Schafer AL, Burghardt AJ, Sellmeyer DE, Palermo L, Shoback DM, Majumdar S, et al. Postmenopausal women treated with combination parathyroid hormone (1-84) and ibandronate demonstrate different microstructural changes at the radius vs. tibia: the PTH and ibandronate combination study (PICS). Osteoporos Int. 2013;24(10):2591–601. PubMed.

Management of Atypical Femoral Fractures

11

Joseph M. Lane, Libi Z. Galmer, David S. Wellman, Abigail L. Campbell, and Jonathan E. Jo

Summary

- Atypical fractures account for a very small percentage of hip and femur fractures.
- Bilateral radiographic findings are encountered 20–40 % of the time, so very important to assess both sides.
- Atypical fractures are typically seen in women with history of at least 8 years of bisphosphonate use.
- History of prior antiresorptive therapy is the most important factor, as the half-life can be up to 10 years.

- Key imaging findings include cortical thickening, marrow edema, or beaking of the cortex.
- Metabolic bone laboratory work-up should be done on all patients; vitamin D and calcium supplemented if low, and bone turnover state assessed with NTX.
- There is some evidence to suggest that anabolic agents such as teriparatide may be useful in the treatment of incomplete fractures.
- For complete deformities, careful examination of anatomy and varus deformity of the femur is crucial to successful reduction and surgical repair.
- Nonunion is a common complication and may warrant revision surgery or further augmentation.
- Incomplete fractures typically present with several months of prodromal pain, but approximately 2 % may be asymptomatic.
- Incomplete fractures with marrow edema on MRI and identifiable fracture line should be treated with surgical fixation with intramedullary nailing for stabilization.
- Patients with fracture line but no marrow edema may be treated conservatively.

J.M. Lane, MD (✉) • L.Z. Galmer, DO
Metabolic Bone Disease Service, Orthopaedics,
Hospital for Special Surgery, 535 E. 70th St.,
New York, NY 10021, USA
e-mail: lanej@hss.edu

D.S. Wellman, MD
Orthopaedic Surgery, Hospital for Special Surgery,
New York Presbyterian Hospital, New York, NY, USA

Orthopaedic Surgery, Weill Cornell Medical College,
New York, NY, USA

A.L. Campbell, MD, MSc, BSE
Orthopaedic Surgery, NYU Hospital for Joint Diseases,
New York, NY, USA

J.E. Jo, BS
Orthopaedic Surgery, Weill Cornell Medical College,
New York, NY, USA

Atypical femoral fractures are relatively uncommon; however, in the setting of a geriatric fracture service, these fractures are encountered regularly. Subtrochanteric and diaphyseal fractures account for approximately 5–10 % of all hip/femur fractures. Of these, only about 17–29 %

© Springer International Publishing Switzerland 2016
S.L. Silverman, B. Abrahamsen (eds.), *The Duration and Safety of Osteoporosis Treatment*, DOI 10.1007/978-3-319-23639-1_11

are classified as atypical [1]. In addition, the high association of bilateral radiographic findings in the order of 20–40 % depending on the series suggests that silent incomplete fractures will also be encountered during thorough evaluation [1, 2].

Other chapters of this monograph have clearly stated the demographics, the purported etiology, and diagnostic hallmarks. The purpose of this chapter is to address the evaluation and both the medical and orthopedic management of complete and incomplete atypical femoral fractures.

The organization for this section is divided into recognition and work-up followed by the treatment of complete fractures and finally the discussion of the more controversial topic incomplete fractures.

Recognition and Work-Up

The recognition of atypical fractures is critical for prompt management. With that consideration, the American Society for Bone and Mineral Research (ASBMR) assembled a task force consisting of multidisciplinary experts to review the pathogenesis, presenting symptomology, and early diagnostic work-up of these fractures [1]. Additionally, clinical studies have evaluated various risk factors and the laboratory data to aid in the diagnosis [3]. In these reports, atypical fractures were more commonly seen in women who are younger than those presenting with typical femoral fractures [1, 3]. The women who suffer atypical femur fractures also have a tendency to relatively healthy with active lifestyles and a history of 8 years of bisphosphonate use on average [4].

Up to 70 % of patients will present with a prodromal period which can last several weeks and even up to a year of thigh pain [1]. It may not be constant, but it is often aggravated by increased activity. The vagueness of the actual pain can be confusing to the physician and is often thought to be related to sciatica, bursitis, or hip arthritis. X-rays of the spine as well as detailed imaging including MRI will often show degenerative arthritis or old residual herniated disks, spinal stenosis, facet arthropathy, or possibly impingement of an exiting nerve root. This often will mislead the physician into suspecting that this is in fact related to radiculopathy and often these patients are treated with epidural or other steroid injections, which can worsen their underlying osteoporosis [5]. Secondly, the diagnosis can often be confusing to the patient and physician, as radiographs to evaluate hip arthritis are typically narrow field and do not capture sufficient length of the femur to elucidate the underlying fracture. These patients will often be started in a physical therapy program directed at arthritis and may miss the opportunity for recognition of these fractures. There is some suggestion that nonsteroidals commonly used for symptomatic relief in arthritis negatively impact fracture healing. When the fracture occurs, it is most often a low-energy event. The patient may report a low-energy small fall from a low height, though a number of these fractures have occurred spontaneously with just twisting motions or changing positions and are followed by the patient falling. During subsequent evaluation, when one couples the transverse nature of the fracture line with the level of energy, the physician should immediately recognize that this is a pathological fracture and requires a more detailed history and evaluation.

The critical elements for the history would involve recognition that the patient may have had osteoporosis or osteopenia that has been treated with antiresorptive therapy in the past. Additional contributing drugs include corticosteroids, long-term nonsteroidals, and proton-pump inhibitors, among others that will be discussed in greater detail in latter chapters.

The most important is the history of prior antiresorptive therapy, since these medications can persist for many years and some having a half-life as long as 10 years [6, 7]. The patient may have stopped the drug a year or two prior to the fracture, and she and her physician may not recognize the association. Careful detailed questions pointing to both the use of antiresorptive agents and the use of steroids and other underlying medical issues that can enhance this process should be carefully performed.

Laboratory tests for patients with these fractures should be directed to preparing the patient for surgery, and this would include a complete chemical profile, CBC, PT, APTT, and coagulation profile, and then some specific assays should include 25-hydroxy vitamin D, intact PTH, and bone markers (urine NTX or serum CTX). Once the surgery has been accomplished, these assays are often diluted due to administration of IV fluids and can be difficult to interpret. Since almost a third of the patients had a prodromal event or partial fracture predating the actual fracture, the bone markers are often elevated. However, if the patient has a very low CTX and NTX despite the fracture, that would be supportive of a low bone turnover state.

The ASBMR task force released a second report addressing additional diagnostic features with detailed descriptions of radiographic findings [26]. They recommend imaging to include at least classical AP and lateral radiographs of the femur as well as the contralateral femur, since at least 28 % of patients have been found to have contralateral radiographic findings [1, 26]. Radiographs should span from the hip to the knee. If there is significant deformity of the femur due to the fracture, mild traction may be beneficial, also allowing the physician to better examine the nature of the fracture line. It is often quite obvious that it should meet the criteria for the second ASBMR task force on atypical femoral fractures [1]. X-ray of the contralateral leg may not be as diagnostic. Some patients may have had a prior fracture that has completely healed and is currently inactive. Any prominence of the femur or cortical thickening should be followed up with further imaging including an MRI with STIR sequence to determine the acuity of the fracture. Marrow edema would suggest that this is an ongoing fracture, while the absence of marrow edema and pain would suggest that this may be inactive or partially healed fracture. In reviewing incomplete fractures, a CT scan is often successful in identifying a clear fracture line that has prognostication as to increased risk of fracture and inability to fully heal spontaneously. Finally, a bone density should have been obtained at some time prior to the fracture or in the early perioperative phase to determine the direction of further therapy. Many of these patients with atypical fractures will in fact have osteopenia, or it may

have been corrected to a normal bone mass from prolonged bisphosphonate therapy. This documentation should be carried out as part of the preoperative evaluation as well as review of other fragility fracture history. Further X-rays of these sites may be necessary to define the nature of the osteoporosis.

The medical management of patients with atypical femoral fractures has not been formalized. Clearly, calcium and the vitamin D intake should be addressed at the very least. Since fracture healing is going to be a significant consideration, it is important to bring the calcium to a normal level, which is somewhere in the order of the 9.5 mg/dl with a target parathyroid hormone (PTH) level between 20 and 50 pg/ml. High PTHs would be suggestive of secondary hyperparathyroidism and indicate that calcium intake may be limited. On the other hand, a very low PTH might suggest that the patient has been oversupplemented with calcium. There is concern over too much calcium intake, particularly if there is history of cardiovascular disease [8]. In terms of vitamin D, the Institute of Medicine has recommended levels of at least 20 ng/ml to be adequate [9]; however, most other organizations have supported values of at least 32 ng/ml [10, 11]. While fracture healing can occur at 30 ng/ml, higher doses of vitamin D may be helpful for the muscular elements [10]. A number of studies have suggested that the higher levels of vitamin D may be translated into better function with less falls [12, 13], so vitamin D somewhere in the order of 40 ng/ml may be more optimal. To achieve this dose patients may either receive 50,000 units of vitamin D twice a week, then lowered when corrected, or start with 6000 IU of vitamin D3 daily and adjusted when vitamin D has achieved the desired level. This often will only take 2–3 weeks at most.

Many questions regarding osteoporotic management have yet to be resolved. Richard Dell, MD of Kaiser Permanente, presented unpublished data at the 2012 Orthopedic Research Society meeting showing that persistence of bisphosphonate use has led to high level of contralateral fractures and that this incidence can be reduced by over 50 % by discontinuing the bisphosphonate. Controversy remains as to whether or not an anabolic agent would be indicated in treatment of these fractures. There have been several studies on fracture healing and in spine fusion using PTH analogs. The study by Aspenberg's group suggests that in Colles' fractures, the osteoporotic dose of 20 μg per day led to about a 1–2-week earlier healing but that doubling the dose to 40 μg was actually no more effective [14]. In Europe, Peischl's group addressed pelvic fractures using repetitive CT scan as their markers of success, and by adding PTH 1-84 and 100 μg^{-1} per day, they were able to demonstrate improvement in healing rates at 2 months from approximately 10 % with calcium and vitamin D alone to 100 % by adding the PTH [15]. This was a semi-randomized controlled study but it had great impact. Further information suggests that the anabolic agents may be beneficial in the spine fusion realm. Ohtori demonstrated that PTH 1-34 given to spine fusion patients led to a higher fusion rate and less instrumentation pull out compared to the non-treated group [16]. In addition, that study compared the use of anabolic agents to bisphosphonates, and the risedronate appears to be comparable to the control population and did not lead to inhibition. The general evolution today is leading toward (1) stopping the bisphosphonates and (2) to seriously consider an anabolic agent to augment healing of these atypical fractures. The data still remains to be resolved at this time.

Complete Atypical Femoral Fractures

Atypical femoral fractures typically occur in the subtrochanteric or diaphyseal area of the femur with a transverse or short oblique fracture line; other features of the fracture include a lack of comminution and thickening of the cortices at the fracture site [17]. These patients have clinical and radiographic evidence of preexisting stress fractures. Most report about 6 months of prodromal pain prior to the fracture event [18]. Strict adherence to surgical principles is critical in this patient population as the fracture healing is slower in the

setting of bisphosphonates. Complications such as delayed union, nonunion, and implant failure are much higher in atypical femur fractures, with up to 46 % of patients requiring revision surgery [18–20] (Fig. 11.1).

Complete fractures are treated most commonly with intramedullary devices; more proximal fractures that are difficult to control with nails are considered for plating [20]. When selecting intramedullary fixation, surgeons must be very careful with the choice of device as fracture union is not as reliable as in the patient without bisphosphonate exposure. Problems with outcomes from atypical fracture nailing can be attributed in part to start point selection, nail design, and shaft/nail mismatch.

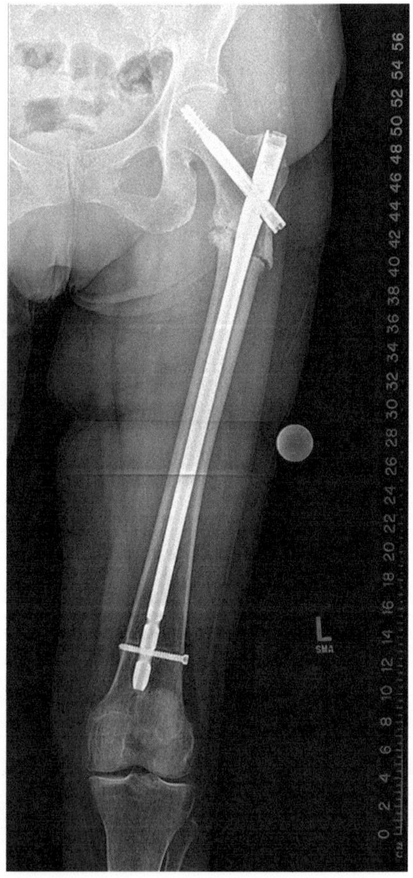

Fig. 11.1 Atypical femur fracture treated with intramedullary nail showing sclerotic margins consistent with nonunion

The insertion point of the nail can be the piriformis fossa or the greater trochanter, and the design of the nail may or may not allow for fixation into the neck. Extension of fixation into the neck (cephalomedullary nailing) theoretically extends the length of bone protected by the device and alleviates the concern of initiating a secondary femoral neck or basal fracture (as with a piriformis entry nail). The difficulty with cephalomedullary devices, however, is that the patients have a thickened proximal cortex and a narrowed canal. The large size of the proximal part of the nail encounters the thickened cortex on insertion and may force a proximal fracture into a varus deformity. If left malreduced, healing time and outcome results suffer significantly in this patient population [18]. In addition to varus deformity, iatrogenic fracture of the proximal femur on nail insertion is more common in patients with atypical fractures [20]. If selecting a greater trochanteric start point, surgeons should stay medial on the trochanter with the guidewire to decrease the chances of this complication, as well as help prevent a varus malreduction. High subtrochanteric fractures may require piriformis nails to avoid the varus driving force that is present in greater trochanteric entry cephalomedullary devices; plate and screw constructs are also a viable option in these difficult patterns.

Once start point and device have been carefully selected, obtaining and maintaining an anatomic reduction are paramount to the success of treatment in atypical femur fractures [18]. If any evidence of malreduction exists after closed reduction attempts, surgeons should be prepared to perform an open reduction, whether on a fracture table or a flat radiolucent table. Reductions should be maintained after passing the guidewire; this leads to symmetrical reaming of the proximal and distal segments of the fracture. Reaming with a malreduction in place reinforces the poor alignment and may prevent future attempts to restore anatomy. As reaming progresses, over-reaming the canal beyond the typical 1.5 mm may be necessary to have ample room for the proximal component of the nail. Over-reaming also helps if there is bowing of the femur. Matching the femur to the curve of the nail is critical to prevent anterior perforation of the shaft on nail insertion. Femoral bowing is related to age and ethnicity; Asian populations in particular have been found to have shorter radii of curvature [21, 22].

The postoperative course with intramedullary devices should allow the patient to bear weight as soon as comfortable. Calcium, vitamin D, and perhaps anabolic agent should be started. There is evidence in the literature that administration of a bone-forming agent such as teriparatide in the postoperative course leads to faster union times [14, 15, 23]. Bisphosphonate drugs should be stopped. The opposite femur should be continuously monitored secondary to the increasing weight requirements in the setting of a healing contralateral limb. Atypical fractures have occurred even when the original screening X-rays were negative at the time of the contralateral fracture.

If there is a delay in healing, further augmentation or revision surgery may be warranted. The Hernigou technique, which applies mesenchymal stem cells possibly coupled with an anabolic agent, or a formal bone grafting procedure can be tried in the setting of delayed union [24]. There is no evidence to suggest that BMP will augment delayed union in this group of patients. If the patient shows no progressive bone formation over a 3-month period, they are diagnosed with nonunion. Usually, the nonunion appears atrophic without appreciable callous formation, likely secondary to the metabolic derangements in the setting of bisphosphonates. Infection should always be considered, and cultures should always be taken at the time of revision. Options for treatment include exchange nailing of the femur or conversion to a plate and screw construct (Fig. 11.2). In either setting, the ability of the body to produce bone, not just the hardware, needs revision and augmentation. Locally, bone grafting should be used to enhance the regional environment; systemically, ensuring proper calcium and vitamin D levels along with consideration for anabolic pharmacologic therapy optimizes the systemic bone-forming capability of the patient.

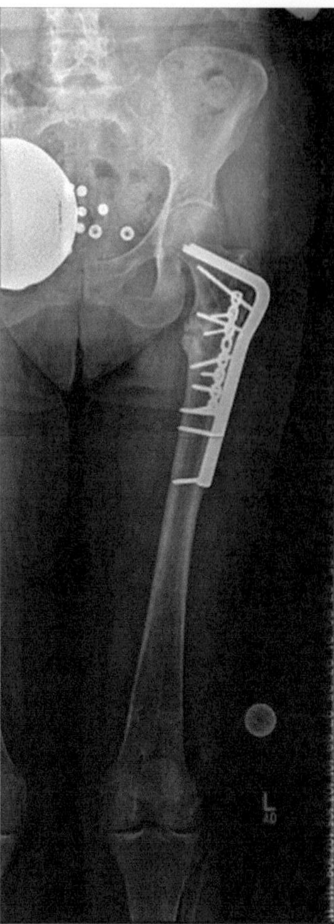

Fig. 11.2 The patient has undergone revision surgery for prior nonunion with blade plate and screws. Also treated with Forteo postoperatively with evidence of periosteal bridging and callous formation

From a surgical standpoint, both exchange nailing and conversion to a plate and screw construct have pitfalls. Exchange nailing should only be considered in the setting of anatomic alignment in the diaphysis. Varus deformity, even if subtle, lengthens the healing time and is a risk factor for nonunion [18]. Correcting a varus nonunion deformity of the proximal femur after a cephalomedullary nailing procedure with an exchange nailing is dangerous because the varus positioning often persists; the new nail falls into the same reamed track as the first device. In the setting of a varus deformity, blade plating with correction of deformity and compression across the fracture is a better option. Bone grafting and systemic anabolic medication should be employed as discussed above. Compression is usually gained through an articulated tensioning device, as the fracture often has a near transverse plane. The downside of plating is the lengthy period of weight-bearing restriction that follows; 3 months of non-weight bearing is advised with plates secondary to lengthy expected union times. Because of this delay, a second plate orthogonal to the first may be added to give additional fixation and torque control to the construct. There is no data as to whether further augmentation with allograft struts would be beneficial at this period of time.

Incomplete Fractures

Patients with an incomplete atypical femoral fracture commonly present with several months of prodromal thigh pain similar to an initial atypical fracture. Prompt diagnosis and management of an incomplete fracture are critical to prevent progression to a complete fracture. However, because approximately 2 % of asymptomatic patients on greater than 3 years of bisphosphonate treatment may have incomplete atypical femoral fractures, careful radiographic screening must be performed in patients with histories of long-term bisphosphonate use [25].

Clinical imaging provides diagnostic information that is essential in planning a treatment strategy. On plain radiographs, the lateral femoral cortex characteristically shows focal thickening as a consequence of the underlying stress reaction (Fig. 11.3). Additionally, a transverse radiolucent line may or may not be present [26]. The presence of this finding, known as the "dreaded black line," portends a poor prognosis for spontaneous healing and suggests the impending progression to complete fracture. MRI and CT can also be used both as a confirmatory test and to detect fracture line, bone marrow, and periosteal edema indicative of an active stress reaction (Fig. 11.4) [26]. Collectively, these radiographic findings can guide whether to manage conservatively or to surgically intervene.

Symptomatic patients presenting with pain, a transverse radiolucent line on plain film, and bone marrow edema on MRI are unlikely to improve

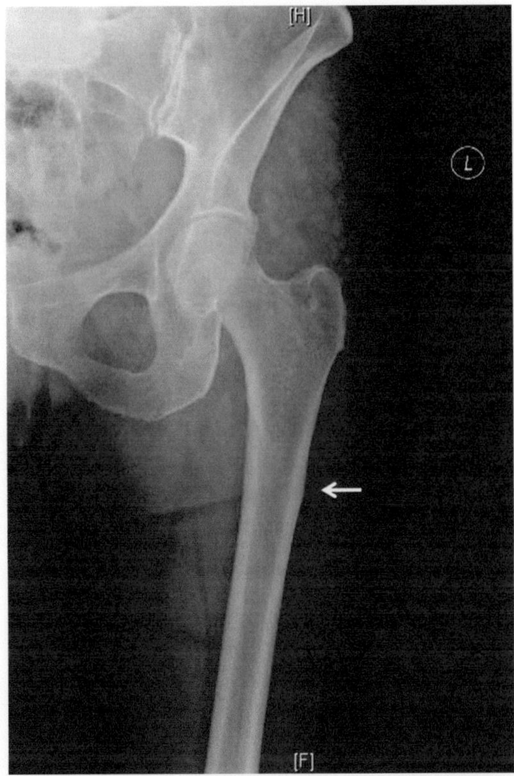

Fig. 11.3 X-ray of the left femur showing thickening of cortex indicative of bisphosphonate-related incomplete fracture

with conservative medical therapy. When managed conservatively, these patients are likely to have persistent pain, poor radiographic evidence of healing, and a high probability of fracture completion within one year. One level III study focused solely on patients with incomplete atypical femoral fractures and saw improved clinical outcomes with prophylactic surgery compared to medical management [27]. Surgical fixation via intramedullary nailing is the recommended treatment due to the high rate of union and rare progression to complete fracture [27–30].

Certain considerations must be addressed regarding surgical technique. Because the fracture is incomplete, it is critical that the nail entry port be on the medial aspect of the trochanter. Furthermore, due to the difficulty in aligning the nail with the anatomic bow of the femur, the medullary canal must be over-reamed to limit nail deformity upon insertion. Over-reaming

also helps to decrease the risk of intraoperative comminuted fracture during nail placement, which is the most common complication of this procedure. Postoperatively, the medical management of these patients is identical to that of complete atypical femoral fractures.

There is no consensus treatment strategy for symptomatic patients without a fracture line who have bone marrow edema on MRI. Conservative medical management may be effective but is highly controversial due to insufficient evidence and the concern for fracture completion [27, 30, 31]. Nonsurgical treatment consists of immediate cessation of the bisphosphonate, calcium, and vitamin D supplementation to correct any abnormalities and non-weight-bearing restriction. There are conflicting reports regarding the use of an anabolic agent such as teriparatide, which may facilitate healing and improve bone quality [32, 33]. Studies supporting the use of teriparatide saw increased bone activity in fragility fractures of the distal radius and tibia compared to conservative or surgical management, which indicates a potential pharmacologic intervention to treat these fractures [33]. Patients managed conservatively must be closely monitored because of the risk for fracture progression. An MRI should be repeated after 2–3 months to assess for diminution of marrow edema. If no improvement is seen on imaging or there is persistent pain, prophylactic intramedullary nailing should be considered. However, conservative therapy should be continued if there is an interval decrease in bone marrow edema and pain reduction. Full weight bearing can be resumed upon complete resolution of marrow edema and pain improvement to less than two out of ten on the visual analog scale. When managed conservatively, incomplete fractures can take up to 1–2 years to fully heal. Patients who are unwilling to endure a prolonged period of limited activity, reduced weight bearing, and medical therapy should be considered for intramedullary fixation.

Asymptomatic patients with the "dreaded black line" on plain film but without marrow edema on MRI can be managed nonoperatively. They should be placed on a regimen of anabolic agents for at least 1 year and advised initially to limit physical activity. After 3 months of treatment, they can

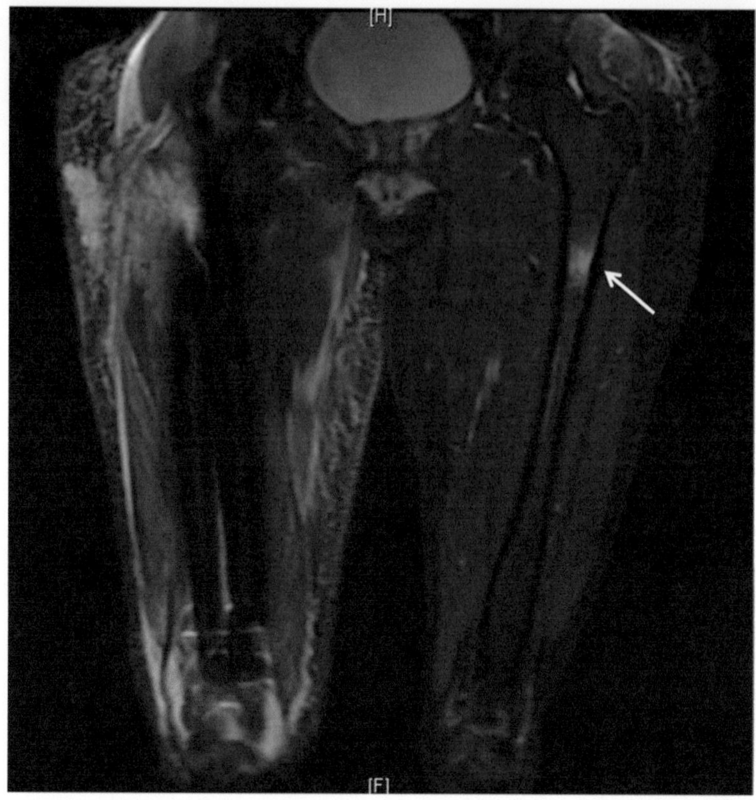

Fig. 11.4 Impending atypical femur fracture demonstrating bone marrow edema pattern on fat suppressed MRI

gradually increase their activity level and may resume sporting activities after 6 months.

Lastly, asymptomatic patients without a transverse radiolucency or marrow edema and patients with healed fractures should be placed on a drug holiday. The use of an anabolic agent should be discussed and normal physical activities can be permitted. However, high-contact activities should be avoided for the duration of any treatment.

The ultimate goal in managing incomplete atypical femoral fractures is preventing the progression to complete fractures. The clinical implications are tremendous, as the surgical treatment of incomplete fractures is less complicated than with complete lesions and has been associated with higher success rates, shorter hospital stays, and more rapid recovery compared to complete atypical femoral fractures [34]. The evidence discussed here suggests that clinical suspicion must be high and the physician providing care for patients on bisphosphonate treatment should consider these lesions even in asymptomatic patients.

References[1]

1. *Shane E, Burr D, Abrahamsen B, Adler RA, Brown TD et al. Atypical subtrochanteric and diaphyseal femoral fractures: Second report of a task force of the American Society for Bone and Mineral Research. J Bone Miner Res 2014;29: 1-23. *A task force that defines atypical fractures, diagnosis, pathophysiology and treatment.
2. **Dell R, Abrams A, Greene D, Funahashi T, Silverman S, Eisemon E, et al. Incidence of atypical nontraumatic diaphyseal fractures of the femur. J Bone Miner Res. 2012;27(12):2544–50. **Note association of prolonged bisphosphonate treatment and atypical femoral fracture.
3. *Markman L, Allison M, Rosenberg Z, Vieira R, Babb J, Tejwani N, et al. A retrospective review of patients with atypical femoral fractures while on long-term bisphosphonates: including pertinent biochemical and imaging studies. Endocr Pract. 2013;19(3): 456–61. *Define characteristics of patients obtaining an AFF.

[1] *Important References
**Very Important References

4. La **Rocca VR, Rosenberg Z, Allison M, Im S, Babb J, Peck V. Frequency of incomplete atypical femoral fractures in asymptomatic patients on long-term bisphosphonate therapy. AJR Am J Roentgenol. 2012;198(5):1144–51. **Further confirmation on patients with complete and incomplete AFF.

5. **Kang S, Hwang B, Son H, Cheong I, Lee S, Chung T. Changes in bone mineral density in post menopausal women treated with epidural steroid injections for lower back pain. Pain Phys. 2012;15(3):229–36. **Define spine alteration in patients receiving epidural injections.

6. **Khan S, Kanis J, Vasikaran S, Kline W, Matuszewski B, McCloskey E, et al. Elimination and biochemical responses to intravenous alendronate in postmenopausal osteoporosis. J Bone Miner Res. 1997;12(10):1700–7. **The prolonged presence of bisphosphonate in bone.

7. **Lin J. Bisphosphonates: a review of their pharmacokinetic properties. Bone. 1996;18(2):75–85. **Detailed pharmacokinetic properties of bisphosphonates in bone.

8. **Bolland M, Avenell A, Baron J, Grey A, MacLennan G, Gamble G, et al. Effect of calcium supplements on risk of myocardial infarction and cardiovascular events: meta-analysis. Br Med J. 2010;341:C3691. **High calcium intake may result in cardiac disease.

9. **Ross A, Manson J, Abrams S, Aloia J, Brannon P, Clinton S, et al. The 2011 report on dietary reference intakes for calcium and vitamin D from the institute of medicine: what clinicians need to know. J Clin Endocrinol Metab. 2011;96(1):53–8. **Institute recommendation of vitamin D for patients.

10. **Dam T, Von Muhlen D, Barrett-Connor E. Sex-specific association of serum vitamin D levels with physical function in older adults. Osteoporos Int. 2009;20(5):751–60. **Challenged vitamin D levels set by Institute of Medicine.

11. **Binkley N, Gemar D, Engelke J, Gangnon R, Ramamurthy R, Krueger D, et al. Evaluation of ergocalciferol or cholecalciferol dosing, 1,600 IU daily or 50,000 IU monthly in older adults. J Clin Endocrinol Metab. 2011;96(4):981–8. **Description of vitamin D supplementation dosing.

12. **Snijder M, Van Schoor N, Pluijm S, Van Dam R, Visser M, Lips P. Vitamin D status in relation to one-year risk of recurrent falling in older men and women. J Clin Endocrinol Metab. 2006;91(8):2980–5. **How vitamin D influences fall rates.

13. **LeBoff M, Hawkes W, Glowacki J, Yu-Yahiro J, Hurwitz S, Magaziner J. Vitamin D-deficiency and post-fracture changes in lower extremity function and falls in women with hip fractures. Osteoporos Int. 2008;19(9):1283–90. **Low vitamin D is associated with falls.

14. **Aspenberg P, Johansson T. Teriparatide improves early callus formation in distal radial fractures. Acta Orthop. 2010;81(2):234–6. **PTH 1-34 improves fracture healing of distal radius in randomized study.

15. **Peichl P, Holzer L, Maier R, Holzer G. Parathyroid hormone 1-84 accelerates fracture-healing in pubic bones of elderly osteoporotic women. J Bone Joint Surg. 2011;93(17):1583–7. **PTH 1-84 markedly enhances pelvic fracture healing.

16. **Ohtori S, Inoue G, Orita S, Yamaguchi K, Equchi Y, Ochiai N, et al. Comparison of teriparatide and bisphosphonate treatment to reduce pedicle screw loosening after lumbar spinal fusion surgery in postmenopausal women with osteoporosis from a bone quality perspective. Spine. 2013;38(8):E487–92. **PTH 1-34 lowers spine fusion failure and prevent pedicle screw pullout.

17. **Unnanuntana A, Saleh A, Mensah KA, Kleimeyer JP, Lane JM. Atypical femoral fractures: what do we know about them?: AAOS exhibit selection. J Bone Joint Surg Am. 2013;95(2):e8 1–13. **Original overview of AFF including treatment options.

18. **Egol KA, Park JH, Rosenberg ZS, Peck V, Tejwani NC. Healing delayed but generally reliable after bisphosphonate-associated complete femur fractures treated with IM nails. Clin Orthop Relat Res. 2013 Apr 20. **Delayed healing of AFF with nailing.

19. **Weil YA, Rivkin G, Safran O, Liebergall M, Foldes AJ. The outcome of surgically treated femur fractures associated with long-term bisphosphonate use. J Trauma. 2011;71(1):186–90. **Complication and results of treating AFF surgically.

20. **Prasarn ML, Ahn J, Helfet DL, Lane JM, Lorich DG. Bisphosphonate-associated femur fractures have high complication rates with operative fixation. Clin Orthop Relat Res. 2012;470(8):2295–301. **A series of AFF's treated with nails and plates – results.

21. **Tang WM, Chiu KY, Kwan MF, Ng TP, Yau WP. Sagittal bowing of the distal femur in Chinese patients who require total knee arthroplasty. J Orthop Res. 2005;23(1):41–5. **Structural deformity associated with AFF – in Chinese patients.

22. **Leung KS, Procter P, Robioneck B, Behrens K. Geometric mismatch of the gamma nail to the Chinese femur. Clin Orthop Relat Res. 1996;323:42–8. **Difficulty of nail geometry and Asian femurs.

23. **Lin TL, Wang SJ, Fong YC, Hsu CJ, Hsu HC, Tsai CH. Discontinuation of alendronate and administration of bone-forming agents after surgical nailing may promote union of atypical femoral fractures in patients on long-term alendronate therapy. BMC Res Notes. 2013;6:11. doi:10.1186/1756-0500-6-11. **Shifting from bisphosphonates to anabolic agents enhances healing of AFF's.

24. **Homma Y, Zimmermann G, Hernigou P. Cellular therapies for the treatment of non-union: the past, present and future. Injury. 2013;44 suppl 1:S46–9. **The rational for cell based therapy in cases of delayed fracture healing.

25. **Allison MB, Markman L, Rosenberg Z, Vieira RL, Babb J, Tejwani N, et al. Atypical incomplete femoral fractures in asymptomatic patients on long term bisphosphonate therapy. Bone. 2013;55(1):113–8. **The problem of treating incomplete AFF's.

26. *Shane E, Burr D, Ebeling PR, Abrahamsen B, Adler RA, Brown TD, et al. Atypical subtrochanteric and diaphyseal femoral fractures: report of a task force of the American society for bone and mineral research. J Bone Miner Res. 2010;25(11):2267–94. *Original task force recommendation for AFF's.

27. *Egol KA, Park JH, Prensky C, Rosenberg ZS, Peck V, Tejwani NC. Surgical treatment improves clinical and functional outcomes for patients who sustain incomplete bisphosphonate-related femur fractures. J Orthop Trauma. 2013;27(6):331–5. *Thorough evaluation of options of care for incomplete AFF's.

28. **Banffy MB, Vrahas MS, Ready JE, Abraham JA. Nonoperative versus prophylactic treatment of bisphosphonate-associated femoral stress fractures. Clin Orthop Relat Res. 2011;469(7):2028–34. **A discussion of operative vs. conservative care of incomplete AFF's.

29. **Ha YC, Cho MR, Park KH, Kim SY, Koo KH. Is surgery necessary for femoral insufficiency fractures after long-term bisphosphonate therapy? Clin Orthop Relat Res. 2010;468(12):3393–8. **Clear benefit for surgical treatment of incomplete AFF's.

30. **Oh CW, Oh JK, Park KC, Kim JW, Yoon YC. Prophylactic nailing of incomplete atypical femoral fractures. ScientificWorldJournal. 2013;2013: 450148. **Advantage of prophylactic nailing of incomplete AFF's.

31. **Saleh A, Hegde VV, Potty AG, Schneider R, Cornell CN, Lane JM. Management strategy for symptomatic bisphosphonate-associated incomplete atypical femoral fractures. HSS J. 2012;8(2):103–10. **Comprehensive medical and surgical approach to incomplete AFF's.

32. **Lee YK, Ha YC, Kang BJ, Chang JS, Koo KH. Predicting need for fixation of atypical femoral fracture. J Clin Endocrinol Metab. 2013;98(7):2742–5. **Breakdown of incomplete AFF's that need surgical fixation.

33. *Chiang CY, Zebaze RM, Ghasem-Zadeh A, Iuliano-Burns S, Hardidge A, Seeman E. Teriparatide improves bone quality and healing of atypical femoral fractures associated with bisphosphonate therapy. Bone. 2013;52(1):360–5. *Role of teriparatide in restoring bone health after bisphosphonate therapy.

34. **Ward WGS, Carter CJ, Wilson SC, Emory CL. Femoral stress fractures associated with long-term bisphosphonate treatment. Clin Orthop Relat Res. 2012;470(3):759–65. **Advantage of timely nailing of incomplete AFF's.

Parish P. Sedghizadeh and Allan C. Jones

Summary

- Osteonecrosis of the jaw (ONJ) is a serious adverse effect associated with a specific subset of antiresorptive therapy (ART) and is referred to as "antiresorptive osteonecrosis of the jaw" or ARONJ.
- There are two distinct clinical types of ARONJ (cases associated with oncologic therapy and cases associated with rheumatologic therapy) that differ in prevalence, severity, and prediction of risk.
- A confirmed case of ARONJ is defined as the persistence of exposed necrotic jawbone in the oral cavity for 8 weeks, despite adequate treatment, in a patient with current or previous history of ART and without local evidence of malignancy or prior radiotherapy to the affected region.

- Staging systems for ARONJ form the basis for diagnosis and help direct appropriate treatment for each stage.
- The pathogenesis of ARONJ is multifactorial and may involve drug-related effects on bone remodeling, angiogenesis, matrix necrosis, tissue toxicity, host immune responses, and infection.
- Several risk factors have been identified for ARONJ, and recent development of risk assessment tools using pharmacometric analytical methods will provide practitioners a quantitative approach for determining drug accumulation in bone to levels associated with ARONJ induction.
- Patients with ARONJ can be asymptomatic in early stage disease or may present with a wide variety of signs and symptoms clinically.
- Histopathologic examination of ARONJ lesions reveals non-vital bone in association with bacterial colonization and inflammation.
- Radiologic examination is essential for accurate diagnosis and staging of ARONJ.
- The differential diagnosis for ARONJ can be broad, so definitive diagnosis requires careful correlation of medical and dental history, medication history, risk factors, presenting signs and symptoms, examination, radiologic findings, and histopathologic findings when available.

P.P. Sedghizadeh, DDS, MS (✉)
Ostrow School of Dentistry, Center for Biofilms, University of Southern California, 925 West 34th Street #4110, Los Angeles, CA 90089, USA
e-mail: sedghiza@usc.edu

A.C. Jones, DDS, MS
A Professional Corporation, Skypark One Professional Building, Torrance, CA, USA

© Springer International Publishing Switzerland 2016
S.L. Silverman, B. Abrahamsen (eds.), *The Duration and Safety of Osteoporosis Treatment*, DOI 10.1007/978-3-319-23639-1_12

Introduction

Soon after the turn of the twenty-first century, dental surgeons began to observe cancer patients presenting with a persistent pattern of nonhealing exposed alveolar bone in the oral cavity. This clinical presentation was initially called "avascular necrosis." It was discovered that the only common etiology shared by all patients with this condition was bisphosphonate (BP) use regardless of medical history, comorbidities, dental procedures, or other potential confounders and risk factors. This ostensible problem with BP drugs, more specifically those with a nitrogenous side chain (nitrogen-containing or "n-BP"), would soon be referred to as "osteonecrosis of the jaw" or "ONJ," which simply means "jawbone death" without specifying underlying causation or risk association. In September of 2004, Novartis gave notice to the medical community, in a broadly distributed written letter, that package inserts for Zometa™ (zoledronate) and Aredia™ (pamidronate) would be updated to contain a precaution regarding the occurrence of ONJ in cancer patients who have undergone invasive dental procedures.

At present, the majority of reported ONJ cases are observed in patients who have received intravenously administered n-BP or antiresorptive (ART) therapy for skeletal malignancies [1, 2]. Oncology patients may be more vulnerable due to compromised health status, jaw metastases, and the immunosuppressive effects of antineoplastics and corticosteroids. However, ONJ is also seen to occur in rheumatologic patients who have received only oral administration or low-dose intravenous infusion of n-BP or subcutaneous injection of denosumab (Dmab) as ART for osteoporosis [3, 4]. Accordingly, there are two distinct clinical types of ONJ—cases associated with oncologic ART and cases associated with rheumatologic ART [5]; these differ in prevalence, severity, and prediction of risk.

ONJ cases associated with oncologic ART can quickly progress to advanced stages and are often unresponsive to conservative therapy or drug discontinuation. Cases associated with rheumatologic dosing of ART are less aggressive and generally respond to non-surgical or conservative surgical therapy. Large epidemiologic studies

conflict regarding whether oral ART therapy is associated with ONJ risk [6, 7]. Generally, studies which review medical records for ONJ case adjudication reveal little or no risk associated with oral ART, while studies that review dental records reveal a significant risk [6, 7]. Epidemiologic studies may underestimate the risk of ONJ because most cases are associated with dental surgery, wherein it was first observed. Therefore, the more accurate population to study is dental patients who have a history of dentoalveolar surgery or oral trauma. This will allow for more accurate generalizability of epidemiologic findings to the population at risk.

It is important to note that in general, ONJ is unique as compared to osteonecrosis at other skeletal sites with respect to epidemiology, etiopathogenesis, risk factors, clinical features, diagnosis, and treatment. For example, osteonecrosis of diaphyseal or endochondral long bones (e.g., femur and tibia) primarily affects men (with a notable exception of cases related to systemic lupus erythematosus, which have a female predominance), usually occurs in the third to fifth decades of life, and is related to known risk factors such as corticosteroid or alcohol use in nontraumatic cases [8]. Conversely, osteonecrosis of the membranous or flat craniofacial bones (e.g., maxilla and mandible) affects both men and women (but predominantly women in the osteoporosis ART setting), usually occurs in the fifth decade of life or higher, and is associated with dental risk factors and oral trauma in most cases [9, 10].

Clinically, many factors or conditions can culminate in ONJ, including head and neck radiation (osteoradionecrosis), jawbone infection (osteomyelitis), dentoalveolar surgery, exposure to certain drugs (e.g., antiangiogenics, n-BP, Dmab) or chemicals (e.g., white phosphorous occupationally, recreational cocaine), and various bone-related pathoses. Additionally, some cases of ONJ are spontaneous or idiopathic, with no known etiology or risk factors. Given the wide range of differential diagnosis for ONJ and the varying international classification of disease (ICD) codes that have been used for case diagnosis and charting historically, the term ONJ has become controversial and somewhat ambiguous. This has made clinical diagnosis challenging in some cases, created confusion in the literature, and made case adjudication in epidemiologic studies and medicolegal settings challenging. For example, cases of ONJ have been referred to as ARONJ (antiresorptive osteonecrosis of the jaw), BRONJ (bisphosphonate-related osteonecrosis of the jaw), BIONJ (bisphosphonate-induced osteonecrosis of the jaw), BAONJ (bisphosphonate-associated osteonecrosis of the jaw), BONJ (bisphosphonate osteonecrosis of the jaw), DIONJ (drug-induced osteonecrosis of the jaw), and DAONJ (drug-associated osteonecrosis of the jaw), and most recently MRONJ (medication-related osteonecrosis of the jaw) to name a few. To avoid nosological debates and to simply discuss ONJ in the context of this specific monograph, we herein use the acronym ARONJ to refer to ONJ observed in the setting of ART.

Definition

Several definitions and staging systems have been proposed for ARONJ. Notably, as proposed by the Advisory Task Forces from both the American Association of Oral and Maxillofacial Surgeons (AAOMS) and the American Society for Bone and Mineral Research (ASBMR), a *confirmed* case of ARONJ is defined as the persistence of exposed necrotic jawbone in the oral cavity for 8 weeks, despite adequate treatment, in a patient with current or previous history of ART and without local evidence of malignancy or prior radiotherapy to the affected region [11, 12]. A *suspected* case of ARONJ is defined as an area of exposed jawbone for less than 8 weeks in a patient with a history of ART and no radiotherapy to the head and neck. However, it is estimated that up to 30 % of ARONJ cases may initially present without clinical evidence of exposed jawbone or characteristic signs and symptoms [13]. Therefore, most working definitions of ARONJ have inherent limitations, particularly the requirement for exposed jawbone of 8 weeks duration given the existence of nonexposed (NE) variants of ARONJ. The absence of characteristic clinical signs and symptoms of ARONJ in NE cases can lead to late diagnosis, prolonged disease course, and refractory treatment. Some of these NE cases

of ARONJ represent advanced stages of the disease process, but without mucosal breakdown and exposed bone on clinical presentation. These cases are usually classified as early stage (stage 0) disease in accordance with the current AAOMS diagnostic and staging criteria and are quite often underdiagnosed and thus undertreated [14]. Therefore, in NE cases of ARONJ, formulating an accurate diagnosis and initiating a proper treatment protocol can be challenging. This is in contrast to ARONJ cases with exposed bone, which can be more readily diagnosed given the overt osseous exposure and characteristic signs or symptoms along with aforementioned case-defining criteria.

Staging

Several staging systems have been proposed for ARONJ. A feature common to all is the progressive severity of disease and increase in associated signs and symptoms with advancing stage. For example, the Marx system is predicated on the number of affected jawbone quadrants and specific clinical features; the more jawbone quadrants involved, the more severe the disease and the higher the stage [15]. The staging system used most commonly in the clinical setting and in the literature is the AAOMS system for ARONJ, which includes four stages (stages 0, 1, 2, and 3) for case classification [11] as summarized in Table 12.1.

Stage 0 cases show no clinical evidence of exposed necrotic bone, but nonspecific clinical or radiographic findings as described in Table 12.1. Figure 12.1 shows an example of stage 0 ARONJ in a patient taking Dmab for osteoporosis. Stage 0 cases can be the most challenging to diagnose clinically given the nonspecific signs and symptoms and the fact that some cases may represent another disease process and not ARONJ. Only with hindsight and disease progression, in the presence or absence of therapy, could it be deemed that indeed a case presumed to be stage 0 actually represents stage 0 ARONJ. For example, one could argue that the patient in Fig. 12.1 has a periodontal abscess only and should be treated as

Table 12.1 ARONJ staging system with clinical and radiographic features for each stage

Stage	Clinical characteristics	Radiographic findings
Stage 0	*No* evidence of necrotic bone, but presence of nonspecific signs or symptoms • Odontalgia not explained by an odontogenic cause • Dull, aching bone pain in the body of the mandible, which may radiate to the temporomandibular joint region • Sinus pain, which may be associated with inflammation and thickening of the maxillary sinus wall • Altered neurosensory function • Loosening of teeth not explained by chronic periodontal disease • Periapical/periodontal fistula or sinus tract that is not associated with pulp necrosis due to caries • Gingival swelling/inflammation with or without crevicular exudate (spontaneous or on palpation)	• Persistence of unremodeled extraction socket • Prominent osteosclerosis in a jawbone region with changes to trabecular pattern • Alveolar bone loss or resorption not attributable to chronic periodontal disease • Thickening/obscuring of the periodontal ligament (thickening of the lamina dura and decreased size of the periodontal ligament space) • Inferior alveolar canal narrowing
Stage 1	• Exposed and necrotic jawbone evident in the oral cavity • Asymptomatic • No soft tissue infection or purulence	• Lytic bone lesion • With or without evidence of sequestrum • No cortical perforation or periosteal bone formation
Stage 2	• Exposed and necrotic jawbone evident in the oral cavity • Inflammatory signs and symptoms • Infection/purulence	• Lytic bone lesion • Sequestrum centrally • Displacement of adjacent anatomic structures such as teeth which may have thickened lamina dura • May have cortical involvement
Stage 3	• Exposed and necrotic bone evident in the oral cavity • Inflammatory signs and symptoms • Infection/purulence • One or more of the following: – Sequestrum extending beyond the alveolar bone area – Pathologic fracture – Extraoral fistula – Oroantral/oronasal communication – Osteolysis extending to the inferior border of the mandible or the antrum of the sinus or zygoma in the maxilla	• Extensive lytic bone lesion • Sequestrum • There may be evidence of cortical expansion, thinning, erosion and perforation, and/or periosteal bone formation • Displacement of adjacent anatomic structures such as teeth, the inferior alveolar nerve canal, or the maxillary sinus • Tooth involvement may appear as thickened lamina dura • Pathologic fracture may be observed

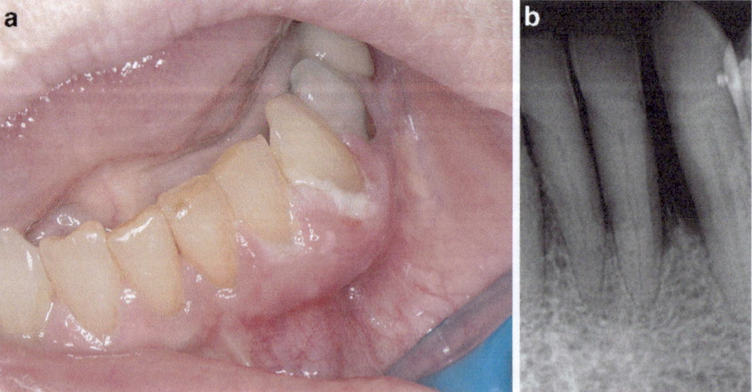

Fig. 12.1 (**a**) Seventy-six-year-old Caucasian female on Dmab therapy for osteoporosis for 2 years duration, presenting with loose teeth and swelling of the left mandibular anterior gingiva and purulent crevicular exudate from the periodontium, but no overt evidence of exposed bone. (**b**) Periapical dental X-ray of the area reveals ill-defined lytic change and bone loss around affected teeth with widening of the lamina dura space (stage 0 ARONJ)

such; subsequently, if there is lesion resolution with appropriate treatment for a periodontal abscess, it would be impossible to definitively diagnose the case as ARONJ unless overt bone exposure were to occur at some point in the future despite the treatment. This is just one example of many with respect to nonspecific presentations of ARONJ and the potentially broader differential diagnosis as experienced by clinicians in evaluating challenging stage 0 cases of disease.

The clinical features of stage 1 cases include the presence of exposed necrotic bone, but no evidence of soft tissue infection or purulence. Figure 12.2 shows an example of stage 1 ARONJ in a patient taking oral ibandronate for osteoporosis. Stage 2 is characterized by exposed necrotic bone that is associated with signs of infection (e.g., pain, erythema, and/or purulence). Figure 12.3 shows an example of stage 2 ARONJ in a patient taking oral alendronate for osteoporosis. Stage 3 cases exhibit more extensive necrotic bone and infection which extend beyond the alveolar region or osteolysis that extends to the inferior border of the mandible or the sinus floor, amenable to pathologic fracture, extraoral fistula, and oroantral or oronasal communication [16]. Figure 12.4 shows a patient with cellulitis involving the right mandible and face, from spread of ARONJ infection.

To address NE variants of ARONJ, which can resemble advanced stages of disease clinically, the AAOMS staging system has been adapted to include the addition of NE variants of ARONJ for each stage [13]. Aside from forming the basis for diagnosis guidelines, staging systems for ARONJ direct appropriate treatment for each stage. However, there is currently no clear consensus on appropriate therapeutics.

Pathogenesis

The pathogenesis of ARONJ is multifactorial and may be different for n-BP cases as compared to Dmab cases; however, similarities or common pathways may also exist. Much more investigation and literature is available on the pathogenesis of n-BP ARONJ and virtually little to none on Dmab ARONJ. Alterations in bone remodeling, antiangiogenic effects, matrix necrosis, tissue toxicity, immunomodulation, and infection have been proposed to play roles in ARONJ pathogenesis. n-BP compounds are known to deposit in the bone compartment, where they inhibit osteoclast activation and promote osteoclast apoptosis by several mechanisms, including inhibition of protein prenylation and blockade of mevalonate metabolism [17]. They also have antiangiogenic properties [18] and inhibit matrix metalloproteinases [19] and in vitro proliferation of oral keratinocytes [20]. The toxic or inhibitory effect on oral epithelial growth by n-BP drugs may explain the delayed wound healing seen in ARONJ cases.

Knowledge of the pharmacology (pharmacokinetics and pharmacodynamics) of n-BP drugs

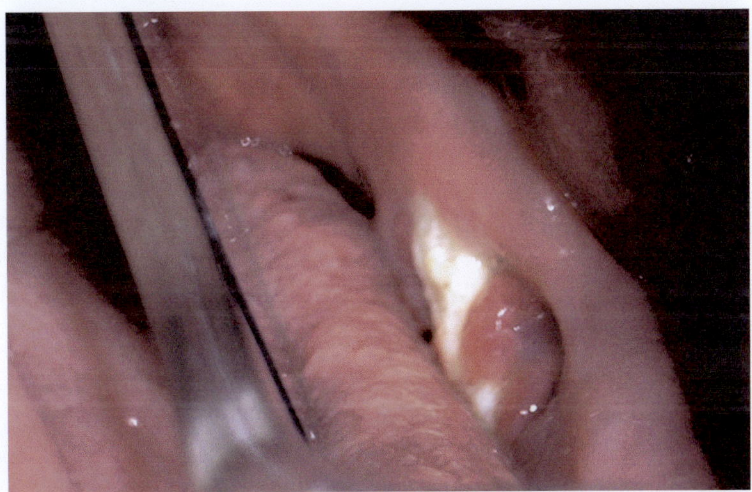

Fig. 12.2 Seventy-one-year-old Caucasian female with a 4-year history of oral ibandronate use for osteoporosis, presenting with an asymptomatic area of exposed bone and associated granulation tissue involving the lingual surface of the left posterior hemimandible (stage 1 ARONJ)

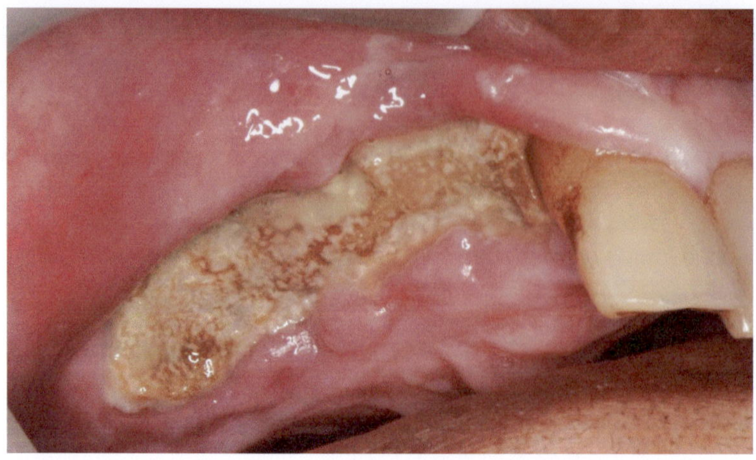

Fig. 12.3 Seventy-eight-year-old Caucasian male with a 6-year history of oral alendronate use for osteoporosis, presenting with a painful area of exposed and infected bone involving the right hemimaxilla (stage 2 ARONJ)

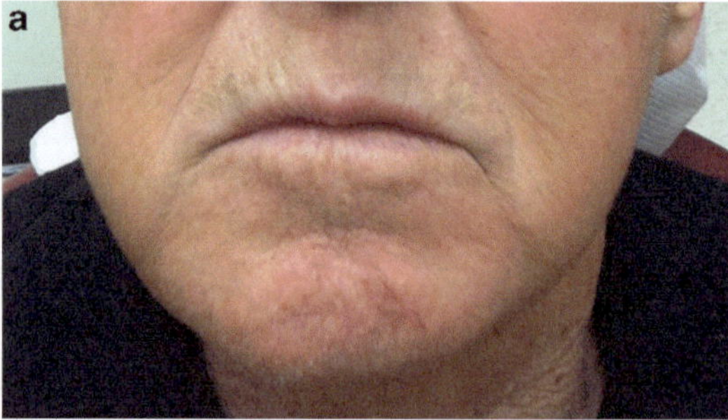

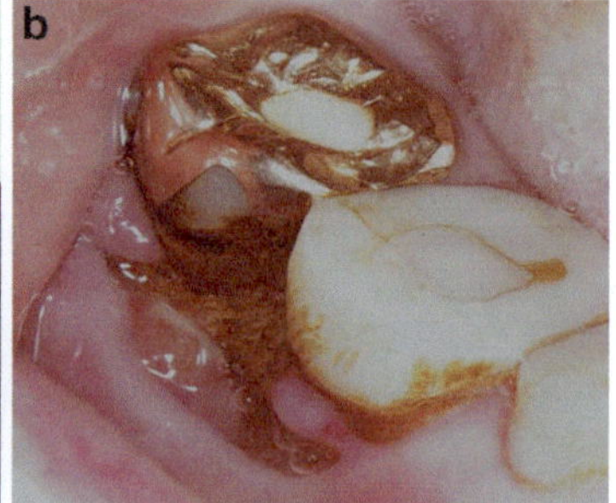

Fig. 12.4 (**a**) 69-year-old male with diffuse right facial swelling, pain, and cutaneous sinus tract formation (see Fig. 12.9) consistent with a stage 3 ARONJ. (**b**) Intraoral photograph of the same patient shows the source of the infection from the exposed bone and inflamed gingiva on the buccal aspect of the posterior right mandibular molars

is essential to understanding most cases of ARONJ disease and pathogenesis. Once resident in bone, n-BP compounds are usually eliminated during bone resorption—a process that can take years [21]. This results in a long half-life in bone, for example, up to 10 years for alendronate [21]. Orally administered n-BP drugs have a very low bioavailability (0.3–6 %), whereas intravenous administration provides much higher bioavailability, allowing for greater drug accumulation in the skeleton; for example, 50 % of an intravenous-administered therapeutic dose of the n-BP pamidronate concentrates selectively in the skeletal compartment from the plasma, while the rest is excreted unchanged in the urine [22]. These differences in oral versus intravenous dosing and bone bioavailability may explain the greater frequency of ARONJ in oncologic versus rheumatologic dosing. Further, there is significant interpatient variability in n-BP pharmacokinetics and biodistribution, but little intrapatient variability [22]. Significant differences also exist in the potency and binding affinities of various n-BP drugs to bone. These differences in the pharmacokinetics and pharmacodynamics of the various n-BP drugs can impact bone binding and release of drug, the observed clinical differences in potency and duration of effect, and complications like ARONJ.

Not only does bone acts as a reservoir for n-BP, but the drug can also be released during bone resorption or trauma and surgery to bone. The concentration of active n-BP drug released into the surrounding jawbone environment by osteoclastic resorption is approximately one-half that of the concentration of drug in bone. In vitro thresholds for toxicity to cells in the local area essential for covering exposed alveolar bone are known. For example, oral mucosal wound healing stops at 0.1 mM of pamidronate [20]. Similar studies with osteoblasts, endothelial cells, fibroblasts, T-cells, and macrophages demonstrate a threshold-dependent toxicity to concentrations of n-BP drugs in vitro [20]. Therefore, after a tooth extraction or oral surgical procedures to bone, which is when most cases of ONJ occur, bound n-BP from both superficial and deep layers of bone is released into the local milieu where it can inhibit oral wound healing in addition to other effects which we discuss shortly and which have been validated in vivo.

Investigators have questioned why the jawbones are predominantly affected by osteonecrosis when n-BP drugs disseminate to all bones of the body. Accordingly, one popular hypothesis for ARONJ pathogenesis is that there is higher bone remodeling in the jawbones as compared to other skeletal sites and greater remodeling in the mandible as compared to the maxilla. Masticatory load and mechanics could potentially result in greater accumulation of n-BP compounds in the mandible versus the maxilla or other osseous sites such as the femur. However, a recent study evaluating bone scintigraphy scans of cancer patients prior to and throughout the course of n-BP therapy revealed a similar bone turnover in the mandible and the femur and a significantly lower bone turnover in the mandible as compared with the maxilla [23]. All investigated bone regions showed no significant changes throughout n-BP administration, and bone remodeling in the jawbones was not overly suppressed by ART [23]. The finding that the mandible has a significantly lower bone turnover than the maxilla, and the fact that most ARONJ cases occur in the mandible, led the authors to suggest that the aforementioned popular hypothesis for ARONJ pathogenesis is not plausible. Additionally, uptake of n-BP has been shown to be higher in the axial skeleton compared with the appendicular skeleton or craniofacial bones; teeth and jawbones show no exceptional differences in drug uptake compared with other hard tissues [24]. Therefore, common notions with respect to pathogenesis—that there is preferential uptake of n-BP drug to jawbones and greater remodeling in the jawbones as compared to other bones in the body—may be unfounded.

There is, however, mounting evidence that the jawbones are unique from other bones in the body mainly in their susceptibility to ARONJ because of the presence of bacteria in the mouth and saliva which have ready access to jawbone [25, 26]. Histopathologic findings indicate that even the healthy edentulous jaw can contain regions of nonviable bone and microbial biofilm formation for more than one year after tooth extraction and normal mucosal healing [27]. Regions of nonviable bone and subclinical infection may contribute to the development of untoward clinical events such as ARONJ. Recent microbiologic findings reveal a characteristic pathogenic profile of organisms in patients with ARONJ compared to patients without disease [28]. This pathogenic profile is dominated by a few phyla, mainly Proteobacteria, Firmicutes, and Actinobacteria and predominantly facultative anaerobes. The same phyla have been shown to dominate symptomatic dental periradicular infections as analyzed by 454-pyrosequencing [29]. These pathogens reside in saliva, infected teeth, and periradicular lesions and can easily gain access to jawbone, especially after invasive dental procedures that expose bone, which is when most cases of ARONJ occur [30]. All studies to date examining ARONJ-affected bone histopathologically report microbial colonization [31].

Recent investigations have also shown that n-BP drugs not only inhibit oral wound healing and bone healing but also facilitate bacterial colonization on bony surfaces where both drug and biofilm bacteria co-localize [32]. Therefore, the clinical problem of ARONJ is essentially a biofilm-mediated osteomyelitis of the jawbones secondary to poor wound healing from toxic accumulation of n-BP [33]. The common role of infection in ARONJ pathogenesis explains the current antimicrobial and surgical approaches to ARONJ therapy, the finding of ONJ with other classes of drugs not related to ART, and the fact that patients are at risk for disease years after discontinuation of n-BP given the long bioavailability of n-BP and of pathogens in jawbone.

The development of animal models has provided additional insights into ARONJ pathogenesis. For example, it has been shown that osteoclasts at different anatomic sites internalize n-BP differentially, but differential uptake does not correlate directly with osteoclastogenesis or osteoclast precursor sensitivity to drug [34]. Propensity to n-BP is site-specific and varies in the jawbones as compared to the femur; jawbone osteoclasts are more susceptible to inhibition of prenylation. Further, n-BP accumulation in bone has been shown, contrary to popular belief, to be an equilibrium-dependent drug–crystalline bone mineral interaction which more accurately explains n-BP biodistribution and pharmacokinetics and may be more relevant to ARONJ pathogenesis [35]. These findings reveal that although the jawbones do not take up more n-BP than other skeletal sites, jawbone osteoclasts may be more sensitive to the effects of n-BP than osteoclasts at other sites. Recent animal studies have also revealed a role for immune dysregulation in ARONJ pathogenesis [36]. Additionally, animal studies provide the opportunity to test novel therapeutics such as molecular and stem cell-based approaches to ARONJ treatment. However, extrapolating data from animal studies directly to humans is problematic as there are considerable differences in bone remodeling, pharmacokinetics, microbiome, immune responses, and oral function. Further studies in humans and higher levels of evidence are necessary before direct translation to humans.

Finally, the "-omics" revolution and advanced molecular methodologies have provided knowledge into ARONJ pathogenesis through evaluation of the salivary proteome [37], the pharmacogenome via genome-wide association studies [38], the microbial metagenome or microbiome [39], and single nucleotide polymorphisms [40, 41] associated with disease. This line of investigation has the potential to reveal differences or unique signatures in patients affected with ARONJ as compared to those without disease, allowing for development of potential clinical biomarkers in the future. Prospective well-controlled studies using a transdisciplinary team of clinicians and basic scientists, with bioinformatic and computation biology analyses and a hypothesis-driven approach, will be essential for advancement in understanding ARONJ pathogenesis and risk, as well as for biomarker development and validation.

Risk

To date, most ARONJ literature represents lower levels of evidence and a weak strength of evidence for direct translation and application to clinical understanding. These publications include editorials, expert opinions, in vitro models, animal models, case reports, case series, and retrospective studies. Few prospective well-controlled human studies exist, which has hindered accurate disease characterization and risk assessment. The available literature that represents relatively higher levels of evidence, such as systematic reviews and case–control, cohort, and controlled longitudinal studies, provides insight into risk factors for ARONJ. Table 12.2 lists potential risk factors that have been reported to be associated with ONJ in general [6, 9, 42–45]. Further studies are needed to more accurately address risk and risk assessment for ARONJ specifically, and many currently proposed risk factors require validation. Additionally, risk factors differ for rheumatologic versus oncologic patients receiving ART.

At currently available levels of evidence, it is difficult to stratify risk (e.g., low to high), and it is more appropriate to identify patients that are potentially at risk. Risk assessment must involve consideration of medical, dental, and medication history, in addition to other clinical parameters. Risk assessment aids in identifying patients unaffected but susceptible to ARONJ, allowing preventative and dental prophylactic measures to be instituted when necessary [46]. Risk reduction efforts may involve restorative or endodontic dentistry to avoid extractions or invasive dental procedures when possible or the implementation of antibiotic prophylactic protocols prior to and after necessary invasive dental procedures, which has been shown to significantly reduce risk and ARONJ incidence [47].

More recently, the application of pharmacometric and bioinformatic analytical tools and predictive modeling to patients with ARONJ has enabled the quantification of drug levels in the bony compartment, allowing determinations of drug accumulation to potentially toxic levels for induction of ARONJ [48]. *Pharmacometrics* is a burgeoning field that has enabled personalized

Table 12.2 Potential risk factors for ONJ

- Dental risk factors (periodontal or periapical disease, oral trauma, extractions, implants)
- Dose and duration of ART therapy
- Cancer
- Osteoporosis
- Corticosteroids
- Chemotherapy
- Antiangiogenics
- Immunotherapy
- Female sex/estrogen therapy
- Advanced age
- Ethnicity (Asian race highest risk)
- Smoking
- Anemia
- Diabetes
- Arthritis
- Hypothyroidism
- Storage diseases
- Systemic lupus erythematosus
- Hypertension
- Hemodialysis
- Blood dyscrasias
- Vascular disorders
- Chemical exposure
- Herpes zoster
- Alcohol abuse
- Coagulation abnormalities
- Gaucher disease
- Human immunodeficiency virus infection
- Hyperlipidemia and embolic fat

medicine and individualized pharmacotherapy and has provided significant clinical insight into drug-associated conditions [49]. In the future, the application of this approach clinically will give practitioners a quantitative pharmacokinetic method for determining drug accumulation in bone without the need for compartmental measurements or invasive procedures, serving as a powerful risk assessment tool to guide clinical decision-making. Pharmacometric modeling of accumulation of n-BP in bone has validated that ONJ is predictable in dental surgery patients who have acquired sufficient concentrations of drug to liberate aqueous solutions concentrated above the 0.1 mM in vitro threshold required to impair cell migration and completely inhibit intracellu-

lar production of isoprenoid lipids. These population-based pharmacometric tools have also identified ethnic predispositions to ARONJ and indicate that Asians have the highest risk due to anthropometric and potentially pharmacogenomic parameters [48], which has been partially validated in large epidemiologic studies [45]. Finally, biomarkers associated with bone physiology (e.g., CTX, NTX, BAP, OC, DPD, PTH) have been investigated for their utility in ARONJ risk assessment, but there is currently insufficient prospective evidence for risk prediction of ARONJ based on biomarkers, and additional research and validation are necessary [50].

Clinical Features

Patients with ARONJ can be asymptomatic or may have a variety of signs and symptoms. Some patients with early stage ARONJ, in both exposed and NE variants, may have no associated symptoms and may be unaware of having disease until diagnosed by a health-care provider. In NE cases at early stage, diagnosis may be delayed until overt signs or symptoms become evident with disease progression. Early symptomatology includes discomfort and an abnormal feeling in the mouth. Most ARONJ cases are associated with precedent oral trauma or infection, such as tooth extraction or an abscess, with delayed wound healing [51]. Therefore, dental consultation and evaluation is prudent prior to the initiation of, or especially during, ART.

A common presentation for ARONJ is a nonhealing ulcer or extraction socket (Fig. 12.5). The mandible is affected more often than the maxilla. When exposed bone or sequestrum is present, patients may feel the ulcerative lesion with their tongue as a rough hard area (the sequestrum) with surrounding irregular soft tissue. Patients with tori or exostoses are particularly susceptible to ARONJ because the overlying mucosa is normally attenuated and prone to trauma and injury. Figure 12.6 shows a typical lesion of ARONJ involving mandibular tori. Epithelialization over tori even at early stage disease without signs of

a

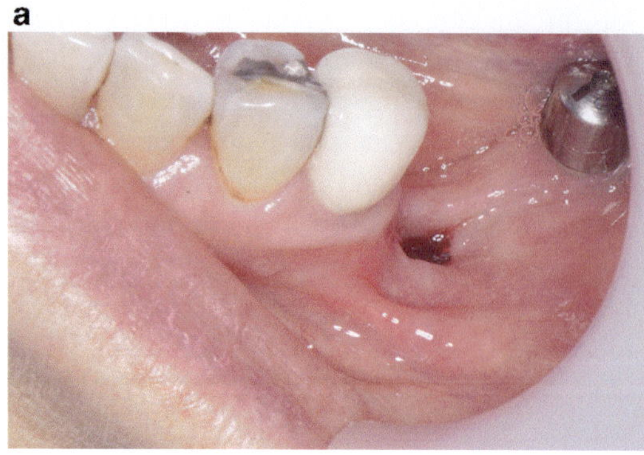

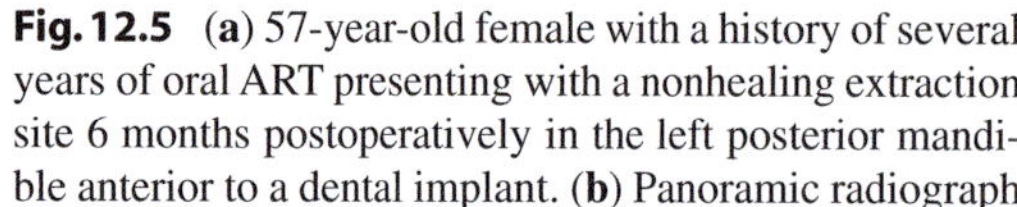

b

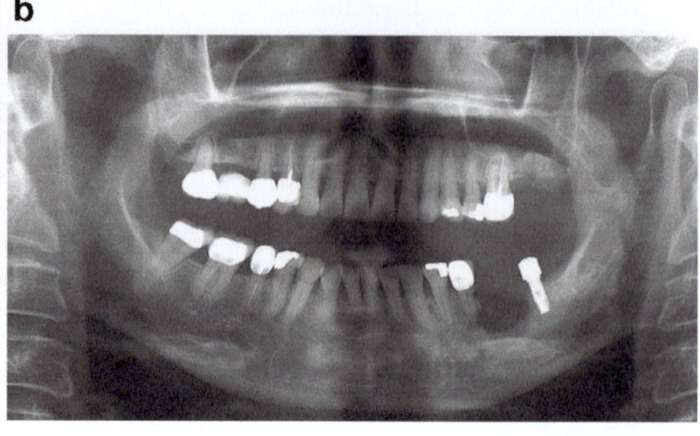

Fig. 12.5 (**a**) 57-year-old female with a history of several years of oral ART presenting with a nonhealing extraction site 6 months postoperatively in the left posterior mandible anterior to a dental implant. (**b**) Panoramic radiograph of the same patient shows a relatively well-defined saucerized radiolucent lesion in the region with suggestion of central sequestrum formation

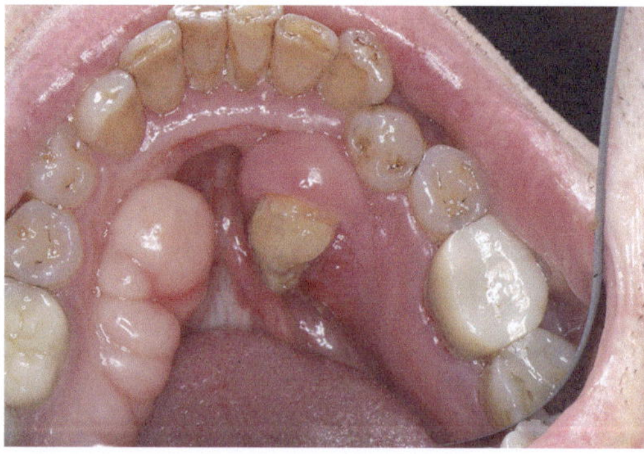

Fig. 12.6 Sixty-four-year-old male with a painless area of exposed bone and stage 1 ARONJ involving mandibular tori

infection is difficult to achieve naturally and may require some surgical intervention.

Inflammatory signs and symptoms such as pain and erythema can be a common finding with ARONJ, usually with progression of disease past stage 1. Inflammation of soft tissues surrounding affected bone may result in the appearance of swollen and/or bleeding gingival tissues as shown in Fig. 12.7. Loosening of teeth may occur due to periodontal involvement of ARONJ. Purulence may be an important finding with disease progression and may be accompanied by malodor or bad breath. Culture of pus from ARONJ lesions with antibiotic sensitivity testing may help guide antimicrobial therapeutics, and notoriously pathogenic oral bacteria are usually cultured. Exposed sequestrum may be sharp, causing irritation and traumatic ulcers of adjacent mucosa such as the tongue or buccal mucosa. Figure 12.8 shows a ventrolateral tongue ulcer secondary to trauma from exposed sharp sequestrum in ARONJ. Patients with prosthodontic or dental appliances may complain of ill-fitting prostheses due to inflammatory changes in underlying affected tissues, and this can be an early symptom of ARONJ. With disease progression, patients may complain of difficulty eating or dysphagia, and weight loss can be observed in such cases. Fever is only seen in more severe cases or advanced-stage disease. With fever or active purulence from lesions, systemic hematology lab values may show increased leukocyte counts, particularly lymphocytosis or neutrophilia with or without evidence of neutrophil bands.

When ARONJ occurs in the mandible and there is inferior alveolar nerve involvement, patients may have sensory complaints such as numbness or tingling in the lower jaw and lip on the affected side of the face. Sensory complaints may represent paresthesia, dysesthesia, allodynia, hypesthesia, or anesthesia. In advanced stages of disease, pathologic fracture of the jawbone, oroantral or oronasal communication, or sinus tract formation to the skin of the face can occur [52]. Figure 12.9 shows a cutaneous sinus tract, which developed from an advanced ARONJ that was

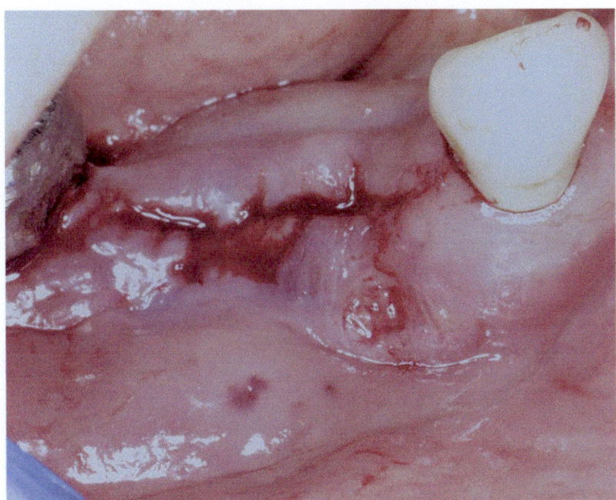

Fig. 12.7 Fifty-nine-year-old female with a stage 2 ARONJ lesion that bleeds spontaneously and has frequent episodes of exudate coming from the lesion, with concomitant malodor. The gingival swelling and bleeding can make it difficult to visualize the exposed subjacent bone; therefore, gentle saline irrigation may be required in order to do so clinically

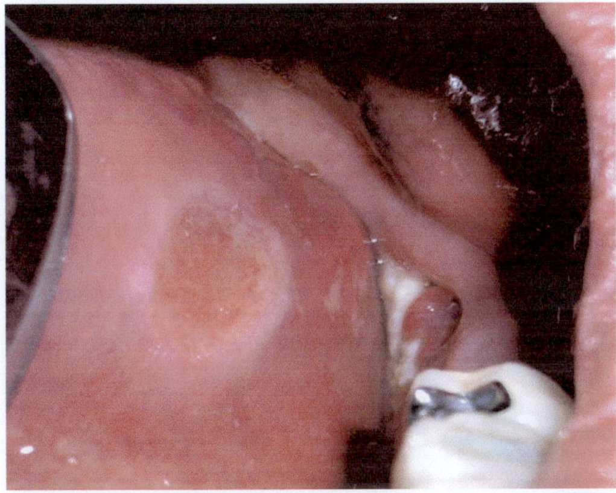

Fig. 12.8 The same patient as shown in Fig. 12.2 with an ulcer of the left ventrolateral tongue due to trauma from the adjacent area of exposed bone. In cases like this, curettage, filing, or debridement of the bone should allow for tongue tissue healing within a few weeks. If healing does not occur after addressing the traumatic etiology, biopsy of the tongue ulcer may be warranted to rule other conditions in the differential diagnosis of ventrolateral tongue ulcers, such as squamous cell carcinoma

associated with facial cellulitis. Cellulitis can be seen in severe cases with infection dissemination through facial spaces; maxillary phlegmon may involve canine or buccal spaces, and mandibular phlegmon may involve submental, sublingual, and submandibular spaces [53]. Further direct or

lymphatic spread may occur to secondary spaces such as pterygomandibular, lateropharyngeal, masseteric, and pterygomaxillary spaces.

Importantly, advanced or severe cases of ARONJ are rarely seen with rheumatologic ART as compared to oncologic ART dosing regimens. ARONJ in the rheumatologic patient follows an indolent course. When severe cases are seen in patients receiving ART for osteoporosis alone, they usually have other risk factors and comorbidities in addition to many years of n-BP therapy to the point that bone concentrations of the drug have potentially reached parity with intravenous dosing concentrations. The most fulminant courses of ARONJ are seen in patients receiving ART concomitant with corticosteroid or antiangiogenic therapy for oncologic care. A recent Food and Drug Administration (FDA) analysis of oral ART and adverse effects noted that the highest prevalence of ARONJ cases occurred after 4 years of n-BP therapy, supporting previous findings that clinical risk for ARONJ is associated with cumulative dose and duration of therapy [54].

The medical history of patients affected with ARONJ may reveal comorbidities other than osteoporosis, such as diabetes, rheumatoid arthritis, and anemia. Therefore, thorough review of systems and investigation into medical and dental history is necessary in all cases. Medication history besides ART is also important as antiangiogenics have been reported to induce ONJ in the absence of ART [55] or exacerbate disease course in the presence of ART [56]. The finding that antiangiogenics alone have been associated with ONJ development has led several investigators to coin terms like "medication-related" or "drug-associated" ONJ to more accurately and broadly capture etiology. Patients that have ARONJ may experience a reduced quality of life with disease progression. It is not unusual for patients to have multiple clinical visits for their condition, often without accurate diagnosis or curative treatment. Some patients may have multiple surgeries to treat the condition without resolution or response, while others have no surgery at all when it is actually needed. Long-term antibiotics and analgesics are not unusual for treatment, whether oral or intravenous, but still may

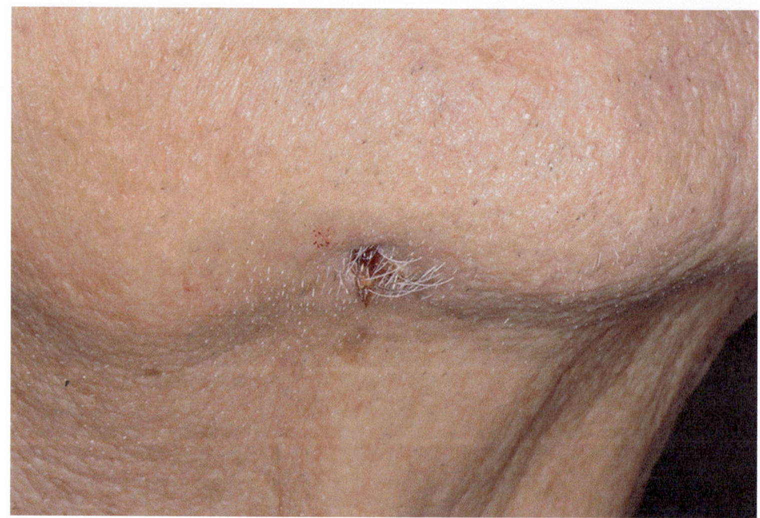

Fig. 12.9 The same patient as shown in Fig. 12.4 with a cutaneous sinus tract from their right mandibular ARONJ lesion

not provide definitive disease resolution. Overall, there can be a significant financial and temporal burden on both patients and the health-care system with respect to ARONJ.

Histopathology

Biopsies of bone in ARONJ patients demonstrate trabeculae of sclerotic lamellar bone with osteocyte dropout from lacunae. The periphery of non-vital bone may have scalloped bone resorption in association with bacterial biofilm colonization on the surface. Most cases of ARONJ reveal *Actinomyces* species on routine microscopic evaluation [57]. Figure 12.10 shows the bone histopathology for a case of ARONJ. Normal bone adjacent to affected bone may demonstrate irregular trabeculae of pagetoid bone, with enlarged osteoclasts containing abundant intracytoplasmic vacuoles. Granulation tissue with occasional presence of multinucleated giant cells and medullary inflammation and fibrosis may also be observed in specimens [58].

Oral soft tissue adjacent to affected bone may demonstrate acute and/or chronic inflammatory cell infiltration. Pseudoepitheliomatous hyperplasia of adjacent mucosa may also be observed, but should not be considered a sign of malignancy [59]. More advanced microscopic evaluation with tools such

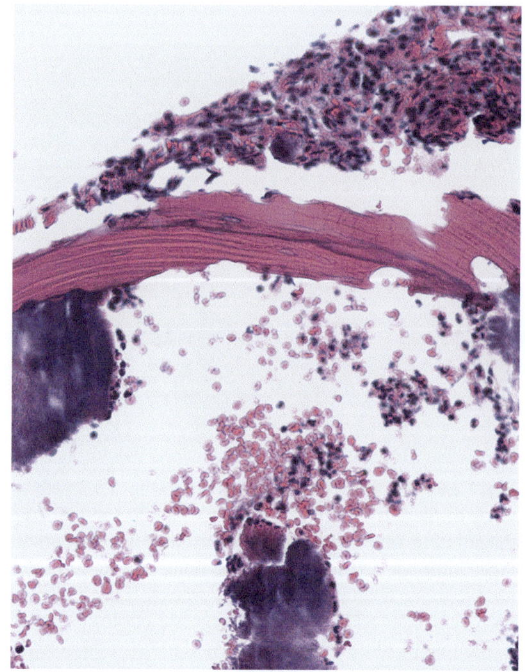

Fig. 12.10 Biopsy of necrotic bone in ARONJ shows areas of non-vital bone or sequestrum characterized by osteocyte dropout from lacunae and scalloped resorption of the surfaces. Biofilm colonization can be seen on the left inferior side of the necrotic bone, and free-floating *Actinomyces*-like colonies can be seen at the bottom of the image. Note the acute/chronic inflammatory cell infiltrates granulation tissue and extravasated erythrocytes (above and below the bone) (H&E, 40× original magnification)

as confocal scanning laser microscopy or scanning electron microscopy has identified multispecies microbial biofilms in association with affected bone. Figure 12.11 shows a scanning electron microscopic image of an *Actinomyces* microcolony from a multispecies bone biofilm in a patient with maxillary involvement of ARONJ. Importantly, microscopic findings in ARONJ can be similar to other conditions in the differential diagnosis, such as osteoradionecrosis or osteomyelitis; therefore, correlation of histopathologic findings with and clinical and radiologic findings and medical history is essential for accurate diagnosis.

Radiology

In conjunction with clinical examination, radiologic examination is essential for (1) jawbone evaluation and determination of the extent of ARONJ lesions, (2) monitoring disease progression or response to treatment, and (3) guiding therapeutics and surgery. In many cases, the clinical picture does not reveal the full extent of jawbone involvement by ARONJ. However, radiologic evaluation alone can rarely provide definitive diagnosis of ARONJ in the absence of clinical evaluation and in most cases should not be used solely for this purpose. In early cases of ARONJ without constitutional signs or symptoms (e.g., AAOMS stage 0 disease) or in NE cases at any stage, imaging studies may be more informative than clinical findings for accurate diagnosis. If previous imaging studies are available for comparison, they should be acquired to serve as a baseline and provide insight into disease progression. Radiologic examination is also useful for excluding jawbone malignancy in patients with cancer and suspected ARONJ.

In the dental setting, dental X-rays such as periapical or panoramic radiographs and/or conebeam CT (CBCT) scans that allow visualization of both jaws are part of a standard initial or preoperative workup of a patient [60]. These imaging modalities are often readily available in dental or oral surgery settings and are cost-effective and associated with less radiation exposure to patients

than conventional medical CT scans. Medical CT scans and MRI are also very useful modalities and appropriate in a hospital setting for ARONJ evaluation and are frequently reported in the literature. Positron emission tomography (PET), PET/ CT, SPECT/CT, planar scintigraphy, optical coherence tomography, and digital subtraction radiography have also been reported for ARONJ evaluation [61–63]. CBCT or CT-based scans can be reconstructed three-dimensionally to allow for further analyses and evaluation of extent of disease, which is critical for accurate staging (Fig. 12.12). To facilitate detection of early stage cases of ARONJ which may have equivocal clinical signs or symptoms, investigators have developed simple methodologies based on radiodensity measurements of jawbone in dental and medical radiographs [64–66]. Importantly, imaging modalities have varying sensitivity and specificity for ARONJ lesion detection, but a systematic analysis directly comparing all modalities has yet to be conducted. Since there are advantages and disadvantages to each imaging modality and each patient and case is unique, patient parameters and clinical judgment should guide appropriate imaging study selection.

Radiographic findings in ARONJ vary depending on stage of disease or degree of jawbone involvement. Prior to overt evidence of disease (e.g., stage 0 or NE early stage), there may be marked radiopacity or osteosclerosis in a region of jawbone (Fig. 12.13) or persistence of unremodeled bone in an extraction socket (Fig. 12.14). With frank bone necrosis, destruction of the trabecular structure of cancellous bone can be observed; these present as lytic, poorly to well-defined radiolucent regions of jawbone spreading from the epicenter of the lesion. Areas of bone lysis with centralized sequestrum formation may be seen with ARONJ progression (Fig. 12.15); these appear as mixed or mottled areas radiographically. There may be evidence of cortical expansion, thinning, erosion and perforation, and/or periosteal bone formation (Fig. 12.16). ARONJ lesions are usually space-occupying, but they can displace adjacent anatomic structures such as teeth, the inferior alveolar nerve canal, or the maxillary sinus.

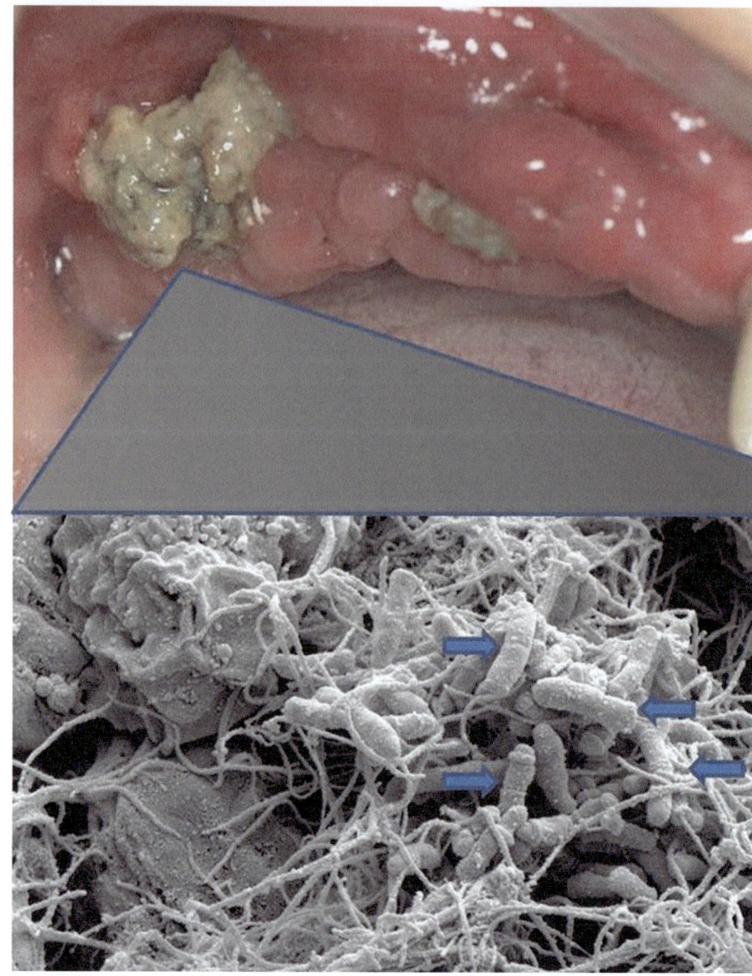

Fig. 12.11 The *top half* of the image shows a patient with maxillary ARONJ, and the *bottom half* shows a scanning electron micrograph (5000× original magnification) of the resected bone specimen with a biofilm microcolony of pleomorphic bacterial rods (*blue arrows*), with some exhibiting the characteristic circumferential ring indicative of *Actinomyces* species

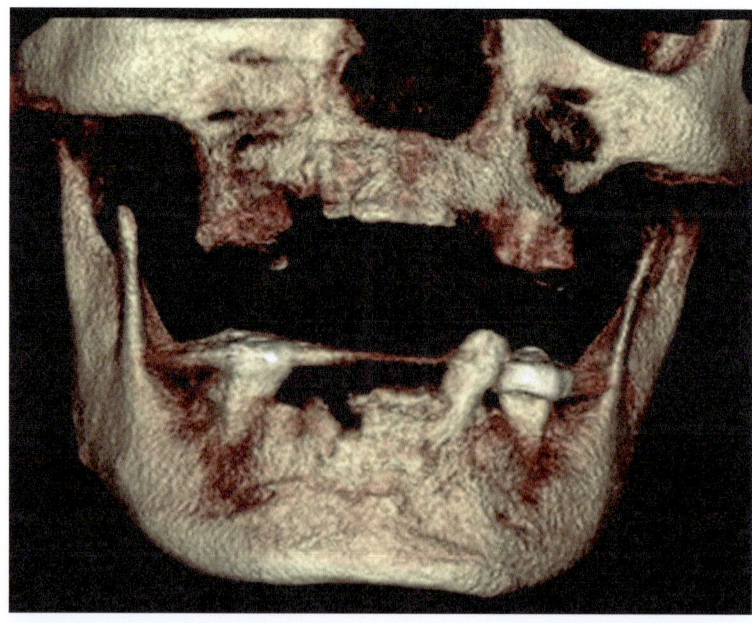

Fig. 12.12 Cone-beam CT with 3D reconstruction of the jaws in a 71-year-old African American male with a history of multiple myeloma and 2 years of intravenous zoledronate therapy. Stage 3 ARONJ is evident with extensive bone necrosis to the inferior alveolar nerve in the mandible and the antrum of the maxillary sinus

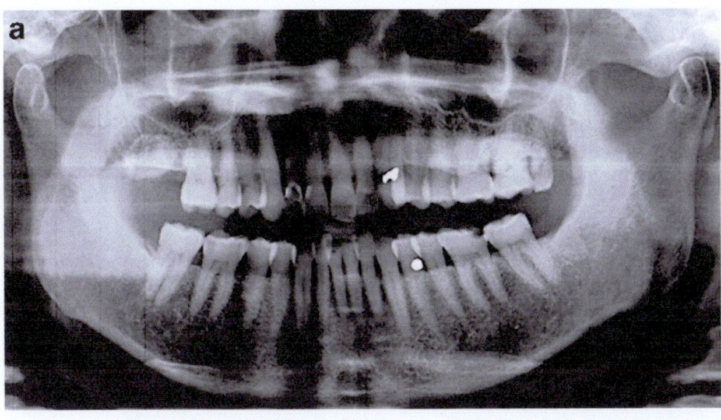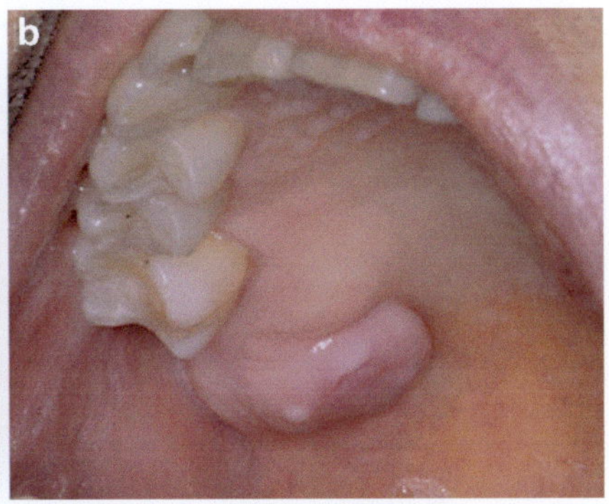

Fig. 12.13 (**a**) Panoramic radiograph of a patient with stage 0 ARONJ of the right posterior maxilla shows an area of well-defined radiopacity or osteosclerosis subjacent to the floor or antrum of the maxillary sinus. (**b**) The same patient has a swollen soft tissue lesion in the same area as the radiographic sclerosis but without evidence of exposed necrotic bone in the oral cavity

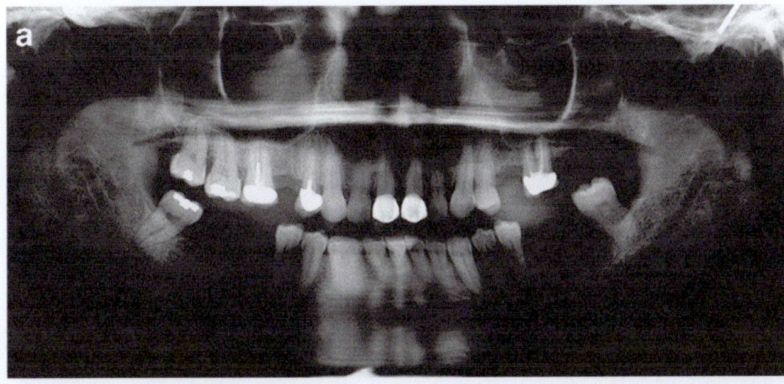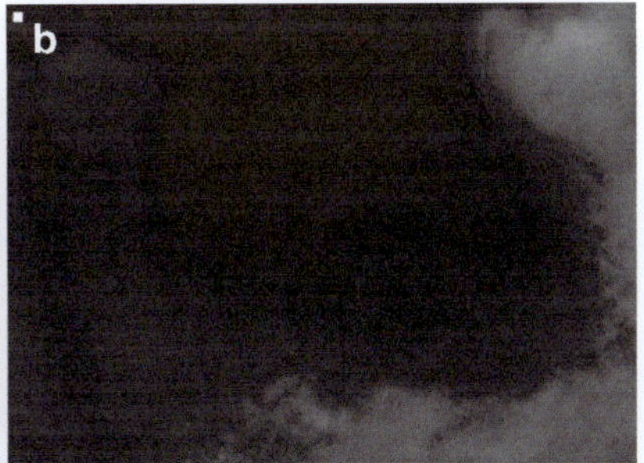

Fig. 12.14 (**a**) Panoramic radiograph showing a nonhealing extraction socket 8 months postoperatively in a patient with stage 0 ARONJ of the left posterior mandible. Compare the ARONJ lesion on the patient's left (*right* of image) to the patient's right mandible (*left* of image) where extractions were performed previously at the same time as the contralateral side but complete healing has occurred with bone fill, trabeculation, and cortication. (**b**) Periapical X-ray of the same case shows how the interseptal bone is developing into sequestrum

Fig. 12.15 Panoramic radiograph of patient with advanced ARONJ affecting the inferior alveolar nerve and appearing as a mixed lesion, with central sequestrum formation and peripheral lytic change

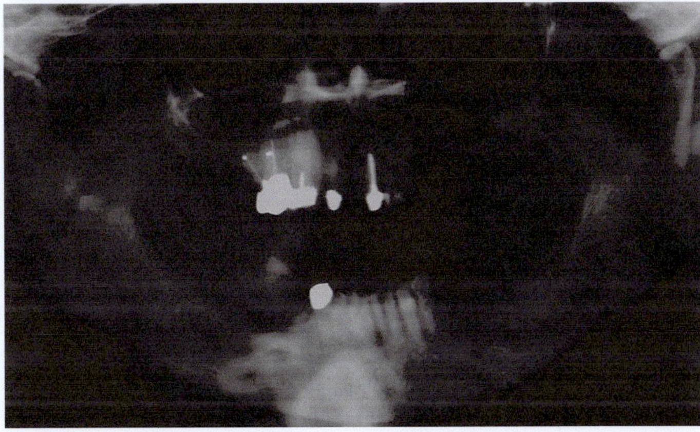

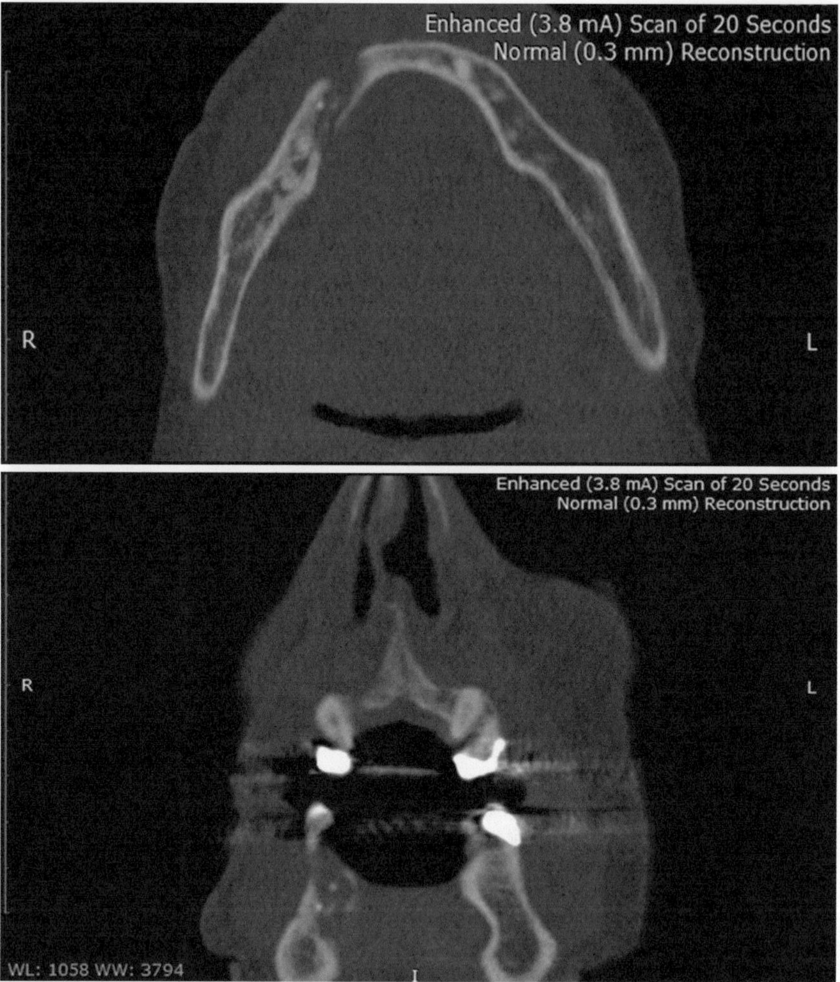

Fig. 12.16 Axial (*top*) and coronal (*bottom*) CBCT images of a 75-year-old male who has ARONJ affecting the right hemimandible, with evidence of cortical erosion and perforation and central sequestrum formation. Compare to the unaffected left hemimandible which appears normal in morphology and cortical outline

Tooth involvement may appear as widened or thickened lamina dura on radiographs. With advanced or late stage cases, pathologic fracture may be observed, but again this is a rare finding with ART in the rheumatologic setting.

On MRI evaluation, ARONJ is identified as regions within jawbone showing decreased signal of the bone marrow on T1-weighted images and increased signal on T2-weighted images. In cases with soft tissue spread of infection, MRI can be useful for evaluation of extent of disease and anatomic localization (Fig. 12.17). Contrast-enhanced MRI can also be useful for such evaluation. Radionuclide-based imaging studies show pathologically increased tracer uptake in affected regions of jawbone, and contralateral jawbone, if normal, may be used as an internal control or reference standard. Importantly, radiologic features of ARONJ can be similar to other conditions in the differential diagnosis, such as cases of osteomyelitis, osteoradionecrosis, or malignancy. Therefore, as with histopathology, definitive diagnosis is difficult with imaging alone in the absence of clinical correlation.

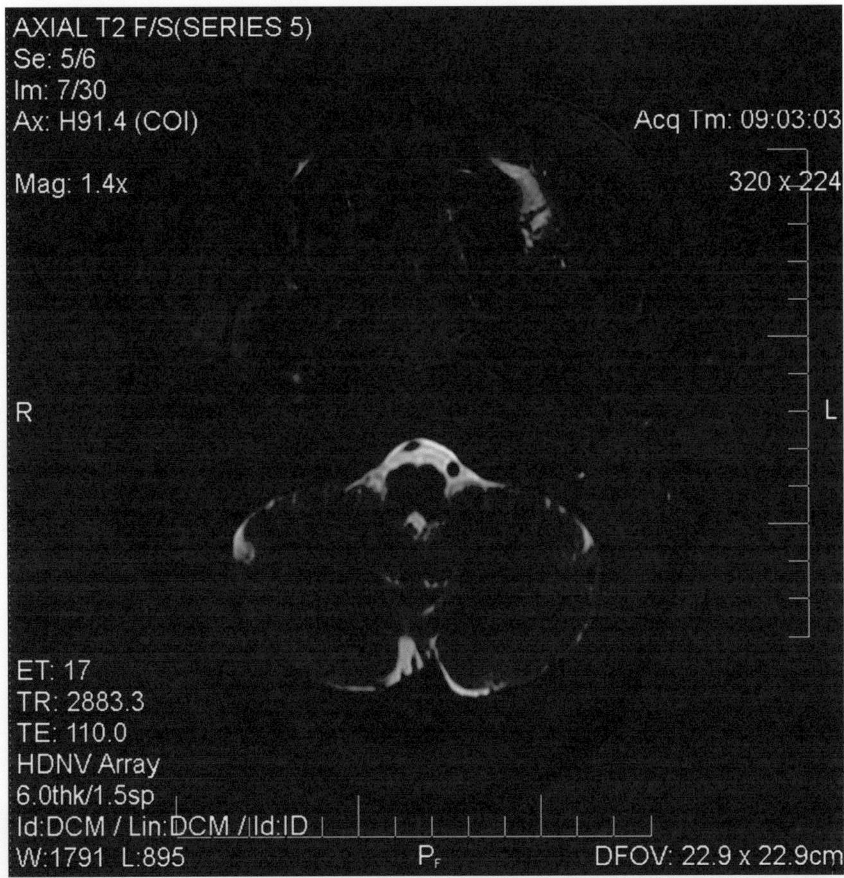

Fig. 12.17 Axial fat suppression T2-weighted MRI of the head and neck in a patient with stage 3 ARONJ and nearly complete replacement of fatty marrow in the right hemimandible, with edema/phlegmon of the adjacent masseter muscle. Note that this is the same patient as shown in Figs. 12.4 and 12.9

Diagnosis

Many conditions may resemble or have overlapping features with ARONJ clinically, radiographically, and/or histopathologically depending on anatomic location of involvement and various clinicopathologic parameters. The differential diagnosis of ARONJ may include osteomyelitis, osteoradionecrosis, and osteonecrosis secondary to herpes zoster infection, osteopetrosis, osteosclerosis, spontaneous lingual sequestration of the mandible, cemento-osseous dysplasia, Paget's disease, fibrous dysplasia, gingivitis/periodontitis, pyogenic granuloma, traumatic ulcer, pulpitis, mucositis, sinusitis, neuropathy or neuralgia, temporomandibular disorders, myofascial syndrome, odontogenic tumors, and primary or metastatic tumors of jawbone. Since there is no single finding or combination of findings that is pathognomonic for ARONJ, clinical diagnosis of ARONJ should be predicated on thorough review of systems, evaluation of medical and dental history, risk factors, medication history, presenting signs and symptoms, examination, radiologic findings, histopathologic findings when available, and exclusion of other conditions within the differential diagnosis. The schematic in Fig. 12.18 represents a useful clinical diagnosis algorithm for ARONJ.

In the clinical setting, many of the conditions in the differential diagnosis of ARONJ such as osteoradionecrosis, osteomyelitis, or osteopetrosis are extremely uncommon for many reasons.

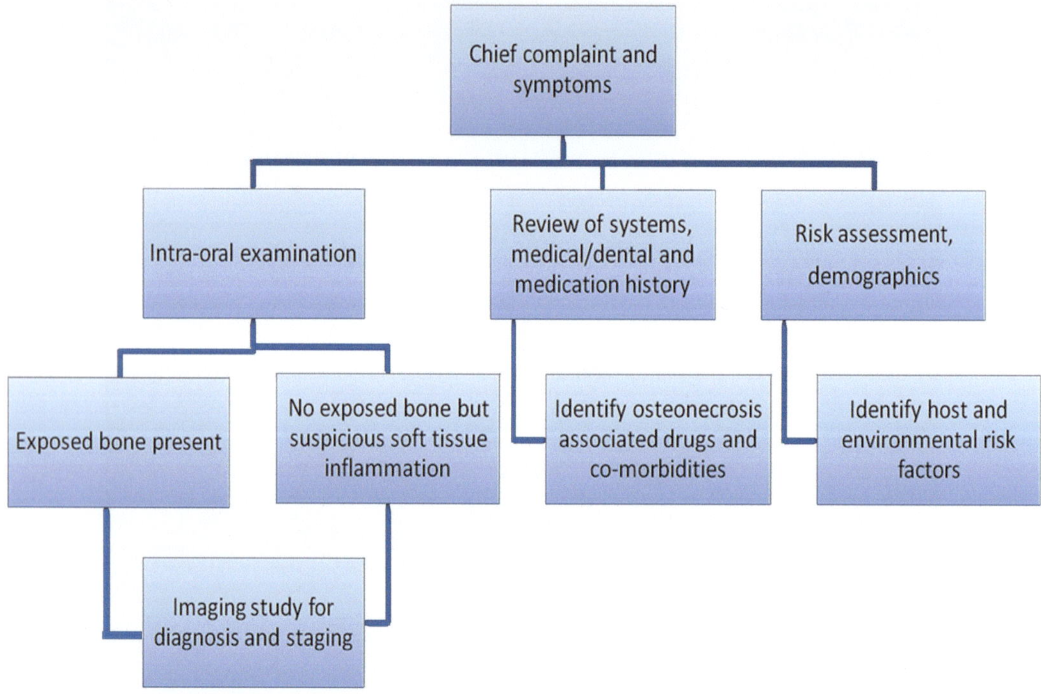

Fig. 12.18 Clinical algorithm for ARONJ diagnosis and staging

For example, osteoradionecrosis of the jaws in irradiated head and neck cancer patients has become less common due to the emergence of more focused delivery of radiation therapy via technological and biological advances in radiation oncology, the use of hyperbaric oxygen for dental preventative and therapeutic measures, and greater clinical awareness of this complication resulting in preventative measures prior to, during, and after radiation therapy. Osteomyelitis of the jaws has also declined in incidence because of antimicrobial therapeutics and in general is rare in the jaws and usually involves long bones [67]. Osteopetrosis is also uncommonly encountered clinically because by definition it refers to a group of rare, heritable disorders of the skeleton [68].

In early 2014, a PubMed or Medline article search of the English language scientific literature from 1800 to 2002 would reveal approximately 120 publications using the Medical Subject Headings (MeSH) search terms "jaw" and "osteonecrosis" in humans, and most of these are case reports of jawbone conditions such as osteoradionecrosis, osteomyelitis, chemical osteonecrosis, and zoster-associated osteonecrosis to name a few. A similar PubMed or Medline article search of the scientific literature with the same MeSH headings and parameters, but from the years 2002 to 2014, would reveal nearly 1500 publications. Most of these are ART-related cases which suggest that ARONJ is a unique and emergent phenomenon. The point being that ONJ unrelated to ART is rarely seen clinically and when it does occur, it responds to established therapies. Conversely, ONJ *is* encountered clinically given the widespread use of ART and has a very distinct presentation and course as compared to other conditions in the differential diagnosis.

Physical examination for ARONJ diagnosis should include an intraoral examination with a mouth mirror and adequate direct lighting (and universal precautions with personal protective equipment) in order to carefully visualize intraoral anatomic structures for abnormalities. Usually, the presence of exposed bone in the mouth meeting the AAOMS criteria for ARONJ definition is sufficient for accurate diagnosis once other conditions in the differential diagnosis are ruled out. In oncologic ARONJ cases, jaw-bone biopsy may ultimately be warranted to rule out metastatic disease which can mimic ARONJ clinically and radiographically [69]. However, biopsy is usually unnecessary in ARONJ cases associated with rheumatologic therapy in non-oncologic patients, especially in early stage cases that respond to conservative or noninvasive measures. In fact, surgical biopsy and further bone exposure may be contraindicated in some cases as this may exacerbate the condition. Clinicians should also systematically approach the diagnosis and management of NE cases of ARONJ, based on the presenting clinical signs and symptoms, an assessment of associated risk factors, radiologic evidence, examination, and history of refractory medical treatment. These findings, in conjunction with medical and dental history and a review of systems, should guide a tentative diagnosis of the NE variant of ARONJ and enable initiation of management prior to the clinical onset of exposed necrotic bone.

References[1]

1. Migliorati CA, Epstein JB, Abt E, Berenson JR. Osteonecrosis of the jaw and bisphosphonates in cancer: a narrative review. Nat Rev Endocrinol. 2011; 7:34–42.
2. Mhaskar R, Redzepovic J, Wheatley K, Clark OA, Miladinovic B, Glasmacher A, Kumar A, Djulbegovic B. Bisphosphonates in multiple myeloma: a network meta-analysis. Cochrane Database Syst Rev. 2012;5, CD003188.
3. *Khan AA, Sándor GK, Dore E, Morrison AD, Alsahli M, Amin F, et al. Bisphosphonate-associated osteonecrosis of the jaw. Canadian task force on osteonecrosis of the Jaw. J Rheumatol. 2009;36(3):478–90. *This systematic review revealed that ARONJ is associated with high-dose n-BP therapy primarily in the oncology patient population.
4. **Papapoulos S, Chapurlat R, Libanati C, et al. Five years of denosumab exposure in women with post-menopausal osteoporosis: results from the first two years of the FREEDOM extension. J Bone Miner Res. 2012;27:694–701. **This study shows data on adverse events from extension of the pivotal FREEDOM trial, and indicates that ARONJ incidence is low (2 cases) in the treatment group and that adverse events did not increase with long-term Dmab administration.
5. Marx RE, Stern D. Oral and maxillofacial pathology: a rationale for diagnosis and treatment. 2nd ed. New Malden: Quintessence Publishing; 2012. ISBN 9780867155129.
6. **Barasch A, Cunha-Cruz J, Curro FA, Hujoel P, Sung AH, Vena D, et al. Risk factors for osteonecrosis of the jaws: a case-control study from the CONDOR dental PBRN. J Dent Res. 2011;90(4):439–44. **This epidemiologic study revealed that dental factors such as suppuration and extractions were independent risk factors for ARONJ in addition to duration of treatment (>2yrs). Both oral and intravenous ART was strongly associated with ONJ.
7. Cartsos VM, Zhu S, Zavras AI. Bisphosphonate use and the risk of adverse jaw outcomes: a medical claims study of 714,217 people. J Am Dent Assoc. 2008;139:23–30.
8. *Firestein GS, Budd RC, Gabriel SE, McInnes IB, O'Dell JR. Kelley's textbook of rheumatology. 8th ed. Elsevier, Philadelphia, PA 2009. p. 1611. *This textbook provides accurate information on osteonecrosis in general and not just limited to the jawbones.
9. Barasch A, Cunha-Cruz J, Curro F, DeRouen T, Gilbert GH, Hujoel P, et al. Dental risk factors for osteonecrosis of the jaws – a CONDOR case-control study. Clin Oral Invest. 2013;17:1839–45.
10. Yarom N, Yahalom R, Shoshani Y, Hamed W, Regev E, Elad S. Osteonecrosis of the jaw induced by orally administered bisphosphonates: incidence, clinical features, predisposing factors and treatment outcome. Osteoporos Int. 2007;18(10):1363–70.
11. *Ruggiero SL, Dodson TB, Assael LA, et al. American association of oral and maxillofacial surgeons position paper on bisphosphonate-related osteonecrosis of the jaws – 2009 update. J Oral Maxillofac Surg. 2009;67:2–12. *This position paper by the AAOMS provides useful information for clinicians on ARONJ diagnosis, risk and management.
12. *Khosla S, Burr D, Cauley J, et al. Bisphosphonate-associated osteonecrosis of the jaw: report of a task force of the American society for bone and mineral research. J Bone Miner Res. 2007;22:1479. *This ASBMR task force reviewed the literature and identified several gaps in the current evidence base in addition to formulating a number of clinical and basic research questions which should help guide research agendas to better understand, prevent and manage ARONJ.
13. *Patel S, Choyee S, Uyanne J, Nguyen AL, Lee P, Sedghizadeh PP, et al. Non-exposed bisphosphonate-related osteonecrosis of the jaw: a critical assessment of current definition, staging, and treatment guidelines. Oral Dis. 2012;18(7):625–32. *This study presents and delineates an accurate approach for the diagnosis and staging of non-exposed variants of ARONJ.

---

[1] *Important References
**Very important References

14. Fusco V, Galassi C, Berruti A, et al. Osteonecrosis of the jaw after zoledronic acid and denosumab treatment. J Clin Oncol. 2011;29:521–2.
15. Marx RE. Oral and intravenous bisphosphonate-induced osteonecrosis of the jaws: history, etiology, prevention, and treatment. New Malden: Quintessence Publishing; 2007. ISBN 9780867154627.
16. Ruggiero SL, Mehrotra B. Bisphosphonate-related osteonecrosis of the jaw: diagnosis, prevention, and management. Annu Rev Med. 2009;60:18.1–2.
17. Russell RG, Rogers MJ, Frith JC, et al. The pharmacology of bisphosphonates and new insights into their mechanisms of action. J Bone Miner Res. 1999;14 Suppl 2:53–65.
18. *Wood J, Bonjean K, Ruetz S, et al. Novel antiangiogenic effects of the bisphosphonate compound zoledronic acid. J Pharmacol Exp Ther. 2002;302(3):1055–61. *This study showed marked anti-angiogenic properties of zoledronate *in vitro* and *in vivo*.
19. Ferretti G, Fabi A, Carlini P, et al. Zoledronic-acid induced circulating level modifications of angiogenic factors, metalloproteinases and proinflammatory cytokines in metastatic breast cancer patients. Oncology. 2005;69(1):35–43.
20. *Landesberg R, Woo V, Cremers S, et al. Potential pathophysiological mechanisms in osteonecrosis of the jaw. Ann N Y Acad Sci. 2011;1218:62–79. *This review provides a comprehensive summary of the proposed mechanisms for ARONJ development.
21. *Wong PK, Borromeo GL, Wark JD. Bisphosphonate-related osteonecrosis of the jaw in non-malignant bone disease. Rheumatol Int. 2013;33(9):2189–98. *This literature review provides useful information on the diagnosis and pathogenesis of ARONJ.
22. Cremers S, Sparidans R, Hartigh JD, Hamdy N, Vermeij P, Papapoulos S. A pharmacokinetic and pharmacodynamic model for intravenous bisphosphonate (pamidronate) in osteoporosis. Eur J Clin Pharmacol. 2002;57:883–90.
23. Ristow O, Gerngroß C, Schwaiger M, Hohlweg-Majert B, Ristow M, Koerdt S et al. Does regular zoledronic acid change the bone turnover of the jaw in men with metastatic prostate cancer: a possible clue to the pathogenesis of bisphosphonate-related osteonecrosis of the jaw? J Cancer Res Clin Oncol. 2014; 140(3):487–93.
24. Weiss HM, Pfaar U, Schweitzer A, Wiegand H, Skerjanec A, Schran H. Biodistribution and plasma protein binding of zoledronic acid. Drug Metab Dispos. 2008;36:2043–9.
25. *Sedghizadeh PP, Kumar SK, Gorur A, Schaudinn C, Shuler CF, Costerton JW. Identification of microbial biofilms in osteonecrosis of the jaws secondary to bisphosphonate therapy. J Oral Maxillofac Surg. 2008;66:767–75. *This article reveals the presence and nature of microbial biofilms in ARONJ specimens and their role in clinical disease and pathogenesis.
26. Hansen T, Kunkel M, Springer E, Walter C, Weber A, Siegel E, Kirkpatrick CJ. Actinomycosis of the jaws: histopathological study of 45 patients shows significant involvement in bisphosphonate-associated osteonecrosis and infected osteoradionecrosis. Virchows Arch. 2007;451:1009–17.
27. *Kassolis JD, Scheper M, Jham B, Reynolds MA. Histopathologic findings in bone from edentulous alveolar ridges: a role in osteonecrosis of the jaws? Bone. 2010;47:127–30. *This study shows that even healthy edentulous jawbones can contain regions of necrotic bone and microbial biofilms, which could contribute to the development of ARONJ.
28. Wei X, Pushalkar S, Estilo C, Wong C, Farooki A, Fornier M, et al. Molecular profiling of oral microbiota in jawbone samples of bisphosphonate-related osteonecrosis of the jaw. Oral Dis. 2012;18:602–12.
29. Saber MH, Schwarzberg K, Alonaizan FA, Kelley ST, Sedghizadeh PP, Furlan M, Levy TA, Simon JH, Slots J. Bacterial flora of dental periradicular lesions analyzed by the 454-pyrosequencing technology. J Endod. 2012;38:1484–8.
30. Pichardo SE, van Merkesteyn JP. Bisphosphonate related osteonecrosis of the jaws: spontaneous or dental origin? Oral Surg Oral Med Oral Pathol Oral Radiol. 2013;116(3):287–92.
31. *Kumar SK, Gorur A, Schaudinn C, Shuler CF, Costerton JW, Sedghizadeh PP. The role of microbial biofilms in osteonecrosis of the jaw associated with bisphosphonate therapy. Curr Osteoporos Rep. 2010;8(1):40–8. *This review describes the role of infection and oral microbial biofilms in the pathogenesis of ARONJ.
32. *Kos M, Junka A, Smutnicka D, Bartoszewicz M, Kurzynowski T, Gluza K. Pamidronate enhances bacterial adhesion to bone hydroxyapatite. Another puzzle in the pathology of bisphosphonate-related osteonecrosis of the jaw? J Oral Maxillofac Surg. 2013;71:1010–6. *This study reveals that oral bacteria have a significantly greater binding affinity to bone in the presence of n-BP than in its absence, providing insight into the infectious nature of pathogenesis.
33. Reid IR. Osteonecrosis of the jaw: who gets it, and why? Bone. 2009;44:4–10.
34. **Vermeer JA, Jansen ID, Marthi M, Coxon FP, McKenna CE, Sun S, et al. Jaw bone marrow-derived osteoclast precursors internalize more bisphosphonate than long-bone marrow precursors. Bone. 2013;57:242–51. **This study shows that osteoclasts at different anatomic sites internalize n-BP differentially, but differential uptake does not correlate directly with osteoclastogenesis, and jawbone osteoclasts are more susceptible to n-BP effects such as inhibition of prenylation.
35. Hokugo A, Sun S, Park S, McKenna CE, Nishimura I. Equilibrium-dependent bisphosphonate interaction with crystalline bone mineral explains anti-resorptive pharmacokinetics and prevalence of osteonecrosis of the jaw in rats. Bone. 2013;53:59–68.
36. Kikuiri T, Kim I, Yamaza T, Akiyama K, Zhang Q, Li Y, et al. Cell-based immunotherapy with mesenchy-

mal stem cells cures bisphosphonate-related osteonecrosis of the jaw-like disease in mice. J Bone Miner Res. 2010;25:1668–79.

37. Thumbigere-Math V, Michalowicz BS, de Jong EP, Griffin TJ, Basi DL, Hughes PJ, Tsai ML, Swenson KK, Rockwell L, Gopalakrishnan R. Salivary proteomics in bisphosphonate-related osteonecrosis of the jaw. Oral Dis 2015;21:46–56.

38. Nicoletti P, Cartsos VM, Palaska PK, Shen Y, Floratos A, Zavras AI. Genomewide pharmacogenetics of bisphosphonate-induced osteonecrosis of the jaw: the role of RBMS3. Oncologist. 2012;17:279–87.

39. *Sedghizadeh PP, Yooseph S, Fadrosh DW, Zeigler-Allen L, Thiagarajan M, Salek H, Farahnik F, Williamson SJ. Metagenomic investigation of microbes and viruses in patients with jaw osteonecrosis associated with bisphosphonate therapy. Oral Surg Oral Med Oral Pathol Oral Radiol. 2012;114:764–70. *This study shows that patients with ARONJ have a unique microbial profile as compared to patients without disease, and describes the role of viruses for the first time in microbial biofilms associated with ARONJ.

40. Ferla FL, Paolicchi E, Crea F, Cei S, Graziani F, Gabriele M, Danesi R. An aromatase polymorphism (g.132810C>T) predicts risk of bisphosphonate-related osteonecrosis of the jaw. Biomark Med. 2012; 6:201–9.

41. Sarasquete ME, Garcia-Sanz R, Marin L, Alcoceba M, Chillon MC, Balanzategui A, et al. Bisphosphonate-related osteonecrosis of the jaw is associated with polymorphisms of the cytochrome P450 CYP2C8 in multiple myeloma: a genome-wide single nucleotide polymorphism analysis. Blood. 2008;112:2709.

42. Ruggiero SL, Gralow J, Marx RE, et al. Practical guidelines for the prevention, diagnosis, and treatment of osteonecrosis of the jaw in patients with cancer. J Oncol Pract. 2006;2:7–14.

43. Assouline-Dayan Y, Chang C, Greenspan A, et al. Pathogenesis and natural history of osteonecrosis. Semin Arthritis Rheum. 2002;32:94–124.

44. Thumbigere-Math V, Tu L, Huckabay S, Dudek AZ, Lunos S, Basi DL, et al. A retrospective study evaluating frequency and risk factors of osteonecrosis of the jaw in 576 cancer patients receiving intravenous bisphosphonates. Am J Clin Oncol. 2012;35:386–92.

45. *Lee JK, Kim KW, Choi JY, Moon SY, Kim SG, Kim CH, et al. Bisphosphonates-related osteonecrosis of the jaw in Korea: a preliminary report. J Korean Assoc Oral Maxillofac Surg. 2013;39(1):9–13. *This multi-center population study in Korea found that the incidence for ARONJ is higher in Korea than other reported countries, confirming previous findings of a higher predilection for ARONJ in Asians.

46. Kyrgidis A, Tzellos TG, Toulis K, Arora A, Kouvelas D, Triaridis S. An evidence-based review of risk-reductive strategies for osteonecrosis of the jaws among cancer patients. Curr Clin Pharmacol. 2013;8: 124–34.

47. *Schubert M, Klatte I, Linek W, Müller B, Döring K, Eckelt U, Hemprich A, Berger U, Hendricks J. The Saxon bisphosphonate register – therapy and prevention of bisphosphonate-related osteonecrosis of the jaws. Oral Oncol. 2012;48:349–54. *This longitudinal study demonstrates that preventative measures, which include pre-operative and post-operative antibiotics in patients receiving ART and undergoing invasive dental surgery, reduce the risk of ARONJ.

48. **Sedghizadeh PP, Jones AC, LaVallee C, Jelliffe RW, Le AD, Lee P, Kiss A, Neely MN. Population pharmacokinetic and pharmacodynamic modeling for assessing risk of bisphosphonate-related osteonecrosis of the jaw. Oral Surg Oral Med Oral Pathol Oral Radiol. 2013;115:224–32. **This clinical case-control study validates in vitro findings of a toxic threshold for n-BP accumulation in jawbone for induction of ARONJ, and introduces for the first time a pharmacometric analytical approach for risk assessment in ARONJ. It also identifies unique risk factors (Asian ethnicity) for the first time based on anthropometric variables.

49. Barrett JS, Fossler MJ, Cadieu KD, Gastonguay MR. Pharmacometrics: a multidisciplinary field to facilitate critical thinking in drug development and translational research settings. J Clin Pharmacol. 2008;48:632–49.

50. Kim JW, Kong KA, Kim SJ, Choi SK, Cha IH, Kim MR. Prospective biomarker evaluation in patients with osteonecrosis of the jaw who received bisphosphonates. Bone. 2013;57(1):201–5.

51. *Borromeo GL, Brand C, Clement JG, McCullough M, Crighton L, Hepworth G, Wark JD. A large case-control study reveals a positive association between bisphosphonate use and delayed dental healing and osteonecrosis of the jaw. J Bone Min Res. 2014; 29:1363–8. *This clinical study supports the hypothesis that delayed wound healing in the oral cavity plays a role in the pathogenesis of ARONJ.

52. Otto S, Pautke C, Hafner S, Hesse R, Reichardt LF, Mast G, Ehrenfeld M, Cornelius CP. Pathologic fractures in bisphosphonate-related osteonecrosis of the jaw – review of the literature and review of our own cases. Craniomaxillofac Trauma Reconstr. 2013;6(3): 147–54.

53. Borgioli VC, Duvina M, Brancato L, Spinelli G, Brandi ML, Tonelli P. Bisphosphonate-related osteonecrosis of the jaw: clinical and physiopathological considerations. Ther Clin Risk Manag. 2009;5: 217–27.

54. Food and Drug Administration (FDA). Background document for meeting of advisory committee for reproductive health drugs and drug safety and risk management advisory committee. Center for Drug Evaluation and Research; 2011. p. 17–20.

55. Sivolella S, Lumachi F, Stellini E, Favero L. Denosumab and anti-angiogenetic drug-related osteonecrosis of the jaw: an uncommon but potentially severe disease. Anticancer Res. 2013;33(5):1793–7.

56. Hoefert S, Eufinger H. Sunitinib may raise the risk of bisphosphonate-related osteonecrosis of the jaw: presentation of three cases. Oral Surg Oral Med Oral Pathol Oral Radiol Endod. 2010;110(4):463–9.
57. Anavi-Lev K, Anavi Y, Chaushu G, Alon DM, Gal G, Kaplan I. Bisphosphonate related osteonecrosis of the jaws: clinico-pathological investigation and histomorphometric analysis. Oral Surg Oral Med Oral Radiol Oral Pathol. 2013;115(5):660–6.
58. Koerdt S, Dax S, Grimaldi H, Ristow O, Kuebler AC, Reuther T. Histomorphologic characteristics of bisphosphonate-related osteonecrosis of the jaw. J Oral Pathol Med. 2014;43:448–53.
59. Zustin J, Reske D, Zrnc TA, Heiland M, Scheuer HA, Assaf AT, Friedrich RE. Pseudoepitheliomatous hyperplasia associated with bisphosphonate-related osteonecrosis of the jaw. In Vivo. 2014;28(1):125–31.
60. Guggenberger R, Winklhofer S, Spiczak JV, Andreisek G, Alkadhi H. Bisphosphonate-induced osteonecrosis of the jaw: comparison of disease extent on contrast-enhanced MR imaging, [18F] fluoride PET/CT, and conebeam CT imaging. Am J Neuroradiol. 2013;34:1242–7.
61. Zaman MU, Nakamoto T, Tanimoto K. A retrospective study of digital subtraction technique to detect sclerotic changes in alveolar bone on intraoral radiographs of bisphosphonate-treated patients. Dentomaxillofac Radiol. 2013;42(10):20130242.
62. Bolouri C, Merwald M, Huellner MW, Veit-Haibach P, Kuttenberger J, Pérez-Lago M, et al. Performance of orthopantomography, planar scintigraphy, CT alone and SPECT/CT in patients with suspected osteomyelitis of the jaw. Eur J Nucl Med Mol Imaging. 2013;40:411–7.
63. Belcher R, Boyette J, Pierson T, Siegel E, Bartel TB, Aniasse E, et al. What is the role of positron emission tomography in osteonecrosis of the jaws? J Oral Maxillofac Surg. 2014;72:306–10.
64. Hamada H, Matsuo A, Koizumi T, Satomi T, Chikazu D. A simple evaluation method for early detection of bisphosphonate-related osteonecrosis of the mandible using computed tomography. J Craniomaxillofac Surg. 2014;42:924–9.
65. Takaishi Y, Ikeo T, Nakajima M, Miki T, Fujita T. A pilot case-control study on the alveolar bone density measurement in risk assessment for bisphosphonate related osteonecrosis of the jaw. Osteoporos Int. 2010; 21:815–25.
66. Torres SR, Chen CS, Leroux BG, Lee PP, Hollender LG, Santos EC, et al. Mandibular cortical bone evaluation on cone beam computed tomography images of patients with bisphosphonate-related osteonecrosis of the jaw. Oral Surg Oral Med Oral Pathol Oral Radiol. 2012;113:695–703.
67. Hudson JW. Osteomyelitis of the jaw: A 50-year perspective. J Oral Maxillofac Surg. 1993;51(12):1294–301.
68. Stark Z, Savarirayan R. Osteopetrosis. Orphanet J Rare Dis. 2009;4:5.
69. *Carlson ER, Fleisher KE, Ruggiero SL. Metastatic cancer identified in osteonecrosis specimens of the jaws in patients receiving intravenous bisphosphonate medications. J Oral Maxillofac Surg. 2013;71:2077–86. *This study describes the importance of accurate diagnosis of ARONJ in patients receiving intravenous ART for oncologic care by histopathologic examination of jawbone lesions to rule out malignancy.

Epidemiology of Osteonecrosis of the Jaws from Antiresorptive Treatment

13

Morten Schiødt

Summary

- Osteonecrosis of the jaws (ONJs) from bisphosphonates was first seen in 2003.
- The numbers have risen since with increasing numbers each year.
- ONJ is still a rare occurrence among patients with osteoporosis
  - The prevalence of ONJ is less than 01 %.
- A new type of ONJ, nonexposed ONJ has been recognized recently.
- Nonexposed may occur in up to one fourth of ONJ cases.
- ONJ may occur from bisphosphonate and from denosumab.
- ONJ is now called antiresorptive medication-related ONJ.
- Important risk factors for ONJ include duration of antiresorptive medication, type and dose of the medication, and infection around teeth and tooth extraction.

M. Schiødt, DDS, Dr.Odont (✉)
Department of Oral and Maxillofacial Surgery,
Copenhagen University Hospital (Rigshospitalet),
9, Blegdamsvej, Copenhagen 2100, Denmark
e-mail: morten.schioedt@regionh.dk;
mschioedt@hotmail.com

Introduction

Osteonecrosis of the jaws (ONJ) was first reported around 2003. Marx et al. [1] reported pamidronate (Aredia)- and zoledronate (Zometa)-induced avascular necrosis of the jaws, and a growing epidemic was foreseen. Shortly after, a number of case series documented the start of a new epidemic. Ruggerio et al. [2] reported 63 cases from the New York area, and Marx et al. [3] published 119 cases of ONJ from Florida. During the last 5 years, anti-angiogenic medications, known as tyrosine kinase inhibitors, have additionally been associated with the development of ONJ. Tyrosine kinase inhibitors inhibit vascular endothelial growth factors and may alone or in combination with BF or denosumab give rise to ONJ. However, this happens only in cancer patients, as osteoporosis patients are usually not treated with these drugs [4, 5]. This was the start of the ongoing and growing epidemic of ONJ, although in 1879, a condition known as "phossy jaws" was discovered among workers exposed to phosphorus in match factories. The environmental work exposure to phosphorus at that time leads to accumulation of phosphorus in the jaw bone giving rise to a condition very similar to the ONJ we know today [6]. This first epidemic ended when importing and working with white phosphorus were banned in many countries in 1912.

© Springer International Publishing Switzerland 2016
S.L. Silverman, B. Abrahamsen (eds.), *The Duration and Safety of Osteoporosis Treatment*, DOI 10.1007/978-3-319-23639-1_13

In the decade since 2003, a number of consensus papers by various organizations have set the stage for updates, guidelines for diagnosis and treatment, risk factors, prevention, and not least many unanswered questions that the research community are to address [7–12]. Experimental studies including animal models as well as cell culture studies have already been implemented [13–15].

Terminology

ONJ has been termed bisphosphonate (BP)-associated or BP-induced ONJ in the consensus papers. However, since the discovery of denosumab-induced ONJ, the nomenclature is insufficient. This applies also to the recently reported ONJ induced by the new antiangiogenetic drugs like tyrosine kinase inhibitors (sunitinib, bevacizumab, etc.) [4, 5]. A consensus paper in 2011 by the American Dental Association Council on Scientific Affairs suggested the term: "antiresorptive agent-induced ONJ" (ARONJ) [11]. Most recently, the American Association of Oral and Maxillofacial Surgeons acknowledged the association of ONJ with various types of medication. The term *medication-related ONJ* was introduced in June 2014 [12]. In the present chapter, this will generally be referred to as "ONJ."

Definition of ONJ

ONJ is a clinical diagnosis defined as the presence of exposed bone for more than 8 weeks in a patient presently or previously on bisphosphonate treatment or other antiresorptive treatment and who has not received irradiation for head and neck cancer [7–12]. Thus, patients treated with denosumab and other new medications are usually included in the definition.

It is important to note that although ONJ is defined officially as the presence of exposed jaw bone, a number of ONJ patients have *no* exposed bone, i.e., there is no area of denuded bone visible in the oral cavity. This group, referred to *as*

nonexposed ONJ, is believed to suffer from the same biologic condition as the exposed ONJ patients [16–18]. The nonexposed ONJ is discussed further below under classification.

Diagnosis and Classification

The diagnosis of ONJ is clinical as defined above [8, 10]. A number of consensus papers by various organizations have presented definition and guidelines for diagnosis and treatment [7–11]. In the paper by Ruggerio et al. [8], ONJ was separated into three stages (Table 13.1). Basically, stage 1 signifies exposed bone in a patient without symptoms. Stage 2 implies symptoms and/or signs of infection, whereas stage 3 includes patients with widespread and/or severe osteonecrosis involving, for example, the maxillary sinus, the mandibular alveolar nerve, or showing spontaneous fracture of the jaws. In 2009, the Ruggerio et al. [10] criteria were revised by the introduction of a stage 0, indicating nonspecific symptoms from the jaws but without exposed bone. In June 2014, the American Association of Oral and Maxillofacial Surgeons consensus paper included the presence of fistula as indicative of "exposed bone" and thus improved the classification [12].

However, the subgroup of nonexposed ONJ (with no fistula) is still not covered by the consensus classification. The nonexposed ONJ has been described in a number of studies [16–18]. The proportion of nonexposed ONJ ranges from 14 to 35 % of an ONJ population [16, 18, 19]. If nonexposed ONJs are not recognized or accepted, it might have a significant consequence for epidemiologic studies potentially leading to underreporting [18]. One should bear in mind that odontologic infectious foci as, for example, a dental periapical infection or sinusitis from a periapical infection close to the sinus, should be excluded as the cause of symptoms before a diagnosis of nonexposed ONJ is made.

Schiodt et al. [18] published suggested criteria for nonexposed ONJ (Table 13.2). Nonexposed ONJ has an overlap with stage 0 (Ruggerio et al. 2009 [10]), and it is suggested to avoid using

Table 13.1 Classification of osteonecrosis of the jaws by Ruggerio et al. (2006) [6] and Ruggerio et al. (2009) [8]

How to classify a patient suspected for ONJ	Criteria by AAOMS Ruggerio et al. (2006) [6] and Ruggerio et al. (2009) [8]
1. Present and/or previous bisphosphonate or other antiresorptive treatment	Yes
2. Previous radiation to the jaws	No
3. Exposed bone for ≥8 weeks	Yes
4. Staging as follows	
Stage 0	Patients with no clinical evidence of necrotic bone, but present with nonspecific symptoms or clinical and radiographic findings *Symptoms* • Odontalgia not explained by an odontogenic cause • Dull, aching bone pain in the body of the mandible, which may radiate to the temporomandibular joint region • Sinus pain, which may be associated with inflammation and thickening of the maxillary sinus wall • Altered neurosensory function *Clinical findings* • Loosening of teeth not explained by chronic periodontal disease • Periapical/periodontal fistula that is not associated with pulpal necrosis due to caries *Radiographic findings* • Alveolar bone loss or resorption not attributable to chronic periodontal disease • Changes to trabecular pattern—dense woven bone and persistence of unremodeled bone in extraction sockets • Thickening/obscuring of periodontal ligament (thickening of the lamina dura and decreased size of the periodontal ligament space) • Inferior alveolar canal narrowing These nonspecific findings, which characterize stage 0, may occur in patients with a prior history of stage 1, 2, or 3 disease who have healed and have no clinical evidence of exposed bone
Stage 1	Exposed bone No symptoms
Stage 2	Exposed bone Symptoms of infection
Stage 3	*Exposed* and necrotic bone in patients with pain, infection, and one or more of the following: • Exposed necrotic bone extending beyond the region of alveolar bone, that is, inferior border and ramus in the mandible, maxillary sinus, and zygoma in the maxilla • Pathologic fracture • Extraoral fistula • Oral–antral/oral–nasal communication • Osteolysis extending to the inferior border of the mandible or sinus floor

Table 13.2 Criteria for classification of exposed and nonexposed osteonecrosis after Schiodt et al. (2014) [18]

How to classify a patient suspected for ONJ	Criteria by Schiodt et al. (2014) [18]	
	Criteria for exposed ONJ (E-ONJ)	Criteria for nonexposed ONJ (NE-ONJ)
1. Present and/or previous bisphosphonate or other antiresorptive treatment	Yes	Yes
2. Previous radiation to the jaws	No	No
3. Exposed bone for ≥8 weeks	Yes	No Accepted as ONJ if 1. Intraoral or extraoral fistula and/or 2. Jaw pain 3. Swelling 4. Sequestrum formation on imaging 5. Necrotic bone on histopathology. If specimen available. Item 5 is mandatory
4. Staging as follows		
Stage 0	NA	NA
Stage 1	Exposed bone No symptoms Name: E-ONJ, stage 1	Not exposed bone No symptoms Name: NE-ONJ, stage 1
Stage 2	Exposed bone Symptoms of infection Name: E-ONJ, stage 2	Not exposed bone Symptoms of infections Name: NE-ONJ, stage 2
Stage 3	As AAOMS stage 3 Name: E-ONJ, stage 3	*Nonexposed* and necrotic bone in patients with pain, infection, and one or more of the following • *Nonexposed* necrotic bone demonstrated on imaging extending beyond the region of alveolar bone, that is, inferior border and ramus in the mandible, maxillary sinus, and zygoma in the maxilla • Pathologic fracture • Extraoral fistula • Oral–antral/oral–nasal communication • Osteolysis extending to the inferior border of the mandible or sinus floor Name: NE-ONJ, stage 3

These criteria can be used as a supplement to Table 13.1

stage 0 and instead use nonexposed ONJ (Table 13.2), and those from the previous stage 0 who do not fulfill criteria for nonexposed ONJ can be classified as "at risk." Examples of "at risk" patients are patients on BP treatment with radiologically widened lamina dura around the teeth but without symptoms from the jaw.

Epidemiology

Since the first description by Marx et al. in 2003 [1], increasing numbers of ONJ have been reported. The literature reports quite varying incidence rates from less than 0.01 to 18.6 % [20–22]. Generally, ONJ occurs more frequently among patients on intravenous treatment with nitrogen-containing bisphosphonates, compared to peroral tablet treatment. The incidence is much higher among cancer patients with skeletal metastases or multiple myeloma compared with that seen in osteoporosis patients. The varying incidence rate may be influenced by study designs, as some studies are retrospective or based on questionnaires without an oral examination possibly underestimating the incidence, and others are based on a detailed oral examination by dental or maxillofacial specialists. Prospective studies of the latter type reveal incidences of more than 10 % [20, 23, 24]. For example, Walter et al. [20] reported an incidence of 18.6 % in zoledronate-treated cancer patients in a prospective design with thorough dental examination of all patients. In contrast, patients with osteoporosis have a much lower risk, around 0.1 % [25].

In a recent large multi-clinic case–control study from Australia involving 4212 patients recruited during a 6-month window period, Borromeo et al. [26] found that odds ratio for osteoporosis patients on bisphosphonate treatment developing delayed healing (including ONJ) was 11.6 (95 % CI 1.9–69.4; $P = 0.01$).

A systematic literature review by Solomon et al. [27] included nine studies and patient populations exceeding 500,000 bisphosphonate-treated patients. They reported an incidence rate for ONJ among osteoporosis patients varying from 0.028 to 4.3 %. The relative risk for ONJ among bisphosphonate-treated osteoporosis patients showed odds ratio of 7.2–9.2 [27]. Another systematic review among osteoporosis patients from 2013 revealed comparable results [28].

A case–control study of ONJ cases diagnosed after January 1st 2003 in the USA involving several NIH-supported private dental practice research networks identified 191 cases of ONJ and allocated 573 controls [29]. Patients with a history of any cancer had odds ratio of 14.3 for ONJ compared with those without cancer. Similarly, patients with osteoporosis (OR = 7.0), diabetes (OR = 1.7), or anemia (OR = 3.1) had higher associations with ONJ compared with individuals without these conditions. Excluding those with cancer, bisphosphonate use of varying length and local risk factors as oral suppuration and dental extraction were highly associated with ONJ [29]. Table 13.3 gives an overview of the findings of Barasch et al. [29], including the odds ratio for ONJ with varying length of oral bisphosphonate treatment.

Table 13.3 Risk factors for osteonecrosis of the jaws among study participants without cancer in case–control study

Risk factor	ONJ cases ($n = 30$)	Controls ($N = 81$)	Odds ratio (95 % CI)	P-value
Oral suppuration	Yes	No	11.9 (2.0–69.5)	0.006
Tooth extraction	Matched extraction	Any extraction	6.6 (1.6–26.6)	0.008
Oral bisphosphonate	Yes	No	7.2 (2.1–24.7)	0.002
Bisphosphonate use any type	<0–2 years		9.9 (2.2–45.6)	0.003
	2–5 years		39.8 (10.0–158.8)	<0.0001
	>5 years		38.6 (9.1–163.6)	<0.0001

Modified after Barasch et al. 2011 [29]

Risk Factors

Risk factors for the occurrence of ONJ may be systemic or local, which may be present both in patients treated for malignant bone involvement or benign conditions including osteoporosis. In the following, the emphasis will be on data from osteoporosis.

Systemic Risk Factors

The basic disease in terms of malignant disease with skeletal metastatic involvement including breast cancer, prostate cancer, and multiple myeloma is associated with a higher risk for ONJ than osteoporosis. In case series of ONJ, the majority of patients are cancer patients. The osteoporosis patients constitute varying proportion from 7 to 70 % [18, 30, 31]. The reasons for the different proportion may be due to referral selection or type of medication in various populations. However, irrespective of basic disease (being malignant or osteoporosis), the risk of ONJ is dependent of the potency of bisphosphonate (nitrogen-containing bisphosphonates carrying a higher risk than other bisphosphonates), the dose of bisphosphonate (risk increasing with dose), the mode of administration (iv higher risk than oral bisphosphonates), and the duration of bisphosphonate treatment (risk increasing with duration).

Other antiresorptive agents, such as the RANKL-inhibitor denosumab, are associated with ONJ [32]. ONJ occurs both associated with high dose (XGEVA) administered subcutaneously monthly for cancer patients and with low dose (Prolia) given subcutaneously half-yearly [18]. Denosumab was introduced rather recently and has not yet been used for sufficient time that solid epidemiologic data on denosumab-induced ONJ have appeared.

Ages older than 65 years and diabetes have been associated with increased risk of ONJ [2, 33, 34]. Corticosteroid treatment was suggested as risk factor, but findings are not consistent [11]. Smoking and obesity were risk factors in a case–control study on cancer patients treated with zoledronic acid, but these factors are unconfirmed in osteoporosis patients [35]. Other systemic risk

> **Important Risk Factors for ONJ Caused by Antiresorptive Treatment**
>
> **Systemic Risk Factors**
> - Type of bisphosphonate: zoledronic acid and pamidronate, higher risk
> - IV administration compared to oral tablets
> - Duration of bisphosphonate
> - Cancer diagnosis (compared to osteoporosis)
> - High age
> - Diabetes
>
> **Local Risk Factors**
> - History of tooth extraction or other dentoalveolar surgery
> - Mandibular and palatal tori
> - Ill-fitting dentures
> - Oral infection with suppuration
> - Periodontitis
> - Insufficient oral hygiene

factors, such as chemotherapy or antiangiogenetic agents, may be of importance for the occurrence of ONJ, but formal statistical evidence is lacking. Recently, tyrosine kinase inhibitors like sunitinib [4] and bevacizumab and other agents used in cancer treatment were reported associated with ONJ, either alone or in association with bisphosphonates [5]. Recently, a number of studies have suggested that might be a genetic predisposition for developing ONJ. This is the subject for a number of ongoing studies [36, 37].

Local Risk Factors

The most important local risk factor is a history of recent tooth extractions. In virtually all published clinical case series, a history of tooth extractions or other dentoalveolar surgical procedures prior to the onset of ONJ has been recorded in more than half of the patients. Reported frequencies range from 38 to 88 % of the cases [11, 18, 20, 38, 39].

In a study by Schiodt et al. (2014) [18] comprising 102 patients including 33 patients with osteoporosis, 61 % had a history of tooth extraction before the onset of ONJ. The mean time from tooth extraction to referral for the ONJ was 7 months with a range of 1–36 months. Thus, there is sometimes a lack of attention to the symptoms and signs of ONJ among the primary health-care providers giving rise to late referrals. Local risk factors may relate to anatomical location of ONJ lesions in the oral cavity.

Clinical Features, Management, and Treatment of ONJ

The reader is referred to Chaps. 12 and 14.

References[1]

1. *Marx RE. Pamidronate (Aredia) and zoledronate (Zometa) induced avascular necrosis of the jaws: a growing epidemic. J Oral Maxillofac Surg. 2003;61(9):1115–7. *This is the first paper describing start of the new epidemic of ONJ related to the use of bisphosphonate. This paper is important and the foundation for many subsequent papers.
2. Ruggiero SL, Mehrotra B, Rosenberg TJ, Engroff SL. Osteonecrosis of the jaws associated with the use of bisphosphonates: a review of 63 cases. J Oral Maxillofac Surg. 2004;62(5):527–34.
3. Marx RE, Sawatari Y, Fortin M, Broumand V. Bisphosphonate-induced exposed bone (osteonecrosis/osteopetrosis) of the jaws: risk factors, recognition, prevention, and treatment. J Oral Maxillofac Surg. 2005;63(11):1567–75.
4. Brunello A, Saia G, Bedogni A, Scaglione D, Basso U. Worsening of osteonecrosis of the jaw during treatment with sunitinib in a patient with metastatic renal cell carcinoma. Bone. 2009;44:173–5.
5. Hopp RN, Pucci J, Santos-Silva AR, Jorge J. Osteonecrosis after administration of intravitreous bevacizumab. J Oral Maxillofac Surg. 2012;70(3):632–5.
6. Jacobsen C, Zemann W, Obwegeser JA, Grätz KW, Metzler P. The phosphorous necrosis of the jaws and what can we learn from the past: a comparison of "phossy" and "bisphossy" jaw. Oral Maxillofac Surg. doi:10.1007/s10006-012-0376-z. Published online 28 Dec 2012.
7. Migliorati CA, Casiglia J, Epstein J, Jacobsen PL, Siegel MA, Woo SB. Managing the care of patients with bisphosphonate-associated osteonecrosis: an American academy of oral medicine position paper. J Am Dent Assoc. 2005;136(12):1658–68.
8. *Ruggiero SL, Fantasia J, Carlson E. Bisphosphonate-related osteonecrosis of the jaw: background and guidelines for diagnosis, staging and management. Oral Surg Oral Med Oral Pathol Oral Radiol Endod. 2006;102(4):433–41. *This paper is the consensus paper of the American Association of Oral & Maxillofacial Surgery. It was the first to establish an overview, which was adopted as a global standard of current knowledge in 2006.
9. AAOMS. American Association of Oral and Maxillofacial Surgeons position paper on bisphosphonate-related osteonecrosis of the jaws. J Oral Maxillofac Surg. 2007;65(3):369–76.
10. **Ruggiero SL, Dodson TB, Assael LA, Landesberg R, Marx RE, Mehrotra B. American association of oral and maxillofacial surgeons position paper on bisphosphonate-related osteonecrosis of the jaw – 2009 update. Aust Endod J. 2009;35(3):119–30. **This paper is an update of the consensus paper from 2006. It introduced stage 0 ONJ and updated the literature.
11. Hellstein JW, Adler RA, Edwards B, et al. Managing the care of patients receiving antiresorptive therapy for prevention and treatment of osteoporosis: executive summary of recommendations from the American dental association council on scientific affairs. J Am Dent Assoc. 2011;142(11):1243–51.
12. Ruggerio SL, Dodson TB, Fantasia J, Goodday R, Aghaloo T, Mehrotra B, et al. Medication-related osteonecrosis of the jaw – 2014 update. In: American Association of Oral and Maxillofacial Surgeons Position Paper (AAOMS).
13. Pautke C, Kreutzer P, Weitz J, Knödler K, et al. Bisphosphonate related osteonecrosis of the jaw: a minipig large animal model. Bone. 2012;51:592–9.
14. Abtahi J, Agholme F, Aspenberg P. Prevention of osteonecrosis of the jaw by mucoperiosteal coverage in a rat model. Int J Oral Maxillofac Surg. 2013;42: 632–6.
15. *Otto S, Pautke C, Opelz C, Westphal I, et al. Osteonecrosis of the jaw: effect of bisphosphonate type, local concentration, and acidic milieu on the pathomechanism. J Oral Maxillofac Surg. 2010;68: 2837–45. *This paper emphasized the importance of concentration and dose of bisphosphonate for ONJ and introduce the potential importance of infection for ONJ.
16. Fedele S, Porter SR, D'Aiuto F, et al. Nonexposed variant of bisphosphonate-associated osteonecrosis of the jaw: a case series. Am J Med. 2010;123(11):1060–4.
17. Patel S, Choyee S, Uyanne J, Nguyen A, Lee P, Sedghizadeh P, et al. Non-exposed bisphosphonate-related osteonecrosis of the jaw: a critical assessment of current definition, staging, and treatment guidelines. Oral Dis. 2012;18:625–32.
18. *Schiodt M, Reibel J, Oturai P, Kofod T. Comparison of nonexposed and exposed bisphosphonate-induced osteonecrosis of the jaws: a retrospective analysis from the Copenhagen cohort and a proposal for an

[1] *Important References
**Very Important References

updated classification system. Oral Surg Oral Med Oral Pathol Oral Radiol. 2014;117:204–13. *This paper demonstrated that non-exposed ONJ is biologically not different from exposed ONJ, and should be included into the definition of ONJ. The paper also suggested new criteria for classification of non-exposed ONJ.

19. *Fedele S, Bedogni G, Scoletta M, Favia G, Colella G, Agrillo A, et al. Up to a quarter of patients with osteonecrosis of the jaw associated with antiresorptive agents remain undiagnosed. Br J Oral Maxillofac Surg. 2014, 10; E-version before print. *This paper demonstrated that a high proportion of ONJ may remain undiagnosed because they are non-exposed, and therefore do not qualify for the current (2009) AAOMS definition of ONJ (ref. [8]).

20. Walter C, Al-Nawas B, Grötz KA, Thomas C, et al. Prevalence and risk factors of bisphosphonate-associated osteonecrosis of the jaw in prostate cancer patients with advanced disease treated with zoledronate. Eur Urol. 2008;54:1066–72.

21. Bamias A, Kastritis E, Bamia C, Moulopoulos LA, et al. Osteonecrosis of the jaw in cancer after treatment with bisphosphonates: incidence and risk factors. Clin Oncol. 2005;23:8580–7.

22. Yamazaki T, Yamori M, Yamanoto K, Saito K, et al. Risk of osteomyelitis of the jaw induced by oral bisphosphonates in patients taking medication for osteoporosis: a hospital-based cohort study in Japan. Bone. 2012;51:882–7.

23. Vahtsevanos K, Kyrgidis A, Verrou E, et al. Longitudinal cohort study of risk factors in cancer patients of bisphosphonate-related osteonecrosis of the jaw. J Clin Oncol. 2009;27(32):5356–62.

24. Boonyapakorn T, Schirmer I, Reichart PA, Sturm I, Massenkeil G. Bisphosphonate-induced osteonecrosis of the jaws: prospective study of 80 patients with multiple myeloma and other malignancies. Oral Oncol. 2008;44:857–69.

25. Lo JC, O'Ryan FS, Gordon NP, et al. Prevalence of osteonecrosis of the jaw in patients with oral bisphosphonate exposure. J Oral Maxillofac Surg. 2010;68(2):243–53.

26. Borrromeo GL, Brand C, Clement JG, McCullough M, Crighton L, Hepworth G, Wark JD. A large Case-control study reveals a positive association between bisphosphonate use and delayed dental healing and osteonecrosis of the jaw. J Bone Miner Res. 2014;Epub. doi:10.1002/JMR.2179

27. Solomon DH, Mercer E, Woo SB, Avorn J, Schneeweiss S, Treister N. Defining the epidemiology of bisphosphonate-associated osteonecrosis of the jaw: prior work and current challenges. Osteoporos Int. 2013;24(1):237–44.

28. Lee S-H. Chang S-S, Lee M, Chan R-C, Lee C-C. Risk of osteonecrosis in patients taking bisphosphonates for prevention of osteoporosis: a systematic review and meta-analysis. Osteoporos Int Online. Published 17 Dec 2013. doi:10.1007/s00198-013-2575-3

29. **Barasch A, Cunha-Cruz J, Curro FA, Hujoel P, Sung AH, Vena D, Voinea-Griffin AE, CONDOR Collaborative Group. Risk factors for osteonecrosis of the jaws: a case-control study from the CONDOR dental PBRN. J Dent Res. 2011;90(4):439–44. **This paper demonstrated a number of risk factors for ONJ including providing odds ratio of risk, which are reported in Table 13.3. Notably, oral suppuration, tooth extraction, and bisphosphonate treatment of long duration are important risk factors.

30. Otto S, Abu-Id MH, Fedele S, et al. Osteoporosis and bisphosphonates-related osteonecrosis of the jaw: not just a sporadic coincidence—a multi-centre study. J Craniomaxillofac Surg. 2011;39(4):272–7.

31. Jacobsen C, Metzler P, Obwegeser JA, Zemann W, Graetz KW. Osteopathology of the jaw associated with bone resorption inhibitors: what have we learned in the last 8 years? A single-centre experience with 110 patients. Swiss Med Wkly. 2012;142:w13605.

32. Otto S, Baumann S, Ehrenfeld M, Pautke C. Successful surgical management of osteonecrosis of the jaw due to RANK-ligand inhibitor treatment using fluorescence guided bone resection. J Cranio Maxiallofac Surg. 2013;41:694–8.

33. Yarom N, Yahalom R, Shoshani Y, Hamed W, Regev E, Elad S. Osteonecrosis of the jaws associated with the use of bisphosphonates: a review of 63 cases. J Oral Maxillofac Surg. 2004;62(5):527–34.

34. Mavrokokki T, Cheng A, Stein B, Goss A. Nature and frequency of bisphosphonate-associated osteonecrosis of the jaws in Australia. J Oral Maxillofac Surg. 2007;65(3):415–23.

35. Wessel JH, Dodson TB, Zavras AI. Zoledronate, smoking, and obesity are strong risk factors for osteonecrosis of the jaw: a case-control study. J Oral Maxillofac Surg. 2008;66(4):625–31.

36. Sarasquete ME, et al. Bisphosphonate-related osteonecrosis of the jaw is associated with polymorphisms of the cytochrome P450 CYP2C8 in multiple myeloma: a genome-wide single nucleotide polymorphism analysis. Blood. 2008;112(7):2709–12.

37. Raje N, et al. Clinical, radiographic, and biochemical characterization of multiple myeloma patients with osteonecrosis of the jaw. Clin Cancer Res. 2008;14(8):2387–95.

38. Otto S, Schreyer C, Hafner S, et al. Bisphosphonate-related osteonecrosis of the jaws – characteristics, risk factors, clinical features, localization and impact on oncological treatment. J Craniomaxillofac Surg. 2012;40(4):303–9.

39. Fede D, Fusco V, Matranga D, Solazzo L, Gabriele M, Gaeta GM, et al. Osteonecrosis of the jaws in patients assuming oral bisphosphonates for osteoporosis: a retrospective multi-hospital-based study of 87 Italian cases. Eur J Int Med. 2013;24:784–90.

Management of Osteonecrosis of the Jaw in Patients Receiving Antiresorptive Treatment

14

Morten Schiødt

Summary

- Osteonecrosis of the jaw (ONJ) most often shows exposed bone, but non-exposed osteonecrosis occurs.
- ONJ occurs most often in the posterior mandible.
- ONJ may sometimes lead to loss of teeth, jaw bone, and masticatory function.
- ONJ can be successfully surgically treated in the majority of cases.
- Always have the teeth examined and fixed before start of antiresorptive treatment.
- If suspicious of osteonecrosis, refer the patient to a central clinic, for example, oral and maxillofacial surgery, with expertise in osteonecrosis.

Introduction

Since the early reports of ONJ [1–3], we have learned a lot on diagnosis and treatment of ONJ. Today (October 2014), a large number of publications are known in the Western world. A number of consensus papers by various organizations have set the stage for updates, guidelines for diagnosis and treatment, risk factors, prevention, and not least many unanswered questions that the research community are to address [4–9]. Experimental studies including animal models as well as cell culture studies have already been implemented [10–12].

See Chap. 13 for terminology, definition, diagnosis and classification, and risk factors of ONJ. In the present chapter, osteonecrosis of the jaw will be generally referred to as "ONJ."

Clinical Features of ONJ

Symptoms of ONJ

Symptoms of ONJ include exposed bone and/or a nonhealing tooth socket after extraction, pain, or swelling of the jaw. Other oral symptoms may be loosening of teeth, oral ulcer of the tongue or gums from a denture or from protruding exposed bone, or in advanced cases a numbness of the lower lip. This latter symptom indicated advanced mandibular osteonecrosis involving the mandibular nerve canal. Rarely, an oral or submandibular abscess formation may be the first symptom of ONJ, and rarely a spontaneous jaw fracture may occur.

M. Schiødt, DDS, Dr.Odont (✉)
Department of Oral and Maxillofacial Surgery,
Copenhagen University Hospital (Rigshospitalet),
9, Blegdamsvej, Copenhagen 2100, Denmark
e-mail: morten.schioedt@regionh.dk;
mschioedt@hotmail.com

© Springer International Publishing Switzerland 2016
S.L. Silverman, B. Abrahamsen (eds.), *The Duration and Safety of Osteoporosis Treatment*, DOI 10.1007/978-3-319-23639-1_14

Clinical Findings

The typical ONJ lesion appears as exposed bone, most often in the alveolar process in mandible or maxilla corresponding to a missing tooth (Figs. 14.1, 14.2, and 14.3). This may occur after tooth extraction with a nonhealing socket. Other clinical presentations are exposed bone on the gums of edentulous patients wearing dentures (Fig. 14.1).

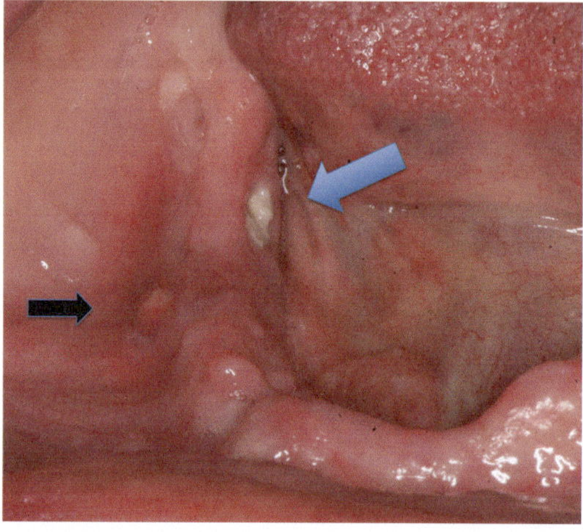

Fig. 14.1 Stage 1 osteonecrosis of edentulous mandible of a 73-year-old woman with osteoporosis treated with alendronate for 10 years. Note exposed bone on the lingual aspect of the mandible (*blue arrow*) and small fistula on the buccal aspect (*black arrow*)

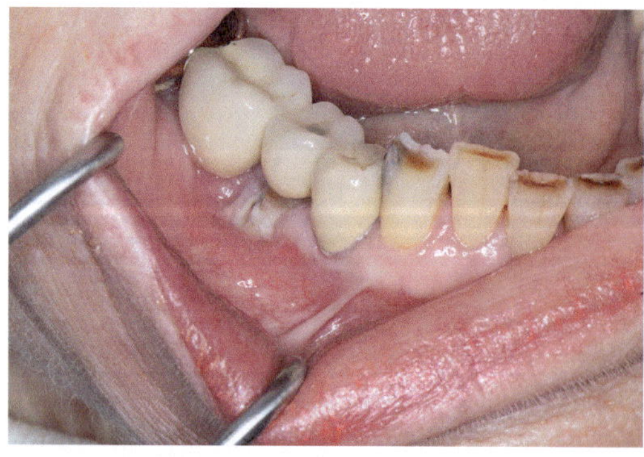

Fig. 14.2 Stage 1 osteonecrosis showing exposed bone around lower premolar in right mandible (*arrow*) in a 81-year-old woman with osteoporosis treated with bisphosphonate for 51 months (48 months alendronate, 3 months Forsteo). She was treated by surgery including small local bone resection and removal of the tooth

Two thirds of ONJ lesions occur in the mandible, one third in the maxilla, and a small percentage occur in both jaws [13–15].

The presences of mandibular exostosis (tori) or maxillary exostosis (palatal tori) are risk locations for ONJ (Fig. 12.6). These cases are often spontaneously occurring. Another local risk area is the lingual aspect of the mandible at the wisdom tooth area, both in dentate and in edentulous patients. It is important to visually inspect these areas carefully, as the lesions are easily overlooked (Fig. 14.1).

When exposed bone after tooth extraction has been left without treatment, the necrotic lesion may expand and involve the neighboring teeth, which then usually cannot be saved (Fig. 14.3).

Another clinical presentation is lack of visible exposed bone but only a fistula, sometimes with pus coming out on pressure, on the alveolar process (Fig. 14.4a). These cases are so-called non-exposed ONJ. Other types of non-exposed ONJ are even more difficult to diagnose as there may be only pain and swelling but no exposed bone and no fistula. Useful imaging techniques in addition to radiograph include CT or cone beam scans and bone scintigraphy, sometimes combined with CT (SPECT–CT) (see Fig. 14.4). These patients should always have a dental examination, and a common periapical infection around a tooth should be excluded; see also diagnostic criteria of non-exposed ONJ (Table 13.2).

A nonhealing socket after tooth extraction presenting with exposed bone is usually without symptoms or sign of infection in the beginning. Other lesions may start at the marginal bone around the tooth (Fig. 14.2). When symptoms and signs of infection occur the lesion is classified as stage 2; see Fig. 14.4.

Stage 3 (cf. Tables 13.1 and 13.2) refers to the advanced cases which are widespread, often with multiple sites of exposed bone (Fig. 14.3) and involvement of the maxillary sinus (Fig. 14.3b), in the mandible extending to the inferior nerve canal, showing extraoral fistula, or present with a spontaneous jaw fracture (see also below).

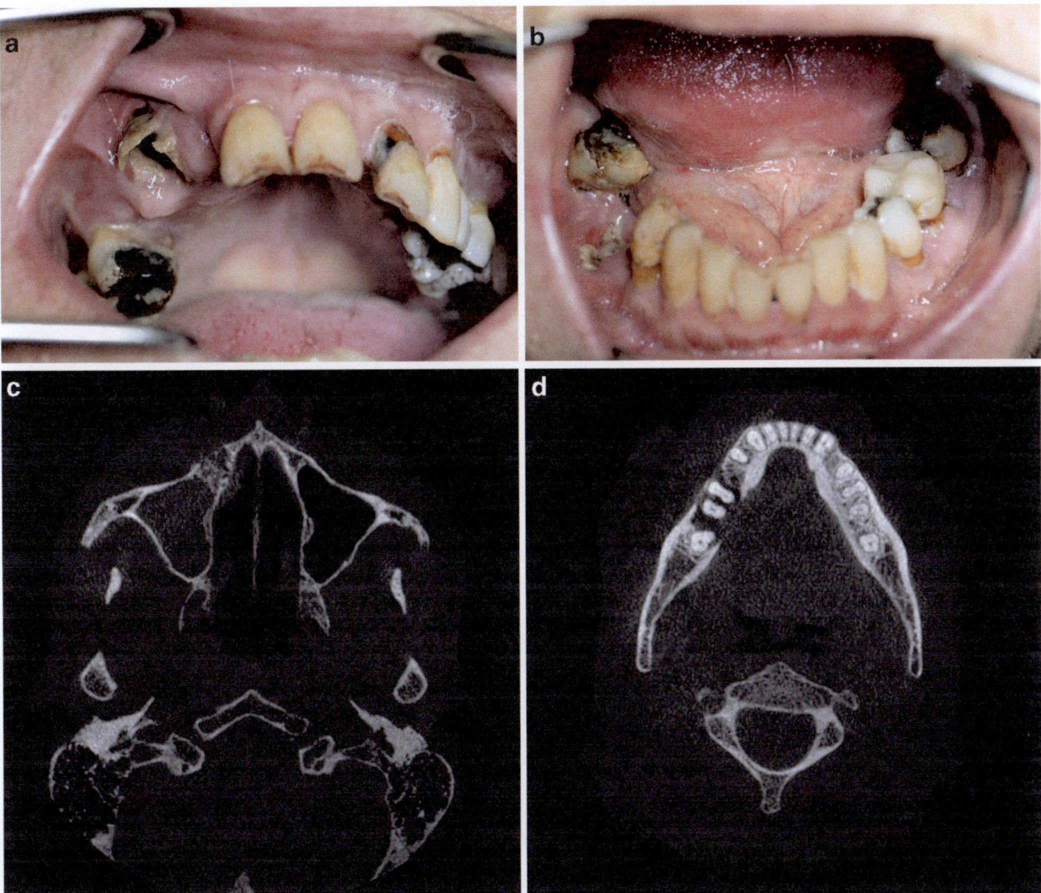

Fig. 14.3 Stage 3 osteonecrosis showing exposed bone in the maxilla and mandible in a 51-year-old woman with osteoporosis, chronic obstructive lung disease, alcohol problem, and liver disease. The patient had severe extraoral fistulas with pus secretion from the mandible. She had been treated with alendronate (36 months), aclasta (18 months), and denosumab (36 months) for a total of 90 months. Notice infection on right maxillary sinus. After hospitalization and feeding until sufficient weight (from 35 kg to 42 kg), she had a continuity resection done in the lower jaw and partial resection in the upper jaw. She became free of symptoms and was cured of her ONJ

Severe Clinical Manifestations

These features only occur by definition in ONJ stage 3 (see Tables 13.1 and 13.2). A number of patients present with a cutaneous fistula as the first sign of ONJ. Fistulas may appear submandibularly or on the chin or cheek. Usually, but not always, fistulas are associated with severe bone exposure intraorally. A submandibular or intraoral abscess as sign of acute infection is another manifestation, which is rarely the first symptom, but during long-term course may occur in 30 % of the cases [13] and thus quite common. There may be varying degree of suppuration from the fistulas. Cutaneous fistulas occur in 5–10 % of ONJ cases [13, 15].

Paresthesia, numbness, or hyposensation of the lower lip indicating mandibular alveolar nerve involvement occur in around 11 % of ONJ at initial examination [13]. During operation, necrosis of the bone surrounding the nerve is often evident. Spontaneous fracture of the mandible is rarely seen (3–4 %) [13, 16]. Severe ONJ lesions of the maxilla often involve the maxillary sinus (Fig. 14.3c).

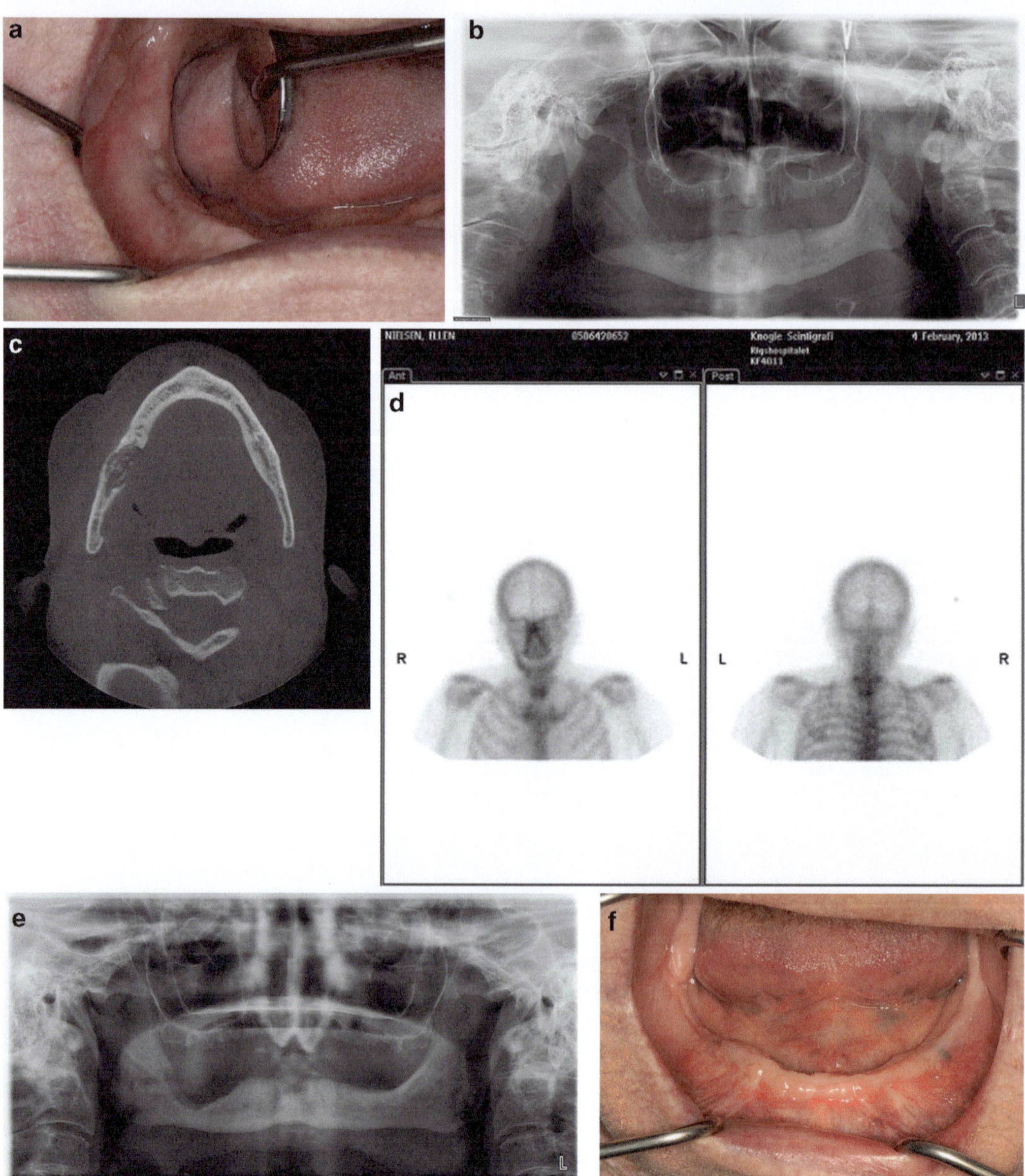

Fig. 14.4 (**a**) Stage 2—non-exposed type of osteonecrosis of the lower jaw in a 70-year-old woman with osteoporosis. She was treated with alendronate 70 mg/week p.o. for 3 years followed by aclasta i.v. yearly for 3 years, thus a total of 6 years of bisphosphonate treatment before onset of osteonecrosis. Notice the fistula with pus on the top of the alveolar process (*arrow*) in the lower right (edentulous) mandible. There is no exposed bone in the jaws. (**b**) Preoperative panoramic radiograph of the patient from Fig. 14.3a showing sequester in the alveolar process of right lower mandible (*arrow*). (**c**) Cone beam CT scan of the mandible of the patient shown in Fig. 14.3a. Notice the extensive necrotic area in the lower mandible extending through the lingual aspect of the jaw (*arrow*). The alveolar nerve was affected by the necrosis. (**d**) Scintigraphy of the jaws showing moderately increased signal in the right mandible. (**e**) Postoperative radiograph after block resection and removal of sequester in right mandible (*arrow*). (**f**) Postoperative healing. The patient was free of symptoms 1 week postoperatively and still without symptoms and without recurrence of osteonecrosis after 1.5 years observation time

Imaging of ONJ

The imaging of ONJ has improved during the last decade (see also Chap. 12). The traditional orthopantomograph is the basis of imaging of the jaws. However, most patients will have a CT scan or cone beam scan of the jaws. Bone scintigraphy is useful, either the traditional type or combined as SPECT–CT or PET–CT. MR scans may have value evaluating the soft tissue changes including suspected abscesses, and other types of imaging will most likely find its way to the diagnostic tools [17, 18]. None of the imaging methods can stand alone. ONJ is still a clinical diagnosis, and it is not expected that imaging will be the gold standard of diagnosis in the near future. However, imaging is tremendously important for evaluating a given ONJ lesion and for the planning of treatment as well as for monitoring natural history and treatment results.

Radiographs

The reader is also referred to Chap. 12. First, ONJ lesions may present on orthopantomograph in several ways. The typical sequester is a demarcated area of radiopaque or normally looking (dead) bone surrounded by an osteolytic zone (Fig. 14.4b). In patients who have had a tooth extracted, the dental socket is not healing within half a year as in normal patients but may stay open for months to years after extraction. This is the effect of the bisphosphonate reducing the remodeling of the bone. A characteristic sign of long-term bisphosphonate treatment is the thickening of the lamina dura surrounding the teeth. The widening of lamina dura is not a sign of ONJ but only indicates the long-term effect of bisphosphonate and places the patient in the "at-risk" classification (Table 13.1). Other manifestations are radiopacities, either focally or more widespread.

Often a mix of radiolucent and radiopaque areas is seen, which may in fact be necrotic. In these cases, additional imaging in the form of a CT scan or cone beam scan should be considered mandatory.

CT Scans

CT scans including cone beam scans give the possibility to map the osteonecrosis in detail including evaluating the involvement of mandibular alveolar canal and the maxillary sinus (Fig. 14.3).

Scintigraphy

Bone scintigraphy utilizing a radioactive technetium tracer alone or combined with CT scans (SPECT–SCAN) may map the extent of the lesions. Often, there is a good correlation between the clinical and radiographic features of a given ONJ lesion (Fig. 14.4d). As the tracer depends on active bone formation, the signal is almost certainly due to the periosteal reaction of the ONJ lesion and is thus not a feature of the dead bone itself. This may also explain why some patients show little signal on scintigraphy. The importance of the scintigraphy is that lesions extending further than the clinical or radiologic lesion may be identified [18].

Pathogenesis of ONJ

The pathogenesis of ONJ is complex and partly unknown (see also Chap. 12). Most likely, the onset of ONJ is based on a multifactorial combination of local and systemic risk factors.

Bisphosphonate and denosumab, although acting through different pathways, both lead to a reduced remodeling of the skeletal bones and increased bone mineral content. The pathogenesis may involve a changed turnover of bone modeling, different response of osteoclasts to cytokine stimuli, as well as genetic factors [19, 20].

It is noticeable that tooth extractions or other oral surgical procedures precede the onset of ONJ in a high proportion (50–75 %) of the cases [13, 21]. However, it has been proposed that it is the infection that leads to the tooth extraction rather than the tooth extraction itself, which may be of importance [12, 16, 21, 22]. Cell culture experiments seem to indicate that the acidic environment in infectious areas as well as release of free BP might be of importance [12]. Epithelial healing following oral ulceration decreased due to alendronate in BP treatment [23].

Recently, the establishment of animal models of ONJ including rodents, beagle dogs, and mini pigs has been published [10, 24]. It seems that ONJ can be reliably established giving a tool for studying the pathogenesis as well as treatment modalities for ONJ [10].

Histopathology of ONJ

The pathology of affected ONJ specimens shows bone necrosis with loss of osteocyte nuclei. Osteocyte lacunae are empty, and the haversian channels reveal necrotic tissue. The jaw bone marrow spaces are necrotic, sometimes showing signs of active infection with pus, i.e. neutrophils and other inflammatory cells (Fig. 14.5). The exposed bone surface is commonly covered with bacteria and colonies of actinomyces colonies, which also may occur in the central bone marrow areas. Operation specimens may show varying degree of necrosis with some vital bone cells or bone marrow at the periphery, indicating a periosteal reaction [25]. Resection specimens may show a considerable periosteal reactive new bone formation on the surface of the central necrotic bone tissue [25].

Principles for Management of ONJ

All new patients should have a thorough medical history taken including basic disease and previous and present medication. Emphasis should be put on dose, type, and method of administration and duration of bisphosphonate and/or denosumab therapy. Also, for cancer patients, the medical history should include specific chemotherapeutic drugs like tyrosine kinase inhibitors (e.g., bevacizumab) known to contribute to ONJ. A dental history should include recent dental treatments especially tooth extractions.

Clinical oral examination should include the presence or absence of extraoral or intraoral fistulas and swollen submandibular lymph nodes and loss of sensation of the lower lips. Intraoral

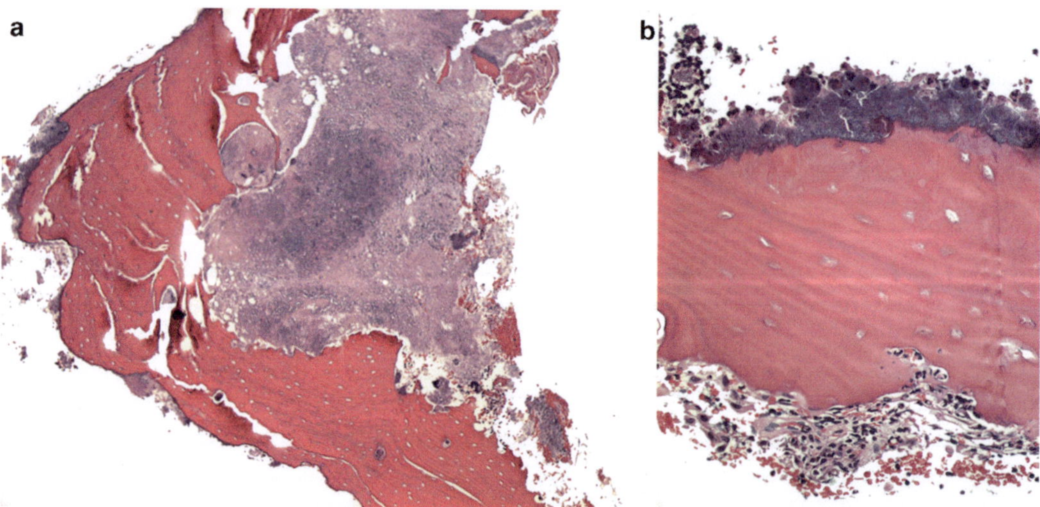

Fig. 14.5 (**a**) Sequester removed from osteonecrosis lesion of the jaw. Notice bacteria on the surface to the *left*. The bone marrow is replaced with inflammatory cells, necrotic tissue, and bacteria. (**b**) High power of histology of sequester removed from the jaws showing dead bone with bacteria on the surface. The osteocyte lacunae are empty and in the marrow space inflammatory cells and erythrocytes are seen (Photos courtesy of Dr. Jesper Reibel, Department of Odontology, University of Copenhagen, Denmark)

examination should include a dental examination as well as check of oral mucosa for fistulas, swellings, redness, abscesses, and exposed bone. The location and extension of exposed bone should be recorded.

Pain from the oral cavity should be assessed by VAS scale.

Based on the medical history, clinical and imaging examination and diagnosis (ONJ) should be made.

The stage of ONJ should be assessed. Hereafter, a treatment plan and decision should be reached.

When a treatment plan for ONJ is done, the patient's endocrinologist or oncologist should be consulted and informed. There should be a close and continuous collaboration between the dentist/oral maxillofacial surgeon on one side and the medical health-care provider (endocrinologist/oncologist/physician) on the other side. Matters of drug holiday should also be discussed between the parties (see later).

Treatment of ONJ

The consensus papers [5–9, 26] have set up recommendations for treatment. Basically, stage 1, the asymptomatic stage, is treated conservatively with chlorhexidine rinsing and is observed. Stage 2 (the stage with symptoms/infection) is often treated with antibiotics, superficial sequestrectomy, or more radical sequestrectomy, whereas stage 3 (advanced symptomatic stage) may need antibiotic and surgical treatment. At the start of the epidemic, the trend was rather conservative, but in recent years, many centers have discovered the advantage of more aggressive surgical treatment [27–30].

Thus, today, if a patient with stage 1 ONJ is bothered by the rough surface of the exposed bone and wants to be operated, we offer surgery, and they usually heal and the patient get cured [30]. However, most stage 1 ONJ patients are treated conservatively. Stage 2 patients are always offered antibiotic treatment and local sequestrectomy with block resection into clinical healthy bone. In stage 3, the surgical treatment may either be block resection or a continuity resection. However, some stage 3 patients are so weak from their general disease (cancer metastases or osteoporosis) that they cannot comply with a bigger operation. These patients are offered conservative treatment with tight control, antibiotics, and palliative treatment. In a study on 50 consecutive ONJ patients by Schiodt et al. (2013) [30], the severity of ONJ stages 1–3 preoperatively (stage 1, 26 %; stage 2, 54 %; stage 3 20 %) was reduced to a postoperative distribution of cured: 88 % (stage 1, 6 %; stage 2, 6 %; stage 3, 0 %). Thus, surgical treatment was successful in this open series, in which two thirds of patients came from an oncology setting, while one third came from an osteoporosis setting. There was at the same time a significant reduction of jaw pain (VAS scale) preoperatively to 13 months postoperatively [30]. Several studies have reported promising results from surgical treatment [28, 31]. Thus, in general, the trend has changed toward more surgery with successful outcomes. This trend may appear in contrast to several consensus papers favoring more conservative approach. The consensus papers are by nature more conservative as it takes time to establish the scientific documentation of surgery. However, the scientific community lacks randomized controlled studies of conservative treatment versus surgical treatment.

C-Terminal Telopeptide Testing

Serum markers for bone remodeling have been suggested, including C-terminal telopeptide (CTX) and N-terminal telopeptide, for use for predicting the risk of ONJ in association with drug holiday [30]. However, CTX has not been scientifically validated in this context, and its value outside osteoporosis management has been questioned by a number of papers. Thus, the American Dental Association Council on Scientific Affairs' consensus paper does not recommend the use of CTX [9], and we conclude that CTX testing does not seem to have a place in management of ONJ patients at this time.

Drug Holiday

Bisphosphonates

Discontinuing thebisphosphonate therapy may not eliminate risk of developing ONJ. The bisphosphonate is build into the bone tissue and has many years of elimination time. When ONJ is diagnosed, many patients have their bisphosphonate treatment discontinued by their oncologist (cancer patients) or by their endocrinologist or private physician (osteoporosis). However, discontinuation may have a negative impact on the outcomes of the low bone mass treatment [9]. It seems that drug holiday is not mandatory to obtain successful outcome of surgical treatment [9]. The decision of discontinuation of bisphosphonate treatment in a patient diagnosed with ONJ should always be a decision between the responsible physician and the ONJ-treating oral and maxillofacial surgeon, based on evaluation of the individual patient. However, there is a scientific need for more studies to address the importance of drug holiday in the management of ONJ.

Denosumab

Denosumab has another mechanism of action than bisphosphonate and can be eliminated from the body much faster than bisphosphonate from the bone when discontinued. It can thus be a consideration to pause denosumab and to postpone a surgical treatment of ONJ or larger oral surgical procedures some months as bone resorption returns to normal or elevated levels less than a year after the last injection. Presently (Feb. 2014), it is not yet documented what the best recommendations are.

Guidelines for the Physician and Dentist Prior to Start of Antiresorptive Treatment

All osteoporosis patients who are going to start bisphosphonate or denosumab treatment for their general condition should be informed about the possible risk of development of a complication, "dead bone" (ONJ). Although the risk is small (<0.1 %), it is a severe jaw disorder carrying a significant morbidity with loss of teeth and masticatory function when it occurs. The risk can be removed or reduced by removing dental infectious foci before the start of therapy [5–9]. All patients should thus be recommended to see their private dentist for the relevant examination and dental treatment. The goal is that the patient should not have a need for tooth extraction or other dentoalveolar surgery in a long period, when antiresorptive therapy is started. The patients should establish good oral hygiene and have lifelong regular dental examinations as the risk of developing ONJ will increase with time during the continued antiresorptive treatment (see Chap. 13).

Guidelines for Dental and Oral Surgical Treatment including Tooth Extractions during Antiresorptive Treatment

Bisphosphonates

The risk for developing ONJ after tooth extraction in a patient who has been treated with bisphosphonate for a period is much higher for those treated with high-dose bisphosphonate for cancer compared to osteoporosis patients treated with common low-dose bisphosphonate, for example, alendronate 70 mg tablet per week [32].

It is important to be aware that the risk in osteoporosis patients of developing ONJ after tooth extraction is very low and extractions can usually be performed in the primary health-care sector. However, the dentist should secure the healing of the socket and refer the patient to a specialized clinic for ONJ if healing has not occurred after 4 weeks [32]. Dental implants are among the reported risk factors in the early studies. However, it seems that the risk of ONJ is low. No cases of ONJ were recorded among 82 patients with dental implants in osteoporosis patients [33]. Thus, dental implants can seemingly be inserted in these patients under the condition of individual risk assessment.

Denosumab

It is assumed that similar guidelines may be used for patients on denosumab treatment, although there is presently no documentation or validation. There are yet no systematic data on dental implants in patients on denosumab treatment.

Guidelines for Dental and Oral Surgical Treatment including Tooth Extractions in Patients Diagnosed with ONJ

The risk of developing a new ONJ lesion is rather high when performing tooth extraction, whether it is a cancer patient or an osteoporosis patient. It is recommended that such patients are referred to a specialized clinic where the ONJ is treated. Tooth extraction should be done under antibiotic cover and as atraumatic as possible and includes alveolectomy and primary closure of the oral mucosa in order not to leave exposed bone.

References[1]

1. *Marx RE. Pamidronate (Aredia) and zoledronate (Zometa) induced avascular necrosis of the jaws: a growing epidemic. J Oral Maxillofac Surg. 2003;61(9):1115–7. *This is the first paper describing start of the new epidemic of ONJ related to the use of bisphosphonate. This paper is important and the foundation for many subsequent papers.
2. Ruggiero SL, Mehrotra B, Rosenberg TJ, Engroff SL. Osteonecrosis of the jaws associated with the use of bisphosphonates: a review of 63 cases. J Oral Maxillofac Surg. 2004;62(5):527–34.
3. Marx RE, Sawatari Y, Fortin M, Broumand V. Bisphosphonate-induced exposed bone (osteonecrosis/osteopetrosis) of the jaws: risk factors, recognition, prevention, and treatment. J Oral Maxillofac Surg. 2005;63(11):1567–75.
4. Jacobsen C, Zemann W, Obwegeser JA, Grätz KW, Metzler P. The phosphorous necrosis of the jaws and what can we learn from the past: a comparison of "phossy" and "bisphossy" jaw. Oral Maxillofac Surg. doi:10.1007/s10006-012-0376-z. Published online 28 Dec 2012.
5. Migliorati CA, Casiglia J, Epstein J, Jacobsen PL, Siegel MA, Woo SB. Managing the care of patients with bisphosphonate-associated osteonecrosis: an American academy of oral medicine position paper. J Am Dent Assoc. 2005;136(12):1658–68.
6. *Ruggiero SL, Fantasia J, Carlson E. Bisphosphonate-related osteonecrosis of the jaw: background and guidelines for diagnosis, staging and management. Oral Surg Oral Med Oral Pathol Oral Radiol Endod. 2006;102(4):433–41. *This paper is the consensus paper of the American Association of Oral & Maxillofacial Surgery. It was the first to establish an overview, which was adopted as a global standard of current knowledge in 2006.
7. AAOMS. American association of oral and maxillofacial surgeons position paper on bisphosphonate-related osteonecrosis of the jaws. J Oral Maxillofac Surg. 2007;65(3):369–76.
8. Ruggiero SL, Dodson TB, Assael LA, Landesberg R, Marx RE, Mehrotra B. American association of oral and maxillofacial surgeons position paper on bisphosphonate-related osteonecrosis of the jaw – 2009 update. Aust Endod J. 2009;35(3):119–30.
9. Hellstein JW, Adler RA, Edwards B, et al. Managing the care of patients receiving antiresorptive therapy for prevention and treatment of osteoporosis: executive summary of recommendations from the American dental association council on scientific affairs. J Am Dent Assoc. 2011;142(11):1243–51.
10. Pautke C, Kreutzer K, Weitz J, Knödler M, Münzel D, Wexel G, Otto S, Hapfelmeier A, Stürzenbaum S, Tischer T. Bisphosphonate related osteonecrosis of the jaw: a minipig large animal model. Bone. 2012;51:592–9.
11. Abtahi J, Agholme F, Aspenberg P. Prevention of osteonecrosis of the jaw by mucoperiosteal coverage in a rat model. Int J Oral Maxillofac Surg. 2013;42:632–6.
12. Otto S, Pautke C, Opelz C, Westphal I, Drosse I, Schwager J, Bauss F, Ehrenfeld M, Schieker M. Osteonecrosis of the jaw: effect of bisphosphonate type, local concentration, and acidic milieu on the pathomechanism. J Oral Maxillofac Surg. 2010;68:2837–45.
13. *Schiodt M, Reibel J, Oturai P, Kofod T. Comparison of nonexposed and exposed bisphosphonate-induced osteonecrosis of the jaws: a retrospective analysis from the Copenhagen cohort and a proposal for an updated classification system. Oral Surg Oral Med Oral Pathol Oral Radiol. 2014;117:204–13. *This paper demonstrated that non-exposed ONJ is biologically not different from exposed ONJ, and should be included into the definition of ONJ. The paper also suggested new criteria for classification of non-exposed ONJ.
14. Fede D, Fusco V, Matranga D, Solazzo L, Gabriele M, Gaeta GM, et al. Osteonecrosis of the jaws in patients assuming oral bisphosphonates for osteoporosis: a retrospective multi-hospital-based study of 87 Italian cases. Eur J Int Med. 2013;24:784–90.

---

[1] *Important References

15. Otto S, Abu-Id MH, Fedele S, et al. Osteoporosis and bisphosphonates-related osteonecrosis of the jaw: not just a sporadic coincidence—a multi-centre study. J Craniomaxillofac Surg. 2011;39(4):272–7.

16. Otto S, Pautke C, Hafner S, Hesse R, Reichardt LF, Mast G, Ehrenfeld M, Cornelius CP. Pathologic fractures in bisphosphonate-related osteonecrosis of the jaw-review of the literature and review of our own cases. Craniomaxillofac Trauma Reconstr. 2013;6(3): 147–54. Epub 2013 May 31.

17. Jacobsen C, Metzler P, Obwegeser JA, Zemann W, Graetz KW. Osteopathology of the jaw associated with bone resorption inhibitors: what have we learned in the last 8 years? A single-centre experience with 110 patients. Swiss Med Wkly. 2012;142:13605.

18. Chiandussi S, Biasotto M, Dore F, Cavalli F, Cova MA, Di Lena R. Clinical and diagnostic imaging of bisphosphonate-associated osteonecrosis of the jaws. Dentomaxillofac Radiol. 2006;35:236–43.

19. Sarasquete ME, et al. Bisphosphonate-related osteonecrosis of the jaw is associated with polymorphisms of the cytochrome P450 CYP2C8 in multiple myeloma: a genome-wide single nucleotide polymorphism analysis. Blood. 2008;112(7):2709–12.

20. Raje N, et al. Clinical, radiographic, and biochemical characterization of multiple myeloma patients with osteonecrosis of the jaw. Clin Cancer Res. 2008; 14(8):2387–95.

21. Otto S, Schreyer C, Hafner S, et al. Bisphosphonate-related osteonecrosis of the jaws – characteristics, risk factors, clinical features, localization and impact on oncological treatment. J Craniomaxillofac Surg. 2012;40(4):303–9.

22. Otto S, Hafner S, Mast G, et al. Bisphosphonate-related osteonecrosis of the jaw: is pH the missing part in the pathogenesis puzzle? J Oral Maxillofac Surg. 2010;68(5):1158–61.

23. Donetti E, Gualerzi A, Sardella A, Lodi G, Carrassi A, Sforza C. Alendronate impairs epithelial adhesion, differentiation and proliferation in human oral mucosa. Oral Dis. 2013 Jun 25. doi:10.1111/odi.12154

24. Allen MR, Burr DB. Mandible matrix necrosis in beagle dogs after 3 years of daily oral bisphosphonate treatment. J Oral Maxillofac Surg. 2008;66(5): 987–94.

25. Young-Ah C, Hye-Jung Y, Lee JI, Hong S-P, Hong S-D. Histopathological features of bisphosphonate-associated osteonecrosis: findings in patients with partial mandibulectomies. Oral Surg Oral Med Oral Pathol Oral Radiol. 2012;114(6):785–91.

26. Ruggerio SL, Dodson TB, Fantasia J, Goodday R, Aghaloo T, Mehrotra B. et al. Medication-related osteonecrosis of the jaw – 2014 update. In: American association of oral and maxillofacial surgeons position paper (AAOMS).

27. *Otto S, Baumann S, Ehrenfeld M, Pautke C. Successful surgical management of osteonecrosis of the jaw due to RANK-ligand inhibitor treatment using fluorescence guided bone resection. J Craniomaxiallofac Surg. 2013;41:694–8. *This paper is one of several demonstrating the successful effect of surgical treatment with localized resections.

28. Holzinger D, Seemann R, Klug C, Ewers R, Millesi G, Baumann A, Wutzl A. Long-term success of surgery in bisphosphonate-related osteonecrosis of the jaws (BRONJs). Oral Oncol. 2013;49:66–70.

29. Voss PJ, Oshero JJ, Kovalova-Müller A, Merino EAV, Sauerbier S, Al-Jamali J, Lemound J, Metzger MC, Schmelzeisen R. Surgical treatment of bisphosphonate-associated osteonecrosis of the jaw: technical report and follow up of 21 patients. J Craniomaxillofac Surg. 2012;40:719–25.

30. Schiodt M, Rostgaard J, Oturai P, Steno S, Kofod T. Surgical treatment of bisphosphonate-induced osteonecrosis of the jaws significantly reduces pain. In: International association for oral & maxillofacial surgery biannual congress, ICOMS13, Barcelona, 24–27 Oct 2013.

31. Lemound J, Eckardt A, Kokemüller H, et al. Bisphosphonate-associated osteonecrosis of the mandible: reliable soft tissue reconstruction using a local myofascial flap. Clin Oral Invest. 2012;16:1143–52.

32. Yazdi P, Schiødt M. Tandekstraktioner på patienter i Bisfosfonat-behandling (Guidelines for tooth extractions on patients in bisphosphonate treatment). Tandlægebladet (Danish Dental Jr). 2013;117: 298–305.

33. Koka S, Babu NMS, Norell A. Survival of dental implants in post-menopausal bisphosphonate users. J Prosthodont Res. 2010;54:108–11.

Socrates E. Papapoulos

Summary

- Osteoporosis is a chronic disease requiring chronic treatment.
- The efficacy and tolerability of available treatments are well established in studies up to 5 years.
- There are rather limited data of their long-term effects.
- The bisphosphonates alendronate, risedronate, and zoledronate and the inhibitor of RANKL denosumab reduce the risk of all osteoporotic fractures, including those of the hip.
- For these agents, long-term data (>5 years) of efficacy and tolerability are available.
- None of the long-term studies was specifically designed to assess antifracture efficacy.
- In general, these agents have a favorable benefit-to-harm profile when given to patients with osteoporosis at increased risk of fractures.
- Knowledge of the mechanism of action, efficacy, and potential risks of individual treatments is essential for the long-term care of patients with osteoporosis.

S.E. Papapoulos, MD, PhD (✉)
Center for Bone Quality, Leiden University Medical
Center, Albinusdreef 2, 2333 ZA, Leiden,
The Netherlands
e-mail: s.e.papapoulos@lumc.nl

Introduction

Fractures, the main clinical consequence of osteoporosis, are frequent, their incidence increases with age, they are associated with significant morbidity and deterioration of the quality of life of affected patients, and they increase the risk of new fractures and mortality. The aim, therefore, of any intervention in osteoporosis is the prevention of fractures in patients who have not yet fractured or of the progression of the disease in patients who have already sustained a fragility fracture. The management of the patient with osteoporosis consists of general measures, non-pharmacological interventions, and pharmacological interventions. Of the general measures, the most important is the correction of deficiencies or insufficiencies of vitamin D and calcium. Vitamin D supplementation with 800 IU/day and adjustment of the daily calcium intake to 1200 mg (diet and supplements) should be the first step of the management [1]. In most clinical trials of antiosteoporotic treatments with fracture endpoints, patients receive vitamin D and calcium supplements, and any effects of pharmacological interventions on fracture prevention are above those that can be obtained by vitamin D and calcium alone. A daily intake of protein 1 g/kg body weight is also recommended, particularly in elderly individuals with a recent hip fracture and should also be part of the management strategy [2].

© Springer International Publishing Switzerland 2016
S.L. Silverman, B. Abrahamsen (eds.), *The Duration and Safety
of Osteoporosis Treatment*, DOI 10.1007/978-3-319-23639-1_15

Non-pharmacological interventions aim mainly at reducing the frequency or impact of falls, for example, with the use of hip protectors in residents of nursing homes at high risk for falling. Approved pharmacological interventions for the prevention of fractures are generally distinguished into inhibitors of bone resorption and turnover such as bisphosphonates, denosumab, estrogens, and selective estrogen receptor modulators (SERMs) and stimulators of bone formation such as teriparatide (PTH 1-34) and PTH 1-84; the effect of strontium ranelate, an agent approved for the treatment of patients with severe osteoporosis in some parts of the world, on bone remodeling is unclear.

Osteoporosis is a chronic disease requiring chronic treatment. While the efficacy and tolerability of available agents are well established, there are uncertainties about their long-term effects owing to the rather limited data and to the specific pharmacology of bisphosphonates. In this chapter, I review the evidence of the efficacy and tolerability of agents used in the management of osteoporosis for which long-term data (>5 years) are available.

General Considerations

Methodological Issues

For the proper interpretation of the results of clinical studies, certain issues need to be considered including the following:

1. The design of the study: randomized clinical trials (RCTs) with blinding of patient and investigator being the optimal design. In addition, the hypotheses to be tested and the type of analyses for the evaluation of efficacy should be prespecified. An intention-to-treat analysis is very conservative but also the most objective and statistically sound.
2. The documentation of fractures should be done in an objective way. Non-vertebral fractures are easier to document because these are associated with complaints that patients present to health-care professionals, and X-rays

are made. This is not the case with vertebral fractures, two thirds of which are asymptomatic. The methods used to define osteoporotic fractures can influence the outcome.

3. The number of patients with fractures rather than the number of fractures should be counted; counting the latter can inflate the result because fractures are interrelated events.
4. The number of patients lost to follow-up. This should be distinguished from dropouts, patients who for various reasons have stopped taking their medication but continue to be followed in a study. For discrete variables, such as fractures, high loss-to-follow-up numbers can lead to loss of the original randomization reducing the reliability of the results. A well-designed and analyzed clinical trial is essential for the proper evaluation of the observed outcome, and in such trial every participant should be accounted for. This is also the reason why all major journals have adopted the CONSORT Statement in reports of clinical trials [3].

There are different ways to express the results of intervention studies. Commonly used are the relative risk (RR = the risk of having a fracture relative to placebo), the relative risk reduction (RRR = the proportion of baseline risk removed by treatment), and the absolute risk reduction (ARR = proportion of patients avoiding a fracture by treatment). In 1988, the number needed to treat (NNT) was introduced as an alternative approach to summarize the effect of treatment [4]. It was thought that NNT would be more useful to clinicians because it refers to patients rather than to probabilities. This term has been extensively used but is very often misused. For proper interpretation of NNT, its determinants need to be considered. NNT is the number of patients needed to take a treatment to avoid a discrete event (for osteoporosis, this is the fracture) within a given time period. NNT can be simply calculated as follows: NNT = 100:ARR, where ARR = risk in the placebo group—risk in the treatment group. NNT is, therefore, a derived term that depends both on the risk of fracture in the population studied and on the efficacy of the intervention. Because of differences in risk of

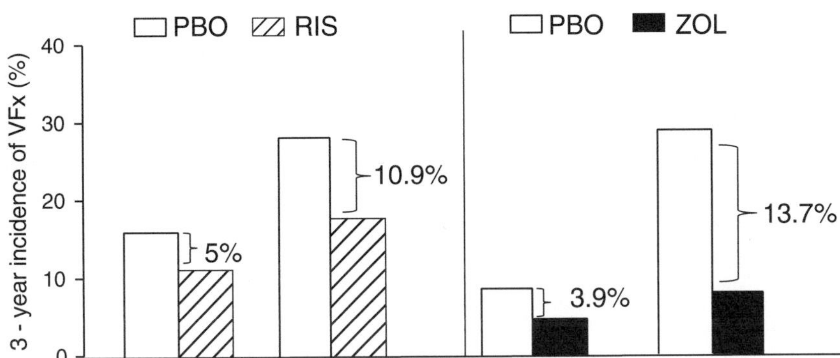

Fig. 15.1 Decrease in absolute risk of new vertebral fractures in patients treated with risedronate in two different clinical trials (*left panel*) and zoledronate in the same clinical trial (*right panel*). (**A**) VERT-NA; (**B**) VERT-MN; (**C**) HORIZON, patients with no prevalent vertebral fractures; (**D**) HORIZON, patients with ≥2 prevalent vertebral fractures; *RRR* relative risk reduction, *NNT* number needed to treat; note the difference in NNT for the same compound in two different clinical trials or in one clinical trial depending on baseline fracture risk. From: Appelman-Dijkstra NM, Papapoulos SE. Prevention of incident fractures in patients with prevalent fragility fractures: Current and future approaches. Best Practice and Research Clinical Rheumatology 2013; 27:805–820

patients included in clinical trials, NNT cannot and should not be used to compare efficacy of interventions obtained in different clinical trials. This is illustrated in Fig. 15.1 for two agents used in the treatment of osteoporosis. Finally, the number needed to harm (NNH) can also be calculated, but, despite its importance, this is rarely used in clinical practice.

The evidence of the antifracture efficacy of pharmacological interventions varies among approved agents, and for treatment decisions, the highest level of available evidence should be selected. Properly designed and performed RCTs and meta-analyses of RCTs are at the top of the hierarchy of evidence. RCTs and meta-analyses provide different perspectives. RCTs address a specific question in a given population, whereas the primary purpose of meta-analysis is to synthesize information from prior studies and provide an estimate of the magnitude of the effect of treatment.

Benefits and Risks of Treatments

An evidence-based approach to treatment of the individual patient with osteoporosis involves the use of the best data available from clinical studies combined with clinical judgment and the patient's preferences and values. The final decision, however, strongly depends on the balance between the benefit and the harm of a given intervention. The fact that any medication, even OTC preparations such as acetaminophen or NSAIDs, may have very serious adverse consequences is frequently overlooked. The best way to achieve zero risk would be never to take a drug, a decision that should be weighed against the price of ignoring the benefit [5]. The benefit of antiosteoporotic treatments is the reduction of the risk of fractures at all skeletal sites including the hip which has the most devastating clinical consequences. In addition, potential extra-skeletal beneficial effects should be considered, but this rarely occurs in clinical practice. It should be appreciated that the true risk of any treatment should be calculated as a fraction, the numerator of which is the number of patients with a given adverse effect and the denominator is the total number of patients who used the medication over the same period of time. Consequently, adverse events are classified as common (1–10 %), uncommon (0.1–1 %), rare (0.01–0.1 %), and very rare (less than 0.01 % or less than 1:10,000). This transparent expression of the risk of a treatment differs from the fear generated by reports in the media of very rare events that may affect the willingness of patients to take or continue a medication but also of physicians to prescribe the medication. Such fear has contributed to the gradual fall of sales of antiosteoporotic agents, particularly bisphosphonates, in recent years [6] despite their efficacy and the generally recognized low uptake of treatments by patients with increased risk of fractures [7, 8]. For example, in the USA, the use of antiosteoporotic medications within one year after a hip fracture fell from 40.2 % in 2002 to 20.5 % in 2011 [9].

There are several examples of the importance of the estimation of the benefits and harms for the approval and use of agents for the management of osteoporosis. Tibolone, an agent with estrogenic, progestogenic, and androgenic effects, has been used for many years for the control of menopausal symptoms and prevention of osteoporosis. In an RCT of 4538 women with postmenopausal osteoporosis, tibolone reduced the risk of vertebral and non-vertebral fractures by 45 % and 26 %, respectively, after a median period of 34 months [10]. In addition, compared with placebo, tibolone reduced the rate of invasive breast cancer by 68 % and that of colon cancer by 69 %, without an increase in the incidence of thromboembolism or coronary heart disease. Women who received tibolone were more likely to report vagi-nal bleeding, endometrial thickness, weight increase, and increases in liver enzymes. However, because of a significantly increased risk of stroke in women treated with tibolone compared with those treated with placebo [HR 2.19 (1.14–4.23)], the study was discontinued. This example, illustrates the importance of the assessment of the risk–benefit balance for the approval of medications for the treatment of osteoporosis. The same also applies to already approved medications for the treatment of osteoporosis, such as intranasal calcitonin which was withdrawn from the market in Europe due to an unfavorable risk–benefit profile.

The risk–benefit balance has also been used to better position approved medications in the treatment of osteoporosis. Hormonal treatment, the dominant intervention for prevention and treatment of osteoporosis in the past, is not any more considered first line of therapy based mainly on the results of the Women's Health Initiative study [11]. In this study, the beneficial effect of hormonal therapy on fractures, including those of the hip, and colon cancer was thought not to clearly exceed the risks of treatment (Fig. 15.2). Another example is the restriction of the use of strontium ranelate, an agent shown to reduce the risk of vertebral and non-vertebral fractures in women with postmenopausal osteoporosis by 24 and 15 % after 5 years [12]. In 2014, the Committee for Medicinal Products for Human Use (CHMP) in Europe recommended that

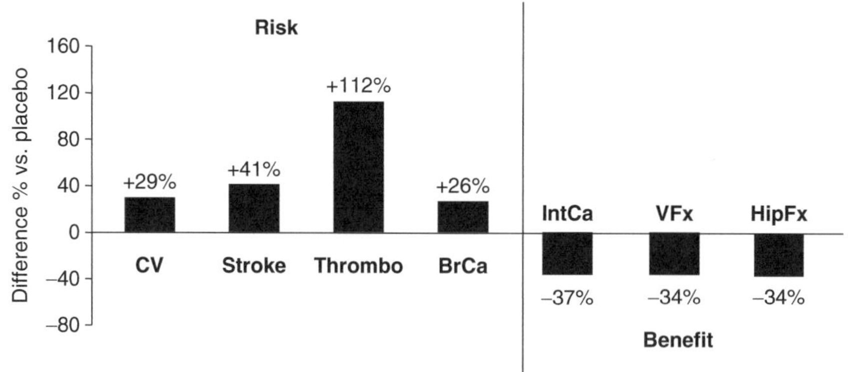

Fig. 15.2 Benefits and risks of HRT relative to placebo in postmenopausal women aged 50–79 years in the Women's Health Initiative Study. *CV* cardiovascular events, *thrombo* thromboembolism, *BrCa* breast cancer, *IntCa* intestinal cancer, *VFx* vertebral fractures, *HipFx* hip fractures. Data from JAMA 2002;288: 321–333

strontium ranelate should only be used to treat severe osteoporosis in postmenopausal women and men at risk of fractures, for which treatment with other medicinal products approved for the treatment of osteoporosis is not possible due to, for example, contraindication or intolerance. Strontium ranelate should further not be used in patients with established, current, or past history of ischemic heart disease, peripheral arterial disease, and/or cerebrovascular disease or uncontrolled hypertension. Decisions should be made on the assessment of the individual patient's risk [13]. This recommendation was based on the assessment of the risk for myocardial infarction and venous, thrombotic, and embolic events in postmenopausal women with osteoporosis treated with this agent.

There are currently four agents that have been shown to reduce the risk of all osteoporotic fractures with variable efficacy; the bisphosphonates alendronate, risedronate, and zoledronate and the RANKL inhibitor denosumab. All these are inhibitors of bone resorption and turnover. Long-term studies are available for these agents and help to better formulate therapeutic decisions. In the absence of head-to-head studies with fracture endpoints, these data together with the safety profiles of these agents should be considered in tailoring therapeutic choices to individuals at risk. Long-term data are also available for other agents [14, 15], but due to either restrictions in their use (Strontium Ranelate) or lack of efficacy in reducing the risk of non-vertebral and hip fractures (SERMs), these as well as PTH peptides, the use of which is restricted to 18–24 months, will not be further discussed.

Rationale for the Use of Inhibitors of Bone Turnover

The definition of osteoporosis, as formulated more than 20 years ago, recognized that low bone mass is not the only determinant of bone fragility and that the strength of the skeleton depends also on other properties of the bone tissue, collectively termed bone quality. As with other materials, the structure and material composition of bone together with its mass will determine its ability to resist structural failure. Bone is, however, different from other materials due to its ability to be continuously renewed throughout life by the process of bone remodeling. The generally higher rates of bone remodeling in osteoporosis combined with the negative balance between bone formation and bone resorption at the basic multicellular unit (BMU) lead to loss of bone mass, an increased number and depth of resorption cavities, perforation of trabecular plates, and loss of trabecular elements of cancellous bone and thinning and porosity of cortical bone [16–19]. They also reduce the degree of mineralization and of the amount of collagen of the bone matrix and may also impair the maturation and cross-linking of collagen fibers [19]. Thus, mass, structure, and material composition of bone can all be affected in patients with osteoporosis compromising bone strength and increasing bone fragility. Currently available inhibitors of bone turnover reduce the rate of bone resorption to different degrees depending on the potency and mechanism of action of the different classes of agents. The decrease of bone resorption is invariably followed by a decrease in the rate of bone formation leading to an overall lower rate of bone turnover. These actions have beneficial effects on bone strength by reducing the remodeling space, maintaining or sometimes improving trabecular or cortical architecture, correcting the hypomineralization of bone tissue, and increasing bone mineral density. The clinically relevant outcome is the reduction in the risk of fractures.

Bisphosphonates

The Benefit

Bisphosphonates reduce the rate of bone resorption and turnover leading after 3–6 months to a new steady state of lower rate of bone turnover that is maintained for at least 10 years of continuous treatment [20]. This response illustrates, in addition, that the accumulation of bisphosphonate in the skeleton is not associated with cumulative effects on bone remodeling. The importance of the reduction of bone resorption and turnover for the antifracture efficacy of bisphosphonates has been suggested by meta-analysis of results of clinical trial [21] and was demonstrated for alendronate by analysis of individual patient data from the Fracture Intervention Trial (FIT) [22]. Bisphosphonates have also been suggested to prolong the life span of osteocytes by reducing their rate of apoptosis by a mechanism different from that of their action in osteoclasts [23].

Antifracture Efficacy of Oral Bisphosphonates

Vertebral fractures, the most representative osteoporotic fractures, are a key outcome in studies of antiosteoporotic treatments. They are less influenced by extrinsic factors (e.g., falls), they increase the risk of new clinical fractures, and they result in more frequent hospitalizations and are associated with increased mortality. The efficacy of alendronate in reducing the risk of vertebral fractures was examined in the FIT study. In the vertebral fracture arm of this trial (FIT1), postmenopausal women with femoral BMD T-score < −1.6 and at least one prevalent vertebral fracture were assigned to placebo ($n=1005$) or alendronate ($n=1022$) for 3 years [24]. The clinical fracture arm (FIT2) included women with femoral neck BMD T-score < −1.6 but without vertebral fractures at baseline of whom 2218 received placebo and 2214 received alendronate for 4 years [25]. The dose of alendronate was initially 5 mg/day and was increased to 10 mg/day after 2 years because other studies suggested that this dose had greater effects than 5 mg on BMD and bone markers with similar tolerability. Spine radiographs were obtained after 2 and 3 years in FIT 1 and after 4 years in FIT2. Alendronate reduced the incidence of new vertebral fractures by 47 % and 44 % in FIT1 and FIT2, respectively.

The VERT study was the pivotal trial that examined the efficacy of risedronate in reducing the risk of vertebral fractures. In VERT North America (NA), women with two or more prevalent vertebral fractures or one prevalent vertebral fracture and low lumbar spine BMD were assigned to placebo ($n=820$) or risedronate 5 mg/ day ($n=821$); in a third group that received risedronate 2.5 mg/day, treatment was discontinued after the first year because data from other trials indicated that this dose was less effective than the 5 mg/day dose [26]. Spine radiographs were obtained after 1, 2, and 3 years. Compared with placebo, risedronate reduced the incidence of vertebral fractures by 41 % after 3 years. VERT International (VERT-MN) included women at higher risk (2 or more prevalent vertebral fractures) who were assigned to placebo ($n=407$) or risedronate 5 mg/day ($n=407$); a third group that received risedronate 2.5 mg/day was discontinued after 2 years [27]. In this study, risedronate reduced the risk of vertebral fractures by 49 % after 3 years.

The consistency of the efficacy of alendronate and risedronate in reducing the risk of vertebral fractures has been demonstrated by meta-analyses of RCTs [28, 29].

The impact of clinical fractures on morbidity, hospitalization, mortality, and health-care costs is immediately obvious. Furthermore, the time of occurrence is easily determined as all these fractures require medical attention and radiographs are made. A treatment effect on the risk of non-vertebral fractures is, however, more difficult to demonstrate, and in no study of oral bisphosphonates was the incidence of non-vertebral fractures a primary efficacy point. Clinical fractures, that included non-vertebral and vertebral fractures, were a primary efficacy outcome in FIT2. A large study with risedronate (HIP) was the only one to assess the efficacy of an oral bisphosphonate on the risk of hip fractures as primary endpoint of the trial [30]. It should be noted that non-vertebral fractures are strongly influenced by extra-skeletal factors, such as trauma, and their definition in clinical trials varies among studied agents which may influence the outcome.

Alendronate reduced the risk of non-vertebral fractures by 20 % and 12 % in FIT1 and FIT2, respectively, both nonsignificant risk reductions. However, in FIT1, alendronate reduced significantly the risk of hip fractures by 51 % and those of the wrist by 48 %, and in post hoc analysis of FIT2, it decreased the risk of any clinical fracture by 34 % and of hip fractures by 56 % in women with osteoporosis (T-score < −2.5). In a pre-planned pooled analysis of women with osteoporosis (prevalent vertebral fracture or BMD T-score < −2.5) of the combined FIT cohorts, alendronate reduced significantly the incidence of non-vertebral fractures by 27 %, of non-vertebral osteoporotic fractures by 36 %, and of hip fractures by 53 % [31].

In the VERT-NA study, risedronate 5 mg/day reduced significantly the cumulative incidence of non-vertebral osteoporotic fractures by 39 % and in the VERT-MN by 33 %, a nonsignificant reduction. The HIP study was designed to assess the efficacy of risedronate on the risk of hip fractures and included 9331 patients, 5445 women 70–79 years old with osteoporosis (femoral neck BMD T-score < −4.0 or < −3.0 plus a nonskeletal risk factor for hip fracture, e.g., poor gait or propensity to fall) and 3886 women ≥80 years old with at least one nonskeletal risk factor for hip fracture or low BMD; the latter group comprised only 16 % of this cohort [30]. The women were randomly assigned to receive treatment with risedronate 2.5 or 5.0 mg/day or placebo for 3 years. In this study, the combined effect of the two risedronate doses was estimated. Compared with placebo, risedronate reduced significantly the incidence of non-vertebral fractures by 20 % due to the effect of the bisphosphonate in the women selected on the basis of osteoporosis. In a post hoc analysis of women with osteoporosis who had, in addition, prevalent vertebral fractures, the risk of non-vertebral osteoporotic fractures was significantly reduced by 30 %. In the whole population of the study, risedronate decreased significantly the incidence of hip fractures by 30 %, 40 % in the women with osteoporosis ($p = 0.009$), and 20 % in the older women with risk factors ($p = 0.35$).

Post hoc analyses, pooled analyses, and meta-analyses of the incidence of non-vertebral and hip fractures during treatment with alendronate and risedronate have been performed [32–37]. Overall, results confirmed the significant effect of these two bisphosphonates in reducing the risk of non-vertebral and hip fractures. For example, a meta-analysis of the Cochrane Collaboration of the efficacy of alendronate and risedronate to reduce the incidence of non-vertebral and hip

fractures in women with osteoporosis reported significant reductions of 23 % (RR 0.77; 95 % CI 0.74–0.94) and 53 % (0.47; 95 % CI 0.46–0.85), respectively, for alendronate and 20 % (RR 0.80; 95 % CI 0.72–0.90) and 26 % (0.74; 95 % CI 0.59–0.94), respectively, for risedronate.

Daily administration of bisphosphonates, though highly efficacious, is inconvenient because of strict dosing instructions and may also be associated with gastrointestinal adverse effects. These reduce adherence to treatment and can diminish the therapeutic potential of bisphosphonates [38]. To overcome these problems, more convenient once-weekly formulations, the sum of seven daily doses, have been developed for alendronate and risedronate and shown to be pharmacologically equivalent to daily formulations and to significantly improve patient adherence to treatment [39–42]. For risedronate, other preparations are also available; a once-monthly preparation of 150 mg (or 75 mg given on two consecutive days once a month) and a 35 mg once-weekly preparation that can be taken after breakfast [43–45].

Antifracture Efficacy of Intravenous Zoledronate

The efficacy of zoledronate in reducing the incidence of osteoporotic fractures was examined in the HORIZON-PFT trial [46]. Postmenopausal women with osteoporosis (femoral neck BMD T-score ≤ −2.5 with or without prevalent vertebral fractures or T-score ≤ −1.5 with at least one moderate or two mild vertebral fractures) were randomized to receive a single 15-min infusion of zoledronate 5 mg ($n = 3889$) or placebo ($n = 3876$) at baseline, at 12 months, and at 24 months. New vertebral fractures (in patients not taking concomitant osteoporotic medications) and hip fractures (in all patients) were primary endpoints, while non-vertebral fractures were a secondary efficacy endpoint. Spine radiographs were taken annually. Compared with placebo, zoledronate reduced the incidence of vertebral fractures by 70 % and that of hip fractures by 41 % after 3 years. The risk of non-vertebral fractures was also significantly reduced by 25 %.

In the HORIZON-RFT [47], men and women with a hip fracture were randomized to receive yearly intravenous zoledronate 5 mg ($n=1065$) or placebo ($n=1062$) within 90 days after surgical repair of the fracture. Patients received also a loading dose of vitamin D (50,000–125,000 IU) 14 days before the first infusion of the bisphosphonate if serum 25-OHD was ≤ 15 ng/ml or if the level was not available. Thereafter, they received vitamin D 800–1200 IU/day and calcium 1000–1500 mg/day. After a median follow-up of 1.9 years, zoledronate decreased the risk of any clinical fracture by 35 % (HR 0.65; 95 % CI 0.50–0.84), of vertebral fractures by 46 % (HR 0.54; 0.32–0.92), of non-vertebral fractures by 27 % (HR 0.73; 95 % CI 0.55–0.98), and of hip fractures by 30 % (HR 0.70; 0.41–1.19). This is a unique study because patients were not selected by the level of BMD or the presence/absence of vertebral fractures; only 41 % of patients had a BMD T-score < -2.5 and 35.3 % had osteopenia, while in 11.4 % BMD was normal and in 12.1 % of patients BMD data were not available. The results of this prospective study demonstrated that not only patients with prevalent vertebral fractures but also patients with hip fractures should receive treatment independently of the level of BMD.

Extra-skeletal Effects of Bisphosphonates

Extra-skeletal effects of bisphosphonates include improvement of aspects of the quality of life, reduction of the incidence of certain cancers, and, more importantly, reduction of the risk of dying. These benefits of bisphosphonate treatment are rarely considered in the choice of a treatment in clinical practice. Alendronate was shown in the FIT trial to reduce the number of days of bed disability and days of limited activity caused by back pain [48]. Similarly, in the HORIZON-PFT trial, zoledronate reduced significantly the number of days that patients reported back pain and limited activity and bed rest due to a fracture [49]. In the HORIZON-RTF trial, compared with placebo, zoledronate decreased significantly all-cause mortality by 28 %. This is a remarkable result, the underlying mechanism of which is unclear at present, but it was not related to the reduction in the incidence

of fractures. It appears that the efficacy of bisphosphonates in reducing mortality is not restricted to zoledronate. Reduction of mortality has also been reported in different cohorts, but not in RCTs, of patients treated with other bisphosphonates [50–52]. In addition, reduction of the incidence of colon cancer and mortality rate, once colon cancer is diagnosed, was reported in alendronate-treated patients [53]. The occurrence of heart failure was investigated in a cohort study of 102,342 bisphosphonate users compared with 307,026 age- and gender-matched controls from the general population [54]. Alendronate users in this cohort showed a dose-dependent, significant reduction in the risk of heart failure. Moreover, in a post hoc analysis of a prospective cohort study of 19281 patients with rheumatoid arthritis in the USA, the adjusted risk of myocardial infarction was 0.72 (0.54–0.96, $p=0.02$) in bisphosphonate users compared with nonusers [55]. A reduction in the risk of myocardial infarction and strokes was also reported in patients with fractures treated with bisphosphonates [56, 57].

Long-Term Effects on Bone Fragility

Skeletal fragility on long-term bisphosphonate therapy has been examined in extensions of four clinical trials (VERT-MN with risedronate, Phase III and FIT with alendronate, and HORIZON with zoledronate) (Fig. 15.3). None of these extension studies were specifically designed to assess antifracture efficacy, but rather safety and efficacy on surrogate endpoints as well as consistency of the effect of bisphosphonates over longer periods were evaluated. Fractures were, however, collected in all studies (Table 15.1).

The first study consisted of two 2-year extensions of the VERT-MN trial [58, 59]. During the first 5 years of the study, two groups of osteoporotic women received either placebo or risedronate 5 mg/day, while in the following 2 years, all patients received active treatment. The annualized incidence of new vertebral fractures during years 6 and 7 was similar in patients who received placebo previously and those who received

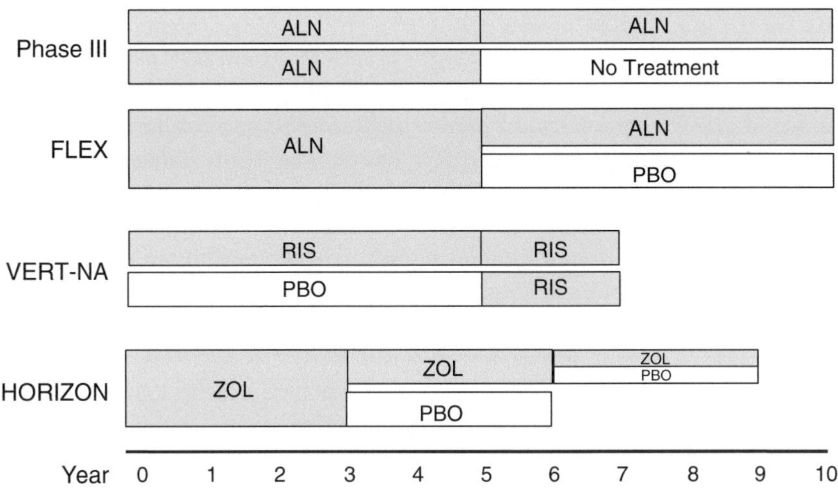

Fig. 15.3 Schematic presentation of the design of long-term controlled studies of bisphosphonates in osteoporosis. *ALN* alendronate, *RIS* risedronate, *ZOL* zoledronate, *PBO* placebo

Table 15.1 Incidence of fractures in long-term studies of bisphosphonates

Study	Patients (nr)	Treatment	Years BP	VFx	NVFx (%)	HFx (%)
Phase III	286	ALN 10 mg/day	10	6.6 %	8.1[a]	n.a.
		ALN	5	5.0 %	12[a]	n.a.
FLEX	1099	ALN	10	2 %[b]	19	3
		ALN/PBO	5	5 %[b]	20	3
VERT-NA	136	RIS	7	3.8 %/year	6[c]	n.a.
		PBO/RIS	2	3.8 %/year	7.4[c]	n.a.
HORIZON	1283	ZOL	6	3.0 %[d]	8.2	1.3
		ZOL/PBO	3	6.2 %[d]	7.6	1.4

[a]Years 8–10
[b]Clinical vertebral fractures
[c]Years 6–7
[d]Morphometric vertebral fractures
BP bisphosphonate, *VFx* vertebral fractures, *NVFx* non-vertebral fractures, *HFx* hip fractures

risedronate continuously (3.8 %/year); the incidence of vertebral fractures in the risedronate group was similar to that observed in years 0–3 (4.7 %/year) and years 4–5 (5.2 %/year). Moreover, the percentage of women with non-vertebral fractures was not significantly different between the two groups during years 6–7 (7.4 vs. 6.0 %). These results indicate consistency of the effect of risedronate on the incidence of fractures with time. Apart from the lack of a placebo group during the whole observation period, an additional limitation of this, as well as of other extension studies, is the substantial decrease in the number of participants with time. For example, 814 patients were initially randomized of whom 473 completed the first 3 years; of these, 260 entered the first extension (4–5 years), 164 the second extension (6–7 years), and 136 completed the study. While loss of patients in such extension studies is expected by the length of the study and the aging of the participants, results should be interpreted with caution.

The second study was an extension of the Phase III clinical trial originally reported by Liberman et al. with alendronate [20]. Patients received alendronate either 5 or 10 mg/day continuously for 10 years or 20 mg/day for 2 years, followed by 5 mg/day for 3 years (providing a total dose equivalent to 10 mg/day for 5 years). The rate of non-vertebral fractures in the pooled alendronate group during years 0–3 was 8.5 %; during years 6–10, this was 11.5 % in patients on 5 mg/day and 8.1 % in those on 10 mg/day, similar, thus, to the initial rates and lower than the estimated rates of the original placebo group adjusted for the effect of aging on the risk. In this study, 247 women of 482 originally assigned to alendronate treatment participated in all three extensions. These results supported the consistency of the long-term effect of alendronate on bone fragility.

In the extension of the FIT trial (FLEX), 1099 patients who participated in the FIT and received on average alendronate for 5 years were randomized to placebo, alendronate 5 mg/day, or alendronate 10 mg/day and were followed for another 5 years [60]. At the end of the 10-year observation period, the incidence of non-vertebral and hip fractures in the ALN/PBO group was similar to that in the ALN/ALN groups (20 % vs. 19 % and 3 % vs. 3 %, respectively), but the incidence of clinical vertebral fractures was significantly reduced in the ALN/ALN groups compared with the ALN/PBO group (2 % vs. 5 %). A post hoc analysis of the FLEX study reported a significant relationship between BMD values at the start of the 5-year extension and incidence of non-vertebral fractures at the end of the study in women with no prevalent vertebral fractures [61]. Compared with placebo, patients on alendronate who entered the extension with BMD T-score $\leq$ −2.5 showed a significant 50 % decrease in the incidence of non-vertebral fractures (RH 0.50; 95 % CI 0.26–0.96), while those who entered the extension with BMD T-score >2.0 showed a 41 % nonsignificant increase. Except BMD and age, no other clinical or biochemical characteristic could identify patients who would benefit from continuation of treatment with alendronate beyond 5 years [62]. In a further analysis, Black et al. reported that patients with vertebral fractures and femoral neck BMD <−2.0 at discontinuation had a lower incidence of clinical vertebral fracture if they continued treatment for another 5 years [63].

The last long-term study was a 3-year extension of the HORIZON-PFT [64]. In this clinical trial, 1233 women who received zoledronate during the first 3 years of the study were randomized to continue yearly infusions of zoledronate or placebo for another 3 years. Compared with women who received 3 years of treatment followed by placebo, those who were treated for 6 years had a significantly lower incident of new morphometric vertebral fractures (OR 0.51; 95 % CI 0.26–0.95). There were no significant differences in the incidence of hip or all clinical fractures between the two groups [HR 0.9 (0.33–2.49) and 1.04 (0.71–1.54), respectively]. In a post hoc analysis, Cosman et al. [65] showed that predictors of fracture in the discontinuation group were an osteoporotic hip BMD at the start of the extension and the presence of incident morphometric vertebral fractures during the initial treatment period. On the other hand, women with total hip BMD >−2.5, no recent incident fractures, and no more than one risk factor for fractures have a low risk for a subsequent fracture if treatment was discontinued. These results are generally similar to those obtained with long-term alendronate treatment.

Taken together, the findings of the long-term extension studies of bisphosphonates are reassuring and indicate that prolonged exposure of bone tissue to bisphosphonate maintains the effect of treatment and is not associated with adverse effects on bone fragility. Whether continuation of treatment offers additional antifracture benefit is not entirely clear, but, within the limitations of the studies, the data strongly suggest that patients with increased fracture risk can benefit from continuation of treatment for up to 6 or 10 years with zoledronate and alendronate, respectively. For clinical decisions, analysis of changes of surrogate endpoints such as BMD and biochemical markers of bone turnover can be of additional value.

Resolution of the Effect of Treatment

Bisphosphonates have the unique properties to be selectively taken up by bone, preferentially at sites of increased bone remodeling, to be embedded in bone for long after completing their action on the surface, and to be slowly released from bone. The capacity of the skeleton to retain bisphosphonate, which is biologically inert, is large, and saturation of binding sites in bone with the doses used in the treatment of osteoporosis is unlikely even if these are given for a very long time [66]. These characteristics differentiate the pharmacodynamics of bisphosphonates from those of all other agents used in the treatment ofosteoporosis and play an important role in the interpretation of their long-term results on bone tissue and their implementation in clinical practice.

Pharmacodynamic responses following cessation of bisphosphonate therapy given for prevention of bone loss were adequately investigated in the Early Postmenopausal Intervention Cohort (EPIC) study [67, 68]. Early postmenopausal women were given alendronate for 2, 4, or 6 years, or placebo, and were followed for 6 years. Cessation of treatment after 2 or 4 years was associated with progressive increases in biochemical markers of bone resorption toward the levels of women treated with placebo, and BMD decreased at a rate similar to that of placebo-treated women. There was, thus, no rapid increase in the rate of bone resorption and no "catch-up" bone loss as observed in a parallel group that received hormone replacement therapy for 4 years.

Bagger and colleagues analyzed the results of studies of 203 women given different daily doses of alendronate or placebo for varying periods for the prevention of postmenopausal bone loss and were followed for up to 9 years [69]. Seven years after withdrawal of treatment, women who received alendronate (2.5–10 mg/day) for 2 years had a 3.8 % higher BMD than those who received placebo. The residual effect was proportionally larger in women who received treatment for 4 or 6 years (5.9 % and 8.6 %, respectively), but the largest residual effect was observed in women who received alendronate 20 mg/day for 2 years (9.7 %). Similar to the EPIC study, bone turnover markers tended to revert back to placebo levels, and the rate of bone loss following cessation of alendronate treatment was comparable to the bone loss observed in the placebo group. This study provides information additional to that

obtained in EPIC. It shows that alendronate has a residual effect on bone metabolism that is proportional to the length of treatment with doses between 2.5 and 10 mg/day. The highest residual effect was obtained with the dose of 20 mg/day, although this was given for only 2 years, corresponding to 4 years of treatment with 10 mg/day or 8 years of treatment with 5 mg/day.

About 20 years ago, in exploratory studies of women and men with osteoporosis treated with daily oral pamidronate for 6.5 years, we reported that cessation of treatment was not associated with decreases of bone mineral density of the spine and the femoral neck and that the rate of vertebral fractures remained stable during 2 years of follow-up without bisphosphonate [70]. We hypothesized that resumption of bone remodeling after stopping treatment led to release of bisphosphonate previously embedded in bone. The concentration of the released bisphosphonate was probably sufficient to correct the imbalance between bone resorption and bone formation and to protect skeletal integrity, but insufficient to maintain the decrease of bone resorption to the same level and to further increase BMD. In a later study, we showed that pamidronate can be released in the circulation of humans for at least 8.0 years after stopping treatment [71]. The long-term responses of women with osteoporosis treated with other nitrogen-containing bisphosphonates are in agreement with these early observations. For example, cessation of alendronate after 5 years of treatment was followed by modest increases in biochemical markers of bone turnover to levels lower than those before any treatment was given [20]. The lack of a control group receiving placebo during the whole period of observation precludes any conclusions about the precise magnitude of this response. Spine BMD remained stable during 5 years off treatment, while it increased further on continuing treatment. Importantly, BMD of hip sites showed some decrease, but not back to baseline. In the FLEX study, patients who received placebo after 5 years of alendronate therapy showed a gradual increase in biochemical markers of bone resorption that remained within premenopausal values during the following 5 years without bisphosphonate [60].

Changes in BMD were similar to those in the extension of the Phase III study, with the exception of total hip BMD, which reached pretreatment values after 5 years off treatment. McNabb et al. performed a detailed analysis of the BMD changes of patients who received placebo following alendronate in the FLEX and found that in these untreated elderly women with osteoporosis, total hip and femoral neck BMD decreased by only 3.6 % and 1.7 %, respectively, after 5 years [62]. However, in 29 % of the women, total hip BMD decreased by more than 5 % after 5 years. In an attempt to identify prognostic markers for this BMD loss, the authors examined a number of risk factors for bone loss and fractures including bone turnover markers but failed to identify women at risk of higher rates of bone loss. They concluded that risk factors are currently of limited utility for predicting bone loss following discontinuation of alendronate treatment after 5 years of continuous administration of the bisphosphonate.

Resolution of the effect of long-term risedronate treatment on biochemical bone markers and BMD was examined in 61 patients with postmenopausal osteoporosis who participated in the three extension studies of the VERT-NA [72]. In patients who received PBO/RIS or RIS/RIS, the bone resorption marker NTx/Cr increased to the same extent by about 20 % after one year remaining clearly below baseline values. The resolution of the effect of risedronate was not different between the two groups with different exposures to therapy (2 vs. 7 years). This finding may be related to the lower affinity of risedronate for bone mineral. These changes were associated with decreases in total hip BMD, but lumbar spine and femoral neck BMD were maintained or increased off treatment. Results of bone markers and BMD longer than 1 year after treatment arrest of risedronate are not available.

In the extension of the HORIZON study, levels of markers of bone turnover changed slightly; serum CTX was 0.16 ng/ml in the ZOL/ZOL group and 0.18 ng/ml in the ZOL/PBO group ($p=0.45$), and serum P1NP was 28.6 ng/ml and 25.8 ng/ml ($p=0.0001$), after 6 years, respectively [64]. Compared with the ZOL/ZOL group, BMD of the total hip and the femoral neck

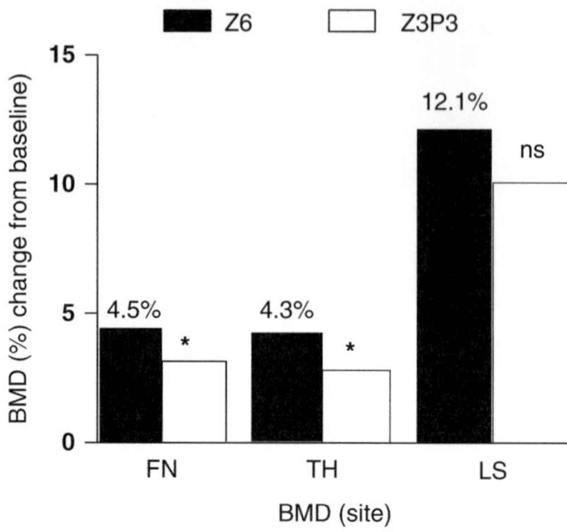

Fig. 15.4 Bone mineral density (BMD) changes after 6 years treatment with yearly infusions of zoledronate 5 mg (Z6) or 3 years treatment with zoledronate followed by 3 years with placebo (Z3P3); *FN* femoral neck, *TH* total hip, *LS* lumbar spine; *ns* nonsignificant, *$p<0.05$. Data from Journal of Bone and Mineral Research 2012; 27: 243–54

decreased significantly in the ZOL/PBO group after 3 years but did not reach pretreatment values (Fig. 15.4).

The combined observations of the long-term studies of bisphosphonates allow some treatment recommendations based on the risk of fracture of the individual patient. In patients with low fracture risk, zoledronate or alendronate treatment may be stopped after 3 or 5 years, respectively; such approach can also have economic implications. Patients should be followed regularly, but reported data do not allow a precise definition of the length of follow-up intervals, and decisions should be based on clinical judgment; yearly clinical assessments with measurements of BMD and markers of bone turnover can be recommended. In patients at high risk of fracture, treatment should be continued beyond 3 and 5 years for zoledronate and alendronate, respectively, as this may offer additional therapeutic benefits. Alendronate treatment may be continued at a dose of 70 mg every 2 weeks as in the FLEX study 5 mg/day was sufficient to fully maintain the responses of biochemical markers of bone turnover and BMD. This suggestion is based, however, on theoretical considerations as no data supporting a similar efficacy of 5 mg/day and 70 mg every 2 weeks are available. Decisions about long-term therapy should not only be based on these efficacy data but also on potential harm associated with prolonged administration of bisphosphonates.

The Risk

Considering the different molecules, doses, routes of administration, and multiple indications for their use, bisphosphonates are generally safe compounds (reviewed in [73, 74]).

General Toxicity

Short-term adverse effects of bisphosphonate treatment are discussed in detail in Chap. 20. In brief, these include *upper GI side effects* with nitrogen-containing bisphosphonates that occur more frequently with daily oral dosing; *ulcerative esophagitis* that occurs rarely and is usually associated with improper use of the bisphosphonates; *acute phase response*, mainly with intravenous nitrogen-containing bisphosphonates after the first treatment; *ophthalmic reactions* (e.g., conjunctivitis, uveitis, scleritis, and keratitis) that occur infrequently and are usually attributed to the acute phase response; *renal toxicity* associated mainly with intravenous administration of bisphosphonate to patients with impaired renal function [75]; *hypocalcemia* especially in patients with increased rates of bone turnover, concurrent vitamin deficiency, and/or impairment of renal function treated with intravenous bisphosphonate; *defective mineralization* of bone tissue, an earlier concern of treatment with etidronate, has not been observed with nitrogen-containing bisphosphonates.

The abovementioned adverse events were identified and thoroughly investigated because of the known pharmacology and targets of bisphosphonate action and metabolism. During the course of clinical trials and long-term pharmacovigilance, however, unexpected adverse effects potentially associated with bisphosphonate use were identified and extensively studied. These are atrial fibrillation (discussed in Chap. 20), osteonecrosis of the jaw (ONJ), and atypical femoral fractures (AFF).

Osteonecrosis of the Jaw

In 2003, a report brought attention to an unexpected and previously unrecognized potential adverse effect of bisphosphonate treatment in the jaws of patients suffering mainly from malignant diseases [76]. This was initially termed "avascular necrosis of the jaws" and later "osteonecrosis of the jaws" (ONJ) [77] in analogy with the condition osteoradionecrosis of the jaw resulting from radiotherapy of patients with head and neck cancers. The original publications were followed by a large number of case reports and case series describing an association between bisphosphonate treatment and ONJ (discussed in detail in Chaps. 12–14). A causal relationship between bisphosphonate treatment and ONJ has not been established [78–81], there is no generally accepted pathogenetic mechanism of ONJ in bisphosphonate-treated patients, and an appropriate animal model of ONJ is not available [82]. An International Classification of Diseases code (ICD) and a working definition for ONJ were introduced for the first time in 2006–2007.

The American Association of Oral and Maxillofacial Surgeons (AAOMS) and the American Society of Bone and Mineral Research (ASBMR) proposed in 2007 the following definition of ONJ:

1. Current or previous treatment with bisphosphonates
2. Exposed necrotic bone in the maxillofacial region, which has been present for at least 8 weeks
3. No history of radiation therapy to the jaws

This definition was widely accepted and formed the basis of studies that examined the frequency and pathogenesis of ONJ. The definition was revised in 2014 by AAOMS as follows:

1. Current or previous treatment with antiresorptive or antiangiogenic agents
2. Exposed bone or bone that can be probed through an intraoral or extraoral fistula(e) in the maxillofascial region that has persisted for more than 8 weeks
3. No history of radiation therapy to the jaws or obvious metastatic disease to the jaw

The main difference of this from the earlier definition of ONJ is the recognition that the disorder does not occur only in bisphosphonate-treated patients, as was widely believed. Patients at risk or with established medication-related ONJ can also present with other common clinical conditions not to be confused with medication-related ONJ. Commonly misdiagnosed conditions include alveolar osteitis, gingivitis/periodontitis, carries, fibro-osseous lesions, and chronic sclerosing osteomyelitis [81]. Importantly, ONJ occurs also in patients not exposed to antiresorptive or antiangiogenic agents. The pathophysiology of ONJ has not been fully elucidated, and various hypotheses have been proposed to explain the unique localization in the jaws including altered bone remodeling, inhibition of angiogenesis, constant microtrauma, vitamin D deficiency, soft tissue bisphosphonate toxicity, and inflammation or infection.

Initial surveys, using different ways to define ONJ, revealed that the condition was much more frequent in patients treated with bisphosphonates for malignant diseases, particularly multiple myeloma and breast cancer. The incidence of ONJ in patients with malignant diseases treated with intravenous zoledronate in clinical trials is approximately 1.0 % [83]. It should be noted that the dose of zoledronate given to patients with malignant diseases for prevention of skeletal-related events is 4 mg every 3–4 weeks accounting for a total yearly dose of about 50 mg; this dose is tenfold higher than the dose of zoledronate used for the treatment of osteoporosis. The estimated prevalence of ONJ in patients with osteoporosis treated with bisphosphonates range between 10 cases per 10,000 and <1 case per 100,000 patients exposed [84]. In clinical trials of oral bisphosphonates in osteoporosis, no cases of ONJ were identified in more than 60,000 patient-years, while in the HORIZON-PFT, the only study of bisphosphonates in osteoporosis in which cases of ONJ were prospectively collected and adjudicated, two documented cases were reported: one in the placebo-treated group and one in the zoledronate-treated group; another case was documented in the zoledronate group of the extension study [46, 64]. Overall, the risk of

ONJ among patients treated with either zoledronate or alendronate for osteoporosis approximates the risk of ONJ in patients treated with placebo [81]. The risk appears to increase with time on treatment and is 100 times lower than in cancer. The studies of ONJ in patients treated with bisphosphonates have identified other risk factors that contribute to the development of the condition, the most common being a dental procedure and the use of glucocorticoids. In contrast to malignant diseases, there are no specific recommendations for dental procedures in patients with osteoporosis on treatment with bisphosphonates. A dental procedure should not be deferred because the risk of ONJ is extremely low. An advice to temporarily stop treatment, for example, 2–3 months, before and after the procedure is more for reassurance of the patient and the dentist and is not based on scientific evidence. Various treatment strategies are used by dental surgeons depending on the stage of ONJ (see Chap. 14). PTH treatment has been reported to have a quick, favorable effect in some cases. In conclusion, the risk of ONJ in patients with osteoporosis treated with bisphosphonate is very low and does not affect the favorable benefit-to-risk balance of bisphosphonate treatment of osteoporosis.

Atypical Fractures of the Femur (AFF)

In recent years, there has also been concern about the potential relation between fractures of the femur below the lesser trochanter deemed to be unusual for patients with osteoporosis on the basis of their localization and radiographic characteristics and long-term use of bisphosphonate. These fractures were termed AFF and were reported to occur as a result of no or minimal trauma, and they may be complete, extending across the entire femoral shaft, or incomplete affecting only the lateral cortex of the femur. They are morphologically transverse or short oblique, often in areas of thickened femur cortices, and they are not comminuted (Fig. 15.5). They are often preceded by prodromal pain and can be bilateral, and healing may be delayed. The first report of AFF in patients treated with oral bisphosphonate [84] for osteoporosis was fol-

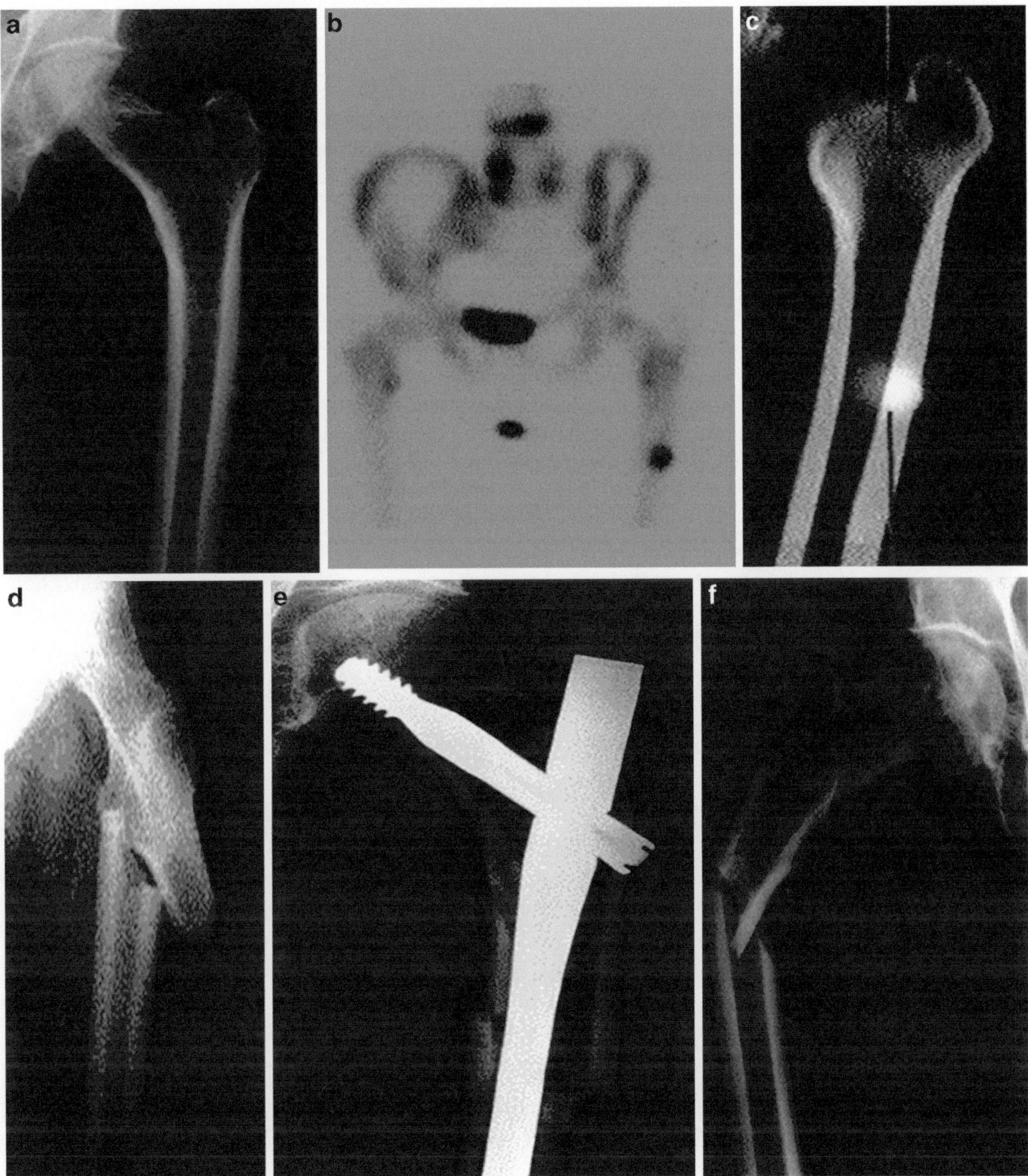

Fig. 15.5 Bilateral atypical femoral fractures of a patient with rheumatoid arthritis and multiple risk factors for fractures (including glucocorticoids and methotrexate) after alendronate for 8 years. *Upper panel*: imaging studies during presentation with prodromal symptoms; (**a**) plain radiograph, (**b**) bone scintigraphy, (**c**) SPECT. *Lower panel*: (**d**) development of complete fracture, (**e**) delayed healing following operation, (**f**) spontaneous frac-ture of the right femur 7 months after the first fracture. Note the lack of scintigraphic evidence of stress fracture in the right femur at presentation. From: Somford MP, et al. Bilateral fractures of the femur diaphysis in a patient with rheumatoid arthritis on long-term treatment with alendronate: clues to the mechanism of increased bone fragility. Journal of Bone and Mineral Research 2009; 24: 1736–1740

lowed by case reports and case series of patients with AFF while on treatment with oral bisphos-phonates (reviewed in [85–87]). In 2010, a Task Force of the ASBMR proposed criteria for the identification and diagnosis of AFF which were revised in 2014 as shown in Table 15.2 [88]. It is now generally accepted that AFF are stress frac-tures that may proceed to complete fractures.

Table 15.2 Atypical fractures of the femur

Major features	Minor features
1. The fracture is associated with minimal or no trauma as in a fall from standing height or less	1. General increase in cortical thickness of the femoral diaphysis
2. The fracture line originates at the lateral cortex and is substantially transverse in its orientation, although it may become oblique as it progresses medially across the femur	2. Unilateral or bilateral prodromal symptoms such as dull or aching pain in the groin or thigh
3. Complete fractures extend through both cortices and may be associated with a medial spike; incomplete fractures involve only the lateral cortex	3. Bilateral incomplete or complete femoral diaphysis fractures
4. The fracture in noncomminuted or minimally comminuted	4. Delayed fracture healing
5. Localized periosteal or endosteal thickening of the lateral cortex is present at the fracture site ("beaking" or "flaring")	*None of these features are required for diagnosis but have been sometimes associated with typical femoral fractures*

The fracture must be located along the femoral diaphysis from just distal to the lesser trochanter to just proximal to the supracondylar flare. At least 4/5 major features must be present

Data from American Society for Bone and Mineral Research Task Force; J Bone Miner Res 2014; 29:1–23 (Ref. [88])

Subtrochanteric and femoral shaft fractures represent 4–10 % of all fractures of the femur, but in elderly residents of nursing homes, the incidence of femoral shaft fractures can be as high as that of hip fractures [89]. Up to 75 % of complete subtrochanteric/femoral shaft, fractures are associated with major trauma, and in elderly patients, they may occur below the prosthesis after total hip replacement. After the age of 60 years, however, subtrochanteric/femoral shaft fractures are more common in women than in men; their incidence increases steeply with age, parallel to that of hip fractures; and they occur mainly after low-energy trauma, similar to typical osteoporotic fractures. Radiographically, they are mainly spiral or longitudinal, but transverse fractures have also been reported, some of which with a radiographic pattern indistinguishable from that reported in patients treated with bisphosphonates.

Compared with hip fractures, the incidence of subtrochanteric/femoral shaft fractures is low and stable over time, ranging between 20 and 34.2/100,000 person-years versus 400 and 694.4/100,000 person-years for hip fractures in large cohorts in the USA (see also Chap. 6). A classification code for AFF is not available, and epidemiological studies report subtrochanteric fractures independently of the presence or not of radiographic features of atypia. In addition, misclassification of femur fractures by ICD coding can be high which may lead to considerably different estimates due to their low incidence.

The association between rates of subtrochanteric/femoral shaft fractures and bisphosphonate use has been examined in large cohort studies. The majority of these studies found that the rates of subtrochanteric/femoral shaft fractures were not higher among patients exposed to bisphosphonates. Similarly, data of clinical trials of bisphosphonates in patients with osteoporosis showed no difference in the low incidence of subtrochanteric/femoral shaft fractures between patients receiving bisphosphonate and those receiving placebo [90, 91].

The main limitation of epidemiological studies was the absence of radiographic adjudication of atypical fractures. The first publication of the prevalence of AFF and their association to the use of bisphosphonates in a cohort of patients with femur fractures with examination of radiographs for signs of atypia was published by Giusti et al. [92]. This was followed by a number of similar studies (reviewed in [88]). The results of these studies showed that AFFs represent only a small fraction of subtrochanteric/femoral shaft fractures (about 1 % of all fractures of the femur). They occur more frequently in bisphosphonate-treatedpatients than in patients never treated with bisphosphonates, and their prevalence increases with prolonged treatment. The reported risk varies widely. While some differences in methodology among these studies may contribute to this large variation, it should also be recognized that the confidence intervals of the estimates are very large and, due to the low frequency of these fractures, inclusion or exclusion of a few cases may have a significant effect on the estimated risk. More importantly, these studies also showed that a substantial proportion of patients with atypical fractures were never treated with bisphosphonates (e.g., 124 of 411 reported in 11 studies). This finding is in full agreement with reports of subtrochanteric/femoral shaft fractures with characteristic radiographic features of atypia both before and after approval of bisphosphonates for osteoporosis [93–98] and suggests that there may be a small group of patients with osteoporosis with a specific predisposition to these fractures.

Causal association between bisphosphonate use and AFFs and a reliable pathogenetic mechanism have not been established [86–88, 99]. Strictly scientifically, a causal relationship between a drug and an event cannot be inferred from retrospective studies. The rarity, however, of the event will never permit the planning of prospective studies specifically designed to test the hypothesis that bisphosphonate use is causally related to the development of AFFs in patients with osteoporosis. The occurrence, however, of AFFs in a substantial number of bisphosphonate-naive patients makes a direct causal relationship between bisphosphonate use and AFFs unlikely. In addition, most studies with radiographic review of the fractures have reported significant associations between glucocorticoid use and AFFs. Moreover, recent studies provide evidence that lower limb geometry contributes significantly to the risk of developing an AFF. To address this issue further, we investigated the association between low-energy trauma fragility fractures of the humeral shaft that share common radiographic features with AFF and bisphosphonate use [100]. The humerus is anatomically a long bone closely resembling the femur but is subjected to different mechanical loads compared to the subtrochanteric region of the femur. We found that "atypical" fractures of the shaft of the humerus occur with a low frequency, similar to that reported for AFF, and that these fractures are not associated with bisphosphonate use. Consistent with the finding that a number of patients with AFF never used bisphosphonates, these findings illustrate that not every fracture of a long bone with radiographic

features of "atypia" should be readily attributed to bisphosphonate use if the patient happens to use one of these agents.

The pathogenesis of AFFs remains unclear. Various hypotheses have been proposed to explain potential adverse effect of bisphosphonates on bone tissue that might explain the increased fragility. These include excessive decrease of bone remodeling, hypermineralization of bone tissue, and microdamage accumulation. Existing evidence does not support any of these hypotheses, and there is insufficient, scientifically reliable evidence to conclude that bisphosphonates cause AFFs. Detailed analysis of existing data and new reports helps, however, to understand the pathogenesis of AFFs in a, currently, small number of patients. For example, in a review of published cases of AFFs, 6 of 77 reported patients treated with bisphosphonates had already sustained a femoral shaft fracture before starting treatment with bisphosphonates [85] indicating preexistent increased fragility of this bone. Sutton et al. [101] described a 55-year-old woman with AFF after 4 years treatment with alendronate followed by intravenous zoledronate. By any current criteria, this patient would have been included in the list of cases with bisphosphonate-associated AFF. However, these authors performed additional investigations and identified a mutation in the gene of alkaline phosphatase establishing the diagnosis of adult hypophosphatasia, a condition associated with increased bone fragility and radiographic features of femur fractures that are indistinguishable from those of AFF in patients receiving bisphosphonates. How many similar cases have already been reported or are included in cohort studies is unknown, and there may be other patients with not yet identified pathology that needs to be further investigated.

Physicians should be alert of the possibility of AFF in patients on long-term bisphosphonate treatment presenting with pain in the hip/femur area with weight bearing which is relieved by unloading. If there are signs of an AFF, treatment should be stopped, and there is epidemiological evidence that the incidence of AFF decreases within 2 years after stopping treatment [102]. There is no general agreement about the management of patients with incomplete fractures, whereas that of complete fractures should be surgical (for details, see Chap. 11). Improvement, no change, or deterioration with PTH treatment have been reported.

The calculation of the benefit (prevention of hip fractures)-to-risk (induction of AFF) balance is in favor of the benefit even if we assume that all AFFs are due to bisphosphonate.

Denosumab

The discovery of the RANK–RANKL–OPG signaling pathway in osteoclasts identified the essential role of RANKL in the formation, function, and survival of osteoclasts [103]. A fully human monoclonal antibody to RANKL (denosumab or Dmab) was developed for the treatment of diseases characterized by absolute or relative increase in bone resorption including osteoporosis. Dmab binds with high specificity to human RANKL to reduce osteoclast number and activity and thereby inhibits bone resorption [104]. This action is followed by a decrease in bone formation and bone turnover and an increase in BMD at all skeletal sites. These actions were confirmed in bone biopsies of patients treated with Dmab for up to 5 years showing marked and sustained inhibition of activation frequency and bone turnover, while the bone formed under treatment was lamellar and mineralized normally [105, 106]. Consistent with the action of other antiosteoporotic treatments, but different from bisphosphonates, the effect of Dmab on bone resorption is quickly reversed following treatment discontinuation. The pharmacokinetic/dynamic background of this response is illustrated in Fig. 15.6. Following a subcutaneous injection of Dmab 60 mg, there is a rapid increase in blood levels which progressively decrease and disappear from the circulation after about 6 months. The elimination of Dmab from the circulation does not involve the kidney and is achieved, as with other antibodies, by the reticuloendothelial system. The increases in blood levels of Dmab are associated with a dramatic decrease in the marker of bone resorption serum CTX which starts to increase again concurrently with the disappearance of Dmab from the circulation.

The Benefit

The efficacy of Dmab in the treatment of osteoporosis was investigated in the FREEDOM study. In this study, 7808 women with postmenopausal

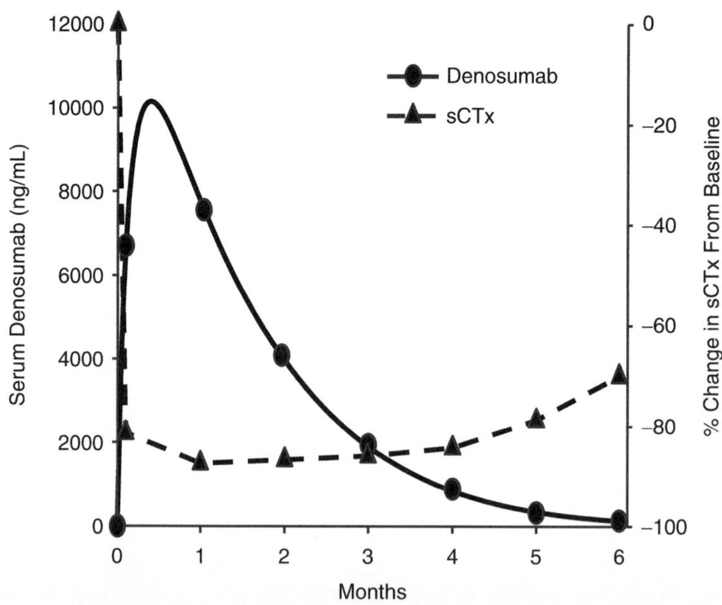

Fig. 15.6 Serum denosumab (*closed circles, solid line*) and CTX (*triangles, interrupted line*) values following a single subcutaneous injection of denosumab 60 mg

osteoporosis (T-score<−2.5 in the spine or total hip and not <−4 at either site) were randomized to receive Dmab 60 mg subcutaneously once every 6 months or placebo [107]. Compared with placebo, Dmab significantly reduced the incidence of new vertebral, hip, and non-vertebral fractures by 68 % (RR 0.32; 95 % CI 0.26–0.41), 40 % (RR 0.60; 95 % CI 0.0.37–0.97), and 20 % (RR 0.80; 95 % CI 0.67–0.95), respectively. Importantly, increases in total hip BMD over 3 years could explain about 80 % of the reduction in the risk of non-vertebral fractures [108]. In the past, there has been much controversy about the contribution of BMD increases to the antifracture efficacy of antiresorptive treatments for osteoporosis. The data obtained with Dmab, supported by data obtained with zoledronate [109], strongly suggest that the reduced potency and the unreliable long-term oral delivery of earlier used preparations are probably responsible for the failure to detect such association. The effect of Dmab in the hip was exerted at all compartments relevant for bone strength (trabecular, subcortical, and cortical) [110, 111].

In the FREEDOM study, a prespecified subgroup analysis of women with prevalent vertebral or non-vertebral fractures was performed [112, 113]. Of a total of 2340 women with mild vertebral deformities (grade 1), 1163 (29.8 %) received Dmab and 1177 (30.1 %) received placebo. After 3 years of treatment, 13.6 % women in the placebo group versus 4.6 % in the Dmab group developed new vertebral fractures (RR 0.34; 95 % CI 0.24–0.48). In women with non-vertebral fractures before entry to the study, 9.4 % in the placebo group sustained a new vertebral fracture versus 3.5 % in the Dmab group (RR 0.38; 95 % CI 0.26–0.54). In both subgroups, the decrease in the incidence of non-vertebral fractures was not significant: HR 1.06 (0.78–1.44) and 0.84 (0.65–1.09) in women with prevalent vertebral and non-vertebral fractures, respectively.

In a post hoc analysis of patients at high risk of fractures selected on the basis of BMD or age (femoral neck BMD ≤−2.5 or age ≥75 years), Dmab, compared with placebo, reduced the incidence of hip fractures by 47 % and 62 %, respectively [114].

Long-Term Effects on Bone Fragility

The FREEDOM study was extended in an open-label design for an additional 7 years during which all women receive Dmab (Fig. 15.7). The extension includes two populations: those who received Dmab for 3 years during the core study (long-term group) and those who received placebo for 3 years during the core study (crossover group). All women who completed the core study (i.e., completed their 3 year visit, did not discontinue investigational product, and did not miss >1 dose of Dmab) were eligible to enter the extension. The primary objective of the extension is to describe the long-term safety and tolerability of Dmab. Secondary objectives include changes in bone turnover markers, BMD, and incidence

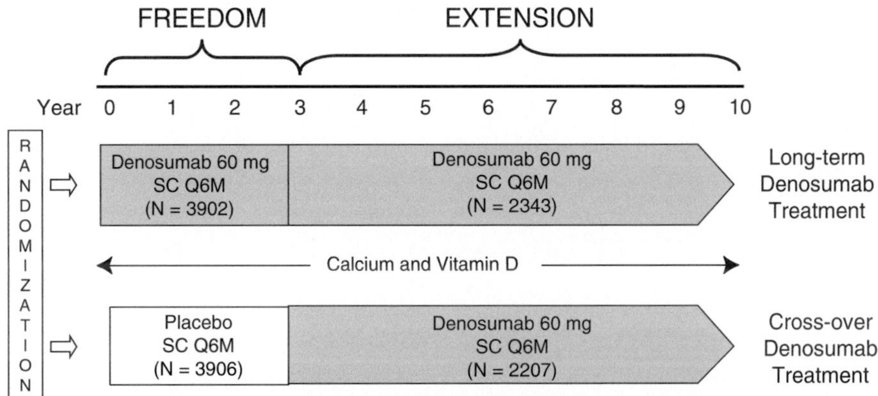

Fig. 15.7 Schematic presentation of FREEDOM and its long-term extension

of vertebral and non-vertebral fractures [115, 116]. At the time of writing this chapter, the FREEDOM Extension study had not been completed, but results up to a total of 8 years of treatment were available [117].

Of the 7808 women enrolled in the FREEDOM trial, 5928 (76 %) were eligible for enrollment in the extension and 4550 (77 %) enrolled (2343 long-term, 2207 crossover group). Of those who entered the extension, 66 % in each group completed Year 5 (long-term group 8 years, crossover group 5 years) totaling 3004 participants. Treatment with Dmab for 8 years resulted in sustained reductions in serum CTX and P1NP. In the crossover group, following the initial administration of Dmab, median values of serum CTX and P1NP were rapidly reduced to levels similar to those observed in the Dmab group in the FREEDOM parent trial. The reduction of the levels of both markers were sustained through 5 years of Dmab treatment, and over time the bone turnover profile was consistent with that of the long-term group during the first 5 years of denosumab exposure. The mean percent changes in BMD from the beginning of FREEDOM through Year 5 of the extension, totaling 8 years of treatment, showed increases of 18.4 % at the lumbar spine, 8.3 % at the total hip, 7.8 % at the femoral neck, and 3.5 % at the one-third radius. During the extension, the BMD gains at each visit for the lumbar spine, total hip, and femoral neck were statistically greater compared with the gains at the previous visit. These changes were very similar to those observed in a small number of women treated for 8 years in a Phase II study. BMD increased also rapidly in the crossover group after the first year of Dmab treatment and mirrored the changes observed in the long-term group indicating consistency of the effect of Dmab on BMD at all skeletal sites. For the lumbar spine, total hip, and femoral neck, gains were statistically greater at each visit compared with the previous time point measured during the extension.

During the extension, fracture rates remained low in an aging population and were below the rates reported in the placebo group of the FREEDOM. Because there was no placebo group in the extension, a simulation method, developed for such an extension study, was used to estimate expected fracture rates in a hypothetical cohort of placebo controls (virtual twin). This method modeled fracture risk for a theoretical placebo-treated population matched to actual study participants with regard to characteristics that were predictive of fracture risk in the participants in the original FREEDOM placebo group. This analysis also showed that the incidence of new vertebral and non-vertebral fracture was lower than the incidence that would have been expected if extension participants had received placebo [116] (Fig. 15.8). These observations are consistent with maintenance of the effect of Dmab to reduce fractures for at least up to 6 years. One inherent limitation of the study is that not all qualified FREEDOM participants enrolled in the extension, so long-term efficacy and safety observations were limited to those who were eligible and chose to participate. However, demographic and clinical characteristics of patients who were not enrolled in the extension did not differ from those of the patients who participated. In addition, the open-label design of the study and the lack of a continuing placebo group precluded direct comparisons of results from Dmab-treated participants and placebo-treated participants for all measures.

The Risk

Dmab has an overall favorable risk–benefit balance. The incidence of serious adverse events in FREEDOM was similar between patients treated with placebo (24.3 %) and those treated with Dmab (25.3 %), and there was a trend for reduced mortality with Dmab treatment (HR 0.76; 95 % CI 0.50, 1.03; $p = 0.08$).

In addition to expression by bone cells, RANKL and RANK are expressed by cells of the immune system including activated T lymphocytes, B cells, and dendritic cells raising the possibility that RANKL inhibition might alter immune function [118]. Gene deletion in rodents showed that the absence of RANK or RANKL during embryogenesis leads to the absence of lymph nodes and changes in thymus architecture, whereas dendritic cells and macrophages remain

a Long-term Denosumba: New Vertebral Fractures

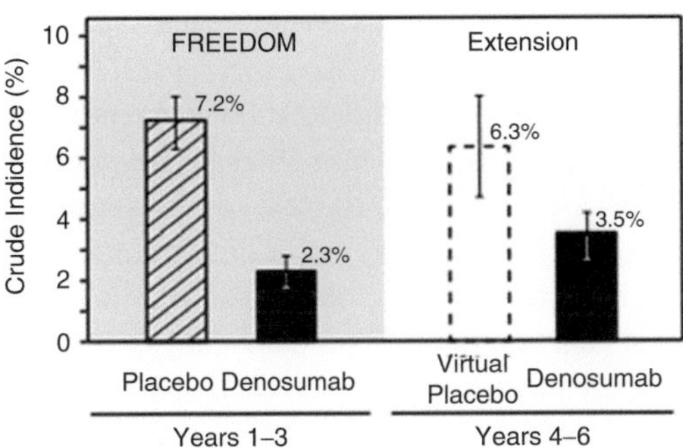

b Long-term Denosumba: Nonvertebral Fractures

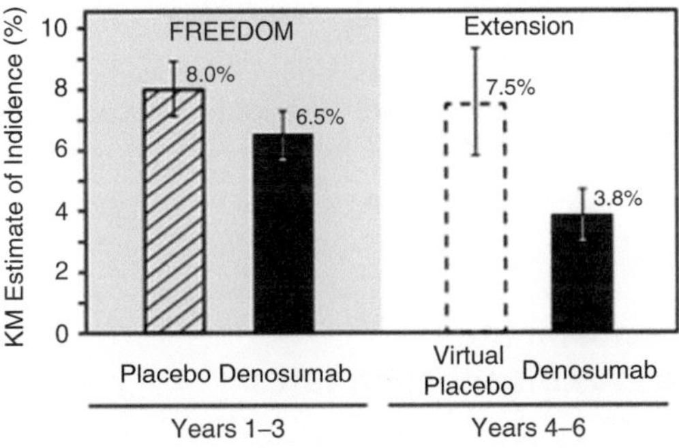

c Cross-over Denosumba: New Vertebral Fractures

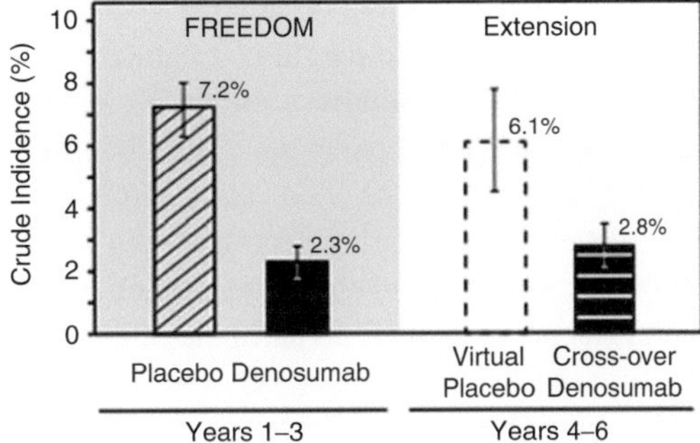

d Cross-over Denosumba: Nonvertebral Fractures

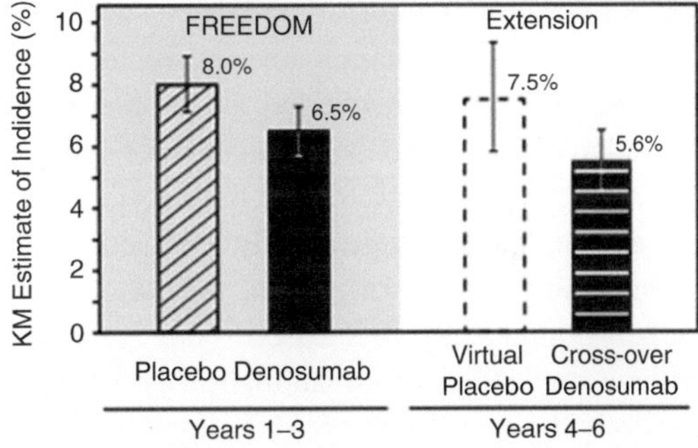

Fig. 15.8 Incidence of vertebral and non-vertebral fractures in FREEDOM and its extension after 6 years. From: Bone HG, et al. The Effect of 3 or 6 Years of Denosumab Exposure in Women With Postmenopausal Osteoporosis: Results From the FREEDOM Extension. Journal of Clinical Endocrinology and Metabolism 2013; 98: 4483–4492

normal [119, 120]. In contrast, in humans with osteopetrosis due to loss-of-function mutations of RANKL, there are hardly any effects on immune system development and function [121]. In addition, in studies of genetically modified rodents and in cynomolgus monkeys, inhibition of RANKL did not have any consequences on basal immune parameters, generation of T or B cell immune responses or response to immunization, or other immune challenges [122–124]. Finally, in a dose-ranging study of Dmab in healthy postmenopausal women, no clinically meaningful differences in overall lymphocyte counts, T cells or B cells, were observed in those treated with Dmab [125]. In the FREEDOM study, the incidence of serious adverse events of infection was similar between placebo-treated (3.4 %) and Dmab-treated (4.1 %) women, but there were some numeric imbalances in specific events particularly those involving the skin.

Serious adverse events in the skin occurred in 3 women (<0.1 %) on placebo and in 15 women (0.4 %) on Dmab ($p < 0.05$). In most of the cases, these were *cellulitis* or *erysipelas* (1 vs. 12 cases) of the lower extremities that bore no relation to the length of treatment and resolved with antibiotics [126]. During the extension, there was no evidence of an increase in these or other infections with increased exposure to Dmab [115–117]. Importantly, in patients who received Dmab following 3 years of treatment with placebo, the incidence of cellulitis or erysipelas did not differ from that of the initial treatment period, one case during 3 years of Dmab treatment [116]. *Gastrointestinal infections* occurred as serious adverse events in 28 placebo-treated women (0.7 %) and in 36 (0.9 %) Dmab-treated women with no consistent pattern in the type of infection. There were no differences in the incidence of respiratory tract infections or osteomyelitis between the two groups, while two cases of endocarditis occurred in Dmab-treated women; these bore no relation to the length of treatment or to the time of Dmab administration, and in both cases no causative pathogen was identified. Finally, the incidence of *opportunistic infections*, a subject of concern during treatment with TNF-α inhibitors, was low and similar in women treated with placebo and Dmab. In particular, tuberculosis was reported as serious adverse event in three and as nonserious adverse event in four women treated with placebo and only as serious adverse event in two women treated with Dmab. Furthermore, in preclinical models of inflammatory arthritis and inflammatory bowel disease, RANKL inhibition decreased bone resorption while having no effect on parameters of inflammation [127, 128]. The former finding was confirmed in a Phase II clinical study of patients with rheumatoid arthritis in whom treatment with Dmab dramatically decreased bone erosions without any effect on inflammation [129]. It is currently thought that the RANK signaling pathway is redundant having a secondary role in the immune response. Whether this is also the case in immunocompromised individuals remains to be studied before Dmab is administered to such patients. Consistent with the effect of Dmab on infections, there was no increase in the incidence of *malignant neoplasms* with prolonged exposure for up to 8 years [117].

While no cases of ONJ or AFF were documented in FREEDOM, eight and two events, respectively, were identified by adjudication during the extension up to 8 years, 5 ONJ cases in the long-term group, and three in the crossover group, one AFF case in each group. *Fracture healing* was neither impaired nor promoted by Dmab treatment [130].

Following the approval of Dmab in several countries worldwide, a pharmacovigilance program was established to supplement data collection from clinical trials. Despite its limitations, this approach helps to assess the safety profile of a medication in clinical practice and in a much larger population than that of clinical trials. During 1,960,405 patient-years exposure, five cases of AFFs (all previously treated with bisphos-

phonates) and 47 cases of ONJ (38 previously treated with bisphosphonates) were reported; these correspond to an incidence of <1/100,000 patient-years and 2.3/100,000 patient-years, respectively. The incidence of *severe symptomatic hypocalcemia* was 5.2/100,000 patient-years; this occurred within 30 days after Dmab administration, and the majority of patients had impaired renal function or were on hemodialysis. As discussed earlier in this chapter, caution is needed in the treatment of patients with renal failure with potent antiresorptives. This is particularly relevant for Dmab, the use of which is not contraindicated in such patients. The rate of severe *anaphylaxis* was 1.5/100,000 patient-years. This occurred within minutes to hours after the first injection and required emergency measures; no fatalities were reported.

Denosumab versus Bisphosphonates

The antifracture efficacy of Dmab cannot be compared with that of the bisphosphonates because of the difference in fracture risk of patients included in pivotal clinical trials (Fig. 15.9). A post hoc analysis of a head-to-head study of Japanese women and men with osteoporosis reported Dmab to be superior to alendronate 35 mg once-weekly in decreasing the incidence of vertebral fractures [131]. It should be noted that the doses of oral bisphosphonates used in Japan are usually half of those approved for the treatment of osteoporosis in Europe and the USA due to higher absorption of bisphosphonates in Japanese individuals. There are, however, other head-to-head studies with intermediate efficacy outcomes which illustrate the differences between the two classes of antiresorptive treatments.

In two double-blind RCTs, the efficacy and safety of Dmab and alendronate were compared in treatment-naïve patients or patients previously treated with alendronate [132, 133]. In both studies, Dmab decreased the levels of bone turnover markers significantly more than alendronate associated with significant greater increases in BMD at all skeletal sites. The superior efficacy of

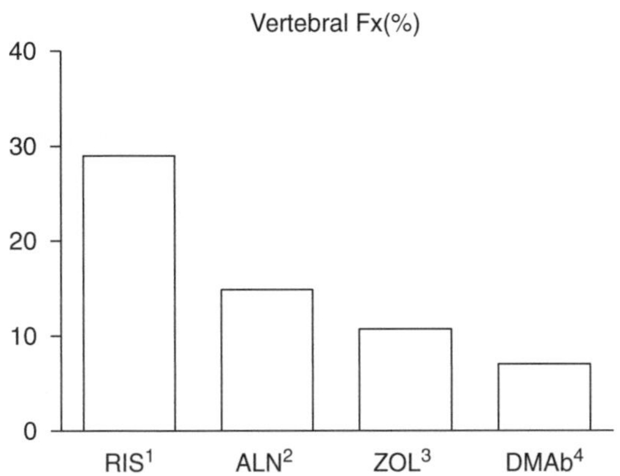

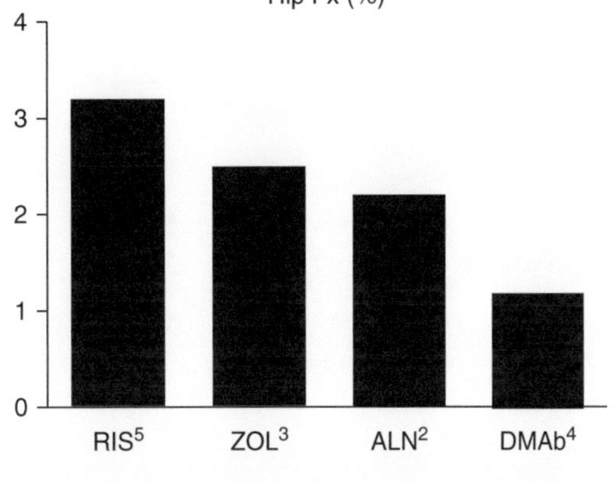

Fig. 15.9 Incidence of vertebral and hip fractures after 3 years of treatment with placebo in pivotal clinical trials of antiresorptive treatments. *RIS* risedronate, *ALN* alendronate, *ZOL* zoledronate, *Dmab* denosumab. Data from: 1. Osteoporosis International 2000; 11:83, 2. Lancet 1996; 348:1535, 3. New England journal of Medicine 2007; 356:1809, 4. New England Journal of Medicine 2009; 361:765, 5. New England Journal of Medicine 2001; 344:333

Dmab against oral bisphosphonates in reducing bone turnover and increasing BMD was further demonstrated in studies of similar design with oral risedronate and ibandronate [134, 135].

The differences in the offset of the action between Dmab and alendronate were examined and confirmed in the Phase II study which demonstrated the fast reversal of the effect of Dmab discontinuation on bone turnover markers and BMD and their slow progressive reversal after discontinuation of alendronate. The results obtained with Dmab raised also the question whether the fast activation of remodeling sites following discontinuation of Dmab may have an adverse effect on bone fragility. Brown et al. [136] examined fracture rates in patients who participated in FREEDOM but discontinued treatment after 2–5 doses and continued participation in the study for ≥7 months. Fracture rates were 13.5/100 patient-years in placebo-treated women and 9.7/100 patient-years in Dmab-treated women indicating that treatment cessation is not associated with excess in fracture risk up to 24 months.

Prevention of microarchitectural deterioration of cortical and trabecular bone by Dmab or alendronate was examined in a placebo-controlled study by HR-pQCT. Both agents prevented the loss of vBMD, increased cortical thickness, and improved estimated bone strength. The effect of Dmab on all these parameters was superior to that of alendronate [137]. In a more recent analysis of images obtained in this study with a new software, the effects of the two agents and placebo on intracortical porosity were measured [138]. Dmab reduced remodeling more rapidly and more completely and decreased porosity more than alendronate. This may be due to easier access of Dmab compared with alendronate to intracortical sites and may lead to better protection of skeletal integrity at sites with predominantly cortical bone. This needs, however, to be proven in head-to-head studies with fracture outcomes.

Increases in hip BMD with bisphosphonates, and other antiresorptives, are not observed beyond 3 years of treatment. In contrast, in all studies with Dmab given for more than 3 years, up to 8 years, a continuous increase in hip BMD has been observed (Fig. 15.10). In addition, in a subset of patients, radial BMD increased significantly up to 8 years of treatment; this response of a primarily cortical bone site contrasts the findings obtained so far with other antiosteoporotic treatments. Although the mechanism(s) underlying this unique pattern of BMD increases remains to be fully elucidated, hypotheses based on previous observations may help explain the continued year-by-year gains in BMD without therapeutic plateau and the low fracture incidence over time. As seen with other antiresorptives, early effects of Dmab may include closing of the remodeling space and improvement in bone mineralization.

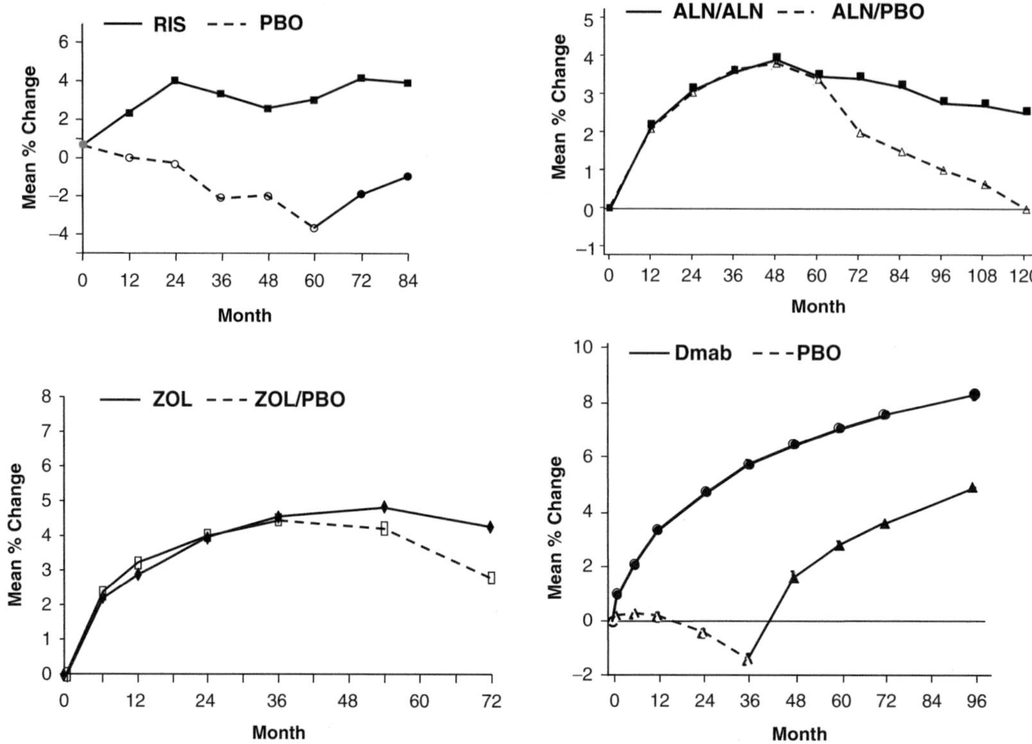

Fig. 15.10 Changes of total hip BMD of women with osteoporosis treated with antiresorptive agents (*solid lines*) or placebo (*interrupted lines*). *RIS* risedronate, *ALN* alendronate, *ZOL* zoledronate, *Dmab* denosumab, *PBO* placebo

Unique attributes may include decreases in cortical porosity and transient increases in PTH after each dose of Dmab. Most recently, modeling-based bone formation was observed in the femoral neck of ovariectomized cynomolgus monkeys treated with Dmab for 16 months at a dose that fully inhibited remodeling [139]. Although further studies are needed to determine if this effect is exerted also in humans, ongoing modeling-based bone formation in the presence of reduced resorption may help explain the continued improvements in bone mass, as well as the low rate of fractures, observed through 8 years of treatment with denosumab.

Conclusion

Pharmacological agents used in the management of patients with osteoporosis are generally efficacious and well tolerated, but there are differences among them. Agents that reduce the risk of all osteoporotic fractures, including those of the hip, have a favorable benefit-to-harm profile especially when given to patients with osteoporosis at increased risk of fractures. Knowledge of the mechanism of action, efficacy, and potential risks of every treatment prescribed is essential for proper care of patients with osteoporosis.

References[1]

1. Bouillon R, Van Schoor NM, Gielen E, Boonen S, Mathieu C, Vanderschueren D, et al. Optimal vitamin D status: a critical analysis on the basis of evidence-based medicine. J Clin Endocrinol Metab. 2013;98:E1283–304.
2. Mithal A, Bonjour JP, Boonen S, Burckhardt P, Degens H, El Hajj Fuleihan G, et al. Impact of nutri-

---

[1] *Important References
**Very Important References

tion on muscle mass, strength, and performance in older adults. Osteoporos Int. 2013;24:1555–66.

3. Moher D, Schulz KF, Altman D. The CONSORT statement: revised recommendations for improving the quality of reports of parallel-group randomized trials. JAMA. 2001;285:1987–91.

4. *Laupacis A, Sackett DL, Roberts RS. An assessment of clinically useful measures of the consequences of treatment. N Engl J Med. 1988; 318:1728–33. *First report of NNT.

5. Jones KW. Medication risk must be balanced with benefit, not fear. Ann Pharmacother. 2010;44:737–9.

6. Wysowski DK, Greene P. Trends in osteoporosis treatment with oral and intravenous bisphosphonates in the United States, 2002–2012. Bone. 2013;57:423–4288.

7. Rabenda V, Vanoverloop J, Fabri V, Mertens R, Sumkay F, Vannecke C, et al. Low incidence of anti-osteoporosis treatment after hip fracture. J Bone Joint Surg Am. 2008;90:2142–8.

8. Roerholt C, Eiken P, Abrahamsen B. Initiation of anti-osteoporotic therapy in patients with recent fractures: a nationwide analysis of prescription rates and persistence. Osteoporos Int. 2009;20:299–307.

9. Solomon DH, Johnston SS, Boytsov NN, McMorrow D, Lane JM, Krohn KD. Osteoporosis medication use after hip fracture in U.S. patients between 2002 and 2011. J Bone Miner Res. 2014;29:1929–37.

10. Cummings SR, Ettinger B, Delmas PD, Kenemans P, Stathopoulos V, Verweij P, et al. The effects of tibolone in older postmenopausal women. N Engl J Med. 2008;359:697–708.

11. *Writing group for the Women's Health Initiative Investigators. Risks and benefits of estrogen plus progestin in healthy postmenopausal women. Principal results from the women's health initiative randomized controlled trial. JAMA. 2002;288:321–32. *Description of the benefit-risk profile of hormonal therapy.

12. Reginster JY, Felsenberg D, Boonen S, Diez-Perez A, Rizzoli R, Brandi ML, Spector TD, Brixen K, Goemaere S, Cormier C, Balogh A, Delmas PD, Meunier PJ. Effects of long-term strontium ranelate treatment on the risk of nonvertebral and vertebral fractures in postmenopausal osteoporosis. Results of a five-year, randomized, placebo-controlled trial. Arthritis Rheum. 2008;58:1687–95.

13. European Medicines Agency/84749/2014.

14. Reginster JY, Kaufman JM, Goemaere S, Devogelaer JP, Benhamou CL, Felsenberg D, Diaz-Curiel M, Brandi ML, Badurski J, Wark J, Balogh A, Bruyère O, Roux C. Maintenance of antifracture efficacy over 10 years with strontium ranelate in postmenopausal osteoporosis. Osteoporos Int. 2012;23:1115–22.

15. Siris ES, Harris ST, Eastell R, Zanchetta JR, Goemaere S, Diez-Perez A, Stock JL, Song J, Qu Y, Kulkarni PM, Siddhanti SR, Wong M, Cummings SR. Skeletal effects of raloxifene after 8 years: results from the continuing outcomes relevant to Evista (CORE) study. J Bone Miner Res. 2005;20:1514–24.

16. Recker R, Lappe J, Davies KM, et al. Bone remodeling increases substantially in the years after menopause and remains increased in older osteoporosis patients. J Bone Miner Res. 2004;19:1628–33.

17. Parfitt AM. High bone turnover is intrinsically harmful: two paths to a similar conclusion. The Parfitt view. J Bone Miner Res. 2002;17:1558–9.

18. Bouxsein ML. Determinants of skeletal fragility. Best Pract Res Clin Rheumatol. 2005;19:897–911.

19. Seeman E, Delmas PD. Bone quality—the material and structural basis of bone strength and fragility. N Engl J Med. 2006;354:2250–61.

20. *Bone HG, Hosking D, Devogelaer JP, et al. Ten years' experience with alendronate for osteoporosis in postmenopausal women. N Engl J Med. 2004;350:1189–99. *First report of long-term use of alendronate.

21. Hochberg MC, Greenspan S, Wasnich RD, et al. Changes in bone density and turnover explain the reductions in incidence of nonvertebral fractures that occur during treatment with antiresorptive agents. J Clin Endocrinol Metab. 2002;87:1586–92.

22. Bauer DC, Black DM, Garnero P, et al. Change in bone turnover and hip, non-spine, and vertebral fracture in alendronate-treated women: the fracture intervention trial. J Bone Miner Res. 2004;19:1250–8.

23. Bellido T, Plotkin LI. Novel actions of bisphosphonates in bone: preservation of osteoblast and osteocyte viability. Bone. 2011;49:50–5.

24. Black DM, Cummings SR, Karpf DB, et al. Randomised trial of effect of alendronate on risk of fracture in women with existing vertebral fractures. Fracture intervention trial research group. Lancet. 1996;348:1535–41.

25. Cummings SR, Black DM, Thompson DE, et al. Effect of alendronate on risk of fracture in women with low bone density but without vertebral fractures: results from the fracture intervention trial. JAMA. 1998;280:2077–82.

26. Harris ST, Watts NB, Genant HK, et al. Effects of risedronate treatment on vertebral and nonvertebral fractures in women with postmenopausal osteoporosis: a randomized controlled trial. Vertebral efficacy with risedronate therapy (VERT) study group. JAMA. 1999;282:1344–52.

27. Reginster J, Minne HW, Sorensen OH, Hooper M, Roux C, Brandi ML, et al. Randomized trial of the effects of risedronate on vertebral fractures in women with established postmenopausal osteoporosis. Vertebral efficacy with risedronate therapy (VERT) study group. Osteoporos Int. 2000;11:83–91.

28. Cranney A, Wells G, Willan A, et al. Meta-analyses of therapies for postmenopausal osteoporosis. II. Meta-analysis of alendronate for the treatment of postmenopausal women. Endocr Rev. 2002;23:508–16.

29. Cranney A, Tugwell P, Adachi J, et al. Meta-analyses of therapies for postmenopausal osteoporosis. III. Meta-analysis of risedronate for the treatment of postmenopausal osteoporosis. Endocr Rev. 2002;23:517–23.

30. McClung MR, Geusens P, Miller PD, et al. Effect of risedronate on the risk of hip fracture in elderly women. Hip intervention program study group. N Engl J Med. 2001;344:333–40.

31. Black DM, Thompson DE, Bauer DC, et al. Fracture risk reduction with alendronate in women with osteoporosis: the fracture intervention trial. FIT research group. J Clin Endocrinol Metab. 2000; 85:4118–24.

32. Wells GA, Craneey A, Peterson J, et al. Alendronate for the primary and secondary prevention of osteoporotic fractures in postmenopausal women. Cochrane Database Syst Rev. 2008;23:CD00115.

33. Wells G, Cranney A, Peterson J, et al. Risedronate for the primary and secondary prevention of osteoporotic fractures in postmenopausal women. Cochrane Database Syst Rev. 2008;23:CD004523.

34. Karpf DB, Shapiro DR, Seeman E, et al. Prevention of nonvertebral fractures by alendronate. A meta-analysis. Alendronate osteoporosis treatment study groups. JAMA. 1997;277:1159–64.

35. Papapoulos SE, Quandt SA, Liberman UA, et al. Meta-analysis of the efficacy of alendronate for the prevention of hip fractures in postmenopausal women. Osteoporos Int. 2005;16:468–74.

36. Boonen S, Laan RF, Barton IP, et al. Effect of osteoporosis treatments on risk of non-vertebral fractures: review and meta-analysis of intention-to-treat studies. Osteoporos Int. 2005;16:1291–8.

37. Nguyen ND, Eisman JA, Nguyen TV. Anti-hip fracture efficacy of bisphosphonates: a Bayesian analysis of clinical trials. J Bone Miner Res. 2006;21:340–9.

38. Siris ES, Harris ST, Rosen CJ, et al. Adherence to bisphosphonate therapy and fracture rates in osteoporotic women: relationship to vertebral and nonvertebral fractures from 2 US claims databases. Mayo Clin Proc. 2006;81:1013–22.

39. Schnitzer T, Bone HG, Crepaldi G, et al. Therapeutic equivalence of alendronate 70 mg once-weekly and alendronate 10 mg daily in the treatment of osteoporosis. Alendronate once-weekly study group. Aging (Milano). 2000;12:1–12.

40. Brown JP, Kendler DL, McClung MR, et al. The efficacy and tolerability of risedronate once a week for the treatment of postmenopausal osteoporosis. Calcif Tissue Int. 2002;71:103–11.

41. Cramer JA, Amonkar MM, Hebborn A, et al. Compliance and persistence with bisphosphonate dosing regimens among women with postmenopausal osteoporosis. Curr Med Res Opin. 2005;21:1453–60.

42. Recker RR, Gallagher R, MacCosbe PE. Effect of dosing frequency on bisphosphonate medication adherence in a large longitudinal cohort of women. Mayo Clin Proc. 2005;80:856–61.

43. Delmas PD, Benhamou CL, Man Z, Tlustochowicz W, Matzkin E, Eusebio R, Zanchetta J, Olszynski WP, Recker RR, McClung MR. Monthly dosing of 75 mg risedronate on 2 consecutive days a month: efficacy and safety results. Osteoporos Int. 2008;19(7):1039–45.

44. Delmas PD, McClung MR, Zanchetta JR, Racewicz A, Roux C, Benhamou CL, Man Z, Eusebio RA, Beary JF, Burgio DE, Matzkin E, Boonen S. Efficacy and safety of risedronate 150 mg once a month in the treatment of postmenopausal osteoporosis. Bone. 2008;42:36–42.

45. McClung MR, Miller PD, Brown JP, Zanchetta J, Bolognese MA, Benhamou CL, Balske A, Burgio DE, Sarley J, McCullough LK, Recker RR. Efficacy and safety of a novel delayed-release risedronate 35 mg once-a-week tablet. Osteoporos Int. 2012;23:267–76.

46. Black DM, Delmas PD, Eastell R, et al. Once-yearly zoledronic acid for treatment of postmenopausal osteoporosis. N Engl J Med. 2007;356:1809–22.

47. **Lyles KW, Colon-Emeric CS, Magaziner JS, et al. Zoledronic acid and clinical fractures and mortality after hip fracture. N Engl J Med. 2007;357:1799–809. **Selection of patients with a hip fracture and not BMD for treatment; significant reduction of all-cause mortality with active treatment.

48. Nevitt MC, Thompson DE, Black DM, Rubin SR, Ensrud K, Yates AJ, Cummings SR. Effect of alendronate on limited-activity days and bed-disability days caused by back pain in postmenopausal women with existing vertebral fractures. Fracture intervention trial research group. Arch Intern Med. 2000;160:77–85.

49. Cauley JA, Black D, Boonen S, Cummings SR, Mesenbrink P, Palermo L, Man Z, Hadji P, Reid IR. Once-yearly zoledronic acid and days of disability, bed rest, and back pain: randomized, controlled HORIZON pivotal fracture trial. J Bone Miner Res. 2011;26:984–92.

50. Center JR, Bliuc D, Nguyen ND, Nguyen TV, Eisman JA. Osteoporosis medication and reduced mortality risk in elderly women and men. J Clin Endocrinol Metab. 2011;96:1006–14.

51. Beaupre LA, Morrish DW, Hanley DA, Maksymowych WP, Bell NR, Juby AG, Majumdar SR. Oral bisphosphonates are associated with reduced mortality after hip fracture. Osteoporos Int. 2011;22:983–91.

52. *Sambrook PN, Cameron ID, Chen JS, March LM, Simpson JM, Cumming RG, Seibel MJ. Oral bisphosphonates are associated with reduced mortality in frail older people: a prospective five-year study. Osteoporos Int. 2011;22:2551–6. *Reduced mortality with oral bisphosphonates.

53. Pazianas M, Abrahamsen B, Eiken PA, Eastell R, Russell RG. Reduced colon cancer incidence and mortality in postmenopausal women treated with an oral bisphosphonate—Danish national register based cohort study. Osteoporos Int. 2012;23:2693–701.

54. Grove EL, Abrahamsen B, Vestergaard P. Heart failure in patients treated with bisphosphonates. J Intern Med. 2013;274:342–50.

55. Wolfe F, Bolster MB, O'Connor CM, Michaud K, Lyles KW, Colón-Emeric CS. Bisphosphonate use is associated with reduced risk of myocardial infarction in patients with rheumatoid arthritis. J Bone Miner Res. 2013;28:984–91.

56. Kang JH, Keller JJ, Lin HC. Bisphosphonates reduced the risk of acute myocardial infarction: a 2-year follow-up study. Osteoporos Int. 2013;24:271–7.

57. Kang JH, Keller JJ, Lin HC. A population-based 2-year follow-up study on the relationship between bisphosphonates and the risk of strokes. Osteoporos Int. 2012;23:2551–7.

58. Sörensen OH, Crawford GM, Mulder H, et al. Long-term efficacy of risedronate: a 5-year placebo-controlled clinical experience. Bone. 2003;32:120–6.

59. *Mellström DD, Sörensen OH, Goemaere S, Roux C, Johnson TD, Chines AA. Seven years of treatment with risedronate in women with postmenopausal osteoporosis. Calcif Tissue Int. 2004;75:462–8. *Long-term use of risedronate.

60. **Black DM, Schwartz AV, Ensrud KE, et al. Effects of continuing or stopping alendronate after 5 years of treatment: the fracture intervention trial long-term extension (FLEX): a randomized trial. JAMA. 2006;296:2927–38. **Long-term use of alendronate.

61. Schwartz AV, Bauer DC, Cummings SR, Cauley JA, Ensrud KE, Palermo L, Wallace RB, Hochberg MC, Feldstein AC, Lombardi A, Black DM. Efficacy of continued alendronate for fractures in women with and without prevalent vertebral fracture: the FLEX trial. J Bone Miner Res. 2010;25:976–82.

62. McNabb BL, Vittinghoff E, Schwartz AV, Eastell R, Bauer DC, Ensrud K, Rosenberg E, Santora A, Barrett-Connor E, Black DM. BMD changes and predictors of increased bone loss in postmenopausal women after a 5-year course of alendronate. J Bone Miner Res. 2013;28:1319–27.

63. Black DM, Bauer DC, Schwartz AV, Cummings SR, Rosen CJ. Continuing bisphosphonate treatment for osteoporosis—for whom and for how long? N Engl J Med. 2012;366:2051–3.

64. **Black DM, Reid IR, Boonen S, Bucci-Rechtweg C, Cauley JA, Cosman F, Cummings SR, Hue TF, Lippuner K, Lakatos P, Leung PC, Man Z, Martinez RL, Tan M, Ruzycky ME, Su G, Eastell R. The effect of 3 versus 6 years of zoledronic acid treatment of osteoporosis: a randomized extension to the HORIZON-pivotal fracture trial (PFT). J Bone Miner Res. 2012;27:243–54. **Long-term use of zoledronate.

65. *Cosman F, Cauley JA, Eastell R, Boonen S, Palermo L, Reid IR, Cummings SR, Black DM. Reassessment of fracture risk in women after 3 years of treatment with zoledronic acid: when is it reasonable to discontinue treatment? J Clin Endocrinol Metab. 2014;99:4546–54. *Selecting patients for continuing treatment with zoledronate.

66. Papapoulos SE. Bisphosphonate actions: physical chemistry revisited. Bone. 2006;38:613–6.

67. McClung MR, Wasnich RD, Hosking DJ, et al. Prevention of postmenopausal bone loss: six-year results from the early postmenopausal intervention cohort study. J Clin Endocrinol Metab. 2004;89:4879–85.

68. Wasnich RD, Bagger YZ, Hosking DJ, et al. Changes in bone density and turnover after alendronate or estrogen withdrawal. Menopause. 2004;11:622–30.

69. Bagger YZ, Tanko LB, Alexandersen P, et al. Alendronate has a residual effect on bone mass in postmenopausal Danish women up to 7 years after treatment withdrawal. Bone. 2003;33:301–7.

70. *Landman JO, Hamdy NA, Pauwels EK, et al. Skeletal metabolism in patients with osteoporosis after discontinuation of long-term treatment with oral pamidronate. J Clin Endocrinol Metab. 1995;80:3465–8. *First report of changes in BMD and bone markers after discontinuation of long-term bisphosphonate treatment.

71. Papapoulos SE, Cremers SC. Prolonged bisphosphonate release after treatment in children. N Engl J Med. 2007;356:1075–6.

72. Eastell R, Hannon RA, Wenderoth D, Rodriguez-Moreno J, Sawicki A. Effect of stopping risedronate after long-term treatment on bone turnover. J Clin Endocrinol Metab. 2011;96:3367–73.

73. Suresh E, Pazianas M, Abrahamsen B. Safety issues with bisphosphonate therapy for osteoporosis. Rheumatology. 2014;53:19–31.

74. *Pazianas M, Abrahamsen B. Safety of bisphosphonates. Bone. 2011;49:103–11. *Comprehensive review of the safety of bisphosphonate therapy.

75. Miller PD, Jamal SA, Evenepoel P, Eastell R, Boonen S. Renal safety in patients treated with bisphosphonates for osteoporosis: a review. J Bone Miner Res. 2013;28:2049–59.

76. Marx RE. Pamidronate (Aredia) and zoledronate (Zometa) induced avascular necrosis of the jaws: a growing epidemic. J Oral Maxillofac Surg. 2003;61:1115–7.

77. Ruggiero SL, Mehrotra B, Rosenberg TJ, Engroff SL. Osteonecrosis of the jaws associated with the use of bisphosphonates: a review of 63 cases. J Oral Maxillofac Surg. 2004;62:527–34.

78. Khosla S, Burr D, Cauley J, et al. Bisphosphonate-associated osteonecrosis of the jaw: report of a task force of the American Society for Bone and Mineral Research. J Bone Miner Res. 2007;22:1479–91.

79. Rizzoli R, Burlet N, Cahall D, Delmas PD, Eriksen EF, Felsenberg D, Grbic J, Jontell M, Landesberg R, Laslop A, Wollenhaupt M, Papapoulos S, Sezer O, Sprafka M, Reginster JY. Osteonecrosis of the jaw and bisphosphonate treatment for osteoporosis. Bone. 2008;42:841–7.

80. Ruggiero SL, Dodson TB, Assael LA, et al. American Association of Oral and Maxillofacial Surgeons position paper on bisphosphonate-related osteonecrosis of the jaws—2009 update. J Oral Maxillofac Surg. 2009;67(5 Suppl):2–12.

81. *Ruggiero SL, Dodson TB, Fantasia J, Goodday R, Aghaloo T, Mehrotra B, O'Ryan F, American Association of Oral and Maxillofacial. Surgeons position paper on medication-related osteonecrosis of the jaw—2014 update. J Oral Maxillofac Surg. 2014;72:1938–56. *Comprehensive review and new definition of medication-related ONJ.

82. Allen MR, Burr DB. The pathogenesis of bisphosphonate-related osteonecrosis of the jaw: so many hypotheses, so few data. J Oral Maxillofac Surg. 2009;67 Suppl 1:61–70.

83. Saad F, Brown JE, Van Poznak C, Ibrahim T, Stemmer SM, Stopeck AT, Diel IJ, Takahashi S, Shore N, Henry DH, Barrios CH, Facon T, Senecal F, Fizazi K, Zhou L, Daniels A, Carrière P, Dansey R. Incidence, risk factors, and outcomes of osteonecrosis of the jaw: integrated analysis from three blinded active-controlled phase III trials in cancer patients with bone metastases. Ann Oncol. 2012;23:1341–7.

84. *Goh SK, Yang KY, Koh JS, Wong MK, Chua SY, Chua DT, Howe TS. Subtrochanteric insufficiency fractures in patients on alendronate therapy: a caution. J Bone Joint Surg (Br). 2007;89:349–53. *First report of AFF in bisphosphonate-treated patients.

85. Giusti A, Hamdy NAT, Papapoulos SE. Atypical fractures of the femur and use of bisphosphonates: a systematic review of cases/case studies. Bone. 2010;47:169–80.

86. **Shane E, Burr D, Ebeling PR, Abrahamsen B, Adler RA, Brown TD, Cheung AM, Cosman F, Curtis JR, Dell R, Dempster D, Einhorn TA, Genant HK, Geusens P, Klaushofer K, Koval K, Lane JM, McKiernan F, McKinney R, Ng A, Nieves J, O'Keefe R, Papapoulos S, Sen HT, van der Meulen MC, Weinstein RS, Whyte M. Atypical subtrochanteric and diaphyseal femoral fractures: report of a task force of the American Society for Bone and Mineral Research. J Bone Miner Res. 2010;25:2267–94. **Comprehensive review of AFF and diagnostic criteria.

87. Rizzoli R, Akesson K, Bouxsein M, Kanis JA, Napoli N, Papapoulos S, Reginster JY, Cooper C. Subtrochanteric fractures after long-term treatment with bisphosphonates: a European Society on clinical and economic aspects of osteoporosis and osteoarthritis, and international osteoporosis foundation working group report. Osteoporo Int. 2011;22:373–90.

88. *Shane E, Ebeling PR, Abrahamsen B, Adler RA, Brown TD, Cheung AM, Cosman F, Curtis JR, Dell R, Dempster DW, Einhorn TA, Genant HK, Geusens P, Klaushofer K, Lane JM, McKiernan F, McKinney R, Ng A, Nieves J, O'Keefe R, Papapoulos S, Tetsen H, van der Meulen MC, Weinstein RS, Whyte MP. Atypical subtrochanteric and diaphyseal femoral fractures: Second report of a task force of the American Society for Bone and Mineral Research. J Bone Miner Res. 2014;29:1–23. *Follow-up review of AFF and revised diagnostic criteria.

89. Martin-Hunyadia C, Heitz D, Kaltenbacha G, Pfitzenmeyer P, Mourey F, et al. Spontaneous insufficiency fractures of long bones: a prospective epide-

90. Bilezikian J, Klemes A, Silverman S, Cosman F. Subtrochanteric fracture reports coincident with risedronate use. J Bone Miner Res. 2009;24 Suppl 1. http://www.asbmr.org/Meetings/AnnualMeeting/AbstractDetail.aspx?aid=0367cfaa-4d0d-47d8-a57a-ff76098839a2

91. Black DM, Kelly MP, Genant HK, Palermo L, Eastell R, Bucci-Rechtweg C, Cauley J, Leung PC, Boonen S, Santora A, de Papp A, Bauer DC. Bisphosphonates and fractures of the subtrochanteric or diaphyseal femur. N Engl J Med. 2010;362:1761–71.

92. *Giusti A, Hamdy NAT, Dekkers OM, Ramautar SR, Dijkstra S, Papapoulos SE. Atypical fractures and bisphosphonate therapy: a cohort study of patients with femoral fractures with radiographic adjudication of fracture site and features. Bone. 2011;48:966–71. *First report of AFF in a defined cohort with radiographic adjudication of fractures.

93. Chalmers J. Subtrochanteric fractures in osteomalacia. J Bone Joint Surg (Br). 1970;52:509–13.

94. Kumm DA, Rack C, Rütt J. Subtrochanteric stress fracture of the femur following total knee arthroplasty. J Arthroplasty. 1997;12:580–3.

95. Salminen ST, Pihlajamäki HK, Avikainen VJ, Böstman OM. Population based epidemiologic and morphologic study of femoral shaft fractures. Clin Orthop Relat Res. 2000;372:241–9.

96. Niimi R, Hasegawa M, Sudo A, Uchida A. Unilateral stress fracture of the femoral shaft combined with contralateral insufficiency fracture of the femoral shaft after bilateral total knee arthroplasty. J Orthop Sci. 2008;13:572–5.

97. Vestergaard P, Schwartz F, Rejnmark L, Mosekilde L. Risk of femoral shaft and subtrochanteric fractures among users of bisphosphonates and raloxifene. Osteoporos Int. 2011;22:993–1001.

98. Tan SC, Koh SBJ, Goh SK, Howe TS. Atypical femoral stress fractures in bisphosphonate-free patients. Osteoporos Int. 2011;22:221–2212.

99. Khosla S, Bilezikian JP, Dempster DW, Lewiecki EM, Miller PD, Neer RM, Recker RR, Shane E, Shoback D, Potts JT. Benefits and risks of bisphosphonate therapy for osteoporosis. J Clin Endocrinol Metab. 2012;97:2272–82.

100. Yavropoulou MP, Giusti A, Ramautar SR, Dijkstra S, Hamdy NA, Papapoulos SE. Low-energy fractures of the humeral shaft and bisphosphonate use. J Bone Miner Res. 2012;27:1425–31.

101. Sutton RA, Mumm S, Coburn SP, Ericson KL, Whyte MP. "Atypical femoral fractures" during bisphosphonate exposure in adult hypophosphatasia. J Bone Miner Res. 2012;27:987–94.

102. *Schilcher J, Michaelsson K, Aspenberg P. Bisphosphonate use and atypical fractures of the femoral shaft. N Engl J Med. 2011;364:1728–37. *Large cohort study of AFF with radiographic adjudication.

103. Boyle WJ, Simonet WS, Lacey D. Osteoclast differentiation and activation. Nature. 2003;423:337–42.

miological survey in nursing home subjects. Arch Gerontol Geriatr. 2000;31:207–14.

104. Baron R, Ferrari S, Russell RG. Denosumab and bisphosphonates: different mechanisms of action and effects. Bone. 2011;48:677–92.

105. Reid IR, Miller PD, Brown JP, Kendler DL, Fahrleitner-Pammer A, Valter I, Maasalu K, Bolognese MA, Woodson G, Bone H, Ding B, Wagman RB, San Martin J, Ominsky MS, Dempster DW. Effects of denosumab on bone histomorphometry: the FREEDOM and STAND studies. J Bone Miner Res. 2010;25:2256–65.

106. Brown JP, Reid IR, Wagman RB, Kendler D, Miller PD, Jensen JE, Bolognese MA, Daizadeh N, Valter I, Zerbini CA, Dempster DW. Effects of up to 5 years of denosumab treatment on bone histology and histomorphometry: the FREEDOM study extension. J Bone Miner Res. 2014;29:2051–6.

107. Cummings SR, San Martin J, McClung MR, et al. Denosumab for prevention of fractures in postmenopausal women with osteoporosis. N Engl J Med. 2009;361:756–65.

108. *Austin M, Yang YC, Vittinghoff E, et al. Relationship between bone mineral density changes with denosumab treatment and risk reduction for vertebral and nonvertebral fractures. J Bone Miner Res. 2012;27:687–93. *Increases in total hip BMD explain a large proportion of the reduction in the risk of nonvertebral fractures with denosumab treatment.

109. Jacques RM, Boonen S, Cosman F, Reid IR, Bauer DC, Black DM, Eastell R. Relationship of changes in total hip bone mineral density to vertebral and nonvertebral fracture risk in women with postmenopausal osteoporosis treated with once-yearly zoledronic acid 5 mg: the HORIZON-pivotal fracture trial (PFT). J Bone Miner Res. 2012;27:1627–34.

110. Genant HK, Libanati C, Engelke K, Zanchetta JR, Høiseth A, Yuen CK, Stonkus S, Bolognese MA, Franek E, Fuerst T, Radcliffe HS, McClung MR. Improvements in hip trabecular, subcortical, and cortical density and mass in postmenopausal women with osteoporosis treated with denosumab. Bone. 2013;56:482–8.

111. Keaveny T, McClung M, Genant H, et al. Femoral and vertebral strength improvements in postmenopausal women with osteoporosis treated with denosumab. J Bone Miner Res. 2014;29:158–65.

112. McClung MR, Boonen S, Törring O, Roux C, Rizzoli R, Bone HG, Benhamou CL, Lems WF, Minisola S, Halse J, Hoeck HC, Eastell R, Wang A, Siddhanti S, Cummings SR. Effect of denosumab treatment on the risk of fractures in subgroups of women with postmenopausal osteoporosis. J Bone Miner Res. 2012;27:211–8.

113. Appelman-Dijkstra NM, Papapoulos SE. Prevention of incident fractures in patients with prevalent fragility fractures: current and future approaches. Best Pract Res Clin Rheumatol. 2013;27:805–20.

114. Boonen S, Adachi JD, Man Z, Cummings SR, Lippuner K, Törring O, Gallagher JC, Farrerons J, Wang A, Franchimont N, San Martin J, Grauer A, McClung M. Treatment with denosumab reduces the incidence of new vertebral and hip fractures in postmenopausal women at high risk. J Clin Endocrinol Metab. 2011;96:1727–36.

115. Papapoulos S, Chapurlat R, Libanati C, et al. Five years of denosumab exposure in women with postmenopausal osteoporosis: results from the first two years of the FREEDOM extension. J Bone Miner Res. 2012;27:694–701.

116. **Bone HG, Chapurlat R, Brandi ML, et al. The effect of three or six years of denosumab exposure in women with postmenopausal osteoporosis: results from the FREEDOM extension. J Clin Endocrinol Metab. 2013;98:4483–92. **Prolongation of denosumab treatment and use of the virtual twin analysis.

117. Papapoulos S, Lippuner K, Roux C, et al. Eight years of denosumab treatment in postmenopausal women with osteoporosis: results from the first five years of the FREEDOM extension Osteoporos Int 2015; Jul 23 (Epub ahead of print).

118. Ferrari-Lacraz S, Ferrari S. Do RANKL inhibitors (denosumab) affect inflammation and immunity? Osteoporos Int. 2011;22:435–46.

119. Kong YY, Yoshida H, Sarosi I, et al. OPGL is a key regulator of osteoclastogenesis, lymphocyte development and lymph-node organogenesis. Nature. 1999;28(397):315–23.

120. Li J, Sarosi I, Yan XQ, Morony S, et al. RANK is the intrinsic hematopoietic cell surface receptor that controls osteoclastogenesis and regulation of bone mass and calcium metabolism. Proc Natl Acad Sci U S A. 2000;15(97):1566–71.

121. Sobacchi C, Frattini A, Guerrini MM, et al. Osteoclast-poor human osteopetrosis due to mutations in the gene encoding RANKL. Nat Genet. 2007;39:960–2.

122. Stolina M, Dwyer D, Ominsky MS, et al. Continuous RANKL inhibition in osteoprotegerin transgenic mice and rats suppresses bone resorption without impairing lymphorganogenesis or functional immune responses. J Immunol. 2007;179:7497–505.

123. Miller RE, Branstetter D, Armstrong A, Kennedy B, Jones J, Cowan L, Bussiere J, Dougall WC. Receptor activator of NF-kappa B ligand inhibition suppresses bone resorption and hypercalcemia but does not affect host immune responses to influenza infection. J Immunol. 2007;179:266–74.

124. Stolina M, Kostenuik PJ, Dougall WC, Fitzpatrick LA, Zack DJ. RANKL inhibition: from mice to men (and women). Adv Exp Med Biol. 2007;602:143–50.

125. Bekker PJ, Holloway DL, Rasmussen AS, et al. A single-dose placebo-controlled study of AMG 162, a fully human monoclonal antibody to RANKL, in postmenopausal women. J Bone Miner Res. 2004;19:1059–66.

126. Watts NB, Roux C, Modlin JF, et al. Infections in postmenopausal women with osteoporosis treated with denosumab or placebo: coincidence or causal association? Osteoporos Int. 2012;23:327–37.

127. Stolina M, Schett G, Dwyer D, et al. RANKL inhibition by osteoprotegerin prevents bone loss without affecting local or systemic inflammation parameters in two rat arthritis models: comparison with anti-

TNF-alpha or anti-IL-1 therapies. Arthritis Res Ther. 2009;11(6):R187.

128. Byrne FR, Morony S, Warmington K, et al. CD4 + CD45RBHi T cell transfer induced colitis in mice is accompanied by osteopenia which is treatable with recombinant human osteoprotegerin. Gut. 2005;54:78–86.

129. Cohen SB, Dore RK, Lane NE, et al. Denosumab treatment effects on structural damage, bone mineral density, and bone turnover in rheumatoid arthritis: a twelve-month, multicenter, randomized, double-blind, placebo-controlled, phase II clinical trial. Arthritis Rheum. 2008;58:1299–309.

130. Adami S, Libanati C, Boonen S, et al. Denosumab treatment in postmenopausal women with osteoporosis does not interfere with fracture-healing: results from the FREEDOM trial. J Bone Joint Surg Am. 2012;94:2113–9.

131. Nakamura T, Matsumoto T, Sugimoto T, et al. Clinical trials express: fracture risk reduction with denosumab in Japanese postmenopausal women and men with osteoporosis: denosumab fracture intervention randomized placebo controlled trial (DIRECT). J Clin Endocrinol Metab. 2014;99: 2599–607.

132. Kendler DL, Roux C, Benhamou CL, et al. Effects of denosumab on bone mineral density and bone turnover in postmenopausal women transitioning from alendronate therapy. J Bone Miner Res. 2010; 25:72–81.

133. Brown JP, Prince RL, Deal C, et al. Comparison of the effect of denosumab and alendronate on BMD and biochemical markers of bone turnover in postmenopausal women with low bone mass: a

randomized, blinded, phase 3 trial. J Bone Miner Res. 2009;24:153–61.

134. Roux C, Hofbauer LC, Ho PR, et al. Denosumab compared with risedronate in postmenopausal women suboptimally adherent to alendronate therapy: efficacy and safety results from a randomized open-label study. Bone. 2014;58:48–54.

135. Brown JP, Roux C, Ho PR, et al. Denosumab significantly increases bone mineral density and reduces bone turnover compared with monthly oral ibandronate and risedronate in postmenopausal women who remained at higher risk for fracture despite previous suboptimal treatment with an oral bisphosphonate. Osteoporos Int. 2014;25:1953–61.

136. Brown JP, Roux C, Törring O, et al. Discontinuation of denosumab and associated fracture incidence: analysis from the fracture reduction evaluation of denosumab in osteoporosis every 6 months (FREEDOM) trial. J Bone Miner Res. 2013;28: 746–52.

137. Seeman E, Delmas PD, Hanley DA, et al. Microarchitectural deterioration of cortical and trabecular bone: differing effects of denosumab and alendronate. J Bone Miner Res. 2010;25:1886–9.

138. Zebaze RM, Libanati C, Austin M, et al. Differing effects of denosumab and alendronate on cortical and trabecular bone. Bone. 2014;59:173–9.

139. *Ominsky M, Libanati C, Boyce RW, et al. Sustained modeling-based bone formation during adulthood in cynomolgus monkeys may contribute to continuous BMD gains with denosumab. J Bone Miner Res. 2015;30:1280–9. *Possible contributing factor to the continuous increase in BMD during long-term treatment with denosumab.*

Management of Drug Holidays

16

Christian Roux and Karine Briot

Summary

- Bisphosphonates are effective in reducing osteoporotic fracture risk.
- Concerns were raised recently about long-term bone retention of bisphosphonates.
- The rationale for a drug holiday (temporary discontinuation) is the high affinity of bisphosphonates for bone.
- A drug holiday could be considered after 3–5 years of treatment, providing that the patient is not at persistent high risk.
- There is no evidence-based data about benefit and risks of such drug holidays.

Introduction

A drug holiday is a temporary discontinuation of a drug. In the context of osteoporosis, this concept has been proposed insistently because of safety concerns about long-term administration of bisphosphonates. The incidence of these bisphosphonate-related adverse events is low, but their perception is high. The rationale for this concept is the property of bisphosphonates to be accumulated in bone over time and released after treatment is stopped. That means that the patient can be exposed to the drug, after the discontinuation of treatment.

There is a controversy over the duration of treatments and duration of drug holidays, and there are no evidence-based data to determine when and whether to resume treatment. Moreover, each bisphosphonate has a unique profile of bone affinity, and a difference in the speed of offset is highly expected within the bisphosphonates. Finally, the concept of drug holidays cannot be applied for drugs for which the effect resolves immediately after discontinuation.

Effect of Stopping Treatments

Bisphosphonates are the most popular treatment of osteoporosis and are widely prescribed. They are unique in their capacity to bind to bone matrix. Alendronate, ibandronate, risedronate, and zoledronate are different in the strength for binding to bone and in their potency for inhibiting farnesyl pyrophosphate synthase, their enzyme target. The high affinity of all bisphosphonates for bone is however a common property. When treatment is stopped, it is actually released from bone; because this release is function of the level

C. Roux, MD, PhD (✉) • K. Briot, MD, PhD
Service de Rhumatologie, Hôpital Cochin,
27 rue du Faubourg Saint Jacques,
75014 Paris, France

INSERM U1153, Paris-Descartes University,
Paris, France
e-mail: christian.roux@cch.aphp.fr

© Springer International Publishing Switzerland 2016
S.L. Silverman, B. Abrahamsen (eds.), *The Duration and Safety of Osteoporosis Treatment*, DOI 10.1007/978-3-319-23639-1_16

of turnover, which is decreased by the presence of the bisphosphonate itself, this release can occur over months or years. This skeletal persistence can be associated with persistence of the clinical effect, for an unpredictable period of time. Whether or not the discontinuation is effective in avoiding side effects has been suggested in a large study, showing that the risk of atypical femur fractures associated with bisphosphonate use decreases immediately and significantly after discontinuation [1].

Long-term prospective extension trials are available for risedronate, alendronate, and zoledronic acid [2–4]. Hip and spine BMD decreases following discontinuation but remains above pretreatment levels after 1, 5, and 3 years of follow-up, respectively. Bone loss looks more rapid with risedronate than with the two other bisphosphonate, and this is in accordance to pharmacological properties.

The fracture risk after discontinuation of risedronate has been assessed after 3 years of treatment [2]. Initially 1628 patients were randomized to receive either placebo or risedronate 5 mg, and 759 entered a 1-year follow-up study; 599 completed the 1-year follow-up. The relative risk of morphometric vertebral fractures was still reduced by 46 % in the former risedronate group (incidence 6.5 %) compared to the former placebo group (incidence 11.6 %). In contrast, there was a −0.8 and −1.23 % decrease in lumbar spine and femoral neck BMD, in the previous risedronate-treated patients. Lumbar spine BMD, but not femoral neck BMD, was significantly higher than the former placebo group at the end of the extension year. For both lumbar spine and femoral neck, BMD values remained significantly higher than placebo at the end of year 4. Urinary NTX as a marker of bone resorption was available at the end of the follow-up in 89 patients of the former risedronate group: it increased from 30 to 51 nmol BCE/nmol creatinine. These data suggest that there is still a risk of fracture immediately after 3 years of treatment with risedronate but that this risk is lower than in untreated women. Surrogate markers, i.e., changes in BMD or biochemical markers over 1 year, cannot help to decide when to resume risedronate treatment, as their changes (decrease in BMD, increase in bone resorption) are not those expected in parallel to the persistent anti-fracture effect.

In FLEX study [3], patients previously treated by alendronate over 5 years were randomized to receive placebo or 5 additional years of alendronate. Those switched to placebo had a 1.5 % increase in lumbar spine BMD and a 3.38 % decrease in the hip BMD over 5 years. Biochemical markers were assessed in a subgroup of 87 patients, but data following immediately the discontinuation were not available: the first point of assessment of biochemical markers was at 3 years. A gradual rise in markers was measured: at 5 years, their value was 50–60 % higher than in patients who continued alendronate. Data on fractures were available in 1071 patients. There was no difference between placebo- and alendronate-treated patients for vertebral and non-vertebral fractures, except for clinical vertebral fractures with a lower incidence in the treated group than in the placebo group: 2.4 versus 5.3 %, respectively, over 5 years. This incidence is low and actually expected in this population, because of the selection at study entry, patients with a hip T score<−3.5 or with a decrease in hip BMD during the previous treatment period were excluded from this study. As a result, mean T score at baseline of the study were −1.3, −1.9, and −2.2 at the lumbar spine, total hip, and femoral neck, respectively. Only 30 % of the patients had osteoporosis based on a T score<−2.5 at the femoral neck; roughly 35 % of the population had a baseline vertebral fracture. Thus data were obtained in a population with a moderate risk of facture.

In the extension of HORIZON study [4], patients who switched to placebo after 3 years of zoledronic acid treatment had (after 3 years of follow-up) a BMD slightly lower than patients who continued treatment (with differences from 1.36 % to 2.06 % at the femoral neck and lumbar spine, respectively). There was no difference in markers of bone turnover at year 6 between patients who were continuously treated over 6 years or switched to placebo after 3 years of treatment. There was no difference in the incidence of vertebral and non-vertebral fractures between the two groups, except for morphometric vertebral fractures: 3 % versus 6.2 % over 3 years, respectively.

These results with bisphosphonates are different from those with other antiresorptive treatments, as their cessation results in immediate and large decrease in BMD. This is well known for estrogens, as hormone replacement therapy (HRT). After 2 years of treatment with conjugated estrogen 0.625 mg/day, women who switched to placebo experienced a 4.5 % and 2.4 % decrease at the spine and trochanter, respectively, over 1 year [5]. The post-intervention follow-up of the Women's Health Initiative (WHI) trial showed that the risk of fractures was comparable among women in the previous HRT and placebo groups; this suggests a greater increase in the annualized risk of fractures in women after HRT therapy [6]. One year of discontinuation of raloxifene (after 5 years of administration) results in 2.4 % decrease in lumbar spine BMD [7].

An accelerated bone loss, with a rebound phenomenon, has been observed after withdrawal of denosumab. In an off-treatment extension of a randomized, double-blind study, 128 patients were followed for 2 years after a 2-year treatment period [8]. After 2 years off-treatment, BMD was not different to pretreatment value at the spine and hip, but lower at the radius. At month 48, the group previously treated with denosumab maintained higher spine hip and femoral neck BMD than patients from the placebo group. After denosumab discontinuation, bone resorption marker increases immediately, above baseline values, peaks 6 months after discontinuation, and returns to pretreatment values. The peak median percentage change from baseline of follow-up was 63 % and 47 % for CTX and P1NP, respectively. Post hoc analysis showed significant association between the percentage change in lumbar spine BMD after denosumab discontinuation and the peak of CTX, an observation which has not been made with bisphosphonates. The huge increase in markers of resorption is worrisome if relationship between the increase in these markers and decrease in BMD and increase in fracture risk, which has been established in untreated women, is true also in previously treated patients. The key issue of potential effect of these variations on fracture risk has been assessed in 797 subjects (470 placebo, 327 denosumab) in the FREEDOM study who discontinued treatment after receiving 2–5 doses of either denosumab or placebo [9]. They were followed for a median of 0.8-year per subject; 42 % and 28 % of the previous placebo and denosumab groups respectively received an anti-osteoporotic treatment during the follow-up. There was no difference in fracture occurrence pattern between the groups during the off-treatment period (9 % placebo, 7 % denosumab). Time to first osteoporotic fracture was not different between the two groups. These data have been obtained in a population with a mean baseline T score of −2.8 and −2.1 at the lumbar spine and hip, respectively, and only 26 % of patients had prevalent vertebral fractures. Thus these reassuring data do not apply to a higher risk population.

Prediction of Effect of Discontinuation

All these data suggest that the changes in bone markers and BMD after discontinuation are not relevant enough to be used solely in the decision to resume the treatment by bisphosphonate. Thus the question is: is there any parameter assessable at the time of discontinuation which could be used to decide about the relevance of a drug holiday?

Analyses have been conducted in order to assess the determinants of long-term anti-fracture effects based on bone evaluation at the time of discontinuation. Data are from post hoc analysis and thus limited by methodological issues precluding any definitive conclusion on fracture effect. They suggest that BMD measurements of the femoral neck could be used to select patients for prolonged therapy. In the FLEX study, among women without vertebral fracture at baseline, continuation of alendronate reduced non-vertebral fractures in those having still a femoral neck T score of −2.5 or less. Such a benefit was not observed in those having a higher T score. There was no statistically significant interaction with lumbar spine

T scores and incident fractures [10]. These results cannot be applied to patients with vertebral fractures at baseline, though it is the most likely population to treat. Reanalysis of FLEX data shows that the number of patients needed to treat to prevent a fracture (after 5 years of initial alendronate treatment) is 24 if T score <-2.5 and 102 if T score >-2, in the population without prevalent vertebral fracture. The predictive value of a T score <-2.5 at the femoral neck has been confirmed at the end of a 3-year period of zoledronate treatment [11]; in this post hoc analysis, an incident morphometric vertebral fracture during the initial treatment period was also a predictor of a benefit of a prolonged treatment.

The other determinant is adherence to the treatment. Using a large US administrative database, the rate of hip fracture was examined in women who discontinued bisphosphonates, compared to those who remained on therapy [12]. For women compliant for 3 years, there was no significant difference in risk associated with discontinuation. However, in women with low medication possession ratio, discontinuation of 1 year or longer was associated with a two- to threefold increased relative risk of hip fracture. These data suggest that cumulative bisphosphonate exposure provides greater fracture protection. No BMD data were available is this study. Non-adherent patients should be managed cautiously as far as a drug holiday is discussed.

Management of Drug Holidays

There are strong differences among drugs in bone parameter changes after cessation of treatment: the answer to the question about the consequences of stopping treatment must be drug-specific. With bisphosphonates, data suggest that patients without hip osteoporosis at the end of 3–5 years of treatment may not suffer from a "drug holiday." Any benefits, even if persisting for some time, are not permanent, and this "drug holiday" is usually only a temporary suspension of treatment.

In the context of very limited evidence regarding the incidence of fractures with the discontinuation of the treatments, an operational proposal is:

- Recommendation for discontinuation and drug holiday should be limited to bisphosphonates.
- The discontinuation is based on an individual assessment of risk after 3 (risedronate, zoledronic acid) or 5 (alendronate) years, based on incident fracture during treatment, new risk factor, and final femoral neck T score.
- If patient is not at high risk, treatment is stopped. Then the drug holiday can be continued till:
  - A new fracture
  - A significant decrease of BMD

There is lack of data on risk of fracture related to decrease in BMD in previously treated patients. However, it is a mean of assessing the residual pharmacological effect of the bisphosphonate. One may consider in clinical practice that a decrease in BMD means the end of the drug effect on bone remodeling. Because each bisphosphonate has its own offset, BMD can be measured after 2–3 years for alendronate and zoledronic acid and 1–2 years after risedronate.

A rising marker of resorption could be an earlier indicator of a decrease in BMD, but the relationship of this marker with changes in BMD after bisphosphonate discontinuation has not been studied. It could be an alert to decide for an earlier BMD assessment.

Conclusion

The concept of drug holiday is not applicable to most chronic diseases and in the treatment of osteoporosis can be used only for bisphosphonates. There are very limited data available actually, and the decision must be individualized, based on expert opinion. The perception of risk of adverse event is high, although their incidence is low, and should not preclude unbiased assessment. Decision must be shared with the patient and reasons for discontinuation clearly explained; otherwise, medicolegal implications could occur if a patient has a fracture in the year after intentional discontinuation of the treatment. Patients at high risk should receive long-term treatment [13–16]. Others may not suffer from a drug holiday, and treatment will be restarted after some time off.

References[1]

1. Schilcher J, Michaëlsson K, Aspenberg P. Bisphosphonate use and atypical fractures of the femoral shaft. N Engl J Med. 2011;364:1728–37.
2. Watts NB, Chines A, Olszynski P, McKeever CD, Mc Clung MR, Zhou X, et al. Fracture risk remains reduced one year after discontinuation of risedronate. Osteoporos Int. 2008;19:365–72.
3. *Black DM, Schwartz AV, Ensrud KE, Cauley JA, Levis S, Quandt SA, et al. Effects of continuing or stopping alendronate after 5 years of treatment. The fracture intervention trial long-term extension (FLEX): a randomized trial. JAMA. 2006;296:2927–38. *Large study assessing bone effects of discontinuation of alendronate.
4. *Black DM, Reid IR, Boonen S, Bucci-Rechtweg C, Cauley JA, Cosman F, et al. The effect of 3 versus 6 years of zoledronic acid treatment of osteoporosis: a randomized extension to the HORIZON-pivotal fracture trial (PFT). J Bone Miner Res. 2012;27:240–2. *Large study assessing bone effects of discontinuation of zoledronate.
5. Greenspan SL, Emkey RD, Bone III HG, Weiss SR, Bell NH, Downs RW, et al. Significant differential effects of alendronate, estrogen, or combination therapy on the rate of bone loss after discontinuation of treatment of postmenopausal osteoporosis. A randomized, double-blind, placebo-controlled trial. Ann Intern Med. 2002;137:875–83.
6. Heiss G, Wallace R, Anderson GL, Aragaki A, Beresford SAA, Brzyski R, et al. Health risks and benefits 3 years after stopping randomized treatment with estrogen and progestin. JAMA. 2008;299:1036–45.
7. Neele SJ, Evertz R, De Valk-De Roo G, Roos JC, Netelenbos JC. Effect of 1 year of discontinuation of raloxifene or estrogen therapy on bone mineral density after 5 years of treatment in healthy post menopausal women. Bone. 2002;30:599–603.
8. Bone HG, Bolognese MA, Yuen CK, Kendler DL, Miller PD, Yang YC, et al. Effects of denosumab treatment and discontinuation on bone mineral density and bone turnover markers in postmenopausal women with low bone mass. J Clin Endocrinol Metab. 2011;96:972–80.
9. Brown JP, Roux C, Törring O, Ho RR, Beck-Jensen JE, Gilchrist N, et al. Discontinuation of denosumab and associated fracture incidence: analysis from the FREEDOM trial. J Bone Miner Res. 2013;28:746–52.
10. **Schwartz AV, Bauer DC, Cummings SR, Cauley JA, Ensrud KE, Palermo L, et al. Efficacy of continued alendronate for fractures in women with and without prevalent vertebral fracture: the FLEX trial. J Bone Miner Res. 2010;25:976–82. **This study supports the concept of using femoral neck T score at the time of discontinuation of a treatment as a tool to assess fracture risk.
11. Cosman F, Caulin F, Eastell R, Boos N, Palermo L, Reid KR et al. Who is at highest risk for new vertebral fractures after 3 years of annual zoledronic acid and who should remain on treatment? (internet). J Bone Miner Res. 2011;26 suppl 1:Abstract 1248 (cited 12 Feb 2012).
12. Curtis JR, Westfall AO, Cheng H, Delzell E, Saag KG. Risk of hip fracture after bisphosphonate discontinuation: implications for a drug holiday. Osteoporos Int. 2008;19:1613–20.
13. Whitaker M, Guo J, Kehoe T, Benson G. Bisphosphonates for osteoporosis. Where do we go from here? N Engl J Med. 2012;366:2048–51.
14. Seeman E. To stop or not to stop, that is the question. Osteoporos Int. 2009;20:187–95.
15. Diab DL, Watts NB. Bisphosphonate drug holiday: who, when and how long. Ther Adv Musculoskelet Dis. 2013;5(3):107–11.
16. McClung M, Harris ST, Miller PD, Bauer DC, Davison KS, Dian L, Hanley DA, Kendler DL, Yuen KY, Lewiecki EM. Bisphosphonate therapy for osteoporosis, benefits, risk, and drug holiday. Am J Med 2013;126:13–20

---

[1] *Important References
**Very important References

Patients Who Do Not Take Their Osteoporosis Medications: Can We Help Them Become Compliant?

17

Deborah T. Gold

Summary

- Compliance and persistence with osteoporosis medications are poor.
- Terminology used in discussions of medication behaviors is confusing and inconsistent.
- Patients with osteoporosis and the physicians who treat them have widely differing perspectives on patient medication behavior.
- The Health Belief Model (HBM), a theory about patients and medication behaviors, is useful in trying to understand why osteoporosis patients do not take medication as directed.
- Perceived susceptibility and perceived severity influence whether patients take medications appropriately.
- Medication side effects have been well publicized, leading to even poorer compliance and persistence.
- The HBM can be used to illustrate patients' attitudes toward medications.
- It appears that the disease threat of osteoporosis is less important than the medication threat which appears to drive patient behavior.
- As long as compliance and persistence with osteoporosis medications remain poor, we are not truly treating this disabling and deforming disease.

D.T. Gold, PhD (✉)
Duke University Medical Center,
Post Box 3003, Durham, NC 27710, USA
e-mail: deborah.gold@duke.edu

Introduction

Many pages in peer-reviewed journals over the last 10–15 years have been filled with data and commentary on medication-taking behaviors of individuals with chronic illnesses. From cancer to epilepsy, from HIV to end-stage renal disease [1], scientific evidence confirms the fact that patients rarely take their medicine as it was prescribed for them. This evidence has been gathered from administrative billing data [2], focus groups [3], observational studies [4], and clinical trials [5].

Although these studies have used varied methodologies, samples, time frames, and data collection methods, they virtually all agree on one topic: the majority of people do not take their medications as directed. This is true for acute illnesses as well as chronic ones but is especially true with those chronic conditions which are asymptomatic such as hypertension, hyperlipidemia, and early-stage Type II diabetes. After all, if people feel no overt discomfort, have no disability or limitations, and neither feel nor see medication actions, they lack positive reinforcement that might provide support for medication-taking behaviors.

© Springer International Publishing Switzerland 2016
S.L. Silverman, B. Abrahamsen (eds.), *The Duration and Safety of Osteoporosis Treatment*, DOI 10.1007/978-3-319-23639-1_17

However, most such studies have taken a provider perspective and, unfortunately, have not provided a useful answer to the question, "Why do patients with chronic disease (in this case, osteoporosis)—with access to effective medications and therapies (exercise, calcium/vitamin D supplementation)—not take those medications as directed?" In this chapter, I will begin by briefly reviewing issues of terminology in research on compliance and persistence and examine the differences in patient and provider perspectives on medication behaviors. In addition I will review several studies which have attempted to change these medication behaviors in patients. Ultimately I will explain the HBM, a psychological framework with which to examine these medication-related behaviors and show how it can also be used to explain noncompliance and nonpersistence. Finally, I will close with recommendations for future research and interventions in this extremely important research and clinical area. After all, if patients do not take their osteoporosis medication as directed, we are not really treating osteoporosis at all.

Note: A Caution About Terminology

Virtually every article or chapter on the topic of medication-taking behaviors begins by defining relevant terminology [6]. One might think this a good strategy that would lead to concordance among researchers in this area. Unfortunately, that is not the case. Confusion abounds with the three most frequently used terms: compliance, persistence, and adherence. The International Society of Pharmacoeconomics and Outcomes Research (ISPOR) has made a valiant effort to standardize language use in this area. Cramer and colleagues [7] established terminology in the following way after reviewing the empirical literature. First, they did a literature review from 1966 through 2005, looking for the commonly used terms used to describe medication behavior. Basing their decisions on the frequency of use in the literature, they defined compliance as the percent of doses taken as prescribed and persistence as the number of days taking the medication.

They also noted that these two words should be the primary terms, noting that adherence should be used as a synonym of compliance (and not to mean a combination of compliance and persistence). Even though this paper has been cited over 580 times, the nomenclature problems still remain. Several articles, in fact, state that they used the ISPOR definitions but in fact, did not do so [8, 9].

In addition to those mentioned above, let me clarify two additional terms: primary and secondary nonadherence. Primary nonadherence occurs when a prescriber orders a medication, but the patient does not pick it up. Secondary nonadherence occurs when the patient has the medication but, for whatever reason or reasons, does not take it as directed.

As a final effort to be sure that readers understand the many dichotomies within the compliance/persistence/adherence literature, we take a moment to differentiate between *unintentional* and *intentional* nonadherence, concepts that reflect whether a patient forgets to take medication (unintentional) or actively chooses not to take it (intentional).

Standardizing terminology has been so difficult because of the historical language chaos in this research area. A researcher can choose to follow the ISPOR guidelines or another protocol, but many other publications will not have done so. Despite their attempts to sort these definitions out, even new articles and chapters on compliance and persistence add to the existing confusion. For this chapter, I will rely on the ISPOR definitions as much as possible. That said, the preferred terms used in this chapter will be compliance and persistence.

Osteoporosis Perspective: Why Physicians and Patients Have Different Perspectives

For decades, physicians have assumed that their patients with virtually any chronic illness are taking their medications as they were directed [10]. For that reason, many physicians rarely ask the basic question, "Are you taking your medications as directed?" nor do they examine refill records—unless they are easily available—to determine compliance. When asked about how compliant their own patients are with medications, physicians almost always overestimate their patients' compliant behavior, and it is rare to find physicians and their patients agreeing about medication behavior.

Such beliefs are widely held by those prescribers who are treating osteoporosis [11, 12]. The literature is rife with study after study of administrative databases that show that patients who were prescribed virtually any osteoporosis medications are not complying with those prescriptions. The three studies mentioned below provide empirical evidence of the facts that osteoporosis patients are not taking their medications as directed and that the gap between physician beliefs and actual compliance behavior is substantial.

Curtis and colleagues [11] compared the adherence ratings of physicians about their patients with pharmacy refill data from the HealthCare Integrated Research Database (covers 43 million people in 14 states). They selected all women who filled prescriptions for an oral bisphosphonate (weekly or monthly), calcitonin, SERM, or teriparatide and their physicians. Those physicians prescribing osteoporosis medications for five or more sample patients were invited to respond to survey questions on adherence (defined as compliance plus persistence). They were asked separately by medication what percentage of their patients adhered to that medication at least 80 % of the time. These estimates were compared to actual refill data of their patients.

Probably not surprisingly, physicians believed on average that 67.2 % of their patients adhered to their medication protocols; pharmacy claims data showed that only 40.0 % of these physicians' patients adhered to prescribed medications. The researchers identified two subgroups of physicians: those who overestimated by at least 10 % (the *optimistic* physicians) and those who underestimated patients' medication behaviors by 7.7 % (the *non-optimistic* physicians). Over 74 % of physicians were *optimistic* (MDs rated adher-

ence as 71.9 %, while claims data showed patient adherence to be 32.2 %); 26 % of physicians were *non-optimistic* (MDs rated adherence as 54 %, while claims data showed patient adherence to be 62 %). The fact that physicians overestimated patient adherence suggests that little if anything is being done by those physicians to improve adherence.

In another study in France, investigators randomly identified 684 physicians (420 GPs, 154 rheumatologists, and 11 gynecologists) and 785 of their patients with osteoporosis. Both physicians and patients completed questionnaires. Physicians were asked if each of the patients was compliant, and patients reported their compliance on the Morisky Medication-Taking Adherence Scale (MMAS). Physicians estimated that almost all of their patients were fully compliant (95.4 %). On the other hand, 65.5 % of the women reported that they were compliant with their osteoporosis medications. Obviously, the correlation between physician and patient compliance ratings was very poor ($p = <0.001$) [12].

Finally, Copher and colleagues [13] studied 412 physicians (a 22 % response rate out of 2000 invited physicians) via questionnaire data to determine their perceptions of compliance and persistence of patients with prescribed osteoporosis medications. They looked as well at insurance coverage of these patients. Physicians estimated that 70 % of patients would comply with their medication prescriptions. Pharmacy claims data showed that nearly 49 % of patients had medications available for compliance and persistence (although we know that having medication and taking medication are often different concepts). Thus, the findings from this study support those from the others. Physicians appear not to know when their patients are being noncompliance and/or nonpersistence. If they don't know, how can they remediate this problem? If anything, it may be that physicians spend little time talking to their patients about a medication, its side effects, how to take it correctly, or why it is so important. In addition, physicians may be unaware if patients have financial difficulties in paying for the medication, if they do not believe that they have osteoporosis or believe that osteoporosis is insignificant, or if they do not believe in the efficacy of the medication in question. Perhaps physicians and other prescribers (physician assistants and nurse practitioners) would be able to assist in the war on nonadherence if they were aware of why patients are not taking their osteoporosis medications as directed.

Given that the evidence of noncompliance and nonpersistence is overwhelming, prescribers and public health officials have tried to design interventions to change osteoporosis medication behavior. Hiligsmann and colleagues [14] in *Osteoporosis International* completed a thorough review of published interventions to improve osteoporosis medication behaviors. Prospective studies reviewed occurred between 1/1/1999 and 6/30/2012. Using a Delphi consensus methodology, the researchers selected the studies to include. Out of 113 possible articles, 20 studies were included in the analysis. After reviewing these studies, the authors noted in the discussion that the "efficacy of patient education was still uncertain" (p. 2911). Although several studies reported showing improvements in compliance or persistence [15], results appeared to be non-generalizable or the quality of the study was such that its findings were questionable. Some suggested that simplifying dosing or decision aids might help a little, but most resulted in only marginal improvement. A later study similar to those reviewed here [16] tested nursing monitoring as a way of enhancing compliance and found that two telephone interventions over 12 months did not improve adherence significantly.

Many of the usual educational interventions for improving medication behaviors are not effective in helping patients take their osteoporosis medication as directed. Why? In a 2011 review of problems with compliance and persistence, Silverman and colleagues [17] made an intriguing suggestion about future strategies. "First, we need to better understand the process by which patients form intentions to take or not take recommended medication. Secondly, we need to understand the roles of patient time preference in patient decision-making, which refers to the degree that patients are willing to expend resources such as time, money, or bother now to prevent adverse events such as fracture which may or may not happen in the future. We also need to understand patient risk preferences in terms of fracture risk and side effects." (p. 24) Applying the HBM to what we know about osteoporosis patient challenges with medication behaviors will help us identify ways in which we can improve medication compliance and persistence in patients with this disease.

Setting the Framework for Improvement: The Health Belief Model

The HBM [18, 19] is a psychological model which explains and predicts human behavior around compliance and persistence with health-related tasks. First introduced in the 1950s to explain why widespread screening programs for tuberculosis failed [20], it has remained a key part of research on health behaviors and health beliefs. Although it was originally designed to examine preventive health behavior, it has been used to study illness behavior as well [21]. In general, it has been found useful for both of these tasks, although it does support a medical perspective on compliance and persistence rather than a broader biopsychosocial one. However, no other theoretical model seems to come close to explaining the health and medication behavior of women with osteoporosis.

The original HBM focused on four basic attitudes and beliefs of people about a particular disease or condition [22]. Each of these components relates to how individuals view certain disease aspects and how that view (or perspective) influences their health behaviors [22]. These four central constructs are as follows: *perceived susceptibility, perceived severity, perceived benefits,* and *perceived barriers.* In other words, how much does the patient feel that the disease threatens her well-being and how will the benefits of acting (i.e., taking medications, beginning exercise, avoiding poor lifestyle behaviors) improve overall outcomes [23]? If the benefits exceed the threats, then the patient will be more likely to engage in positive health behaviors. These appear to be the components relevant to use of osteoporosis medication.

Table 17.1 Features of the health belief model

Construct	Definition	Application
Perceived susceptibility	Individual assessment of vulnerability to the condition or disease	Individual believes that she/he has some likelihood of developing the index disease
Perceived severity	Individual's belief that the condition/disease has serious consequences	Individual believes that this disease has unpleasant aspects—pain, dysmobility, and deformity—that can cause suffering
Perceived benefits	Belief that taking action will reduce the negative disease impact	Individual believes that behavior change will improve or prevent negative consequences such as pain and suffering
Perceived barriers	Belief that taking action has tangible and/or psychological costs	Individual sees how barriers can be overcome through reassurance and assistance

Table adapted from [22]

In Table 17.1 below are the 4 HBM constructs with general definitions and applications of each.

The HBM, as a guiding theory in research about chronic illnesses, focuses on two issues: patient attitudes and beliefs about the disease and patient benefits and barriers to carrying out appropriate treatment. When asked about perceived susceptibility and perceived severity in this model, patients respond with their perceptions of the susceptibility and severity of the disease itself [23]. This model is relevant for people undergoing dialysis [24], diabetes [25], and cancer [26]. As noted in Table 17.1, this means asking questions such as, "How vulnerable am I to this disease? Will I contract it? What are the odds? If I do, how serious will it be? Are there ways to manage it?"

HBM and Osteoporosis: Susceptibility and Severity

Osteoporosis, like many other asymptomatic chronic illnesses, has unique challenges and barriers. Researchers have used the HBM to examine different health-related behaviors for both prevention and treatment [27]. Remember that the focus of the model here is specifically to examine issues around compliance and persistence with prescription medications. Certainly other osteoporosis-related behaviors such as calcium and vitamin D, exercise, and avoidance of harmful lifestyle behaviors might also be framed in this model.

Table 17.2 includes the HBM framework but includes osteoporosis-specific issues. Column 4 contains specific osteoporosis applications of the first four constructs from the perspective of a Caucasian postmenopausal woman on corticosteroids with a family history of osteoporosis which is at high risk of this disease. Column 5 lists specific challenges to medication compliance and persistence that research has shown to be important potential causes of noncompliance. Again, the focus is on the original constructs of *perceived susceptibility*, *perceived severity*, *perceived benefits*, and *perceived barriers*.

Many studies of the HBM focus on the disease as the driving issue: What is perceived susceptibility to the disease? What is the perceived severity of the disease? What are the benefits of taking medication (or engaging in other positive health behaviors) to treat the disease? What are the perceived barriers to completing those important health behaviors? But I believe that, in the area of osteoporosis and its medications, patients have a different perspective. They wonder about certain aspects of osteoporosis (e.g., is it really a disease? is it unavoidable?) but do not concentrate on the answers to these items. Instead, they ask, "How susceptible am I to side effects of medications for osteoporosis? What are the consequences of taking the medications?" In terms of severity, patients ask, not about the disease but about the severity of medication side effects: "What harm can this medication do? How serious is this?" They are caught up in the popular press

Table 17.2 HBM and osteoporosis

Construct	Definition	Application	OP application	OP example
Perceived susceptibility	Individual assessment of vulnerability to the condition or disease	Individual believes that she/he has some likelihood of developing the index disease	Postmenopausal white women and glucocorticoid users are at higher risk; mother had a hip fracture	According to Hsieh et al. [28], most women do not perceive a personal risk of OP. Believe it is a part of normal aging, not a disease
Perceived severity	Individual's belief that the condition/disease has serious consequences	Individual believes that this disease has unpleasant aspects—pain, dysmobility, and deformity—that can cause suffering	People die of hip fractures; women develop dowager's hump from spinal fractures; nursing homes are filled with women with OP	According to McHorney et al. [29], side effects, cost, and uncertainty about necessity of treatment were important in noncompliance
Perceived benefits	Belief that taking action will reduce the negative disease impact	Individual believes that behavior change will improve or prevent negative consequences such as pain and suffering	Taking CA, vitamin D, doing exercise, and taking medications reduce the risk of experiencing a fracture	Unclear what benefits exist because the side effect profiles have been so dominant in the news
Perceived barriers	Belief that taking action has tangible and/or psychological costs	Individual sees how barriers can be overcome through reassurance and assistance	I don't like taking medicine; OP medicine causes terrible side effects; I hate needles; I need my coffee first thing in the morning	Dosing regimen too difficult; dosing intervals too frequent or too difficult to remember

myths about medication side effects and forget about the osteoporosis itself and the significant negative consequences such as pain, deformity, and reduced quality of life [30].

Perceived Susceptibility: *Osteoporosis: Is it a disease?* Since the first pharmaceutical agent designed specifically to treat osteoporosis appeared in the marketplace (alendronate, 1995), consumers and some general healthcare providers have questioned the validity of the diagnosis of osteoporosis. The question is not whether it exists; people with multiple vertebral fractures or a hip fracture are evidence of bone thinning and fracture. The question is more whether osteoporosis is a disease (i.e., medical diagnosis) or simply a natural consequence of aging. Many women believe that because their mothers and grandmothers had dowager's humps or broken hips and seemed unable to avoid its progression. So believing that osteoporosis is truly a pathological condition and neither a figment of big pharmaceutical companies' imaginations nor a normal consequence of aging is essential. If this is not a disease process, then why bother with diagnostic testing and pharmaceutical treatments? Only a disease to which someone is vulnerable should be treated with medications.

If women search the Internet to determine whether osteoporosis is truly a disease, they will find oppositional opinions. On sites sponsored by the National Osteoporosis Foundation (NOF), the American Society of Bone and Mineral Research (ASBMR), the National Institutes of Health (NIH), or other science-based organization, they will find strong support for the disease perspective on osteoporosis and the need for prescription medications to prevent future disease deterioration or fracture. However, they need only ask, "Is osteoporosis REALLY a disease?" to be given links to sites such as Save Our Bones (http://saveourbones.com/osteoporosis-is-not-a-disease/) or a natural way to health site with bone information (https://w3.newsmax.com/newsletters/brownstein/osteo.cfm) which tells readers that Big Pharma is lying to them in order to make a profit.

In short, many women read these websites and other sources of the "osteoporosis is not a disease" paradigm and believe that their primary susceptibility is to believing the medicalization of osteoporosis. In other words, they view osteoporosis medicines, not osteoporosis, as the threat.

Osteoporosis: My mother and grandmother had it. That means I'll get it… right?

Perceived Severity: *Do potential side effects cause people to become noncompliant with all osteoporosis medications?* Women hear the message that osteoporosis medications are dangerous in and of themselves. Early postmarketing use of bisphosphonates revealed a substantial number of GI problems (especially in the esophagus) that hadn't been seen in the randomized Phase III trials. However, the trials had excluded people with GI disease, so the investigators had no way of knowing how or whether this medication could have such consequences. Patients and providers became concerned about these outcomes but initially had few options because other medications were not available. Recent studies suggest that oral bisphosphonates increase the risk of upper- and lower-GI side effects [31]. However, it is credible that these reports have consistently contributed to the reduction in compliance and persistence with alendronate treatment.

As time went on and more bisphosphonates were brought to market, additional side effects were identified. The three most significant side effects received media coverage and became so frightening that many women elected not to take antifracture medication at all rather than take a chance that they would experience of these. The first, *osteonecrosis of the jaw (ONJ)*, appeared in the scientific literature as potentially caused by bisphosphonates in 2003 when Ruggiero and colleagues [32] published the first peer-reviewed article in which they described 63 case studies of patients who had received bisphosphonates and also presented with ONJ. This article has subsequently been cited by over 1500 additional articles on the same topic. Because this caused a maelstrom of concern by patients and dentists alike, the ASMBR established a Task Force on ONJ and ultimately published a report from it in 2007 [33]. This Task Force noted that the risk of ONJ was estimated to be between 1 in 10,000 and <1 in 100,000 patient-treatment years. They also stated that patients with cancer who received high-dose IV bisphosphonate therapy had a substantially higher risk (1–10 per 100 patients) depending on the duration of the therapy. Subsequent research supported these findings, but the media ran headlines such as, "Drug for Bones Is Newly Linked to Jaw Disease" (*New York Times*, 6/2/2006) or "Study Links Osteoporosis Drugs to Jaw Trouble" (*Washington Post*, 1/1/2009). Not surprisingly, people on or contemplating taking these drugs expressed concern about their impact, and many never started them or quit immediately.

A second major and potentially frightening side effect of bisphosphonates that has contributed substantially to the reduced number of bisphosphonate users is the atypical femur fracture. Atypical subtrochanteric fractures were identified in women who had been on long-term bisphosphonates [34]. The first reports came out in the early 2000s, and ASBMR had established a Task Force on this topic as well, and its report was published in 2010 [35]. In it, the authors noted that these fractures occurred in some people who had been on long-term bisphosphonate therapy (mean duration = 7 years) and appeared more frequently in those people with glucocorticoid-induced osteoporosis than in postmenopausal osteoporosis. Again, like ONJ, these fractures are extremely rare (2 per 100,000 cases per year for 2 years of BP use to 78 per 100,000 cases per year for 8 years of BP use) [36].

Other potential side effects including atrial fibrillation and osteosarcoma add to the growing list of potential negative consequences of taking bone strengthening medications as portrayed by the media (see New York Times, Wall Street

Journal). The media have jumped on the bandwagon, telling women that these medications are not safe and implying that the side effects are more prevalent than they really are. In addition, websites such as https://www.lawyersandsettlements.com/lawsuit/bisphosphonates-side-effects-lawsuits.html and http://www.youhavealawyer.com/bisphosphonates/ offer legal services to patients who want to sue the makers of these drugs in class action litigation.

Perhaps, it is no wonder that many osteoporosis patients stop taking their medications as directed (or never start them). Barraged on all sides by conflicting but threatening information about the consequences of these drugs, they hear terms such as "cancer" and "jaw death" and decide not even to listen to the information provided by legitimate prescribers. Although the American Dental Association convened an expert panel which agreed that ONJ was very rare and recommended that dentists not modify routine dental work based only on the fact that a patient was taking a bisphosphonate [37], anecdotal evidence suggests that many community dentists are recommending that patients stop bisphosphonate therapy altogether; some will not treat patients on oral or IV bisphosphonates. Unfortunately, the expert panel advice has not disseminated through the dental community or to dental patients; instead, the communications of some practicing dentists have added confusion and incorrect information to the question of bisphosphonate treatment for osteoporosis.

Thus, it appears to be the severity of *side effects of the medications* rather than osteoporosis itself which influences women in choosing to become noncompliance and nonpersistent. That osteoporosis patients and those at risk of this disease fear the consequences of treatment *more* than they fear the disease itself is remarkable.

Perceived Benefits: *Positive outcomes of taking osteoporosis medications.* Health behaviors are directed by many factors. An obvious example that promotes compliance and persistence with medications are benefits from taking medications. In some areas, this is easy to see. If you have a headache, take a pain medication, and the headache disappears. That is a benefit. If you suffer from diabetes, then insulin prevents your blood sugar from getting too far out of balance to avoid diabetic coma or insulin shock. Because these negative outcomes are obvious to patients, their benefits are easily identified. This is true for many symptomatic problems from colds to constipation.

Unfortunately, the positive changes in bone that result from compliance and persistence with osteoporosis medications are more subtle and cannot be immediately perceived by patients after they take medication. The scientific literature is replete with empirical and review articles that discuss the ways in which antifracture medication works and benefits the patients.

Perceived Barriers: *Complexity of dosing regimens.* According to the HBM, patients who are noncompliance with their medication regimens often make this choice based on insurmountable barriers they see to the successful medication behaviors. In particular, the unusual dosing regimen of oral bisphosphonates inspires many patients to reject these medications before even trying them or shortly after beginning them. The rigid ritual of taking these medications first thing in the morning on an empty stomach with 6–8 ounces of plain water is seen as distasteful. Add to that the delay in eating or drinking anything else for 30–60 min and needing to remain upright (not reclining) for 30 min as the final reason for rejecting these medications. Other medications, including teriparatide, monthly ibandronate, denosumab, and zoledronic acid, require the use of an injection/infusion—sometimes as frequently as daily. Depending on their personal fears and beliefs, those with osteoporosis feel burdened by this regimen and believe that they cannot successfully sustain these rituals over time. Thus, perceived serious side effects and diffi-

Table 17.3 FDA-approved osteoporosis medications by dose duration and delivery method

Medication	Dose frequency	Delivery method	Approval date
Alendronate	Daily[a]	Oral	1995
	Weekly[a]	Oral	2000[b]
Risedronate	Daily[a]	Oral	2000
	Weekly[a]	Oral	2002[c, d]
	Monthly[a]	Oral	2012
Ibandronate	Monthly[a]	Oral	2005[e, f]
	Every 3 months	IV injection	2006
Zoledronic acid	Annually	IV infusion	2007
Raloxifene	Daily	Oral	1997[g]
Teriparatide	Daily	Subcutaneous self-injection	2002
Denosumab	Every 6 months	IV injection	2010

[a]Complex bisphosphonate dosing: first thing in the morning on an empty stomach; take with 6–8 oz. of plain water; wait at least 30 minutes until eating or drinking; do not recline for 30 min
[b]In 2005, weekly alendronate plus vitamin D was FDA approved
[c]In 2005, weekly risedronate with calcium was FDA approved
[d]In 2011, a delayed-release once-weekly tablet of risedronate (could be taken after breakfast) was approved under the brand name of Atelvia
[e]Daily oral ibandronate was approved in 2003 but never marketed in the United States
[f]In 2006, quarterly injectable ibandronate was FDA approved
[g]Approved in 2007 to reduce the risk of invasive breast cancer

cult dosing regimens encourage many patients not to take their osteoporosis medication.

Dosing Interval and Drug Delivery Systems Knowing that the bioavailability of oral bisphosphonates is poor even under the best circumstances and how important it is for patients to take these medicines correctly, pharmaceutical researchers began searching out ways to maximize the likelihood of compliance and persistence. They hypothesized that patients, disliking the dosing regimens of these drugs, would be more likely to follow them if easier dosing options were offered [38].

Given that they could not change the strict regimen for taking oral bisphosphonates, pharmaceutical researchers concentrated on dosing duration as a means by which to enhance patient compliance and persistence. The first two oral bisphosphonates (alendronate and risedronate) went from daily to weekly dosing. Marketers believed that having to delay coffee or breakfast once a week rather than every morning would be viewed as a major improvement. In Table 17.3, osteoporosis medications approved in 1995 or later are listed with frequency of dosing and dosing method, and additional relevant information is provided.

Studies began almost immediately to determine whether the different dosing durations also differed in their compliance and persistence rates. With alendronate and risedronate, weekly dosing showed significant improvement in compliance and persistence over daily dosing [39, 40]. Initially, it appeared that patients preferred a monthly bisphosphonate to weekly dosing [41]. However, when patients were told about efficacy differences in the monthly (ibandronate) as opposed to weekly (alendronate, risedronate), this was no longer the case [42, 43]. Other studies reported that database studies showed better adherence with monthly over weekly dosing intervals [44], but little additional empirical evidence was found.

Although, it was convenient to believe that infrequent dosing would improve compliance and persistence with antifracture medication, Lee and colleagues [45] reviewed published articles between 1970 and 2009 to see if this variable (i.e., time to next dose) was truly making a difference in medication behaviors. In an outstanding article, these researchers agreed that there was a clear trend that weekly medications had better compliance and persistence than daily medications but that the longer intervals did not make a significant difference in compliance. They suggest that efficacy, side effects, and administration route are far more important to compliance and persistence than is dosing interval. And some studies show that even the annual dosing of zoledronic acid is no guarantee of persistence with this medicine over time [46]. And the consequences of a single missed dose with a yearly interval are substantially more concerning than those of a daily, weekly, or even monthly medication.

Finally, many healthcare providers believed that patients would prefer any oral dosing over injectable dosing, regardless of the dosing intervals. As noted above, zoledronic acid, the bisphosphonate delivered via a once-yearly infusion, has not solved the problem of noncompliance and persistence with osteoporosis medications [46]. But the other two drugs (teriparatide and denosumab) which are injectable/infusible and have no oral option are not bisphosphonates. Teriparatide is a recombinant human parathyroid hormone analog (1–34) designed to treat osteoporosis. It is the only anabolic or bone-building drug currently available; all others are antiresorptive medications. It requires a daily dose, self-injected by patients. In addition, it can be taken safely for a maximum of 24 months. These factors might well cause patients to be intentionally noncompliant for safety and comfort reasons alone. However, research shows that compliance and persistence with teriparatide are relatively high, especially when compared with oral bisphosphonates [47–49].

Although denosumab is a more recently approved (2010) medication and requires subcutaneous injections every 6 months, compliance and persistence have been positive. The DAPS (Denosumab Adherence Preference Satisfaction) study was a 2-year, open-label study in which patients were randomized to take either alendronate or denosumab for the first year. Patients crossed over to the other drug for the second year. Investigators measured both compliance and persistence and found that both were significantly better with denosumab as a subcutaneous 6-month injection than with oral weekly alendronate [50]. In addition, patients reported preference for denosumab over alendronate for their own long-term treatment. As noted by Freemantle et al. [51], patient preference may have also increased compliance and persistence with this medication. In a subsequent article, Kendler and colleagues [52] compared patient perceptions and adherence between denosumab and alendronate. They found that patients had more positive perceptions of denosumab over alendronate while on treatment and that those positive perceptions were associated with better adherence for every 6-month injectable denosumab than with weekly oral dosing alendronate.

These findings show that extended dosing was not the magic bullet for compliance and persistence with osteoporosis medication. Although compliance and persistence with weekly dosing was better than with daily dosing with oral bisphosphonates, longer dosing intervals did not guarantee improved compliance and persistence and, in some cases, made it worse. Thus, unlike dosing complexity, dosing interval appears not to be a significant barrier to taking osteoporosis medications correctly.

Disease Threat or Medication Threat

The questions above and their answers help individuals understand their risk of their disease and its impact should they receive such a diagnosis. The ultimate conclusion they reach from these answers is called the *disease threat*. With diseases such as cancer or heart disease, the threat seems clear. But as noted in many studies, the vast majority of patients with or at significant risk of osteoporosis view its disease threat as very low. Table 17.4 is modified from Fig. 1 in Jachna et al. [53].

Ordinarily, when someone believes a disease threat is low, that person is unlikely to make preventive efforts. This is certainly true with osteoporosis patients or people with low bone density

Table 17.4 Perceived susceptibility to and severity of osteoporosis

Perceived severity of osteoporosis	Perceived susceptibility to osteoporosis
Part of the normal process of aging Chronic disease with few consequences	Not life-threatening
	Not severe if no kyphosis or pain
	Lack of relationship to fractures
	Not much can be done to avoid it

Low perceived severity and low perceived susceptibility of osteoporosis lead to *low perceived threat of osteoporosis*

Table 17.5 Perceived susceptibility to and severity of osteoporosis medications

Perceived severity of osteoporosis medications	Perceived susceptibility to side effects
Medications cause cancer, ONJ, atypical femoral fractures	My doctor said I already have GERD (60 % of adults), and I am very likely to suffer from GI problems
Chronic use can lead to upper GI problems, blood clots (especially if you have a history of blood clots), and leg pain	Another set of side effects for men taking Prolia: back pain, arthralgia, and nasopharyngitis. I already have back pain from fractures; will this make it worse?
In addition you can have nausea, difficulty swallowing, and hot flashes	A shot every single day? I HATE needles
There are probably worse side effects than we even know about	

Leads to *INCREASED* PERCEIVED THREAT OF OSTEOPOROSIS MEDICATION

Modified from Jachna et al. [53]

who often find it difficult to engage in behaviors like exercise when their disease risk is minimal [54–56]. According to the HBM, the relatively low perceived severity and low perceived susceptibility that women have about osteoporosis suggest that they will be noncompliant and nonpersistent with their medications. One of the few ways that might work is to educate women about the consequences of this disease and especially of fractures.

However, while many women feel that the threat of osteoporosis is low and therefore so are the threats associated with disease consequences (fractures), they have a different perspective toward the medications used to prevent and treat this disease. Throughout the lay and scientific literature, we see that women feel highly threatened by the medications themselves. The specific threats of these medications (and especially of oral bisphosphonates) are documented and discussed below. But if we modify the HBM structure to focus on the threats and severity of osteoporosis medications, we see that perceived risk changes radically. The medications are seen as potentially harmful, unnecessary, and useless. In Table 17.5, we see the same approach with "medications" substituted for "disease."

In an excellent 2013 article, Schousboe [8] examines osteoporosis compliance and persistence using the HBM. He points out a fascinating phenomenon. In five of the six studies using the extended HBM found an important additional predictor that has not previously been included as a part of this model: *concerns about or distrust in medications*. It is this distrust or concern that fuels the poor compliance and persistence with these medications [29, 57–60].

In order to be compliant with medications for a chronic illness, most patients need to believe that (1) they have a health problem that won't go away by itself and will only get worse without treatment, (2) that osteopathic or other nonpharmaceutical treatments will not be effective in treating the disease, and (3) that prescription medication for this condition will not be harmful [8]. In truth, many osteoporosis patients never get to the point of belief that osteoporosis is an illness rather than a part of aging and therefore doesn't need medication. Those who do accept that this is a disease then move into reasoning that leads to the potential conclusions outlined above. When asked what makes them believe that the medicine for osteoporosis is so bad, people usually respond with one of two answers: the media (Internet searches, blogs, e-mails) or friends or relatives who take the medicine or who know someone who took the medicine.

The Future

The field of osteoporosis treatment has moved from estrogen supplementation as the only viable therapy to the virtual panoply of medications that currently exists. Within that panoply, physicians have different delivery systems, dosing regimens, and mechanisms of action. In addition, the pipelines of various pharmaceutical companies have new options that will create other choices for the future. The blossoming of alternatives for the prevention and treatment of this metabolic bone disease has been nothing short of remarkable. And yet, the truth is that, of the 54 million people in the United States who have low bone mass or osteoporosis (http://nof.org/articles/4), only a fraction even receive treatment and fewer still continue to take their medications for an appropriate length of time. Writing a prescription for anti-osteoporosis medications cannot be considered treating these patients, for so many do not follow the treatment regimens their physicians prescribe. Study after study has documented the poor compliance and persistence with these medications, but no one has come close to finding ways to keep those with osteoporosis on their pharmaceutical regimens.

So where to from here? There seems to be little point to finding new medications for this disease as long as patient perceptions about the medications are so negative. Simple—and even complex—educational interventions have not changed those perceptions. Even celebrity spokespersons have not overcome the powerful myths that continue to turn patients away from medications that could—and almost certainly would—improve bone health.

Remember that noncompliance and nonpersistence are NOT unique to osteoporosis. Virtually, any chronic disease that requires ongoing pharmaceutical treatment faces the same challenges to medication behaviors. As the baby boomers continue to move into late life, medical personnel will be faced with the problem of atraumatic fractures and the rigid refusal to comply with physician orders. The answer is almost certainly not to be found in laboratories or via large surveys. Instead, we must dig deeper into individual health beliefs and the ways in which social factors (e.g., education, income, race, and age) and psychological factors (locus of control, anxiety, and self-image) affect those beliefs. In the distant past, researchers believed that the only reason patients were not compliant with medication was that they forgot it. Neupert and colleagues [61, 62] suggest that understanding the context of an individual's life is best for finding out how and when medication behaviors should take place.

Instead of simple forgetfulness, we realize today that noncompliance and nonpersistence are complex phenomena, biopsychosocial in nature. Although we can identify barriers to compliance with great confidence, we have yet to solve this mystery. Future research must be aimed at disentangling those factors which contribute to noncompliance and then, most importantly, finding a way to modify both patients' behaviors and patients' beliefs. Only then will we truly be treating osteoporosis and other chronic illnesses.

References[1]

1. Loghman-Adham M. Medication noncompliance in patients with chronic disease: issues in dialysis and renal transplantation. Am J Manag Care. 2003;9(2): 155–71.
2. Fan T, Zhang Q, Sen SS. Persistence with weekly and monthly bisphosphonates among postmenopausal women: analysis of a US pharmacy claims administrative database. Clinicoecon Outcomes Res. 2013;5:589–95.
3. Iversen MD, Vora RR, Servi A, Solomon DH. Factors affecting adherence to osteoporosis medications: a focus group approach examining viewpoints of patients and providers. J Geriatr Phys Ther. 2011;34(2):72–81.
4. Cramer JA, Gold DT, Silverman SL, Lewiecki EM. A systematic review of persistence and compliance with bisphosphonates for osteoporosis. Osteoporos Int. 2007;18(8):1023–31.
5. Solomon DH, Iversen MD, Avorn J, Gleeson T, Brookhart MA, Patrick AR, Rekedal L, Shrank WH, Lii J, Losina E, Katz JN. Osteoporosis telephonic intervention to improve medication regimen adherence: a large, pragmatic, randomized controlled trial. Arch Intern Med. 2012;172(6):477–83.

[1] *Important References
**Very important References

6. Gold DT. Understanding patient compliance and persistence with osteoporosis therapy. Drugs Aging. 2011;28(4):249–55.

7. Cramer JA, Roy A, Burrell A, Fairchild CJ, Fuldeore MJ, Ollendorf DA, Wong PK. Medication compliance and persistence: terminology and definitions. Value Health. 2008;11(1):44–7.

8. *Schousboe JT. Adherence with medications used to treat osteoporosis: behavioral insights. Curr Osteoporos Rep. 2013;11(1):21–9. *This is an excellent review of the literature on adherence with osteoporosis medications and highlights social and behavioral factors that influence behavior.

9. Hiligsmann M, Gathon HJ, Bruyère O, Ethgen O, Rabenda V, Reginster JY. Cost-effectiveness of osteoporosis screening followed by treatment: the impact of medication adherence. Value Health. 2010;13(4): 394–401.

10. Osterberg L, Blaschke T. Adherence to medication. N Engl J Med. 2005;353(5):487–97.

11. *Curtis JR, Cai Q, Wade SW, Stolshek BS, Adams JL, Balasubramanian A, Viswanathan HN, Kallich JD. Osteoporosis medication adherence: physician perceptions vs. patients' utilization. Bone. 2013;55(1):1–6. *This article examines differences between patient and physician perceptions of adherence to osteoporosis medications.

12. Huas D, Debiais F, Blotman F, Cortet B, Mercier F, Rousseaux C, Berger V, Gaudin AF, Cotté FE. Compliance and treatment satisfaction of post menopausal women treated for osteoporosis. Compliance with osteoporosis treatment. BMC Womens Health. 2010;10:26.

13. Copher R, Buzinec P, Zarotsky V, Kazis L, Iqbal SU, Macarios D. Physician perception of patient adherence compared to patient adherence of osteoporosis medications from pharmacy claims. Curr Med Res Opin. 2010;26(4):777–85.

14. Hiligsmann M, Salas M, Hughes DA, Manias E, Gwadry-Sridhar FH, Linck P, Cowell W. Interventions to improve osteoporosis medication adherence and persistence: a systematic review and literature appraisal by the ISPOR medication adherence & persistence special interest group. Osteoporos Int. 2013;24(12):2907–18.

15. Nielsen D, Ryg J, Nielsen W, Knold B, Nissen N, Brixen K. Patient education in groups increases knowledge of osteoporosis and adherence to treatment: a two-year randomized controlled trial. Patient Educ Couns. 2010;81(2):155–60.

16. Naseem S, Linton S, Wiles J, Jones G. 'Keep taking the tablets': does brief telephone nurse-led intervention improve adherence to osteoporosis therapy? Age Ageing. 2014;43:i15.

17. Silverman SL, Gold DT. Healthy users, healthy adherers, and healthy behaviors? J Bone Miner Res. 2011;26(4):681–2.

18. Rosenstock IM. Why people use health services. Milbank Mem Fund Q. 1966;44(Spring):94–127.

19. Becker MH, editor. The health belief model and personal health behavior: health education monograph. San Francisco: Society for Public Health Education; 1974.

20. Rosenstock IM. The health belief model and preventive health behavior. Health Educ Behav. 1974;2(4):354–86.

21. Becker MH, Radius SM, Rosenstock IM, Drachman RH, Schuberth KC, Teets KC. Compliance with a medical regimen for asthma: a test of the health belief model. Public Health Rep. 1978;93(3):268–77.

22. Rosenstock I. Historical origins of the health belief model. Health Educ Behav. 1974;2(4):328–35.

23. Khdour MR, Hawwa AF, Kidney JC, Smyth BM, McElnay JC. Potential risk factors for medication non-adherence in patients with chronic obstructive pulmonary disease (COPD). Eur J Clin Pharmacol. 2012;68(10):1365–73.

24. Theofilou P. Quality of life and mental health in hemodialysis and peritoneal dialysis patients: the role of health beliefs. Int Urol Nephrol. 2012;44(1): 245–53.

25. Gherman A, Schnur J, Montgomery G, Sassu R, Veresiu I, David D. How are adherent people more likely to think? A meta-analysis of health beliefs and diabetes self-care. Diabetes Educ. 2011;37(3): 392–408.

26. Tanner-Smith EE, Brown TM. Evaluating the health belief model: a critical review of studies predicting mammographic and pap screening. Soc Theory Health. 2010;8(1):95–125.

27. *McLeod KM, Johnson CS. A systematic review of osteoporosis health beliefs in adult men and women. J Osteoporos. 2011;2011:197454. doi:10.4061/ 2011/197454. *This is an excellent explanation of ways in which the Health Belief Model is relevant to osteoporosis.

28. Hsieh C, Novielli KD, Diamond JJ, Cheruva D. Health beliefs and attitudes toward the prevention of osteoporosis in older women. Menopause. 2001;8(5):372–6.

29. McHorney CA, Schousboe JT, Cline RR, Weiss TW. The impact of osteoporosis medication beliefs and side-effect experiences on non-adherence to oral bisphosphonates. Curr Med Res Opin. 2007;23(12): 3137–52.

30. Gold DT. The clinical impact of vertebral fractures: quality of life in women with osteoporosis. Bone. 1996;18 Suppl 3:185S–9S.

31. Peng YL, Hu HY, Luo JC, Hou MC, Lin HC, Lee FY. Alendronate, a bisphosphonate, increased upper and lower gastrointestinal bleeding: risk factor analysis from a nationwide population-based study. Osteoporos Int. 2014;25(5):1617–23.

32. Ruggiero SL, Mehrotra B, Rosenberg TJ, Engroff SL. Osteonecrosis of the jaws associated with the use of bisphosphonates: a review of 63 cases. J Oral Maxillofac Surg. 2004;62(5):527–34.

33. Khosla S, Burr D, Cauley J, Dempster DW, Ebeling PR, Felsenberg D, Gagel RF, Gilsanz V, Guise T, Koka S, McCauley LK, McGowan J, McKee MD, Mohla S, Pendrys DG, Raisz LG, Ruggiero SL, Shafer DM, Shum L, Silverman SL, Van Poznak CH,

Watts N, Woo SB, Shane E, American Society for Bone and Mineral Research. Bisphosphonate-associated osteonecrosis of the jaw: report of a task force of the American society for bone and mineral research. J Bone Miner Res. 2007;22(10):1479–91.

34. Goh SK, Yang KY, Koh JS, Wong MK, Chua SY, Chua DT, Howe TS. Subtrochanteric insufficiency fractures in patients on alendronate therapy: a caution. J Bone Joint Surg (Br). 2007;89(3):349–53.

35. **Shane E, Burr D, Ebeling PR, Abrahamsen B, Adler RA, Brown TD, Cheung AM, Cosman F, Curtis JR, Dell R, Dempster D, Einhorn TA, Genant HK, Geusens P, Klaushofer K, Koval K, Lane JM, McKiernan F, McKinney R, Ng A, Nieves J, O'Keefe R, Papapoulos S, Sen HT, van der Meulen MC, Weinstein RS, Whyte M, American Society for Bone and Mineral Research. Atypical subtrochanteric and diaphyseal femoral fractures: report of a task force of the American society for bone and mineral research. J Bone Miner Res. 2010;25(11):2267–94. **This task force report provides critical information on atypical subtrochanteric fractures.*

36. Dell RM, Adams AL, Greene DF, Funahashi TT, Silverman SL, Eisemon EO, Zhou H, Burchette RJ, Ott SM. Incidence of atypical nontraumatic diaphyseal fractures of the femur. J Bone Miner Res. 2012;27(12):2544–50.

37. American Dental Association Council on Scientific Affairs. Dental management of patients receiving oral bisphosphonate therapy: expert panel recommendations. J Am Dent Assoc. 2006;137(8):1144–50.

38. Cramer JA, Lynch NO, Gaudin AF, Walker M, Cowell W. The effect of dosing frequency on compliance and persistence with bisphosphonate therapy in postmenopausal women: a comparison of studies in the United States, the United Kingdom, and France. Clin Ther. 2006;28(10):1686–94.

39. Kendler D, Kung AW, Fuleihan G-H, González González JG, Gaines KA, Verbruggen N, Melton ME. Patients with osteoporosis prefer once weekly to once daily dosing with alendronate. Maturitas. 2004;48(3):243–51.

40. Sunyecz J, Gallagher R, MacCosbe P. Persistence with medication in women taking daily versus weekly bisphosphonates for osteoporosis. Female Patient. 2006;31:21–8.

41. Emkey R, Koltun W, Beusterien K, Seidman L, Kivitz A, Devas V, Masanauskaite D. Patient preference for once-monthly ibandronate versus once-weekly alendronate in a randomized, open-label, cross-over trial: the Boniva alendronate trial in osteoporosis (BALTO). Curr Med Res Opin. 2005;21(12):1895–903.

42. Keen R, Jodar E, Iolascon G, Kruse HP, Varbanov A, Mann B, Gold DT. European women's preference for osteoporosis treatment: influence of clinical effectiveness and dosing frequency. Curr Med Res Opin. 2006;22(12):2375–81.

43. Gold DT, Safi W, Trinh H. Patient preference and adherence: comparative US studies between two bisphosphonates, weekly risedronate and monthly ibandronate. Curr Med Res Opin. 2006;22(12):2383–91.

44. Silverman SL, Cramer JA, Sunyecz JA, Sarawate C, Harley C, Blumentals WA, Poston S, Lewiecki EM. Women are more persistent with monthly bisphosphonates therapy compared to weekly bisphosphonates: 12-month results from 2 retrospective databases. J Bone Miner Res. 2007;22 Suppl 1:S454.

45. Lee S, Glendenning P, Inderjeeth CA. Efficacy, side effects and route of administration are more important than frequency of dosing of anti-osteoporosis treatments in determining patient adherence: a critical review of published articles from 1970 to 2009. Osteoporos Int. 2011;22(3):741–53.

46. Curtis JR, Yun H, Matthews R, Saag KG, Delzell E. Adherence with intravenous zoledronate and intravenous ibandronate in the United States medicare population. Arthritis Care Res (Hoboken). 2012;64(7):1054–60.

47. Adachi JD, Hanley DA, Lorraine JK, Yu M. Assessing compliance, acceptance, and tolerability of teriparatide in patients with osteoporosis who fractured while on antiresorptive treatment or were intolerant to previous antiresorptive treatment: an 18-month, multicenter, open-label, prospective study. Clin Ther. 2007;29(9):2055–67.

48. Arden NK, Earl S, Fisher DJ, Cooper C, Carruthers S, Goater M. Persistence with teriparatide in patients with osteoporosis: the UK experience. Osteoporos Int. 2006;17(11):1626–9.

49. Mulgund M, Beattie KA, Wong AK, Papaioannou A, Adachi JD. Assessing adherence to teriparatide therapy, causes of nonadherence and effect of adherence on bone mineral density measurements in osteoporotic patients at high risk for fracture. Ther Adv Musculoskelet Dis. 2009;1(1):5–11.

50. Kendler DL, McClung MR, Freemantle N, Lillestol M, Moffett AH, Borenstein J, Satram-Hoang S, Yang YC, Kaur P, Macarios D, Siddhanti S, DAPS Investigators. Adherence, preference, and satisfaction of postmenopausal women taking denosumab or alendronate. Osteoporos Int. 2011;22(6):1725–35.

51. Freemantle N, Satram-Hoang S, Tang ET, Kaur P, Macarios D, Siddhanti S, Borenstein J, Kendler DL, DAPS Investigators. Final results of the DAPS (Denosumab adherence preference satisfaction) study: a 24-month, randomized, crossover comparison with alendronate in postmenopausal women. Osteoporos Int. 2012;23(1):317–26.

52. Kendler DL, Macarios D, Lillestol MJ, Moffett A, Satram-Hoang S, Huang J, Kaur P, Tang ET, Wagman RB, Horne R. Influence of patient perceptions and preferences for osteoporosis medication on adherence behavior in the denosumab adherence preference satisfaction study. Menopause. 2014;21(1):25–32.

53. Jachna CM, Forbes-Thompson S. Osteoporosis: health beliefs and barriers to treatment in an assisted living facility. J Gerontol Nurs. 2005;31(1):24–30.

54. Boulware LE, Carson KA, Troll MU, Powe NR, Cooper LA. Perceived susceptibility to chronic

kidney disease among high-risk patients seen in primary care practices. J Gen Intern Med. 2009;24(10): 1123–9.

55. Gao X, Nau DP, Rosenbluth SA, Scott V, Woodward C. The relationship of disease severity, health beliefs and medication adherence among HIV patients. AIDS Care. 2000;12(4):387–98.

56. Gerend MA, Aiken LS, West SG, Erchull MJ. Beyond medical risk: investigating the psychological factors underlying women's perceptions of susceptibility to breast cancer, heart disease, and osteoporosis. Health Psychol. 2004;23(3):247–58.

57. Yood RA, Mazor KM, Andrade SE, Emani S, Chan W, Kahler KH. Patient decision to initiate therapy for osteoporosis: the influence of knowledge and beliefs. J Gen Intern Med. 2008;23(11):1815–21.

58. Schousboe JT, Dowd BE, Davison ML, Kane RL. Association of medication attitudes with non-persistence and non-compliance with medication to prevent fractures. Osteoporos Int. 2010;21(11): 1899–909.

59. Cline RR, Farley JF, Hansen RA, Schommer JC. Osteoporosis beliefs and antiresorptive medication use. Maturitas. 2005;50(3):196–208.

60. Schousboe JT, Davison ML, Dowd B, Thiede Call K, Johnson P, Kane RL. Predictors of patients' perceived need for medication to prevent fracture. Med Care. 2011;49(3):273–80.

61. McGuire LC. Remembering what the doctor said: organization and adults' memory for medical information. Exp Aging Res. 1996;22(4):403–28.

62. *Neupert SD, Patterson TR, Davis AA, Allaire JC. Age differences in daily predictors of forgetting to take medication: the importance of context and cognition. Exp Aging Res. 2011;37(4):435–48. *This article tests the importance of cognition and busyness in older and younger adults and shows that less busy older adults remember medication more fully.*

Fractures and Healing on Antiresorptive Therapy

Eli Kupperman and Susan V. Bukata

Summary

- Patients with osteoporosis are more likely to suffer fragility fracture.
- Medications to treat osteoporosis decrease risk of future fracture.
- What is effect of osteoporosis medications on fracture healing?
- No osteoporosis medications have been shown to delay fracture healing with the exception of bisphosphonates after stress fractures.
- Anabolic agents (PTH, anti-sclerostin antibody) may accelerate fracture healing.
- It is safe to start osteoporosis medications immediately after fracture with the exception of IV bisphosphonates, which should be started after a 2-week holiday.
- New drugs are currently being studied in animal and clinical trials for their safety and efficacy.

E. Kupperman, MD • S.V. Bukata, MD (⊠)
Department of Orthopaedics, UCLA, 1250 16th St.,
Suite 23100, Santa Monica, CA 90404, USA
e-mail: SBukata@mednet.ucla.edu

Introduction

Fragility fracture prevention is the primary purpose of osteoporosis treatment [1]. While some patients are already taking medications for osteoporosis at the time of their fragility fracture, many patients are first diagnosed with osteoporosis after a fragility fracture. One of the greatest predictors for future fragility fractures is prior fracture, and therefore it is imperative that patients be placed on medications for osteoporosis as quickly as possible after their fragility fracture [2]. There are many good treatment options available for osteoporosis, but because these medications act on bone metabolism and decrease the risk of fracture, it is reasonable to believe that their mechanism of action could also affect fracture healing. So which drugs are safe to use during fracture healing and how soon after a fracture should they be started?

In this chapter, we review the current literature surrounding osteoporosis medications and their effect on fracture healing in the osteoporotic patient. Many of the questions surrounding antiresorptive and anabolic therapies in the period immediately surrounding a fracture are still unanswered, but it is clear that these medications help to prevent the occurrence of future fractures. Therefore, it is imperative that we understand how these medications effect fracture healing, as our patients should be given the opportunity to

© Springer International Publishing Switzerland 2016
S.L. Silverman, B. Abrahamsen (eds.), *The Duration and Safety
of Osteoporosis Treatment*, DOI 10.1007/978-3-319-23639-1_18

take their medications as soon as possible once it is safe to do so. As long as the effect on fracture healing is at least neutral, these medications should be restarted or begun immediately following a fracture. If the effect on fracture healing is negative, then it must be determined how long patients must wait before their medications can be safely begun.

How Fracture Healing Occurs

The three main stages of fracture healing are (1) inflammation, (2) repair, and (3) remodeling [1]. All fractures pass through these three stages, but the mechanisms used to achieve fracture healing can vary depending upon the size of the fracture gap and the stability of the fracture. The inflammatory phase begins within the first 24 h after a new fracture. First, a hematoma emerges around the site of the fracture which carries with it hematopoietic cells including macrophages, neutrophils, and platelets. These cells each release their own hormones and growth factors that aid in attracting more cells to the region and beginning the reparative process. Later in the inflammatory phase, fibroblasts and mesenchymal cells migrate to the fracture in order to begin the formation of granulation healing tissue. Finally, osteoblasts and fibroblasts dominate as new matrix is laid down.

In the reparative phase, fracture healing can occur by one of two pathways. Primary fracture healing occurs when the two sides of a fracture are in direct contact with each other on a microscopic level, and the fracture is essentially mechanically stable. Primary bone healing in many ways resembles normal bone remodeling. Osteoclasts directly cross the fracture site with cutting cones, and osteoblasts follow, essentially remodeling away the fracture site. Healing that occurs with stress fractures is a good example of this. Most fractures heal in a way that resembles development, with endochondral bone formation. A fracture with a material gap has some micromotion, and a cartilage callus forms at the fracture site replacing the hematoma and fibrous tissue, often within the first 2 weeks after fracture.

This is called the soft callus. As the cartilage gradually becomes calcified over the next few weeks, it begins to be overlaid with bone. This is called the hard callus. Finally, the entire callus is gradually remodeled to bone to complete healing. Much of this remodeling occurs via osteoblasts and osteoclasts and is governed by Wolff's law, meaning the remodeling occurs in response to mechanical stress. This remodeling stage of fracture healing begins only a few weeks after the fracture but is sustained for many months until the fractured bone realizes its final structure.

Effect of Specific Antiresorptive Therapies on Fracture Healing

Antiresorptives

Bisphosphonates

Bisphosphonates are one of the most widely used of the osteoporosis medications. Their main mechanism of action is through the inhibition of osteoclastic activity, thereby slowing bone resorption and remodeling [2]. The interaction between bisphosphonates and fracture healing is widely studied in animal models, but there are few human studies, so clinical decision-making should still be made with care. Bisphosphonates do not appear to have a major effect on the initial phases of fracture healing, including the ability to form cartilage callus. However, bisphosphonates do effect the remodeling phases of fracture healing, both from cartilage callus to bony callus and then the final remodeling to lamellar bone. Both human and animal studies have shown that fracture healing while on bisphosphonate therapy leads to a larger callus volume, and because there is a greater quantity of cartilage present compared to the callus seen in control subjects, there is concern that it may be weaker. Biomechanical testing of this callus shows that on a microscopic level, the strength of a section of the callus is decreased compared to a similar sized section of normal callus, but macroscopically because there is a larger quantity of callus, the entire callus is biomechanically equivalent to normal callus. To date, there are no studies that show that short-term administration of bisphosphonates leads to any negative clinical results in fracture healing [3]. Below, we summarize some of the seminal publications pertaining to particular bisphosphonates and how they affect fracture healing.

Zoledronate

Of the bisphosphonates, zoledronate is the most efficient inhibitor of osteoclastic bone resorption, making it an ideal candidate for aiding in fracture healing. Zoledronate was shown in a randomized prospective blinded study by Lyles et al. to be associated with decreased risk of fracture as well as decreased mortality following osteoporotic hip fracture surgically repaired. Those patients receiving an infusion of zoledronate within 90 days of surgery had a 35 % risk reduction of fracture in the follow-up period of the study as well as a 28 % reduction in all-cause death [4].

The role of zoledronate in fracture healing has also been studied but is not as promising as its role in reducing future fractures. In a model of fibular osteotomies in rabbits, Matos et al. demonstrated that rabbits receiving a single dose of zoledronate demonstrated increased stimulation of primary bone production, but with decreased remodeling [5]. These rabbits treated with zoledronate had smaller areas of callus formation at 1 week and increased trabecular bone volume, increased woven bone quantity, and decreased periosteal fibrosis when compared to control rabbits at 4 weeks. McDonald et al. showed similar findings in a rat femur fracture model with increased callus volume and delayed remodeling. This study did not demonstrate any delay in endochondral ossification, just a delay in remodeling [6].

Studies following fracture healing in humans have shown that zoledronate does not accelerate or enhance fracture healing. Patients receiving a single dose of zoledronate after osteoporotic hip fracture were shown to have a reduced risk of subsequent fracture as well as all-cause mortality, but their time to healing was not significantly reduced. Healing time was also not found to be delayed. In a study by Colon-Emeric et al. the risk of delayed union was identical between those receiving the infusion and those receiving a

normal saline infusion [7]. In an article by Harding et al., patients who had high tibial osteotomies were placed in one of two groups: a single infusion of zoledronate 4 weeks after surgery or a placebo group who received an infusion of normal saline. No differences were observed between the two groups in terms of time to healing, bone mineral density (BMD), or retention of angular correction. These results were different than those seen in a previous animal model [8].

Pamidronate

Pamidronate is a bisphosphonate used primarily in the care of patients with moderate to severe osteogenesis imperfecta (OI). There are a number of studies assessing fracture healing of patients on pamidronate, but this is in a specialized population, not necessarily generalizable to those with osteoporosis. One study by Munns et al. found that pediatric patients with OI who were on pamidronate had no statistically significant difference in rates of healing of fractures but did demonstrate a delayed healing of surgical osteotomy sites [9]. A study in a similar population by Pizones et al. showed that pamidronate also did not interfere with fracture healing in pediatric OI patients [10].

While its primary use is in patients with OI, pamidronate has also been studied for its biomechanical effects on fracture healing in rats. A study by Amanat et al. of rats given an open osteotomy was divided into four arms: saline control, systemic pamidronate, and two different dosages of local pamidronate and then assessed for healing at 6 weeks. In these rats, those with the single systemic dose of pamidronate had larger volume of callus, higher bone mineral content (BMC) of callus, and 60 % greater strength than the saline control group [11]. This result, of course, is not indicative of faster healing, simple increased bony growth.

Clodronate

Studies on the bisphosphonate clodronate have also been performed. Studies of osteotomies on rats were done by Madsen et al. and demonstrated increased BMD around the fracture site for those rats taking clodronate, but they did not find any significant difference between the groups when it came to callus area, volume, strength, or stiffness [12]. Similar results were obtained in a study of osteoporotic women with distal radius fracture who were given clodronate in a paper by Adolphson et al. They found that BMD was also increased in the experimental group but interestingly that the BMD in a more proximal aspect of the injured radius was significantly reduced in those receiving the drug [13].

Alendronate

Alendronate is the most widely studied of the bisphosphonates in models of fracture healing. It has shown increased volume of callus and BMC when compared to controls in mouse models, as well as greater strength and stiffness [14].

A study of a mouse mid-shaft femoral osteotomy by Saito et al. looked at callus formation and type of bone present at 12 weeks in four groups of animals: sham surgery, ovariectomy, ovariectomy with calcitriol, and ovariectomy with alendronate. They found that those with alendronate had a larger volume of callus, increased enzymatic cross-linking, and greater strength, but had delay in converting woven bone into lamellar bone causing no new cortical shell to appear [15]. Similar to the Saito study, Lu et al. looked at ovariectomized rats which were treated with alendronate before and after osteotomy. They also found an increased volume of callus in the treated group with improved strength but with a lower density of bone and a delay of conversion from woven to lamellar bone [16].

A study by Uchiyama et al. evaluated whether early administration of alendronate slowed healing by causing a delay in conversion to cortical bone. Half of the osteoporotic patients with distal radius fractures were randomized to receive alendronate within days of surgery and half were held without the medication for 4 months following surgery and then given alendronate. There were no significant differences found between the two groups in terms of any of the endpoints assessed including time to cortical bridging, tenderness, grip strength, or range of motion [17]. Alendronate is considered safe for administration in the period immediately following a fracture, but although it does increase callus volume, it does not lead to faster time to complete healing.

General Bisphosphonates

Some studies on fracture healing do not specify by type of bisphosphonate as they are retrospective, but they still may draw noteworthy conclusions, and we wanted to be able to share them here. Rozental et al. compared radiographic healing of distal radius fractures on those who were taking a bisphosphonate at the time of injury and those who were not. They found a statistically significant increase in time to healing of about 1 week in those on antiresorptive therapy versus those not on medical therapy [18]. While their result was statistically significant, it may not be clinically relevant.

Similar to the Uchiyama study, a paper by Gong et al. looked at elderly patients with distal radius fractures treated with locking plate fixation and assessed if there was any difference in healing or clinical outcomes with either early (2 weeks after surgery) or late (3 months after surgery) administration of bisphosphonates. They, too, found no differences with respect to either radiographic or clinical outcomes of healing [19]. The same result was found in a paper by Kim et al. looking at risedronate treatment after fixation of intertrochanteric femoral fractures [20]. Savaridas et al. looked at a rat model with rigid fixation of a tibial osteotomy specifically to evaluate if ibandronate administration delayed primary bone healing, the type of healing that occurs in stress fractures. The study showed more cartilaginous like tissue and undifferentiated mesenchymal tissue present in the fracture site with delayed healing in the bisphosphonate-treated animals, suggesting that bisphosphonates do delay the healing of stress fractures [21]. No randomized trials looking specifically at human healing of stress fractures with bisphosphonate administration have been published to date.

Estrogens

Estrogen has potentially favorable effects on fracture healing, being both anabolic as well as anti-catabolic. Like bisphosphonates, estrogen and selective estrogen receptor modulators

(SERM) are a common medication used in the treatment of osteoporosis, and therefore studying their effects on fracture healing is imperative. Also like bisphosphonates, no studies are currently in print demonstrating negative effects on fracture healing from short-term use of estrogen or estrogen-modifying compounds [3].

Estrogen

It has been previously demonstrated that estrogen-deficient mice, primarily by way of ovariectomy, have increased osteoclastic bone resorption. Estrogen replacement, on the other hand, has reversed this effect and caused these ovariectomized mice to return to normal levels of osteoclast bone resorption [22]. A study by Beil et al. took mice and performed femoral fractures. These mice were then separated into three groups: those which received estrogen, those which were made estrogen-deficient by way of ovariectomy, and those which were left alone to heal as the control group. Those mice that had an ovariectomy were found to have impaired periosteal callus formation, a smaller area of chondrocytes, and less distinctive mineralization, as well as a thinner and more porous cortex. Those mice that received extra estrogen in the form of a continuous infusion had the opposite effect (better fracture healing, increased area of chondrocytes, more distinct mineralization, and thicker cortex) [22].

Raloxifene

Raloxifene, a SERM, has shown similar effects on bone metabolism and fracture healing as estrogen due to its role as an estrogen agonist on bone. In a retrospective database analysis by Foster et al., those osteoporotic patients receiving raloxifene had lower rates of vertebral fractures at all time points studied (1, 3, 5, and 7 years) and had lower rates of non-vertebral fractures at 1 and 5 years [23]. More recent studies have examined raloxifene's role in fracture healing in addition to its role simply as a treatment for osteoporosis.

Stuermer et al. were the first to study the effect of raloxifene on fracture healing in a model of an osteoporotic mouse. They performed tibial metaphyseal osteotomies that were then plated with a T-type fixation device for biomechanical stability. Their mice were placed in one of four groups, namely, ovariectomy, raloxifene-treated after ovariectomy, estrogen-treated after ovariectomy, or no treatment at all after a sham operation, and subsequently were evaluated for healing of the tibial metaphyseal osteotomy. In their study, the researchers found that the fractures in both estrogen- and raloxifene-treated mice could withstand higher loads than the ovariectomized mice. In addition, raloxifene treatment was associated with significantly greater total callus formation [24].

Similar to the previous study, Spiro et al. performed a femoral diaphyseal osteotomy in mice which were then separated into one of four groups: ovariectomy, raloxifene-treated, estrogen-treated, or no treatment at all as controls [25]. They demonstrated that at 10 days after fracture, raloxifene treatment had improved fracture healing significantly more than any of the other three subgroups and that by day 20, all mice treated with raloxifene or estrogen had healed adequately, whereas none of the control mice nor the ovariectomized mice had complete cortical bridging across the fracture site. This demonstrated that raloxifene has no negative effects on fracture healing and in fact may actually be advantageous in the healing of fractures. No randomized clinical trials have been performed in humans to look at fracture healing with raloxifene.

Denosumab

Denosumab is a human monoclonal antibody to RANKL, blocking its binding to RANK. It inhibits osteoclasts, leading to decreased bone resorption and greater bone density. Based on its mechanism of action, denosumab has been studied for its potential usefulness both with osteoporosis and with fracture healing. To date, however, there are no articles that particularly comment on fracture healing during treatment with denosumab in human subjects [2] nor are there any reports documenting deleterious effects from short-term use on fracture healing [3].

A study of osteoporotic women by Cummings et al. showed that those women treated with denosumab had significantly decreased risk of fracture. They showed a 68 % decreased relative risk of vertebral fracture, 40 % decrease for hip fractures, and 20 % decrease for non-vertebral fractures [26]. In addition to fracture prevention, however, denosumab has also been shown to increase strength and BMD after a fracture. Using data from the FREDOM trial, McCloskey et al. showed again that denosumab decreased risk of fracture in osteoporotic women, especially in those with moderate to high risk as measured by FRAX [27].

The article by Gerstenfeld et al., which compared alendronate-treated mice to denosumab-treated mice to controls after femoral fractures, showed that those treated with denosumab had significantly higher BMD and percent bone volume at the fracture site than the other treatment arms. In addition, fracture sites in mice receiving denosumab also had increased biomechanical strength and stiffness compared to controls, but similar to those treated with alendronate. This is in contrast to what one might have expected as denosumab, like bisphosphonates, also delays remodeling [14].

In another analysis using the FREEDOM trial, Adami et al. demonstrated that administration of denosumab in osteoporotic patients within a 6-week period before or after a non-vertebral fracture did not affect fracture healing. In fact, there was a trend toward fewer delayed unions in those receiving denosumab versus those who did not receive the medication [28].

Anabolics

Parathyroid Hormone

Unlike the previously discussed medications, all of which are antiresorptive agents, parathyroid hormone (PTH) is the first drug whose main mechanism of action is anabolic in nature. PTH's effect on bone metabolism differs based on its exposure: a continuous infusion of PTH causes bone resorption through a dominant increase in osteoclastic activity, but intermittent exposure to PTH exerts an anabolic effect and induces bone building by a dominant increase in osteoblast activity [2]. In the United States, the drug used as an analog to PTH is recombinant PTH (1–34), which is the first 34 N-terminal amino acid peptides of human PTH [29]. This form has been shown to prevent the risk of future fractures as well as to increase BMD in osteoporotic patients [29].

Studies in animals and evaluation of human fracture sites have shown that recombinant PTH leads to increased callus volume and BMC [2]. Andreassen et al. exposed rats with tibial fractures to 1-34 PTH or placebo. Rats were evaluated at 3 weeks and 8 weeks after fracture. At 3 weeks, rats receiving drug demonstrated an increased maximum load during biomechanical testing of 160 % and radiographically an increased callus volume of 208 %. By 8 weeks, the maximal load borne was increased by 270 % and callus volume by 135 %. BMC also increased by 190 % at 3 weeks and 388 % by 8 weeks [30].

Animal studies have also clearly demonstrated faster healing times while on recombinant PTH as well. Alkhiary et al. performed osteotomies in rat femora and then subjected them to placebo, low-dose daily PTH, or high-dose daily PTH and measured their response at 3, 5, and 12 weeks. Already by week 3, the high-dose daily PTH rats were significantly improved over the placebo group in terms of strength, stiffness, BMD, BMC, and cartilage volume. By 5 weeks, both PTH subgroups had significantly higher BMD, BMC, and osseous volume than placebo. By the end of the experiment, the high-dose PTH subgroup still had significantly increased BMD and strength compared to the controls, leading to the conclusion that repair occurred faster in the rats receiving PTH [31]. Manabe et al. tested midshaft femoral fractures on cynomolgus monkeys and treated them with low-dose PTH, high-dose PTH, or placebo and then tested the femora at 26 weeks after fracture. By this point after fracture, the bone had healed in all of the monkeys, but the PTH groups had smaller callus, and the high-dose PTH group also had significantly higher BMD than the other groups, leading the authors to conclude that those monkeys receiving PTH had actually accelerated the time of remodeling during fracture healing [32].

Clinical trials in humans have also been done to test the hypotheses shown in the animal studies. In one prospective, randomized, double-blinded study by Aspenberg et al., over 100 women with distal radius fractures not requiring operative fixation were randomized to one of three arms for daily injections for 8 weeks: low-dose PTH (20 µg), high-dose PTH (40 µg), or placebo. They were then assessed for time to radiographic healing defined as bridging across three of four cortices. The time to heal was 7.4, 8.8, and 9.1 weeks for low-dose PTH, high-dose PTH, and placebo, respectively. This was significant between low-dose PTH and control, but not with high-dose PTH [33]. The same authors then looked post hoc at callus formation in a subset of the conservatively managed distal radius fracture patients located at one center. Based on radiographs, they blindly qualified the callus formation as rich, intermediate, or poor at 5 weeks to determine if they would have found more substantial results if they had looked at earlier time points of healing. Of those studied, nine received ratings of "rich" (0 controls, 3 low-dose PTH, 6 high-dose PTH), nine received ratings of "intermediate" (1 control, 5 low-dose PTH, 3 high-dose PTH), and nine received ratings of "poor" (7 controls, 1 low-dose PTH, 1 high-dose PTH), which were highly statistically significant. This led the authors to conclude that it was possible that radiographic quality at an earlier time point may have been more sensitive of a variable than cortical bridging and that therefore recombinant PTH not only accelerated healing but in a dose-dependent manner [34].

More evidence for the benefits of recombinant PTH in humans in terms of fracture healing was seen in a paper by Peichl et al. which randomized elderly patients with pelvic fractures to receive PTH (1–81) versus placebo and then assessed them on time to radiographic healing, pain, and a timed "up and go" test. All three were significantly improved with the patients receiving PTH. Healing was achieved in 7.8 weeks versus 12.6 weeks, pain levels were lower, and the "up and go" test was faster in patients treated with PTH. The authors concluded that not only did PTH accelerate fracture healing but also improved clinical outcomes in this study population [35].

Anti-sclerostin Antibody

As a novel therapy in the treatment of osteoporosis, anti-sclerostin antibody functions by way of a monoclonal antibody directed against sclerostin, an osteocyte-produced inhibitor of bone formation. There is very little literature currently on this new therapeutic in terms of its effectiveness with fracture healing, but one study currently published by Agholme et al. paralyzed a single hind limb in rats with botulinum toxin to create a limb without mechanical loading. The rats then had screws drilled into their proximal tibias. Rats were then randomized to either receive anti-sclerostin antibody or placebo twice weekly for 4 weeks. At 4 weeks, the force necessary to pull out the screws was measured. Rats receiving anti-sclerostin antibody required higher pullout force to remove the screws than those receiving placebo [36]. In a recent study by Suen et al., rats with a femoral diaphyseal osteotomy received anti-sclerostin antibody or placebo for 3, 6, or 9 weeks. Those rats receiving the drug had a higher proportion of their callus mineralized earlier, with higher BMD as well as ultimate load on mechanical testing than those rats which did not receive the medication. Histology also demonstrated increased bone formation in treated animals [37].

Cathepsin K Inhibitors

Another novel treatment for osteoporosis under development utilizes the inhibition of the cathepsin K protease in the osteoclast that is necessary to dissolve the collagen component of the bone matrix during bone remodeling. Inhibition of cathepsin K pathways causes the osteoclast to detach from the bone, but not go through apoptosis or cell death. At the same time, bone formation rates by osteoblasts do not seem to be effected. Soung et al. reported a study of mouse femoral fractures with animals treated with cathepsin K inhibitor, the bisphosphonate alendronate, or placebo for 21 days. Both alendronate and the cathepsin K inhibitor delayed callus remodeling compared to the placebo group, but bone formation was similar between the cathepsin K inhibitor group and placebo group, while bone formation was decreased with alendronate. No mechanical testing was reported [38].

Discussion

The primary purpose of the treatment of osteoporosis is to prevent fragility fractures, as they are associated with high morbidity and mortality in older patients. Once a fracture occurs, there is substantial cost to the healthcare system and the economy, not to mention the cost to the individual and family in terms of pain, disability, and worsening of overall functional status. Since having a fragility fracture significantly increases an individual's risk of subsequent fragility fractures, it is essential to provide treatment for osteoporosis as soon as possible after fracture. It is also important to insure that these fractures heal in a timely manner in order to restore as much functional status in these patients as possible. Many patients sustain fractures while on anti-osteoporosis medications, while many others' first presentation of osteoporosis is at the time of a fragility fracture. It is important for the physician to recognize the effects these medications have on bone metabolism, particularly in the setting of fracture healing, in order to make an informed decision about which medications to prescribe, when to stop medications the patient is taking, and when to start or restart medications after a fragility fracture. This chapter aims to elucidate some of the research publications on this subject matter of anti-osteoporosis medications and their effects on fracture healing.

Of the medications we looked at in this chapter, none were shown to cause delayed healing of fractures, and the anabolic medications including PTH and anti-sclerostin antibody show some evidence supporting their role in potential acceleration of fracture healing. The one exception to this summary is that bisphosphonates may cause a delay in the healing of stress fractures and these medications may need to be stopped during the treatment of stress fractures. This is a very specific type of fracture that relies principally on remodeling to heal, and bisphosphonates have been shown to slow remodeling rates in bone.

Therefore, while these statements have not been definitively proven, we feel that it is safe to start anti-osteoporosis medications for patients as soon as possible after fracture. The possible exception to this is at least a 2-week delay in the administration of IV bisphosphonate, not because of an issue with fracture healing but because the osteoporosis and fracture prevention benefits of the medication are lost if it is administered within the first two weeks after fracture. At this time, there is a plethora of fracture healing data studying osteoporosis drugs in animal models but very limited clinical studies. It is clear that more data is needed for clinicians to best use these medication and to not fear their use in the setting of an acute fracture.

There are some promising new drugs that may hold the key to successfully accelerate the rate of fracture healing safely. Recombinant PTH has shown great success in building bone mineral and preventing fractures in patients with osteoporosis and in both animal models and human clinical trials has had success in accelerating healing. New medications such as anti-sclerostin antibody are still in the early stages of research and have not progressed to the point of clinical trials yet, but show promise in the early animal studies. There is certainly a lot of potential for this space of research, and with new and exciting medications lurking around the corner, the future of osteoporosis care and fracture healing intervention is bright.

References[1]

1. *Goldhahn J, Féron JM, Kanis J, Papapoulos S, Reginster JY, Rizzoli R, Dere W, Mitlak B, Tsouderos Y, Boonen S. Implications for fracture healing of current and new osteoporosis treatments: an ESCEO consensus paper. Calcif Tissue Int. 2012;90(5):343–53. *This is important as a consensus article from the European Society on Osteoporosis regarding a broad selection of osteoporosis medications.
2. *Larsson S, Fazzalari NL. Anti-osteoporosis therapy and fracture healing. Arch Orthop Trauma Surg. 2014;134(2):291–7. *This is important as a surgeon's perspective on fracture healing on osteoporosis medications.
3. Jørgensen NR, Schwarz PS. Effects of anti-osteoporosis medications on fracture healing. Curr Osteoporos Rep. 2011;9(3):149–55.

---

[1] *Important References

4. *Lyles KW, Colón-Emeric CS, Magaziner JS, Adachi JD, Pieper CF, Mautalen C, Hyldstrup L, Recknor C, Nordsletten L, Moore KA, Lavecchia C, Zhang J, Mesenbrink P, Hodgson PK, Abrams K, Orloff JJ, Horowitz Z, Eriksen EF, Boonen S, HORIZON Recurrent Fracture Trial. Zoledronic acid and clinical fractures and mortality after hip fracture. N Engl J Med. 2007;357(18):1799–809. *This is a seminal paper from a large well-run trial that garnered international attention.

5. Matos MA, Tannuri U, Guarniero R. The effect of zoledronate during bone healing. J Orthop Traumatol. 2010;11(1):7–12.

6. McDonald MM, Dulai S, Godfrey C, Amanat N, Sztynda T, Little DG. Bolus or weekly zoledronic acid administration does not delay endochondral fracture repair but weekly dosing enhances delays in hard callus remodeling. Bone. 2008;43(4):653–62.

7. *Colón-Emeric C, Nordsletten L, Olson S, Major N, Boonen S, Haentjens P, Mesenbrink P, Magaziner J, Adachi J, Lyles KW, Hyldstrup L, Bucci-Rechtweg C, Recknor C, HORIZON Recurrent Fracture Trial. Association between timing of zoledronic acid infusion and hip fracture healing. Osteoporos Int. 2011;22(8):2329–36. *Another seminal paper from a well-run trial that garnered attention and is influential in the timing of when IV bisphosphonates can safely be started.

8. Harding AK, W-Dahl A, Geijer M, Toksvig-Larsen S, Tägil M. A single bisphosphonate infusion does not accelerate fracture healing in high tibial osteotomies. Acta Orthop. 2011;82(4):465–70.

9. Munns CF, Rauch F, Zeitlin L, Fassier F, Glorieux FH. Delayed osteotomy but not fracture healing in pediatric osteogenesis imperfecta patients receiving pamidronate. J Bone Miner Res. 2004;19(11): 1779–86.

10. Pizones J, Plotkin H, Parra-Garcia JI, Alvarez P, Gutierrez P, Bueno A, Fernandez-Arroyo A. Bone healing in children with osteogenesis imperfecta treated with bisphosphonates. J Pediatr Orthop. 2005;25(3):332–5.

11. Amanat N, Brown R, Bilston LE, Little DG. A single systemic dose of pamidronate improves bone mineral content and accelerates restoration of strength in a rat model of fracture repair. J Orthop Res. 2005;23(5): 1029–34.

12. Madsen JE, Berg-Larsen T, Kirkeby OJ, Falch JA, Nordsletten L. No adverse effects of clodronate on fracture healing in rats. Acta Orthop Scand. 1998; 69(5):532–6.

13. Adolphson P, Abbaszadegan H, Bodén H, Salemyr M, Henriques T. Clodronate increases mineralization of callus after Colles' fracture: a randomized, double-blind, placebo-controlled, prospective trial in 32 patients. Acta Orthop Scand. 2000;71(2):195–200.

14. Gerstenfeld LC, Sacks DJ, Pelis M, Mason ZD, Graves DT, Barrero M, Ominsky MS, Kostenuik PJ, Morgan EF, Einhorn TA. Comparison of effects of the bisphosphonate alendronate versus the RANKL inhibitor denosumab on murine fracture healing. J Bone Miner Res. 2009;24(2):196–208.

15. Saito M, Shiraishi A, Ito M, Sakai S, Hayakawa N, Mihara M, Marumo K. Comparison of effects of alfacalcidol and alendronate on mechanical properties and bone collagen cross-links of callus in the fracture repair rat model. Bone. 2010;46(4):1170–9.

16. Fu LJ, Tang TT, Hao YQ, Dai KR. Long-term effects of alendronate on fracture healing and bone remodeling of femoral shaft in ovariectomized rats. Acta Pharmacol Sin. 2013;34(3):387–92.

17. Uchiyama S, Itsubo T, Nakamura K, Fujinaga Y, Sato N, Imaeda T, Kadoya M, Kato H. Effect of early administration of alendronate after surgery for distal radial fragility fracture on radiological fracture healing time. Bone Joint J. 2013;95-B(11):1544–50.

18. Rozental TD, Vazquez MA, Chacko AT, Ayogu N, Bouxsein ML. Comparison of radiographic fracture healing in the distal radius for patients on and off bisphosphonate therapy. J Hand Surg [Am]. 2009; 34(4):595–602.

19. *Gong HS, Song CH, Lee YH, Rhee SH, Lee HJ, Baek GH. Early initiation of bisphosphonate does not affect healing and outcomes of volar plate fixation of osteoporotic distal radial fractures. J Bone Joint Surg Am. 2012;94(19):1729–36. *This is a good paper from an orthopaedic surgeon's perspective showing that early treatment with bisphosphonates does not slow healing.

20. Kim TY, Ha YC, Kang BJ, Lee YK, Koo KH. Does early administration of bisphosphonate affect fracture healing in patients with intertrochanteric fractures? J Bone Joint Surg (Br). 2012;94(7):956–60.

21. Savaridas T, Wallace RJ, Salter DM, Simpson AH. Do bisphosphonates inhibit direct fracture healing?: a laboratory investigation using an animal model. Bone Joint J. 2013;95-B(9):1263–8.

22. Beil FT, Barvencik F, Gebauer M, Seitz S, Rueger JM, Ignatius A, Pogoda P, Schinke T, Amling M. Effects of estrogen on fracture healing in mice. J Trauma. 2010;69(5):1259–65.

23. Foster SA, Shi N, Curkendall S, Stock J, Chu BC, Burge R, Diakun DR, Krege JH. Fractures in women treated with raloxifene or alendronate: a retrospective database analysis. BMC Women's Health. 2013;13:15.

24. Stuermer EK, Sehmisch S, Rack T, Wenda E, Seidlova-Wuttke D, Tezval M, Wuttke W, Frosch KH, Stuermer KM. Estrogen and raloxifene improve metaphyseal fracture healing in the early phase of osteoporosis. A new fracture-healing model at the tibia in rat. Langenbecks Arch Surg. 2010; 395(2):163–72.

25. Spiro AS, Khadem S, Jeschke A, Marshall RP, Pogoda P, Ignatius A, Amling M, Beil FT. The SERM raloxifene improves diaphyseal fracture healing in mice. J Bone Miner Metab. 2013;31(6):629–36.

26. *Cummings SR, San Martin J, McClung MR, Siris ES, Eastell R, Reid IR, Delmas P, Zoog HB, Austin

M, Wang A, Kutilek S, Adami S, Zanchetta J, Libanati C, Siddhanti S, Christiansen C, FREEDOM Trial. Denosumab for prevention of fractures in postmenopausal women with osteoporosis. N Engl J Med. 2009;361(8):756–65. *This is a well-run trial that was published in NEJM showing the benefit of RANK-L inhibitors on the treatment of osteoporosis.

27. McCloskey EV, Johansson H, Oden A, Austin M, Siris E, Wang A, Lewiecki EM, Lorenc R, Libanati C, Kanis JA. Denosumab reduces the risk of osteoporotic fractures in postmenopausal women, particularly in those with moderate to high fracture risk as assessed with FRAX. J Bone Miner Res. 2012;27(7):1480–6.

28. *Adami S, Libanati C, Boonen S, Cummings SR, Ho PR, Wang A, Siris E, Lane J, FREEDOM Fracture-Healing Writing Group, Adachi JD, Bhandari M, de Gregorio L, Gilchrist N, Lyritis G, Möller G, Palacios S, Pavelka K, Heinrich R, Roux C, Uebelhart D. Denosumab treatment in postmenopausal women with osteoporosis does not interfere with fracture-healing: results from the FREEDOM trial. J Bone Joint Surg Am. 2012;94(23):2113–9. *This is another paper out of the large FREEDOM trial published in the orthopaedic literature that shows that the RANK-L inhibitors do not interfere with fracture healing.

29. Zhang D, Potty A, Vyas P, Lane J. The role of recombinant PTH in human fracture healing: a systematic review. J Orthop Trauma. 2014;28(1):57–62.

30. Andreassen TT, Fledelius C, Ejersted C, Oxlund H. Increases in callus formation and mechanical strength of healing fractures in old rats treated with parathyroid hormone. Acta Orthop Scand. 2001;72(3):304–7.

31. *Alkhiary YM, Gerstenfeld LC, Krall E, Westmore M, Sato M, Mitlak BH, Einhorn TA. Enhancement of experimental fracture-healing by systemic administration of recombinant human parathyroid hormone (PTH 1-34). J Bone Joint Surg Am. 2005;87(4):731–41. *This is a good study that shows, at least experimentally, that anabolic agents can accelerate the rate of fracture healing.

32. Manabe T, Mori S, Mashiba T, Kaji Y, Iwata K, Komatsubara S, Seki A, Sun YX, Yamamoto T. Human parathyroid hormone (1-34) accelerates natural fracture healing process in the femoral osteotomy model of cynomolgus monkeys. Bone. 2007;40(6):1475–82. Epub 2007 Feb 2.

33. *Aspenberg P, Genant HK, Johansson T, Nino AJ, See K, Krohn K, García-Hernández PA, Recknor CP, Einhorn TA, Dalsky GP, Mitlak BH, Fierlinger A, Lakshmanan MC. Teriparatide for acceleration of fracture repair in humans: a prospective, randomized, double-blind study of 102 postmenopausal women with distal radial fractures. J Bone Miner Res. 2010;25(2):404–14. *Similar to the Alkhiary study, this too shows that Teriparatide can accelerate fracture healing, this time in a human study.

34. *Aspenberg P, Johansson T. Teriparatide improves early callus formation in distal radial fractures. Acta Orthop. 2010;81(2):234–6. *This article is important as it shows how acceleration can occur, in this instance through the improvement in early callus formation.

35. Peichl P, Holzer LA, Maier R, Holzer G. Parathyroid hormone 1-84 accelerates fracture-healing in pubic bones of elderly osteoporotic women. J Bone Joint Surg Am. 2011;93(17):1583–7.

36. Agholme F, Isaksson H, Li X, Ke HZ, Aspenberg P. Anti-sclerostin antibody and mechanical loading appear to influence metaphyseal bone independently in rats. Acta Orthop. 2011;82(5):628–32.

37. Suen PK, He YX, Chow DH, Huang L, Li C, Ke HZ, Ominsky MS, Qin L. Sclerostin monoclonal antibody enhanced bone fracture healing in an open osteotomy model in rats. J Orthop Res. 2014;32(8):997–1005.

38. Soung DY, Gentile MA, Doung LT, Drissi H. Effects of pharmacological inhibition of cathepsin K on fracture repair in mice. Bone. 2013;55(1):248–55. Epub 2014 Feb 26.

Peter Vestergaard

Summary

- Overall, ART may not reduce mortality, as only a minor part of deaths can be attributed to fractures.
- Mortality reductions from fracture prevention may only be achieved in populations at high risk of both fractures and death.
- Besides the well-known breast cancer preventive effect of the selective estrogen receptor modulators (SERM), no general increase or decrease in the risk of cancer seems to exist for antiresorptive therapies.

Antiresorptive Therapy

This is by nature drugs which inhibit bone resorption and thus the osteoclasts, which leads to an increase in bone mineral density (BMD) and thus bone biomechanical competence resulting in a reduction in fracture risk.

P. Vestergaard, MD, PhD, Dr Med Sc (✉)
Department of Endocrinology, Aalborg University, Molleparkvej 4, Aalborg 9000, Denmark
e-mail: p-vest@post4.tele.dk

These drugs include:

1. Bisphosphonates [1, 2]
2. SERM [3]
3. Strontium ranelate [4]
4. Denosumab
5. Activated vitamin D [5, 6]

Some may also include calcium and vitamin D as these may lower parathyroid hormone (PTH) and thus indirectly lower osteoclast activity and are associated with an increase in BMD and a reduction in fracture risk [7]. These will not be considered here as they warrant special consideration and may not be considered true antiresorptive agents [8–10].

Estrogen and estrogen-like compounds [estrogen therapy (ET)] alone or combined with progestogen-like compounds [estrogen progesterone therapy (EPT)] also possess antiresorptive properties, increase BMD [11], and decrease fracture risk [12, 13]. However, these will not be considered in this chapter, as they are not first-line therapy for osteoporosis [14].

Bone anabolic agents such as teriparatide and other PTH analogues will also not be considered here. Also, the use of bisphosphonates to treat skeletal complications to malignancy will not be included here.

© Springer International Publishing Switzerland 2016
S.L. Silverman, B. Abrahamsen (eds.), *The Duration and Safety of Osteoporosis Treatment*, DOI 10.1007/978-3-319-23639-1_19

Mortality

Mortality may be affected by antiresorptive therapy (ART either directly or indirectly:

(a) Directly by interfering with major causes of mortality as was seen with the increase in cardiovascular events and breast cancer [15] with EPT
(b) Indirectly by reducing fracture risk and thus preventing the excess deaths associated with say hip fractures [16, 17]

A drug may thus have opposing effects on mortality by reducing fracture risk but increasing the risk of say cardiovascular events. Other more complex interactions may also be seen as say smoking may increase the risk of cancer and atherosclerosis and thus the risk of death, but smoking may also be associated with osteoporosis and fracture risk [18]. ART may thus by accident be associated with an adverse effect of the underlying disease being treated or a common risk factor such as smoking. Figure 19.1 shows an example on how smoking may be associated with both cardio-

vascular events and osteoporosis and how bisphosphonates by confounding by indication may be erroneously associated with say atrial fibrillation or other cardiovascular events or cancer.

In the industrialized world, the major causes of death are cardiovascular (including stroke) and cancer. Cancer will be described in a separate chapter below. A number of systematic searches were conducted using the PRISMA guidelines (http://www.prisma-statement.org/) for each of the ART categories (bisphosphonates, SERM, strontium ranelate, activated vitamin D) using the search term "mortality" or "cancer" and the drug in question. Extending the search to "survival" instead of mortality yielded more studies, but these were on cell lines. Studies on the use of these drugs to treat malignancy-related complications such as hypercalcemia or bone metastases [19] were excluded.

Bisphosphonates

A systematic search in PubMed using "bisphosphonates" and "mortality" per July 14, 2013 yielded 859 results.

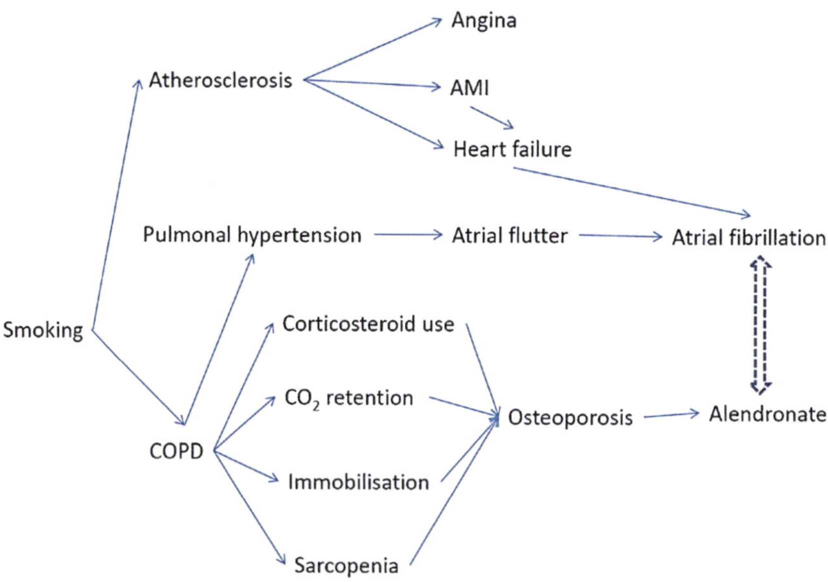

Fig. 19.1 Possible interactions between common causes of osteoporosis and fractures and cardiovascular events

Mortality in General in Users of Drugs against Osteoporosis

Bolland et al. performed a systematic review and meta-analysis of mortality in patients on drugs against osteoporosis [20]. The authors searched Medline and the Cochrane Central Register of Trials prior to September 2008, as well as the 2000–2008 American Society for Bone and Mineral Research conference abstracts.

Study Selection: Eligible studies were randomized placebo-controlled trials of approved doses of medications with proven efficacy in preventing both vertebral and non-vertebral fractures, in which the study duration was longer than 12 months and there were more than 10 deaths. Trials of estrogen and SERM were specifically excluded.

Data Extraction: Data were extracted from the text of the retrieved articles, published meta-analyses, or the Food and Drug Administration web site.

Data Synthesis: Eight eligible studies of four agents (risedronate, strontium ranelate, zoledronic acid, and denosumab) were included in the primary analysis. During two alendronate studies, the treatment dose changed, and those studies were only included in secondary analyses. In the primary analysis, treatment was associated with an 11 % reduction in mortality (relative risk, 0.89, 95 % confidence interval, 0.80–0.99, $p=0.036$). In the secondary analysis, the results were similar (relative risk, 0.90, 95 % confidence interval, 0.81–1.0, $p=0.044$). Mortality reduction was not related to age or incidence of hip or non-vertebral fracture, but was greatest in trials conducted in populations with higher mortality rates. However, this was the results of the combined drugs—for the individual bisphosphonates, no significant reduction was seen (alendronate, $n=2$ studies; risedronate, $n=2$ studies; and zoledronate, $n=2$ studies). See also the sections for the individual bisphosphonates below [20].

Prior to this meta-analysis, several studies were identified that were not included. Cree et al. [21] performed an observational study. This study examined post-fracture osteoporosis drug treatment in hip fracture patients and the association of treatment with mortality and morbidity. Pre- and post-fracture demographic/health information was collected on a cohort of hip fracture patients aged 65+ years. Post-fracture administrative data on prescription drug use and health-care utilization was linked to the cohort data. Five classes of osteoporosis drugs were available during the study period: hormone replacement therapy, bisphosphonates, calcitonin, SERM, and vitamin D. Pre-fracture, 38 of 449 patients (8 %) were on osteoporosis medications. Post-fracture, 81 of 356 patients (23 %) were treated, and 63 of these patients were untreated prior to fracture. Both treated and untreated patients had similar rates of subsequent hip fracture (6 % and 4 %, respectively) and Colles fracture (2 %). Regardless of treatment status, patients were also equally likely to be hospitalized, both in the short-term (28 % in treated, 27 % in untreated) and in the long-term (43 % vs. 37 %). However, mortality was significantly lower in the treated group (long-term, OR=0.34; 95 % CI: 0.17–0.70) [21]. These results, however, raise suspicion that "healthy drug user" effects may be in place. Those taking a drug may be healthier than those not adhering to a prescription. Steinbuch et al. [22] assessed mortality among users of risedronate enrolled in the North American Postmenopausal Osteoporosis Studies and reported no reduction in overall mortality (RR=0.89, 95 % CI: 0.73–1.09)—see also below under risedronate.

Subsequent to the meta-analysis [20], a number of trials have been published. Sharma et al. [23] analyzed the risk of serious atrial fibrillation but also analyzed cardiovascular mortality in a meta-analysis and found no such excess (OR=0.92, 95 % CI: 0.68–1.26). One study by Center et al. [24] using the Dubbo cohort (1223 women and 819 men aged 60+ years) reported that users of drugs against osteoporosis of whom there were 325 women (106 using bisphosphonates, 77 using hormone therapy, and 142 using calcium and vitamin D) and 37 men (15 on bisphosphonates, 22 on calcium and vitamin D) had a reduced risk of death compared to nonusers. In women, mortality rates were lower with bisphosphonates (0.8/100 person-years, 95 % CI: 0.4–1.4) and hormone therapy (1.2/100 person-years, 95 % CI: 0.7, 2.1) but not with calcium and vitamin D (3.2/100 person-years, 95 % CI: 2.5, 4.1) versus no treatment (3.5/100 person-years, 95 % CI: 3.1, 3.8) [24]. Accounting for age, fracture occurrence, comorbidities, quadriceps strength, and BMD, mortality risk remained lower for women on bisphosphonates [hazard ratio (HR) 0.3 (0.2, 0.6)] but not hormone therapy [HR 0.8 (0.4, 1.8)]. For the 429 women with fractures, mortality risk was still reduced in the bisphosphonate group [adjusted HR 0.3 (0.2, 0.7)], not accounted for by a reduction in subsequent fractures [24]. In men, lower mortality rates were observed with bisphosphonates but not calcium and vitamin D [BP 1.0/100 person-years (0.3, 3.9) and calcium and vitamin D 3.1/100 person-years (1.5, 6.6) versus no treatment 4.3/100 person-years (3.9, 4.8)] [24]. After adjustment, mortality was similar, although not significant [HR 0.5 (0.1, 2.0)] for men [24]. The main weakness of this study was the low number of treated especially among the men and the inability to adjust for adherence to the drugs. A study by Sambrook et al. [25] using frail elderly institutionalized subjects ($n=2005$) showed a reduction in overall mortality among the oral bisphosphonate users ($n=78$). Over 5 years of follow-up, 1596 participants (80 %) died. Use of bisphosphonates was associated with a 27 % reduction in risk of death compared to nonusers after adjusting for age, gender, type of institution, immobility, number of medications, weight, cognitive function, comorbidities, and hip fracture incidence during the follow-up period (hazard ratio 0.73, 95 % CI, 0.56–0.94, $p=0.02$) [25]. Again the main limitation was the low number and the inability to adjust for adherence to the drugs and the type of bisphosphonate.

Mortality related to cancer will be described below in the section on cancer.

Prevention of Mortality following a Hip Fracture

Patients with a hip fracture have a high risk of subsequent death and a significant excess risk compared to the background population [16].

A randomized controlled trial in patients with a hip fracture showed a reduction in mortality with zoledronic acid (HR = 0.72, 95 % CI: 0.56–0.93) [26]. A subgroup analysis of patients from the HORIZON trial also using zoledronic acid in men with a recent hip fracture showed a similar trend toward a reduction in mortality [32/255 (13.1 %) vs. 51/261 (19.5 %), OR = 0.62, 95 % CI: 0.38–1.00, $p=0.05$] but no reduction in cardiovascular events [27]. An observational study from Denmark showed that patients on bisphosphonates prior to a hip fracture had a reduced risk of death following the hip fracture compared to patients not on a bisphosphonate (OR, 0.68, 0.59–0.77) [28]. Also patients who began BP after the fracture (2.6 %) had significantly decreased mortality, both for patients who filled only one prescription (adjusted hazard ratio, HR 0.84, 0.73–0.95) and for patients who filled multiple prescriptions HR 0.73 (0.61–0.88) [28].

Myocardial Infarction and Cardiovascular Mortality

Some observational studies have suggested a reduced risk of myocardial infarction with the use of bisphosphonates in observational studies [29–31]. However, this was especially seen with high compliance [30]. The findings have to be confirmed from randomized controlled trials. Overall, no reduction in cardiovascular mortality was seen [22, 23].

Individual Bisphosphonates

Alendronate

A systematic search using "alendronate" and "mortality" produced 97 citations in PubMed. Two studies were included in the meta-analysis by Bolland et al. [20], the FIT trial by Black et al. [32] in postmenopausal women with prior spine fractures and the study by Cummings et al. [33] in postmenopausal women without spine fractures. None of the studies showed significant reductions in mortality, and the pooled estimate was 1.00, 95 % CI: 0.70–1.41 [20].

Clodronate

A systematic search using "clodronate" and "mortality" produced 105 citations in PubMed, but no studies fulfilled the inclusion criteria.

Etidronate

A systematic search using "etidronate" and "mortality" produced 64 citations, but no studies fulfilled the inclusion criteria.

Ibandronate

A systematic search using "ibandronate" and "mortality" produced 43 citations, but no studies fulfilled the inclusion criteria.

Pamidronate

A systematic search using "pamidronate" and "mortality" produced 101 citations, but no studies fulfilled the inclusion criteria.

Risedronate

A systematic search using "risedronate" and "mortality" produced 62 citations. Four studies reported on mortality, but these were partly overlapping.

The meta-analysis by Bolland et al. [20] included three RCTs, a study by Harris et al. [34] in postmenopausal women, a study by Reginster et al. [35] also including women, and a study by McClung et al. [36] including elderly women. The pooled estimate of the three trials was 0.88, 95 % CI: 0.70–1.10 for mortality with risedronate versus placebo. Besides the meta-analysis by Bolland et al. [20], Steinbuch et al. [22] studied 5303 patients exposed to either risedronate 2.5 or 5 mg daily and 2678 placebo-treated postmenopausal women included in the North American part of the risedronate registration studies. This study overlapped with the studies reported in the meta-analysis by Bolland et al. but also reported on causes of death. The study by Steinbuch et al. [22] did not find a reduction in overall (RR = 0.89, 95 % CI: 0.73–1.09), any cancer (0.89, 95 % CI: 0.59, 1.34), lung cancer (RR = 0.93, 95 % CI: 0.49–1.79), GI tract cancer (0.54, 95 % CI: 0.25–1.19), cardiovascular (0.54, 95 % CI: 0.25–1.19), coronary artery (1.15, 95 % CI: 0.72–1.84), stroke (0.50, 95 % CI: 0.29–0.88), or other cause mortality (0.97, 95 % CI: 0.66–1.42). Please also refer to the chapter on cancer below.

Zoledronate

A systematic search using "zoledronate" and "mortality" produced 224 citations and two original studies.

The meta-analysis by Bolland et al. [20] included both these studies, i.e., the study by Black et al. [37] and the study by Lyles et al. [26]. The combined estimate for mortality was 0.90, 95 % CI: 0.76–1.08. A number of subgroup analyses have been performed on the RCT of zoledronate following a hip fracture [26]. Eriksen et al. [38] performed a subgroup analyses by 2-week intervals of the time when the zoledronate infusion was administered after the hip fracture. For the times ≤2 weeks and 2–4 weeks after the hip fracture, no trend toward a reduction in mortality was seen [38]. For the time intervals 4–12 weeks, nonsignificant trends toward a reduction were seen, but the sample sizes were small, and from >12 weeks after the hip fracture, the risk reduction was statistically significant [38]. Upon pooling the results, patients treated >2 weeks following the hip fracture had a significant reduction in mortality, whereas those treated within two weeks did not. Patients dosed within 2 weeks were older and exhibited a higher baseline prevalence of hypertension, coronary artery disease, diabetes, atrial fibrillation, and stroke. These patients were also more likely to have come from an institutional setting before hospitalization for hip fracture and return to an institution after fracture compared with the subgroups dosed after the first 2 weeks [38]. Only 8 % of the reduction in mortality seemed attributable to the reduction of overall fracture risk after a hip fracture (tertiary prevention [39]) with zoledronic acid [40]. Other factors seemed to be reduced number of pneumonias and arrhythmias [40].

The excess risk of death following a hip fracture [16] is especially high within the first 6 months following the hip fracture owing to the frail nature of the patients sustaining hip fractures and the impact of the trauma. This may explain the absence of an effect of early administration of the drug in patients with a high general

Table 19.1 Potentially preventable deaths in percent of all deaths at different levels of absolute fracture risk and absolute risk of death, if the risk of death following a fracture is twice that of the background population and the fracture risk reduction is 50 %

	Absolute fracture risk %				
Absolute risk of death	3	5	10	15	20
5	1.5	2.4	4.5	6.5	8.3
10	1.5	2.4	4.5	6.5	8.3
15	1.5	2.4	4.5	6.5	8.3
20	1.5	2.4	4.5	6.5	8.3

At an absolute fracture risk of 20 % and an absolute risk of death of 20 % only 8.3 % of all deaths were potentially preventable at a death rate twice that of the background population among fracture patients. As can be seen, the proportion of deaths prevented is independent of the absolute risk of death (however, the absolute number of deaths potentially preventable increases)

risk of death not particularly attributable to modifiable causes. Patients with hip fractures are very likely to sustain recurrent hip fractures [41], and this may explain why some of the reduction in mortality is linked to the prevention of recurrent hip fractures and thus death from these. A theoretical computation may be performed using the numbers from the trial by Lyles et al. [26]. In the placebo group, 33/1062 sustained a second hip fracture within the 3-year study period (and were thus alive at the time of fracture), while 141 died. In the zoledronate arm of the trial, 23/1065 sustained a second hip fracture, and 101 died. If it is assumed that the mortality following a hip fracture is double that of the background population [16], then the preventable deaths by avoiding a second hip fracture are 2.1 % (see also Table 19.1; the higher estimate by Colon-Emeric et al. [40] was due to the inclusion of other fractures besides hip fractures). Thus, even highly effective fracture preventing agents may only reduce overall mortality slightly if the reduction should come from hip fracture prevention alone.

SERM

Raloxifene

A systematic search using the terms "raloxifene" and "mortality" produced 126 citations. Grady et al. [42] reported a pooled analysis of mortality data using two large clinical trials of raloxifene (60 mg/day) versus placebo, including the Multiple Outcomes of Raloxifene Evaluation/ Continuing Outcomes Relevant to Evista studies (7705 postmenopausal osteoporotic women followed for 4 years and a subset of 4011 participants followed for an additional 4 years, 110 deaths) and the Raloxifene Use for the Heart trial (10,101 postmenopausal women with coronary disease or multiple risk factors for coronary disease followed for 5.6 years, 1149 deaths). Cause of death was assessed by blinded adjudicators. Cox proportional hazards regression models compared mortality by treatment assignment in a pooled analysis of trial data from the Multiple Outcomes of Raloxifene Evaluation/Continuing Outcomes Relevant to Evista and Raloxifene Use for the Heart trials. All-cause mortality was 10 % lower among women assigned to raloxifene 60 mg/day versus placebo (HR 0.90, 95 % CI: 0.80–1.00, $p=0.05$). Lower overall mortality was primarily due to lower rates of non-cardiovascular deaths, especially a lower rate of non-cardiovascular, non-cancer deaths. This may be due to the fact that although raloxifene reduced breast cancer, this may be too rare an event for total mortality to be significantly decreased. However, it seems strange that a reduction was seen in non-cardiovascular, non-cancer deaths.

One epidemiological study [43] has suggested a potential excess of fatal strokes as have the Raloxifene Use for the Heart trial [44]. However, this could not be confirmed in another epidemiological study [45].

Bazedoxifene

One RCT in postmenopausal women reported no difference in mortality between bazedoxifene (17/1886 with 20 mg and 13/1872 with 40 mg), raloxifene (19/1849 with 60 mg), and placebo (11/1885) after 3 years [46].

Arzoxifene

One RCT in postmenopausal women reported no difference in mortality between arzoxifene (105/4676) and placebo (98/4678) [47].

Denosumab

A systematic search using "denosumab" and "mortality" yielded 61 citations, but only one included mortality data and was included in the meta-analysis by Bolland et al. [20]. The study by Cummings et al. [48] in postmenopausal women reported a RR for mortality of 0.78, 0.57–1.06 with denosumab versus placebo.

Strontium Ranelate

A systematic search in PubMed using the terms "strontium ranelate" and "mortality" yielded 24 citations. Two studies were identified as included in the meta-analysis by Bolland et al. [20], the study by Meunier et al. [49] mostly including older women and the study by Reginster et al. [50] also including postmenopausal women. The combined estimate for mortality with strontium ranelate versus placebo was 0.94, 95 % CI: 0.77–1.15 [20].

Activated Vitamin D

A systematic search in PubMed using the terms "activated vitamin D" and "mortality" yielded 54 citations, but only provided papers on the survival in end-stage renal failure patients.

Theoretical Considerations

It is possible to simulate the proportion of all deaths in a population that in theory could be prevented by reducing the number of fractures. If assumptions are made in actual death rates, fracture rates, and the increased risk of death following a fracture, the theoretical proportion of all deaths potentially preventable through fracture prevention can be computed.

One may consider an example: say 20 % of a population fractures within a given time interval, i.e., 20 out of 100 suffer a fracture, whereas 80 do not. Suppose that 10 % of the no fracture cases dies (eight subjects) within that time frame and 20 % of the fracture cases dies (four cases as 20 % of 20 is 4). In total $8 + 4 = 12$ or 12 % dies.

If fracture risk is reduced by 50 %, only 10 will fracture while 90 will not. With unchanged mortality rates, 10 % of 90 or 9 will die among the non-fracture cases, while 20 % of the 10 fracture cases or two subjects will die. In total, $9 + 2 = 11$ will thus die although fracture risk is reduced by 50 %. The total mortality is thus reduced by $1/12 = 8.25$ %. The relative risk of death thus is $11/12 = 0.92$.

Tables 19.1 and 19.2 show simulations of the percent of all deaths that could be avoided by preventing fractures at various levels of absolute fracture risk and risk of death. Even at high fracture risk and risk of death, only a minor fraction of total mortality could be prevented. As can be seen, the proportion of deaths prevented is independent of the absolute risk of death (however, the absolute number of deaths potentially preventable of cause increases). A mortality reduction may thus only be achieved with long-term treatment, and here adherence with ART over prolonged time intervals may be an issue [51].

In the studies that allowed evaluation of both mortality risk and risk of any fracture [26, 32, 33, 37, 47], the absolute risk of any fracture was 13 % in the placebo group, and the risk of death was 3 %, i.e., in theory 5.8 % of the deaths were preventable with a 50 % reduction in fracture risk and a doubling of mortality risk following a fracture. This would equal an RR of death of 0.94. If the scenario was altered to a 30 % reduction in fractures, 3.5 % of deaths could be prevented or an RR of 0.96. This is actually in the range observed by Bolland et al. for most drug categories [20]. Only in the study by Lyles et al. [26] was a reduction in the risk of death seen, but this

Table 19.2 Same scenario as in Table 19.1, but with a 70 % reduction in fracture risk

Absolute risk of death	Absolute fracture risk %				
	3	5	10	15	20
5	2.0	3.3	6.4	9.1	11.7
10	2.0	3.3	6.4	9.1	11.7
15	2.0	3.3	6.4	9.1	11.7
20	2.0	3.3	6.4	9.1	11.7

was also a study with a very high mortality rate (13 % in the placebo group) and a high fracture rate (13 % in the placebo group). The other studies may have high fracture rates, but had low mortality rates, i.e., there were few deaths to prevent. In the combined MORE/CORE study on raloxifene, a reduction in mortality was reported despite an absence in a reduction in overall fracture rates, but this may have been related to effects on other factors including cancer deaths (see below) [42]. Bolland et al. [20] suggested an 11 % reduction in mortality, the estimate being independent of hip and non-vertebral fracture rates, but higher at higher mortality rates [52]. This may be due to the fact that hip and vertebral fracture rates in general were low and the number of preventable fracture-related deaths thus low. Prevention of non-fracture-related deaths may be a possibility, but besides the raloxifene-related breast cancer deaths (which were not included in the meta-analysis by Bolland et al. [20]), none of the studies have pinpointed specific causes of death that were preventable by ART.

Conclusions

Overall ART may not reduce mortality, as only a minor part of deaths can be attributed to fractures. Mortality reductions from fracture prevention may only be achieved in populations at high risk of both fractures and death (i.e., typically the elderly and especially subjects with a prior hip fracture). Unless ART have effects on other causes of death, mortality reductions may thus not be seen. Studies to address the effects of dose and duration as well as adherence to ART and effects of ART on other causes of mortality are warranted. Almost no studies have included men as the majority has dealt with postmenopausal women.

Cancer Incidence

A number of the ART may also be used in oncology to treat bone-related events such as hypercalcemia and skeletal metastases (the bisphosphonates and denosumab) and to antagonize estrogen receptor-positive breast cancer (raloxifene and other SERMs such as tamoxifen). However, this is not the focus of this review, which will focus on the effects on cancer incidence by the drugs per se.

Calcitonin

A recent report including a meta-analysis has associated salmon calcitonin with an increased risk of cancer (http://www.fda.gov/downloads/ AdvisoryCommittees/CommitteesMeeting Materials/Drugs/ReproductiveHealthDrugs AdvisoryCommittee/UCM341781.pdf).

Also one of the RCT linked salmon calcitonin to an increased risk of cancer (OR = 1.62, 95 % CI: 1.00–2.61) [53]. Only long-term treatment was associated with an increased cancer risk, which may lend credibility to a true biological mechanism. However, no specific mechanism or subtype of cancer linked to salmon calcitonin has at present been revealed.

Two abstracts presented at the ASBMR 2012 [54] and 2013 [55] annual meeting did not support an increased risk of cancer with calcitonin. However, it should be noted under potential conflicts of interest that the authors were associated with a company that manufactures calcitonin.

A recent clinical trial suggested a possible increased risk of prostate cancer with oral calcitonin. There is no preclinical data that suggests an increased malignancy risk with calcitonin. However, although normal prostate cells do not express calcitonin or its receptor, both calcitonin and its receptor are expressed by some prostate cancer cells.

In a recent meta-analysis of all Novartis placebo-controlled clinical trials requested by the FDA, there was no increased incidence of malignancy relative to placebo in the first 6 months of treatment. The relative risk of malignancy over 36 months did increase relative to placebo. The risk of malignancy on calcitonin over the first 6-month time period remained relatively constant over 36 months. However, a decrease in placebo risk was seen after the first 6 months. The malignancies seen were not of any specific type and were of different cellular origins. There was no evidence of a higher incidence rate with increasing dose. Based on these findings of increased malignancy risk, the FDA has recently recommended in the United States the use of calcitonin only for 6 months. Calcitonin is no longer approved by the European Medicines Agency for the treatment of osteoporosis.

Bisphosphonates

Several studies have been performed, mainly observational trials and case reports, some linking oral bisphosphonates to esophageal cancer. A systematic search using PubMed and the terms "bisphosphonates" and "cancer" produced 7027 citations, the majority linked to treatment of cancer.

Gastrointestinal Cancers with Bisphosphonates

Esophagus

A systematic search using the terms "bisphosphonates," "cancer," and "esophageal" yielded 71 citations, all observational trials. Several meta-analyses were available.

A meta-analysis spanning the years until January 2011 by Oh et al. was present including three cohort and three case–control studies [56]. For esophageal cancer, it included five studies and reported no overall trend in the risk of esophageal cancer (RR=0.96, 95 % CI: 0.65–1.42) [56]. A meta-analysis spanning the years until May 2011 by Sun et al. [57] included seven observational trials, but was only partly overlapping with Oh et al. [56], as the study by Solomon et al. [58] was included in the Oh paper [56], but not the Sun paper [57]. Neither for cohort (OR=1.23, 95 % CI: 0.79–1.92) nor for case–control (1.24, 0.98–1.57) studies did the Sun paper find any evidence for an increased risk of esophageal cancer [57]. The Sun paper performed a subgroup analysis for alendronate and did not report any excess risk of esophageal cancer with this drug [57].

A subsequent case–control study using the CPRD and QResearch databases by Vinogradova et al. did not find any excess risk of esophageal cancer with bisphosphonates—adjusted odds ratios (95 % confidence interval) for QResearch and CPRD were 0.97 (0.79–1.18) and 1.18 (0.97–1.43) for esophageal cancer [59].

Additional analyses showed no difference between types of bisphosphonates for risk of esophageal cancers [59]. However, Wright et al. [60] using some of the same data as the study just mentioned reported a slight increase in the risk of esophageal cancers for women (1.54, 95 % CI: 1.27–1.88) but not for men (0.78, 95 % CI: 0.56–1.09). A further study by Lee et al. could not confirm an increased risk of esophageal cancer with alendronate [61]. A cohort study [62] included in the meta-analyses only showed an increased risk of esophageal cancer with alendronate use for less than 2 years and only in those with low adherence, whereas for etidronate an increased risk was seen for more than 5 years of use with a high adherence [63].

A large-scale Danish register-based study actually reported a lower incidence and mortality of esophageal cancer with alendronate [64]. This study suggested that use of endoscopy prior to initiation of alendronate could be an explanation for the lower rates.

The mechanism for the seemingly increased risk for alendronate may thus have been that alendronate may cause GI discomfort, which may lead to discontinuation of alendronate (hence, the reduced adherence) and subsequently an endoscopy which may then reveal a cancer, i.e., a form of Berkson bias.

In general, it seems that no causal relationship exists between bisphosphonate use and risk of esophageal cancer. However, it must be remembered that few studies had long-term exposure data.

Gastric Cancer

In contrast to esophageal cancer, almost all studies agree that no excess risk of gastric cancer is seen with bisphosphonates. Wright et al. using the GPRD found no excess risk of gastric cancer (1.06, 95 % CI: 0.83–1.37 in women and 0.87, 95 % CI: 0.55–1.36 in men) [60]. Vinogradova et al. [59] reported no overall association

(OR = 1.12, 95 % CI: 0.87–1.44, and 0.79, 95 % CI: 0.62–1.01) for gastric cancers. For gastric cancer, alendronate use was associated with an increased risk (1.47, 95 % CI: 1.11–1.95), but only in data from the QResearch database and without any association with duration and with no definitive confirmation from sensitivity analysis [59]. Oh et al., also in their meta-analysis including three studies, did not observe an association with gastric cancer (OR = 0.89, 95 % CI: 0.71–1.13). An additional cohort study [63] reported on increase in gastric cancers with alendronate (HR = 1.16, 95 % CI: 0.54–2.53), but an increase with etidronate (HR = 1.57, 95 % CI: 1.01–2.43). However, no time or dose relationship was present for etidronate.

In general, no excess risk of gastric cancers seems present lending support to an absence of an association with esophageal cancers. However, again few studies had long-term exposure data.

Colon Cancer

Oh et al. in their meta-analysis [55], including two studies, found no excess risk of colon cancer (OR = 0.62, 95 % CI: 0.30–1.29). Vinogradova et al. [59] in their study also found no association with colon cancer (OR = 1.03, 95 % CI: 0.94–1.14 for QResearch, and 1.10, 95 % CI: 1.00–1.22 for CPRD). One additional cohort study analyzed the association between bisphosphonates and colon cancer and found no overall association with alendronate or etidronate [63].

An observational study by Pazianas et al. [65] found that the overall risk of dying from colon cancer was significantly lower in the alendronate-treated cohort than in control subjects despite the greater comorbidity in alendronate-treated patients. Thus, within the observation period, 0.6 % of alendronate-treated women died of colon cancer compared with 0.7 % of control subjects. Cox survival analysis showed a crude HR of 0.69 (0.59–0.81) with an adjusted HR of 0.62 (0.52–0.72).

In general, no association between bisphosphonates and colon cancer seems present. However, duration of follow-up was limited in most studies.

Other GI Tract Cancers

One cohort study examined the association between bisphosphonates and pancreas, bile duct, liver, and small intestinal cancers [63]. Bile duct and small intestinal cancers were not associated with bisphosphonate use, whereas for liver cancer an increased risk was seen for both alendronate (HR = 2.55, 95 % CI: 1.10–5.89) and etidronate (HR = 2.14, 95 % CI: 1.23–3.71) [63]. For pancreas cancer, an association with etidronate (HR = 1.73, 95 % CI: 1.30–2.31) was observed, whereas no such association could be found for alendronate (HR = 1.36, 95 % CI: 0.81–2.29) [63]. For liver cancer, the association with alendronate was only seen with low adherence, whereas for etidronate it was only seen with high adherence, and no particular time trend was present for either drug [63].

Due to the absence of dose and time dependency, an association between bisphosphonates and other GI cancers seems unlikely; however, scare data are available, and further studies are warranted.

Other Cancers and Bisphosphonates

Besides breast cancer, little data are available on other cancer types, and more studies are needed. Some preclinical studies have indicated a potential beneficial effect on breast cancer cells by bisphosphonates [66–68]. One cohort study [69] reported that before the drugs against osteoporosis were started, an excess prevalence of breast cancer was present [69]. This probably stems from the fact that treatments for breast cancer with say aromatase inhibitors increase the risk of fractures [70] and osteoporosis and thus being prescribed drugs against osteoporosis. After correction for this factor, fewer cases of breast cancer were observed after initiation of alendronate (HR = 0.53, 95 % CI 0.38–0.73) or etidronate (HR = 0.80, 95 % CI 0.73–0.89) [69]. However, no dose–response or time effect was observed.

In conclusion, it is uncertain if bisphosphonates may prevent breast cancer if used to treat osteoporosis in women. Further studies are needed.

SERM

Breast Cancer

Several trials involving SERMs have shown a reduction in breast cancer (estrogen receptor-positive breast cancer). This has been shown for raloxifene [44] (HR=0.67, 95 % CI: 0.47–0.96) [71], (RR=0.24, 95 % CI: 0.13–0.44), [72] (HR=0.34, 95 % CI: 0.22–0.50)—which is the most well-documented although several of the trials mentioned overlap—as well as for arzoxifene (HR 0.44, 95 % CI: 0.26–0.76) [47]. For bazedoxifene [46], a nonsignificant trend toward a reduction in breast cancer risk has been observed (9/3758 with 20 or 40 mg bazedoxifene vs. 8/1885—OR=0.56, 95 % CI: 0.22–1.44). A further cohort study showed a reduction in breast cancer with raloxifene for osteoporosis prevention (HR=0.54, 95 % CI: 0.39–0.76) with a strong dose–response relationship (HR=0.14, 95 % CI: 0.03–0.55 with full compliance) [69]. The preventive effect was most pronounced the first 5 years following initiation of raloxifene and was more pronounced in older compared to younger (<50 years) women. A cohort study comparing women aged 45 years or more starting alendronate or raloxifene showed a reduction in breast cancer incidence in women on raloxifene compared to alendronate users [73].

The effects of SERM on breast cancer are thus a natural extension of their estrogen receptor antagonistic properties as for tamoxifen [74].

Other Cancers

A cohort study showed no effect of raloxifene on gastrointestinal cancers [63]. For other cancers, the evidence is scarce except for an absence of an effect on endometrial cancers with raloxifene [71] (HR=0.8, 95 % CI: 0.2–0.7), bazedoxifene [46], and arzoxifene [47]. No overall change in cancer mortality was seen with raloxifene [42]. More studies may thus be warranted.

Denosumab

No excess risk of cancers was reported in the FREEDOM trial [48].

Strontium Ranelate

A systematic search using the terms "strontium ranelate" and "cancer" yielded 18 citations, none of which were clinical trials. None of the original RTCs on strontium [49, 50] specifically reported on cancer incidence. More research is thus needed.

Activated Vitamin D

Vitamin D holds a special position with respect to cancer [75], as activated vitamin D may suppress growth stimulatory signals and potentiate growth inhibitory signals, which lead to changes in cell cycle regulators [76, 77]. A systematic search using the terms "activated vitamin d" and "cancer" yielded 348 citations. However, these were mainly preclinical studies, and none were designed to look at the effects of activated vitamin D for osteoporosis prevention and risk of cancer.

Conclusions

Besides the well-known breast cancer preventive effect of the SERMs, no general increase or decrease in the risk of cancer seems to exist for ART.

References[1]

1. Wells GA, Cranney A, Peterson J et al. Alendronate for the primary and secondary prevention of osteoporotic fractures in postmenopausal women. Cochrane Database Syst Rev. 2008;CD001155.
2. Wells G, Cranney A, Peterson J et al. Risedronate for the primary and secondary prevention of osteoporotic fractures in postmenopausal women. Cochrane Database Syst Rev. 2008;CD004523.
3. Seeman E, Crans G, Diez-Perez A, et al. Antivertebral fracture efficacy of raloxifene: a meta-analysis. Osteoporos Int. 2006;17:313–6.

---

[1] *Important References
**Very important References

4. O'Donnell S, Cranney A, Wells G et al. Strontium ranelate for preventing and treating postmenopausal osteoporosis. Cochrane Database Syst Rev. 2006; CD005326.

5. Richy F, Schacht E, Bruyere O, et al. Vitamin D analogs versus native vitamin d in preventing bone loss and osteoporosis-related fractures: a comparative meta-analysis. Calcif Tissue Int. 2005;76:176–86.

6. Avenell A, Gillespie W, Gillespie L et al. Vitamin D and vitamin D analogues for preventing fractures associated with involutional and post-menopausal osteoporosis (Review). Cochrane Database Syst Rev. 2005;CD000227.

7. Tang BM, Eslick GD, Nowson C, et al. Use of calcium or calcium in combination with vitamin D supplementation to prevent fractures and bone loss in people aged 50 years and older: a meta-analysis. Lancet. 2007;370:657–66.

8. Bolland MJ, Barber PA, Doughty RN, et al. Vascular events in healthy older women receiving calcium supplementation: randomised controlled trial. BMJ. 2008;336:262–6.

9. Bolland MJ, Avenell A, Baron JA, et al. Effect of calcium supplements on risk of myocardial infarction and cardiovascular events: meta-analysis. BMJ. 2010;341:c3691.

10. Bolland MJ, Grey A, Avenell A, et al. Calcium supplements with or without vitamin D and risk of cardiovascular events: reanalysis of the Women's Health Initiative limited access dataset and meta-analysis. BMJ. 2011;342:d2040.

11. Wells G, Tugwell P, Shea B, et al. Meta-analysis of the efficacy of hormone replacement therapy in treating and preventing osteoporosis in postmenopausal women. Endocr Rev. 2002;23:529–39.

12. Torgerson D, Bell-Syer S. Hormone replacement therapy and prevention of nonvertebral fractures. A meta-analysis of randomized trials. JAMA. 2001;285:2891–7.

13. Torgerson D, Bell-Syer S. Hormone replacement therapy and prevention of vertebral fractures: a meta-analysis of randomised trials. BMC Musculoskelet Disord. 2001;2:7–10.

14. EMEA. EMEA public statement on recent publications regarding hormone replacement therapy. http://www.emea.eu.int/pdfs/human/press/pus/3306503en.pdf

15. Risks and benefits of estrogen plus progestin in healthy postmenopausal women: principal results from the Women's Health Initiative randomized controlled trial. JAMA. 2002;288:321–333.

16. Vestergaard P, Rejnmark L, Mosekilde L. Increased mortality in patients with a hip fracture-effect of pre-morbid conditions and post-fracture complications. Osteoporos Int. 2007;18:1583–93.

17. Vestergaard P, Rejnmark L, Mosekilde L. Loss of life years after a hip fracture. Acta Orthop. 2009;80:525–30.

18. Vestergaard P, Mosekilde L. Fracture risk associated with smoking – a meta-analysis. J Intern Med. 2003;254:572–83.

19. Coleman R, Gnant M, Morgan G, et al. Effects of bone-targeted agents on cancer progression and mortality. J Natl Cancer Inst. 2012;104:1059–67.

20. **Bolland MJ, Grey AB, Gamble GD, et al. Effect of osteoporosis treatment on Mortality, ART: a meta-analysis. J Clin Endocrinol Metab. 2010;95:1174–81. ** Pivotal study on mortality and effects of therapy for osteoporosis in mortality.

21. Cree MW, Juby AG, Carriere KC. Mortality and morbidity associated with osteoporosis drug treatment following hip fracture. Osteoporos Int. 2003;14:722–7.

22. Steinbuch M, D'Agostino RB, Mandel JS, et al. Assessment of mortality in patients enrolled in a risedronate clinical trial program: a retrospective cohort study. Regul Toxicol Pharmacol. 2002;35:320–6.

23. Sharma A, Chatterjee S, Arbab-Zadeh A, et al. Risk of serious atrial fibrillation and stroke with use of bisphosphonates: evidence from a meta-analysis. Chest. 2013;144(4):1311–22.

24. *Center JR, Bliuc D, Nguyen ND, et al. Osteoporosis medication and reduced mortality risk in elderly women and men. J Clin Endocrinol Metab. 2011;96:1006–14. *Observational study on mortality reduction with drugs for osteoporosis.

25. *Sambrook PN, Cameron ID, Chen JS, et al. Oral bisphosphonates are associated with reduced mortality in frail older people: a prospective five-year study. Osteoporos Int. 2011;22:2551–6. *Observational study on mortality with use of bisphosphonates. Deals with all types, and does not separate the types of bisphosphonates.

26. **Lyles KW, Colón-Emeric CS, Magaziner JS, et al. Zoledronic acid and clinical fractures and mortality after hip fracture. N Engl J Med. 2007;357:1799–809. **Large scale randomized controlled trial. This is a pivotal study demonstrating mortality reduction with zoledronic acid after a hip fracture.

27. Boonen S, Orwoll E, Magaziner J, et al. Once-yearly zoledronic acid in older men compared with women with recent hip fracture. J Am Geriatr Soc. 2011;59:2084–90.

28. Bondo L, Eiken P, Abrahamsen B. Analysis of the association between bisphosphonate treatment survival in Danish hip fracture patients-a nationwide register-based open cohort study. Osteoporos Int. 2013;24:245–52.

29. Wolfe F, Bolster MB, O'Connor CM, et al. Bisphosphonate use is associated with reduced risk of myocardial infarction in patients with rheumatoid arthritis. J Bone Miner Res. 2013;28:984–91.

30. Vestergaard P. Acute myocardial infarction and atherosclerosis of the coronary arteries in patients treated with drugs against osteoporosis: calcium in the vessels and not the bones? Calcif Tissue Int. 2012;90:22–9.

31. Kang J, Keller JJ, Lin H. Bisphosphonates reduced the risk of acute myocardial infarction: a 2-year follow-up study. Osteoporos Int. 2013;24:271–7.

32. Black D, Cummings S, Karpf D, et al. Randomised trial of the effect of alendronate on risk of fracture in

women with existing vertebral fractures. Lancet. 1996;348:1535–41.

33. Cummings S, Black D, Thompson D, et al. Effect of alendronate on risk of fracture in women with low bone density but without vertebral fractures: results from the fracture intervention trial. JAMA. 1998;280: 2077–82.

34. Harris S, Watts N, Genant H, et al. Effects of risedronate treatment on vertebral and nonvertebral fractures in women with postmenopausal osteoporosis: a randomized controlled trial. JAMA. 1999;282:1344–52.

35. Reginster J, Minne H, Sorensen O, et al. Randomized trial of the effects of risedronate on vertebral fractures in women with established postmenopausal osteoporosis. Osteoporos Int. 2000;11:83–91.

36. McClung M, Geusens P, Miller P, et al. Effect of risedronate on the risk of hip fracture in elderly women. Hip intervention program study group. N Engl J Med. 2001;344:333–40.

37. Black D, Delmas P, Eastell R, et al. Once-yearly zoledronic acid for treatment of postmenopausal osteoporosis. N Engl J Med. 2007;356:1809–22.

38. Eriksen EF, Lyles KW, Colón-Emeric CS, et al. Antifracture efficacy and reduction of mortality in relation to timing of the first dose of zoledronic acid after hip fracture. J Bone Miner Res. 2009;24: 1308–13.

39. Vestergaard P. Antiresorptive therapy for the prevention of postmenopausal osteoporosis: when should treatment begin? Womens Health. 2007;18:13–6.

40. *Colón-Emeric CS, Mesenbrink P, Lyles KW, et al. Potential mediators of the mortality reduction with zoledronic acid after hip fracture. J Bone Miner Res. 2010;25:91–7. *This is a key study on potential mechanisms behind the reduction in mortality. It investigates the potential mechanisms behind the reduction in mortality with zoledronic acid.

41. Ryg J, Rejnmark L, Overgaard S, et al. Hip fracture patients at risk of second hip fracture: a nationwide population-based cohort study of 169,145 cases during 1977–2001. J Bone Miner Res. 2009;24: 1299–307.

42. Grady D, Cauley JA, Stock JL, et al. Effect of raloxifene on all-cause mortality. Am J Med. 2010;123:469. e1–7.

43. Urushihara H, Kikuchi N, Yamada M, et al. Raloxifene and stroke risks in Japanese postmenopausal women with osteoporosis on postmarketing surveillance. Menopause. 2009;16:971–7.

44. Barrett-Connor E, Mosca L, Collins P, et al. Effects of raloxifene on cardiovascular events and breast cancer in postmenopausal women. N Engl J Med. 2006;355:125–37.

45. Vestergaard P, Schwartz K, Pinholt EM, et al. Stroke in relation to use of raloxifene and other drugs against osteoporosis. Osteoporos Int. 2011;22:1037–45.

46. Silverman S, Christiansen C, Genant H, et al. Efficacy of bazedoxifene in reducing new vertebral fracture risk in postmenopausal women with osteoporosis: results from a 3-year, randomized, placebo-, and active-controlled clinical trial. J Bone Miner Res. 2008;23:1923–34.

47. Cummings SR, McClung M, Reginster J, et al. Arzoxifene for prevention of fractures and invasive breast cancer in postmenopausal women. J Bone Miner Res. 2011;26:397–404.

48. Cummings SR, San Martin J, McClung MR, et al. Denosumab for prevention of fractures in postmenopausal women with osteoporosis. N Engl J Med. 2009;361:756–65.

49. Meunier P, Roux C, Seeman E, et al. The effects of strontium ranelate on the risk of vertebral fracture in women with postmenopausal osteoporosis. N Engl J Med. 2004;350:459–68.

50. Reginster J, Seeman E, de Vernejoul M, et al. Strontium ranelate reduces the risk of nonvertebral fractures in postmenopausal women with osteoporosis: Treatment of peripheral osteoporosis (TROPOS) study. J Clin Endocrinol Metab. 2005;90:2816–22.

51. Vieira HP, Leite IA, Araújo Sampaio TM, et al. Bisphosphonates adherence for treatment of osteoporosis. Int Arch Med. 2013;6:24.

52. Grey A, Bolland MJ. The effect of treatments for osteoporosis on mortality. Osteoporos Int. 2013; 24:1–6.

53. Chesnut III C, Silverman S, Andriano K, et al. A randomized trial of nasal spray salmon calcitonin in postmenopausal women with established osteoporosis: the prevent recurrence of osteoporotic fractures study. PROOF study group. Am J Med. 2000;109:267–76.

54. Krause D, Hernandez NAS, Vitagliano M, Gilligan J, Buben C. One year use of oral recombinant salmon calcitonin is not associated with increased risk of cancer. ASBMR 2012 annual meeting. presentation number. JBMR. 2012, abstract LB-MO17. Available at: http://www.asbmr.org/Meetings/AnnualMeeting/AbstractDetail.aspx?aid=15a40a6c-4dd3-4827-bf70-07a3cda03a2e

55. Wells G, Krause D, Chernoff J, Gilligan J. Does calcitonin-salmon cause cancer? ASBMR 2013 Annual Meeting. Presentation. J Bone Miner Res. 2013;28 Suppl 1:FR0401. Available at: http://www.asbmr.org/ItineraryBuilder/PresentationDetail.aspx?pid=869976b0-fe31-4bc3-b4a8-eac74c2ad478&ptag=WebItinerarySearch

56. Oh YH, Yoon C, Park SM. Bisphosphonate use and gastrointestinal tract cancer risk: meta-analysis of observational studies. World J Gastroenterol. 2012;18: 5779–88.

57. Sun K, Liu JM, Sun HX, et al. Bisphosphonate treatment and risk of esophageal cancer: a meta-analysis of observational studies. Osteoporos Int. 2013;24:279–86.

58. Solomon DH, Patrick A, Brookhart MA. More on reports of esophageal cancer with oral bisphosphonate use. N Engl J Med. 2009;360:1789–90. Author reply 1791–2.

59. Vinogradova Y, Coupland C, Hippisley-Cox J. Exposure to bisphosphonates and risk of gastrointestinal cancers: series of nested case-control studies with QResearch and CPRD data. BMJ. 2013;346:f114.

60. Wright E, Schofield PT, Seed P, et al. Bisphosphonates and risk of upper gastrointestinal cancer—a case control study using the general practice research database (GPRD). PLoS One. 2012;7, e47616.

61. Lee W, Sun L, Lin M, et al. A higher dosage of oral alendronate will increase the subsequent cancer risk of osteoporosis patients in Taiwan: a population-based cohort study. PLoS One. 2012;7, e53032.

62. Vestergaard P, Schwartz K, Pinholt EM, et al. Gastric and esophagus events before and during treatment of osteoporosis. Calcif Tissue Int. 2010;86:110–5.

63. Vestergaard P. Occurrence of gastrointestinal cancer in users of bisphosphonates and other antiresorptive drugs against osteoporosis. Calcif Tissue Int. 2011;89:434–41.

64. Abrahamsen B, Pazianas M, Eiken P, Russell R, Graham G, Eastell R. Esophageal and gastric cancer incidence and mortality in alendronate users. J Bone Miner Res. 2012;27(3):679–86.

65. Pazianas M, Abrahamsen B, Eiken PA, Eastell R, Russell R, Graham G. Reduced colon cancer incidence and mortality in postmenopausal women treated with an oral bisphosphonate—Danish national register based cohort study. Osteoporos Int. 2012; 23(11):2693–701.

66. Chlebowski R, Chen Z, Cauley J et al. Oral bisphosphonates and breast cancer: prospective results from the Women's health initiative (WHI) (Presented at the 32nd annual San Antonio breast cancer symposium 2009). Cancer Res. 2009; 69 Suppl 1.

67. Rennert G, Pinchev M, Rennert H. Use of bisphosphonates and risk of postmenopausal breast cancer (Presented at the 32nd annual San Antonio breast cancer symposium 2009). Cancer Res. 2009;69 Suppl 1.

68. Brufsky A, Bundred N, Coleman R, et al. Integrated analysis of zoledronic acid for prevention of aromatase inhibitor-associated bone loss in postmenopausal women with early breast cancer receiving adjuvant letrozole. Oncologist. 2008;13:503–14.

69. Vestergaard P, Fischer L, Mele M, et al. Use of bisphosphonates and risk of breast cancer. Calcif Tissue Int. 2011;88:255–62.

70. Vestergaard P, Rejnmark L, Mosekilde L. Effect of tamoxifen and aromatase inhibitors on the risk of fractures in women with breast cancer. Calcif Tissue Int. 2008;82:334–40.

71. Cummings S, Eckert S, Krueger K, et al. The effect of raloxifene on risk of breast cancer in postmenopausal women: results from the MORE randomized trial. Multiple outcomes of raloxifene evaluation. JAMA. 1999;281:2189–97.

72. Martino S, Cauley J, Barrett-Connor E, et al. Continuing outcomes relevant to Evista: breast cancer incidence in postmenopausal osteoporotic women in a randomized trial of raloxifene. J Natl Cancer Inst. 2004;96:1751–61.

73. Foster SA, Shi N, Curkendall S, et al. Fractures in women treated with raloxifene or alendronate: a retrospective database analysis. BMC Womens Health. 2013;13:15.

74. Vogel V, Costantino J, Wickerham D, et al. Effects of tamoxifen vs raloxifene on the risk of developing invasive breast cancer and other disease outcomes: the NSABP study of tamoxifen and raloxifene (STAR) P-2 trial. JAMA. 2006;295:2727–41.

75. Gissel T, Rejnmark L, Mosekilde L, et al. Intake of vitamin D and risk of breast cancer—a meta-analysis. J Steroid Biochem Mol Biol. 2008;111:195–9.

76. Colston K, Hansen C. Mechanisms implicated in the growth regulatory effects of vitamin D in breast cancer. Endocr Relat Cancer. 2002;9:45–59.

77. Wu-Wong J, Tian J, Goltzman D. Vitamin D analogs as therapeutic agents: a clinical study update. Curr Opin Investig Drugs. 2004;5(3):320–6.

Other Safety Concerns

20

Michael R. McClung

Summary

- Safety cannot be proven in a clinical trial since only common side effects can be observed.
- Most information about drug safety comes from post-marketing surveillance or observational studies or from astute clinicians who recognize a pattern of concern.
- The few serious risks known to be associated with osteoporosis drugs occur very infrequently and, with exception of atypical fractures with bisphosphonates, are usually not related to duration of therapy.
- Being aware of possible safety concerns, therapy for osteoporosis can be individualized to minimize the potential side effects and thereby optimize the balance of risks and benefits.

Regulatory approval of osteoporosis drugs has been based on placebo-controlled trials, usually lasting 3 years but never more than 5 years. The largest clinical registration trials published to date (HORIZON and FREEDOM) were each comprised of less than 12,000 patient-years of follow-up on active treatment versus placebo [1, 2]. These pivotal studies are primarily designed to evaluate efficacy (fracture risk reduction). Safety issues are evaluated by comparing the incidence of clinical and laboratory adverse events between treatment and placebo groups. More recent studies have established prospective plans to evaluate adverse events of special interest.

Because of the size and duration of the studies, only a common adverse event could be clearly identified in such trials, and very few serious safety issues have been observed in the pivotal placebo-controlled osteoporosis studies. On the other hand, statistical differences in specific, uncommon adverse events may be observed by chance, making attribution of an adverse event to the drug treatment especially difficult unless the same adverse event is identified in more than one trial, is related to duration of therapy, and/or has a very strong plausible mechanism of causality [3].

Many of the pivotal trials have been extended beyond the required 3 years, putatively to gain further information about safety. However, for ethical reasons, patients in these extension trials almost always receive active treatment or they are followed after they discontinue active therapy. This results in the loss of an adequate control group, further limiting safety assessment. Attempts to compare adverse events between patients on continuous treatment and those originally treated with placebo are often seriously compromised by the large and possibly differential dropout that occurs as research patients are required to re-consent to enter the extension phase

M.R. McClung, MD (✉)
Oregon Osteoporosis Center, 25 NW 23rd Place,
Suite 6 #175, Portland, OR 97210, USA
e-mail: mmcclung@orost.com

© Springer International Publishing Switzerland 2016
S.L. Silverman, B. Abrahamsen (eds.), *The Duration and Safety of Osteoporosis Treatment*, DOI 10.1007/978-3-319-23639-1_20

of the study. Furthermore, differential dropout may impair the effectiveness of randomization, due to exclusion from the extension of patients who have experienced significant bone loss or fracture during the main phase of the study, resulting in differential dropout between the active and control treatment arms. Few true safety issues have been identified in these extension studies.

Most safety concerns not apparent in clinical trials have been identified as a result of post-marketing surveillance reports, small case report series, or observational studies. Substantial limitations exist in the ability to each of these strategies to unequivocally identify a specific adverse event as being due to the drug.

Upon that background, this review will focus on common and/or serious adverse events and benefits possibly associated with drugs currently approved for osteoporosis treatment in Europe and North America. Given the uncertainty about the incidence of many of these safety concerns or even the causal relationship between the drug and the safety concern, it is very important to keep the overall risk–benefit profile of treatment in perspective [4]. This important issue has been the subject of recent reviews [5–7].

Bisphosphonates

The four nitrogen-containing bisphosphonates approved to treat osteoporosis are analogs of pyrophosphate. They bind to bone mineral from which they are adsorbed into osteoclasts. By inhibiting farnesyl pyrophosphate synthase in osteoclasts, these drugs interfere with important intracellular functions, resulting in decreased osteoclast activity and survival and reduced bone resorption [8]. Bone mineral density increases modestly over the first few years of therapy. Bisphosphonates have consistently reduced the risk of vertebral fractures by 41–70 % [1, 8–14]. Non-vertebral and hip fracture risk reduction has been demonstrated with three of the four drugs, ibandronate being the exception. Importantly, the full effect of fracture protection appears to occur within the first year of therapy, and protection appears to be maintained with long-term treatment.

General Safety and Tolerance

In clinical trials, both oral and intravenous bisphosphonates have been well tolerated [15]. Upper GI intolerance, usually mild or moderate, is observed with oral dosing in daily practice, although such intolerance was not observed in clinical trials [16]. The incidence of upper GI symptoms among patients receiving placebo in the oral bisphosphonate clinical trials was 30–50 %. Such a high background incidence might have blunted the ability to observe GI intolerance in the trials. Poor adherence to the oral bisphosphonate dosing regimen increases the likelihood of upper GI symptoms. It is unclear whether differences exist in the risk of upper GI intolerance among the oral bisphosphonates [17]. GI bleeding and esophageal ulceration or rupture have been described very rarely.

Acute Phase Reaction

Acute phase reactions with fever and myalgia occur with intravenous or high dose oral therapy [18–21]. These symptoms occur in about 30 % of patients after the first intravenous dose of zoledronic acid in bisphosphonate-naïve patients but occur much less frequently after subsequent doses or in patients previously treated with oral bisphosphonates. Pretreatment with antipyretic medications reduces the incidence and intensity of symptoms [22]. Bone and muscle pain, not related to acute phase reaction, has been reported after oral or intravenous dosing. Since these symptoms were not observed in clinical trials, neither the incidence nor the mechanism of this potential side effect is known.

Hypocalcemia

Transient decreases in serum calcium levels occur upon initiating treatment. Hypocalcemia can occur, especially in patients with renal insufficiency, osteomalacia, vitamin D deficiency, or hypoparathyroidism [23–27]. Ensuing adequate intakes of calcium and especially vitamin D prior to treatment is probably protective, and therapy is contraindicated in hypocalcemic patients.

Renal Safety

Bisphosphonates are cleared from the circulation by either binding to the skeleton or by renal excretion. Rapid intravenous infusion of pamidronate or zoledronic acid to patients with cancer-related bone disease has been associated with renal failure due to focal glomerular sclerosis or acute tubular necrosis [28–30]. Based on this knowledge, patients with severely impaired renal function were not included in clinical osteoporosis trials with bisphosphonates. In the studies with oral agents, no effects on renal function were observed. Among the small numbers of patients with CDK3 renal function enrolled in those trials, no adverse effects on renal function or impaired efficacy were observed [31]. However, therapy with oral bisphosphonates is not recommended in patients with estimated GFR <30 cc/min. Individual cases of acute renal impairment related to oral bisphosphonates have been reported. In the pivotal HORIZON studies, transient increases in serum creatinine were observed after intravenous zoledronic acid, but over the course of the studies, the age-related decline in renal function was similar between treatment and placebo groups [32]. Acute renal failure and death after zoledronic acid infusion have been reported in clinical practice, although usually in patients with cancer-related bone diseases. Zoledronic acid is contraindicated in patients with a creatinine clearance of <35 cc/min [33].

Bisphosphonate nephrotoxicity is related to the maximal concentration of drug in the circulation perhaps explaining the paucity of adverse renal effects of oral bisphosphonates [30]. For patients with CDK3, extending the infusion time of zoledronic acid from the usual 15 to 30 min or even 60 min should limit the Cmax achieved with treatment and perhaps minimize the risk of renal injury.

Cardiovascular Risk

Atrial fibrillation associated with hospitalization occurred more frequently (1.3 %) with intravenous zoledronic acid compared to placebo (0.5 %; $p<0.001$) in the HORIZON Pivotal Fracture Trial [2]. Cardiac arrhythmia could theoretically be caused to the transient decrease in serum calcium after infusion. However, the cases of serious adverse events of atrial fibrillation were not temporally related to the annual dose. Furthermore, the incidence of atrial fibrillation, other arrhythmias, or cardiac events and stroke was similar between treatment and control groups. No association of zoledronic acid therapy and atrial fibrillation was observed in the HORIZON Recurrent Fracture Trial [34]. After review of all bisphosphonate studies, the FDA concluded that a causal link between bisphosphonate therapy and atrial fibrillation has not been established [35]. Driven primarily by the HORIZON Pivotal Fracture Trial, recent systematic reviews continue to suggest an increased risk of atrial fibrillation with intravenous bisphosphonates [36].

No other cardiovascular concerns were noted in clinical trials with bisphosphonates. Although observational studies have demonstrated an association between bisphosphonate therapy and decreased risks of hypertension, myocardial infarction, and stroke, recent meta-analyses do not suggest an association between bisphosphonate therapy and cardiovascular or cerebrovascular disease [37, 38].

Cancer Risk

Cases of esophageal cancer have been reported in patients who took oral bisphosphonates [39]. No evidence of this association was observed in placebo-controlled clinical trials or in several observational cohorts [40–42]. One of two analyses of the UK General Practice Research Database suggested an increased risk of esophageal cancer (3 vs. 2.3 % in controls) and especially with treatment for >5 years (RR 2.24, 1.47–3.43) [42]. No relationship between bisphosphonate use and esophageal cancer was observed in the other analysis of that same database [43]. The FDA has stated that evidence is insufficient to evaluate this association but recommends that oral bisphosphonates not be used in patients at risk for esophageal cancer including those with Barrett's esophagus [44].

In contrast to the associations of bisphosphonate therapy with adverse outcomes, decreased risks of breast, prostate, colon, and pancreatic cancer have been reported with bisphosphonates in observational studies. However, a recent analysis of pooled randomized clinical trials found no association between bisphosphonate therapy and breast cancer over an average follow-up of 3 years.

Mortality

Mortality was reduced by 28 % with IV zoledronic acid therapy in the HORIZON Recurrent Fracture Trial [1]. Decreased mortality in patients treated with bisphosphonates has also been noted in observational studies [45–48]. These effects on mortality were greater than could be explained by the anti-fracture effects of therapy.

Miscellaneous Safety Concerns

Rare cases of inflammatory eye disease (uveitis, iritis) have been described in patients receiving oral and IV bisphosphonates including older non-nitrogen-containing agents like etidronate and tiludronate [49, 50]. In a large register-based cohort, the incidence of hospital-treated uveitis was very low (0.05 %) during the first 12 months of prescription therapy for osteoporosis, with no difference observed between patients receiving bisphosphonates or other osteoporosis drugs [51]. Among 1001 patients receiving intravenous zoledronic acid in a clinical trial, eight (0.8 %) developed acute uveitis within the first few days of treatment [52]. Very rare cases of hypersensitivity and anaphylaxis have been reported with bisphosphonate therapy [53, 54].

Estrogen Agonists/Antagonists

These agents, previously described as selective estrogen receptor modulators (SERMs), have beneficial estrogen-like effects on the skeleton while inhibiting the effects of estrogen on reproductive tissues. Raloxifene was the first of these agents registered for the treatment of postmenopausal osteoporosis. Lasofoxifene 0.5 mg daily and bazedoxifene 20 mg daily have recently been approved for this indication in Europe but not in North America, although bazedoxifene, in combination with conjugated estrogen, is approved in the United States for management of menopausal symptoms and the prevention of bone loss.

After 3 years of therapy, each agent reduced the incidence of new vertebral fracture by about 40 % in postmenopausal women with osteoporosis [55–57]. No effect of raloxifene on non-vertebral fracture risk has been observed. Overall, no effect on non-vertebral fracture risk was reported with bazedoxifene, although a significant reduction (HR 0.60; 95 % CI 0.37–0.95) was noted in a post hoc analysis of a high-risk subgroup [56]. After 5 years of treatment with lasofoxifene 0.5 mg daily, a significant reduction (HR 0.76, 95 % CI 0.64–0.91) in the incidence of non-vertebral fracture was observed [57]. Hip fracture risk reduction has not been observed with any of these drugs.

General Safety and Tolerability

In clinical trials, these agents are generally well tolerated [58, 59]. Vasomotor symptoms and muscle cramps, usually of mild to moderate severity, occurred more frequently with each drug compared to placebo.

Venous Thrombotic Events

Estrogen-like increases in the risk of venous thrombotic events (VTE) have been reported with each drug. In the pivotal phase 3 MORE study, the incidence of VTE was increased in patients receiving raloxifene 60 or 120 mg daily for up to 40 months (1.0 %) versus the placebo group (0.3 %; RR 3.1; 95 % CI 1.5–6.2) [55]. The greatest risk occured within the first 4 months of therapy and did not appear to increase with prolonged exposure to the drug during years 5–8 of treatment with raloxifene 60 mg daily (CORE Study) [56]. Over 8 years of follow-up, the incidence rates for venous thromboembolic events were 2.2 and 1.3 events per 1000 woman-years for the raloxifene and placebo groups, respectively. Over 3 years of therapy with bazedoxifene 20 mg daily, the rate per 1000 woman-years was 2.86 versus 1.76 in the placebo group [57]. As with raloxifene, the rate of VTE was highest in the first year (relative risk of 2.69). During the 5 years of the PEARL study, the rate of VTE with lasofoxifene 0.5 mg daily was 2.9/1000 patient-years compared to 1.4 with placebo [HR 2.06 (95 % CI 1.17–3.61)] [58]. These agents are contraindicated in women with a prior history of venous thrombotic event and are to be used with caution in women at risk for VTE. Temporarily stopping treatment is recommended prior to and during prolonged immobilization [60].

Cardiovascular and Cerebrovascular Events

No differences in the incidence of cardiovascular or cerebrovascular events, in complications from those events or in mortality, were observed during the 8 years of the MORE and CORE studies [61, 62]. The RUTH study evaluated the effect of raloxifene versus placebo in postmenopausal women over a median duration of follow-up of 5.6 years in more than 10,000 postmenopausal women, average age 67.6 years, with documented coronary heart disease or at increased risk for coronary events [63]. Although stroke and cardiovascular events occurred similarly in women who received raloxifene 60 mg daily or placebo, death related to stroke did occur more commonly with raloxifene (1.2 %) compared to placebo (0.8 %) (HR 1.49, 95 % CI 1.00–2.24; $p = 0.0499$), an increase from 15 to 22 per 10,000 woman-years. Raloxifene had no significant effect on all-cause mortality [64]. Lasofoxifene 0.5 mg daily was associated with lower rates of myocardial infarction and stroke [56, 65]. Rates of fatal stroke (HR 1.40; 95 % CI 0.44–4.4) and overall mortality (HR 1.12; 95 % CI 0.80–1.56) did not differ significantly between the lasofoxifene 0.5 mg daily and placebo groups. There were no significant differences in the incidence of cardiovascular events or stroke between patients treated with bazedoxifene or placebo [66].

Invasive Breast Cancer

In studies of postmenopausal women with osteoporosis and the RUTH trial, raloxifene has consistently decreased the risk of invasive breast cancer with overall reductions in relative risk of 44–69 % [67–69]. The relative reduction in risk with raloxifene appears to be similar across the spectrum of risks in the various patient groups. In the STAR study, protection from invasive breast cancer was similar in women at high risk for breast cancer receiving tamoxifen or raloxifene [70]. Treatment with lasofoxifene 0.5 mg daily for 5 years reduced the risk of invasive breast cancer by 85 % (95 % CI 50–96 %), and the effect was greater in women with serum estrogen levels above the group mean [71]. These effects are limited to the risk of invasive estrogen receptor-positive breast cancer [72]. No effect of bazedoxifene on breast cancer risk has been reported.

Others

Raloxifene had no effect on cognitive function [73]. Over 5 years, no endometrial safety issues were observed with raloxifene [74]. Compared to placebo, lasofoxifene therapy for 5 years resulted in small increases in frequency of vaginal bleeding, endometrial thickness, and vaginal polyps but no difference in endometrial cancer or gynecological surgery for uterine prolapse [75]. Bazedoxifene therapy for up to 7 years was not associated with endometrial hyperplasia or changes in endometrial thickening, but was associated with a significant decreased risk of endometrial carcinoma (0.1 vs. 0.4 %; $P = 0.020$) [76].

Calcitonin

This peptide hormone is a potent inhibitor of osteoclast activity in vitro, but its clinical effect on bone metabolism is very modest. Administration of salmon calcitonin by nasal spray induces small reductions in bone turnover markers and increases in bone mineral density.

Evidence supporting the effect of nasal calcitonin treatment on fracture risk is weak, and no effect of treatment on non-vertebral fracture was observed in the only fracture endpoint trial with this drug [77]. In that study, no important safety issues were noted over 3 years of observation nor did safety concerns arise in post-marketing surveillance since regulatory approval in 1995.

Cancer Risk

Signals of a possible increased risk of prostate cancer in a clinical trial evaluating an oral preparation of salmon calcitonin in patients with osteoarthritis prompted a thorough review of all clinical trials of nasal and oral salmon calcitonin. A review by the EMA Committee for Medicinal Products for Human Use identified an increased risk of cancer (2.4 % with nasal administration) [78]. A meta-analysis of 17 randomized, controlled clinical trials with nasal spray salmon calcitonin, performed by the FDA, reported that the overall incidence of malignancies reported was higher among calcitonin salmon-treated patients (4.2 %) compared with placebo-treated patients (2.9 %) (OR 1.4; 95 % CI 1.1–1.7) [79]. Similar results were observed in a meta-analysis by independent authors [80]. No specific type of cancer was associated with calcitonin use. The authors of each report conceded that most of the clinical trials were poorly designed to assess new cancer cases but that the weak cancer signal could not be ignored. On the basis of this possible association with cancer risk, coupled with weak evidence of efficacy, European and Canadian regulatory authorities withdrew approval for nasal calcitonin as a treatment for osteoporosis [78]. In the United States, a FDA Advisory Committee recommended that the drug be withdrawn from the market [81]. The FDA decided instead to simply add a caution about the possible association of cancer risk [82]. Salmon calcitonin therapy has been associated with a few cases of serious allergic-type reactions including bronchospasm and anaphylactic shock, including rare reports of death [83].

Denosumab

This fully human monoclonal antibody very specifically binds to RANK ligand, blunting the proliferation and activation of osteoclasts. Biochemical indices of bone resorption are acutely and markedly reduced after subcutaneous dosing. The average values of the bone resorption markers gradually increase before the next dose given at 6 months to levels observed in patients on long-term alendronate therapy [84]. Bone mineral density increases progressively over at least 8 years of therapy [85]. In the pivotal phase 3 FREEDOM study, denosumab reduced the risks of vertebral, hip and non-vertebral fracture over 3 years by 68 %, 40 %, and 20 %, respectively [2]. After 3 years of placebo-control comparisons, all patients who continued in an extension study received open-label denosumab therapy. Results out to 6 years have been published [86]. Compared to the fracture incidence during the first 3 years of FREEDOM, risks of vertebral fracture appeared to remain stable, while the risk of non-vertebral fracture appeared to decrease progressively with continued therapy.

General Safety and Tolerability

The overall safety profile of denosumab has consistently been excellent in multiple clinical trials. The frequencies of adverse events, serious adverse events, and the rate of patients discontinuing therapy because of an adverse event have been similar between treatment and control groups. Among the 7805 women in the FREEDOM study, 90 in the placebo and 70 in the treatment group died ($p=0.08$) [2]. Other than rare cases of ONJ and femoral shaft fracture with atypical features, no additional safety issues were clearly noted in the FREEDOM extension study [86]. A few cases of atypical fracture occurring with the clinical use of denosumab have been reported, but to date, all those patients had been pretreated with bisphosphonates [87]. Too few cases of atypical fracture have occurred to assess whether the risk, if present, is related to duration of therapy.

Skin Rash and Infection

In the 3 years of FREEDOM, skin rash or eczema occurred more frequently with denosumab therapy than placebo [2]. The incidence of serious adverse events related to cellulitis was greater with denosumab (1.2 %) compared to placebo (one case among 3850 patients). These skin events were unrelated to the time or site of the denosumab injection. The cases of cellulitis responded to standard antimicrobial therapy. During the first 3 years of the FREEDOM extension, the incidence of skin rashes or serious adverse events related to cellulitis was very low in patients who continued taking denosumab for 6 years [86]. Importantly, increased risks of infections, eczema, or serious adverse events related to cellulitis were not observed in patients who had received placebo during the first 3 years and then received denosumab for the next 3 years.

Immunologic Safety

RANK ligand is expressed in dendritic cells and some T cells, raising the possibility that immune dysfunction could result from inhibition of RANK ligand with denosumab [88]. The numeric incidence of infections and neoplasms was slightly greater among the denosumab in patients in FREEDOM compared to placebo. However, due to the manner in which adverse events are coded in clinical trials, many of these "infections" were inflammatory conditions such as diverticulitis or labyrinthitis rather than diseases caused by microorganisms [89]. There was no evidence of increased risk of opportunistic infections or immune-related neoplasms. No evidence of a progressive increase risk of either infection or malignancy was observed in the FREEDOM extension study. Rare, isolated cases of anaphylaxis associated with denosumab therapy have been reported [90, 91].

Hypocalcemia

Denosumab, like other potent anti-remodeling agents, has potential to induce hypocalcemia. This complication of therapy was not observed in the FREEDOM study or numerous other phase 2 and phase 3 studies. However, all patients in those studies received calcium and vitamin D, and patients with vitamin D deficiency were excluded. Isolated case reports of hypocalcemia, sometimes severe and prolonged, have been described [92–94]. The risk of hypocalcemia may be greater in patients with significantly impaired renal function or with other metabolic bone diseases, particularly those associated with hypoparathyroidism, osteomalacia, and impaired bone mineralization [95]. Vitamin D deficiency should be corrected prior to starting therapy, and treatment is contraindicated in patients with hypocalcemia.

Parathyroid Hormone Analogs

Intact PTH (PTH 1-84) and teriparatide (PTH 1-34), given by daily subcutaneous injections, increase bone formation and, subsequently, bone resorption. Bone mineral density increases significantly after 1–2 years of treatment. Trabecular microarchitecture and cortical thickness of the iliac crest improved. Vertebral fracture risk was reduced after 18–24 months of treatment with both drugs [96, 97]. Non-vertebral fracture risk was reduced by 35 % after a median of 19 months of treatment with teriparatide. A significant effect on non-vertebral fracture risk was not observed in the 24 months of trial with intact PTH. PTH 1-84 has recently been voluntary withdrawn from the European market by the manufacturer [98].

General Safety and Tolerability

Few safety issues other than hypercalcemia and hypercalciuria were noted during the pivotal clinical trials. Muscle cramps occurred more frequently with teriparatide therapy, sometimes resulting in discontinuation of treatment. Regulatory restriction limits the duration of treatment to 18–24 months, the median length of treatment in pivotal trials, although effects on bone metabolism and fracture risk appear to persist for at least 3 years of teriparatide treatment in patients receiving glucocorticoids [99].

Hypercalcemia and Hypercalciuria

Mild hypercalcemia, usually transient, occurred in 11 % and 28 % of patients who received teriparatide 20 µg or 40 µg daily, respectively, compared to 2 % in the placebo group [96]. With the 20 µg daily dose, 95 % of patients with hypercalcemia had values less than 11.2 mg/dl (2.80 mmol/l). When measured at multiple times over 12 months, teriparatide 20 µg daily was associated with an increase in 24-h urinary calcium excretion from baseline by up to 32 mg/day compared with placebo at the same time point ($P<0.05$) [100]. Hypercalcemia or hypercalciuria infrequently caused discontinuation of treatment. The higher incidence of hypercalcemia in the 40 µg group was the one reason that the 20 µg dose of teriparatide received regulatory approval. This agent is to be used with caution in patients with hypercalcemia or history of renal stones [101].

Risk of Osteosarcoma

In rats receiving large doses of teriparatide for most of their lifetime, a dose-dependent risk of osteosarcoma was observed [102]. This resulted in regulatory warnings about the potential for osteosarcoma with teriparatide. Therapy is contraindicated in patients at risk for osteosarcoma including patients with Paget's disease of bone, unexplained elevations of serum alkaline phosphatase, children and adolescents with open epiphyses, and patients with a history of skeletal radiation [101]. Isolated cases of osteosarcoma have been reported in patients with exposure to teriparatide, but the number of reported cases is not greater than anticipated in untreated older adults [103–105]. The Osteosarcoma Surveillance Study, an ongoing 15-year post-marketing surveillance study initiated in 2003, evaluates the potential association between teriparatide and development of osteosarcoma. After 7 years of surveillance, no signal of a causal association between teriparatide treatment and osteosarcoma in humans has been observed [106]. Because of the possibility of activating skeletal metastases, teriparatide should not be used in patients with malignancies involving or potentially involving the skeleton.

Strontium Ranelate

This drug is an approved treatment for osteoporosis in most of the world except the United States and Canada. Therapy reduced vertebral and nonvertebral fractures in postmenopausal women with osteoporosis [107, 108]. Hip fracture risk reduction was only demonstrated in a post hoc analysis of a high-risk subgroup of patients. Treatment resulted in significant increases in bone mineral density, due primarily to deposition of strontium into skeletal tissue [109]. The effects of strontium ranelate therapy on biochemical markers of bone remodeling are very small or nil [110].

General Safety and Tolerability

In the two major clinical trials, diarrhea, nausea, headache, and skin rashes occurred more often with strontium ranelate than with placebo, most commonly in the first 3 months of treatment. Elevation of serum creatine kinase occurred more frequently with therapy than with placebo [111]. Patients with marked renal impairment of renal function were excluded from the clinical trials, and the drug is not recommended in patients with calculated creatinine clearance of <30 ml/min [112].

Venous Thrombotic Events

An increased risk of venous thrombotic events was noted after 5 years of strontium ranelate therapy [112]. Deep vein thrombosis or pulmonary embolism occurred in 2.1 % of the placebo group and in 2.7 % of treated patients (OR 1.30, 95 % CI 0.90–1.88). Reviews of cohorts in the United Kingdom have not confirmed an increased incidence of venous thromboembolic events (VTE) [113–115]. Therapy is contraindicated in patients with current or previous VTE and those with temporary or permanent immobilization or prolonged bed rest.

Serious Skin Reactions

In post-marketing studies, rare but serious and even fatal cases of skin lesions including DRESS, Stevens–Johnson syndrome, and toxic epidermal necrolysis have been reported with strontium ranelate [116]. The highest risk of these problems appears to be within the first weeks of treatment.

Cardiovascular Risk

In a recent routine evaluation of safety data in pooled randomized placebo-controlled studies of strontium ranelate in postmenopausal women with osteoporosis, an increased risk of cardiovascular events was observed [117]. Myocardial infarction occurred more in strontium ranelate-treated patients (1.7 %) compared to placebo (1.1 %), with a relative risk of 1.6 (95 % CI [1.07, 2.38]). Analyses of other large cohorts have not confirmed this effect [118]. It is not known if this apparent increased risk is truly due to the drug or to other differences between the treated and control populations [119]. In 2013, the EMA suggested that strontium ranelate not be used in patients with risk factors for heart disease [120]. Upon further review, in early 2014, the EMA's Pharmacovigilance Risk Assessment Committee (PRAC) recommended that the drug should no longer be used to treat osteoporosis [121]. However, the EMA chose to allow strontium ranelate to remain on the market but with warnings that the drug not be used in patients with including uncontrolled hypertension or established, current or past history of ischemic heart disease, peripheral arterial disease and/or cerebrovascular disease [122].

Safety of Osteoporosis Drugs in Children and Pregnancy

No studies have specifically evaluated either the efficacy or safety of any osteoporosis drug in children or in women who are pregnant or breast-feeding. No drug is approved for the treatment of osteoporosis in children, pregnancy, or premenopausal women, and there are no or very limited data (with bisphosphonates) about the safety of osteoporosis agents in these populations. Bisphosphonates are used to treat osteogenesis imperfecta in children and for short-term therapy of rare cases of juvenile osteoporosis [123]. In pregnant rats and rabbits, bisphosphonate administration is associated with abortion, stillbirth, and maternal mortality, due principally to hypocalcemia. Rare abnormalities in fetal development in animals have been described with high-dose bisphosphonate exposure, although very limited experience has not demonstrated a problem with human pregnancies [124]. Oral bisphosphonates are to be used with caution in women at risk for pregnancy, while IV zoledronic acid is contraindicated in pregnancy [33]. Estrogen agonists/antagonists induce bone loss in estrogen-replete women and are contraindicated in pregnancy for the may cause interruption of the pregnancy and/or fetal harm [125]. PTH analogs should not be used in pediatric and young adult patients with open epiphyses due to possible risk of osteosarcoma. PTH [101] and denosumab therapy in animals can cause fetal harm [91]. Calcitonin is predicted to have low probability of adverse effects during pregnancy or childhood, but no studies have documented effectiveness in these patients. Oral bisphosphonates, calcitonin, and teriparatide have a Category C label for pregnancy, while IV zoledronic acid and denosumab have Category D and X labels, respectively. There are no data about the use of strontium ranelate in children or in pregnancy.

Conclusion

Making decisions about osteoporosis treatments requires knowledge of both the benefits and the risks or potential complications of treatment options. Osteoporosis medications are generally very effective and very well tolerated. Mild to moderate intolerance (GI distress, muscle cramps) limits acceptance and persistence with therapy in some patients. Serious or life-threatening side effects are very uncommon. In patients with osteoporosis at high risk for fracture (the appropriate candidates for pharmacological therapy), the benefit-to-risk ratio is very favorable, except for perhaps calcitonin. This risk ratio can be improved by avoiding specific treatments in patients at risk for potential complications of that therapy and by monitoring the patients regularly. By appreciating the magnitude of the salutary effects of treatments as well as the frequency and nature of specific safety concerns with individual drugs, physicians can communicate this information more effectively to patients and can make more appropriate therapeutic decisions, thereby improving effectiveness of patient care.

References[1]

1. **Black DM, Delmas PD, Eastell R, Reid IR, Boonen S, Cauley JA, Cosman F, Lakatos P, Leung PC, Man Z, Mautalen C, Mesenbrink P, Hu H, Caminis J, Tong K, Rosario-Jansen T, Krasnow J, Hue TF, Sellmeyer D, Eriksen EF, Cummings SR, HORIZON Pivotal Fracture Trial. Once-yearly zoledronic acid for treatment of postmenopausal osteoporosis. N Engl J Med. 2007;356(18):1809–22. **Pivotal trial.*

2. **Cummings SR, San Martin J, McClung MR, Siris ES, Eastell R, Reid IR, Delmas P, Zoog HB, Austin M, Wang A, Kutilek S, Adami S, Zanchetta J, Libanati C, Siddhanti S, Christiansen C, FREEDOM Trial. Denosumab for prevention of fractures in postmenopausal women with osteoporosis. N Engl J Med. 2009;361(8):756–65. **Pivotal trial.*

3. Singh S, Loke YK. Drug safety assessment in clinical trials: methodological challenges and opportunities. Trials. 2012;13:138. doi:10.1186/1745-6215-13-138.

4. European Medicines Agency: Benefit-risk methodology (Internet); 2011 (cited 2015 Jun 20). Available from: http://www.ema.europa.eu/ema/index.jsp?curl=pages/special_topics/document_listing/document_listing_000314.jsp&mid=WC0b01ac0580223ed6. Accessed 17 July 2012

5. Khosla S, Bilezikian JP, Dempster DW, Lewiecki EM, Miller PD, Neer RM, Recker RR, Shane E, Shoback D, Potts JT. Benefits and risks of bisphosphonate therapy for osteoporosis. J Clin Endocrinol Metab. 2012;97(7):2272–82.

6. McClung M, Harris ST, Miller PD, Bauer DC, Davison KS, Dian L, Hanley DA, Kendler DL, Yuen CK, Lewiecki EM. Bisphosphonate therapy for osteoporosis: benefits, risks, and drug holiday. Am J Med. 2013;126(1):13–20.

7. Lewiecki EM, Miller PD, Harris ST, Bauer DC, Davison KS, Dian L, Hanley DA, McClung MR, Yuen CK, Kendler DL. Understanding and communicating the benefits and risks of denosumab, raloxifene, and teriparatide for the treatment of osteoporosis. J Clin Densitom. 2014;17(4):490–5.

8. Russell RG, Watts NB, Ebetino FH, Rogers MJ. Mechanisms of action of bisphosphonates: similarities and differences and their potential influence on clinical efficacy. Osteoporos Int. 2008;19: 733–59.

9. **Black DM, Cummings SR, Karpf DB, et al. Randomised trial of effect of alendronate on risk of fracture in women with existing vertebral fractures. Fracture intervention trial research group. Lancet. 1996;348:1535–41. **Pivotal trial.*

10. **Cummings SR, Black DM, Thompson DE, et al. Effect of alendronate on risk of fracture in women with low bone density but without vertebral fractures: results from the Fracture Intervention Trial. JAMA. 1998;280:2077–82. **Pivotal trial.*

11. **Harris ST, Watts NB, Genant HK, et al. Effects of risedronate treatment on vertebral and nonvertebral fractures in women with postmenopausal osteoporosis: a randomized controlled trial. Vertebral efficacy with risedronate therapy (VERT) study group. JAMA. 1999;282:1344–52. **Pivotal trial.*

12. **Reginster J, Minne HW, Sorensen OH, et al. Randomized trial of the effects of risedronate on vertebral fractures in women with established postmenopausal osteoporosis. Vertebral Efficacy with Risedronate Therapy (VERT) Study Group. Osteoporos Int. 2000;11:83–91. **Pivotal trial.*

13. *McClung MR, Geusens P, Miller PD, et al. Effect of risedronate on the risk of hip fracture in elderly women. Hip Intervention Program Study Group. N Engl J Med. 2001;344:333–40. *Largest risedronate trial, in elderly women.*

14. **Chesnut III CH, Skag A, Christiansen C, Recker R, Stakkestad JA, Hoiseth A, Felsenberg D, Huss H, Gilbride J, Schimmer RC, Delmas PD, Oral Ibandronate Osteoporosis Vertebral Fracture Trial in North America and Europe (BONE). Effects of oral ibandronate administered daily or intermittently on fracture risk in postmenopausal osteoporosis. J Bone Miner Res. 2004;19(8):1241–9. **Pivotal trial.*

15. Strampel W, Emkey R, Civitelli R. Safety considerations with bisphosphonates for the treatment of osteoporosis. Drug Saf. 2007;30:755–63.

16. Cryer B, Bauer DC. Oral bisphosphonates and upper gastrointestinal tract problems: what is the evidence? Mayo Clin Proc. October. 2002;77:1031–43.

17. Cadarette SM, Katz JN, Brookhart MA, et al. Comparative gastrointestinal safety of weekly oral bisphosphonates. Osteoporos Int. 2009;20:1735–47.

18. Adami S, Bhalla AK, Dorizzi R, Montesanti F, Rosini S, Salvagno G, Lo CV. The acute-phase response after bisphosphonate administration. Calcif Tissue Int. 1987;41(6):326–31.

---

[1] *Important References
**Very Important References

19. Reid IR, Gamble GD, Mesenbrink P, Lakatos P, Black DM. Characterization of and risk factors for the acute-phase response after zoledronic acid. J Clin Endocrinol Metab. 2010;95:4380–7.

20. Delmas PD, Adami S, Strugala C, Stakkestad JA, Reginster JY, Felsenberg D, Christiansen C, Civitelli R, Drezner MK, Recker RR, Bolognese M, Hughes C, Masanauskaite D, Ward P, Sambrook P, Reid DM. Intravenous ibandronate injections in post-menopausal women with osteoporosis: one-year results from the dosing intravenous administration study. Arthritis Rheum. 2006;54(6):1838–46.

21. Reginster JY, Adami S, Lakatos P, Greenwald M, Stepan JJ, Silverman SL, Christiansen C, Rowell L, Mairon N, Bonvoisin B, Drezner MK, Emkey R, Felsenberg D, Cooper C, Delmas PD, Miller PD. Efficacy and tolerability of once-monthly oral ibandronate in postmenopausal osteoporosis: 2 year results from the MOBILE study. Ann Rheum Dis. 2006;65(5):654–61.

22. Silverman SL, Kriegman A, Goncalves J, Kianifard F, Carlson T, Leary E. Effect of acetaminophen and flu-vastatin on post-dose symptoms following infusion of zoledronic acid. Osteoporos Int. 2011;22(8):2337–45. doi:10.1007/s00198-010-1448-2.

23. Schussheim DH, Jacobs TP, Silverberg SJ. Hypocalcemia associated with alendronate. Ann Intern Med. 1999;130(4 Pt 1):329.

24. Rosen CJ, Brown S. Severe hypocalcemia after intravenous bisphosphonate therapy in occult vitamin D deficiency. N Engl J Med. 2003;348(15):1503–4.

25. Maalouf NM, Heller HJ, Odvina CV, Kim PJ, Sakhaee K. Bisphosphonate-induced hypocalcemia: report of 3 cases and review of literature. Endocr Pract. 2006;12(1):48–53.

26. Richmond BK. Profound refractory hypocalcemia after thyroidectomy in a patient receiving chronic oral bisphosphonate therapy. Am Surg. 2005;71(10):872–3.

27. Kreutle V, Blum C, Meier C, Past M, Müller B, Schütz P, Borm K. Bisphosphonate induced hypo-calcaemia – report of six cases and review of the literature. Swiss Med Wkly. 2014;144:w13979. doi:10.4414/smw.2014.13979. eCollection 2014.

28. Markowitz GS, Fine PL, Stack JI, Kunis CL, Radhakrishnan J, Palecki W, Park J, Nasr SH, Hoh S, Siegel DS, D'Agati VD. Toxic acute tubular necrosis following treatment with zoledronate (Zometa). Kidney Int. 2003;64(1):281–9.

29. Chang JT, Green L, Beitz J. Renal failure with the use of zoledronic acid. N Engl J Med. 2003;349(17):1676–9.

30. Perazella MA, Markowitz GS. Bisphosphonate nephrotoxicity. Kidney Int. 2008;74(11):1385–93.

31. Miller PD, Jamal SA, Evenepoel P, Eastell R, Boonen S. Renal safety in patients treated with bisphosphonates for osteoporosis: a review. J Bone Miner Res. 2013;28(10):2049–59.

32. Boonen S, Sellmeyer DE, Lippuner K, Orlov-Morozov A, Abrams K, Mesenbrink P, Eriksen EF, Miller PD. Renal safety of annual zoledronic acid infusions in osteoporotic postmenopausal women. Kidney Int. 2008;74(5):641–8.

33. Reclast (package insert). East Hanover, NJ: Novartis Pharmaceuticals Corp; 2015.

34. *Lyles KW, Colón-Emeric CS, Magaziner JS, Adachi JD, Pieper CF, Mautalen C, Hyldstrup L, Recknor C, Nordsletten L, Moore KA, Lavecchia C, Zhang J, Mesenbrink P, Hodgson PK, Abrams K, Orloff JJ, Horowitz Z, Eriksen EF, Boonen S, HORIZON Recurrent Fracture Trial. Zoledronic acid and clinical fractures and mortality after hip fracture. N Engl J Med. 2007;357(18):1799–809. *Documented decreased mortality.

35. U.S. Food and Drug Administration. Early communication of an ongoing safety review on bisphospho-nates: alendronate (Fosamax, Fosamax Plus D), Etidronate (Didronel), Ibandronate (Boniva), Pamidronate (Aredia), Risedronate (Actonel, Actonel W/Calcium), Tiludronate (Skelid), and Zoledronic acid (Reclast, Zometa) (Internet) 2007 (cited 2015 Jun 20). Available from: http://www.fda.gov/Drugs/DrugSafety/PostmarketDrugSafetyInformationforPatientsandProviders/DrugSafetyInformationforHeathcareProfessionals/ucm070303.htm

36. Sharma A, Einstein AJ, Vallakati A, Arbab-Zadeh A, Walker MD, Mukherjee D, Homel P, Borer JS, Lichstein E. Risk of atrial fibrillation with use of oral and intravenous bisphosphonates. Am J Cardiol. 2014;113(11):1815–21.

37. Kang JH, Keller JJ, Lin HC. A population-based 2-year follow-up study on the relationship between bisphosphonates and the risk of stroke. Osteoporos Int. 2012;23(10):2551–7.

38. Kim DH, Rogers JR, Fulchino LA, Kim CA, Solomon DH, Kim SC. Bisphosphonates and risk of cardiovascular events: a meta-analysis. PLoS One. 2015;10(4):e0122646. doi:10.1371/journal.pone.0122646. eCollection 2015.

39. Wysowski DK. Reports of esophageal cancer with oral bisphosphonate use. N Engl J Med. 2009;360:89–90.

40. Abrahamsen B, Eiken P, Eastell R. More on reports of esophageal cancer with oral bisphosphonate use. N Engl J Med. 2009;360:1789–90.

41. Solomon DH, Patrick A, Brookhart MA. More on reports of esophageal cancer with oral bisphospho-nate use. N Engl J Med. 2009;360:1789–90.

42. Green J, Czanner G, Reeves G, Watson J, Wise L, Beral V. Oral bisphosphonates and risk of cancer of oesophagus, stomach, and colorectum: case-control analysis within a UK primary care cohort. BMJ. 2010;341:c4444. doi:10.1136/bmj.c4444.

43. Cardwell CR, Abnet CC, Cantwell MM, Murray LJ. Exposure to oral bisphosphonates and risk of esophageal cancer. JAMA. 2010;304:657–63.

44. U.S. Food and Drug Administration. Drug Safety Communication: ongoing safety review of oral osteoporosis drugs (bisphosphonates) and potential increased risk of esophageal cancer (Internet); 2011 (cited 2015 Jun 20). Available from: http://www.fda.gov/Drugs/DrugSafety/ucm263320.htm

45. Center JR, Bliuc D, Nguyen ND, Nguyen TV, Eisman JA. Osteoporosis medication and reduced mortality risk in elderly women and men. J Clin Endocrinol Metab. 2011;96:1006–14.

46. Sambrook PN, Cameron ID, Chen JS, et al. Oral bisphosphonates are associated with reduced mortality in frail older people: a prospective five-year study. Osteoporos Int. 2011;22:2551–6.

47. Beaupre LA, Morrish DW, Hanley DA, Maksymowych WP, Bell NR, Juby AG, Majumdar SR. Oral bisphosphonates are associated with reduced mortality after hip fracture. Osteoporos Int. 2011;22(3):983–91.

48. Bolland MJ, Grey AB, Gamble GD, Reid IR. Effect of osteoporosis treatment on mortality: a meta-analysis. J Clin Endocrinol Metab. 2010;95:1174–81.

49. Sharma NS, Ooi JL, Masselos K, Hooper MJ, Francis IC. Zoledronic acid infusion and orbital inflammatory disease. N Engl J Med. 2008;359:1410–1.

50. Fraunfelder FW. Ocular side effects associated with bisphosphonates. Drugs Today (Barc). 2003;39:829–35.

51. Pazianas M, Clark EM, Eiken PA, Brixen K, Abrahamsen B. Inflammatory eye reactions in patients treated with bisphosphonates and other osteoporosis medications: cohort analysis using a national prescription database. J Bone Miner Res. 2013;28(3):455–63.

52. Patel DV, Horne A, House M, Reid IR, McGhee CN. The incidence of acute anterior uveitis after intravenous zoledronate. Ophthalmology. 2013;120(4):773–6.

53. Naniwa T, Maeda T, Mizoshita T, Hayami Y, Watanabe M, Banno S, Ito R. Alendronate-induced esophagitis: possible pathogenic role of hypersensitivity to alendronate. Intern Med. 2008;47(23):2083–5.

54. Isik A, Uras I, Uyar ME, Karakurt F, Kaftan O. Alendronate-induced asthma. Ann Pharmacother. 2009;43(3):547–8.

55. **Ettinger B, Black DM, Mitlak BH, Knickerbocker RK, Nickelsen T, Genant HK, Christiansen C, Delmas PD, Zanchetta JR, Stakkestad J, Glüer CC, Krueger K, Cohen FJ, Eckert S, Ensrud KE, Avioli LV, Lips P, Cummings SR. Reduction of vertebral fracture risk in postmenopausal women with osteoporosis treated with raloxifene: results from a 3-year randomized clinical trial. Multiple outcomes of raloxifene evaluation (MORE) investigators. JAMA. 1999;282(7):637–45. **Pivotal trial*.

56. **Cummings SR, Ensrud K, Delmas PD, LaCroix AZ, Vukicevic S, Reid DM, Goldstein S, Sriram U, Lee A, Thompson J, Armstrong RA, Thompson DD, Powles T, Zanchetta J, Kendler D, Neven P, Eastell R, PEARL Study Investigators. Lasofoxifene in postmenopausal women with osteoporosis. N Engl J Med. 2010;362(8):686–96. **Pivotal trial*.

57. **Silverman SL, Christiansen C, Genant HK, Vukicevic S, Zanchetta JR, de Villiers TJ, Constantine GD, Chines AA. Efficacy of bazedoxifene in reducing new vertebral fracture risk in postmenopausal women with osteoporosis: results from a 3-year, randomized, placebo-, and active-controlled clinical trial. J Bone Miner Res. 2008;23(12):1923–34. **Pivotal trial*.

58. Davies GC, Huster WJ, Lu Y, Plouffe Jr L, Lakshmanan M. Adverse events reported by postmenopausal women in controlled trials with raloxifene. Obstet Gynecol. 1999;93:558–65.

59. de Villiers TJ, Chines AA, Palacios S, Lips P, Sawicki AZ, Levine AB, Codreanu C, Kelepouris N, Brown JP. Safety and tolerability of bazedoxifene in postmenopausal women with osteoporosis: results of a 5-year, randomized, placebo-controlled phase 3 trial. Osteoporos Int. 2011;22(2):567–76.

60. Siris ES, Harris ST, Eastell R, Zanchetta JR, Goemaere S, Diez-Perez A, Stock JL, Song J, Qu Y, Kulkarni PM, Siddhanti SR, Wong M, Cummings SR, Continuing Outcomes Relevant to Evista (CORE) Investigators. Skeletal effects of raloxifene after 8 years: results from the continuing outcomes relevant to Evista (CORE) study. J Bone Miner Res. 2005;20(9):1514–24.

61. Barrett-Connor E, Grady D, Sashegyi A, Anderson PW, Cox DA, Hoszowski K, Rautaharju P, Harper KD, MORE Investigators (Multiple Outcomes of Raloxifene Evaluation). Raloxifene and cardiovascular events in osteoporotic postmenopausal women: four-year results from the MORE (Multiple outcomes of raloxifene evaluation) randomized trial. JAMA. 2002;287(7):847–57.

62. *Ensrud K, Genazzani AR, Geiger MJ, McNabb M, Dowsett SA, Cox DA, Barrett-Connor E. Effect of raloxifene on cardiovascular adverse events in postmenopausal women with osteoporosis. Am J Cardiol. 2006;97(4):520–7. *Long-term follow-up*.

63. **Barrett-Connor E, Mosca L, Collins P, Geiger MJ, Grady D, Kornitzer M, McNabb MA, Wenger NK, Raloxifene Use for the Heart (RUTH) Trial Investigators. Effects of raloxifene on cardiovascular events and breast cancer in postmenopausal women. N Engl J Med. 2006;355(2):125–37. **Important data about fatal stroke risk*.

64. *Ensrud K, LaCroix A, Thompson JR, Thompson DD, Eastell R, Reid DM, Vukicevic S, Cauley J, Barrett-Connor E, Armstrong R, Welty F, Cummings S. Lasofoxifene and cardiovascular events in postmenopausal women with osteoporosis: Five-year results from the Postmenopausal Evaluation and Risk Reduction with Lasofoxifene (PEARL) trial. Circulation. 2010;122(17):1716–24. *Long term followup*.

65. Grady D, Cauley JA, Stock JL, Cox DA, Mitlak BH, Song J, Cummings SR. Effect of raloxifene on all-cause mortality. Am J Med. 2010;123(5):469.e1–7.

66. *Silverman SL, Chines AA, Kendler DL, Kung AW, Teglbjærg CS, Felsenberg D, Mairon N, Constantine GD, Adachi JD, Bazedoxifene Study Group. Sustained efficacy and safety of bazedoxifene in preventing fractures in postmenopausal women with osteoporosis: results of a 5-year, randomized, placebo-controlled study. Osteoporos Int. 2012;23(1):351–63. *Long-term follow-up.

67. Cummings SR, Eckert S, Krueger KA, Grady D, Powles TJ, Cauley JA, Norton L, Nickelsen T, Bjarnason NH, Morrow M, Lippman ME, Black D, Glusman JE, Costa A, Jordan VC. The effect of raloxifene on risk of breast cancer in postmenopausal women: results from the MORE randomized trial. Multiple outcomes of raloxifene evaluation. JAMA. 1999;281(23):2189–97.

68. Cauley JA, Norton L, Lippman ME, Eckert S, Krueger KA, Purdie DW, Farrerons J, Karasik A, Mellstrom D, Ng KW, Stepan JJ, Powles TJ, Morrow M, Costa A, Silfen SL, Walls EL, Schmitt H, Muchmore DB, Jordan VC, Ste-Marie LG. Continued breast cancer risk reduction in postmenopausal women treated with raloxifene: 4-year results from the MORE trial. Multiple outcomes of raloxifene evaluation. Breast Cancer Res Treat. 2001;65(2):125–34.

69. Martino S, Cauley JA, Barrett-Connor E, Powles TJ, Mershon J, Disch D, Secrest RJ, Cummings SR, CORE Investigators. Continuing outcomes relevant to Evista: breast cancer incidence in postmenopausal osteoporotic women in a randomized trial of raloxifene. J Natl Cancer Inst. 2004;96(23):1751–61.

70. Vogel VG, Costantino JP, Wickerham DL, Cronin WM, Cecchini RS, Atkins JN, Bevers TB, Fehrenbacher L, Pajon Jr ER, Wade 3rd JL, Robidoux A, Margolese RG, James J, Lippman SM, Runowicz CD, Ganz PA, Reis SE, McCaskill-Stevens W, Ford LG, Jordan VC, Wolmark N, National Surgical Adjuvant Breast and Bowel Project (NSABP). Effects of tamoxifen vs raloxifene on the risk of developing invasive breast cancer and other disease outcomes: the NSABP Study of Tamoxifen and Raloxifene (STAR) P-2 trial. JAMA. 2006;295:2727–41.

71. LaCroix AZ, Powles T, Osborne CK, Wolter K, Thompson JR, Thompson DD, Allred DC, Armstrong R, Cummings SR, Eastell R, Ensrud KE, Goss P, Lee A, Neven P, Reid DM, Curto M, Vukicevic S, PEARL Investigators. Breast cancer incidence in the randomized PEARL trial of lasofoxifene in postmenopausal osteoporotic women. J Natl Cancer Inst. 2010;102(22):1706–15.

72. Cuzick J, Sestak I, Bonanni B, Costantino JP, Cummings S, DeCensi A, Dowsett M, Forbes JF, Ford L, LaCroix AZ, Mershon J, Mitlak BH, Powles T, Veronesi U, Vogel V, Wickerham DL, SERM Chemoprevention of Breast Cancer Overview Group. Selective oestrogen receptor modulators in prevention of breast cancer: an updated meta-analysis of individual participant data. Lancet. 2013;381(9880):1827–34.

73. Yaffe K, Krueger K, Sarkar S, Grady D, Barrett-Connor E, Cox DA, Nickelsen T, Multiple Outcomes of Raloxifene Evaluation Investigators. Cognitive function in postmenopausal women treated with raloxifene. N Engl J Med. 2001;344(16):1207–13.

74. Jolly EE, Bjarnason NH, Neven P, Plouffe Jr L, Johnston Jr CC, Watts SD, Arnaud CD, Mason TM, Crans G, Akers R, Draper MW. Prevention of osteoporosis and uterine effects in postmenopausal women taking raloxifene for 5 years. Menopause. 2003;10(4):337–44.

75. Goldstein SR, Neven P, Cummings S, Colgan T, Runowicz CD, Krpan D, Proulx J, Johnson M, Thompson D, Thompson J, Sriram U. Postmenopausal evaluation and risk reduction with lasofoxifene (PEARL) trial: 5-year gynecological outcomes. Menopause. 2011;18(1):17–22.

76. Palacios S, Silverman SL, de Villiers TJ, Levine AB, Goemaere S, Brown JP, De Cicco Nardone F, Williams R, Hines TL, Mirkin S, Chines AA, Bazedoxifene Study Group. A 7-year randomized, placebo-controlled trial assessing the long-term efficacy and safety of bazedoxifene in postmenopausal women with osteoporosis: effects on bone density and fracture. Menopause. 2015;22:806–13.

77. Chesnut 3rd CH, Silverman S, Andriano K, Genant H, Gimona A, Harris S, Kiel D, LeBoff M, Maricic M, Miller P, Moniz C, Peacock M, Richardson P, Watts N, Baylink D. A randomized trial of nasal spray salmon calcitonin in postmenopausal women with established osteoporosis: the prevent recurrence of osteoporotic fractures study. PROOF study group. Am J Med. 2000;109(4):267–76.

78. European Medicines Agency. Calcitonin (Internet); 2013 (cited 2015 Jun 20). Available from: http://www.ema.europa.eu/ema/index.jsp?curl=pages/medicines/human/referrals/Calcitonin/human_referral_000319.jsp&mid=WC0b01ac0580024e99

79. U.S. Food and Drug Administration. Background Document for Meeting of Advisory Committee for Reproductive Health Drugs and Drug Safety and Risk Management Advisory Committee (Internet); 2011 (cited 2015 Jun 20). Available from: http://www.fda.gov/downloads/AdvisoryCommittees/CommitteesMeetingMaterials/Drugs/ReproductiveHealthDrugsAdvisoryCommittee/UCM341779.pdf

80. Overman RA, Borse M, Gourlay ML. Salmon calcitonin use and associated cancer risk. Ann Pharmacother. 2013;47(12):1675–84.

81. Traynor K. Experts recommend against calcitonin-salmon for postmenopausal osteoporosis. Am J Health Syst Pharm. 2013;70(8):648–50.

82. Miacalcin (package insert). East Hanover, NJ: Novartis Pharmaceuticals Corp; 2011.

83. Porcel SL, Cumplido JA, de la Hoz B, Cuevas M, Losada E. Anaphylaxis to calcitonin. Allergol Immunopathol (Madr). 2000;28(4):243–5.

84. McClung MR, Lewiecki EM, Cohen SB, Bolognese MA, Woodson GC, Moffett AH, Peacock M, Miller PD, Lederman SN, Chesnut CH, Lain D, Kivitz AJ, Holloway DL, Zhang C, Peterson MC, Bekker PJ, AMG 162 Bone Loss Study Group. Denosumab in postmenopausal women with low bone mineral density. N Engl J Med. 2006;354(8):821–31.

85. McClung MR, Lewiecki EM, Geller ML, Bolognese MA, Peacock M, Weinstein RL, Ding B, Rockabrand E, Wagman RB, Miller PD. Effect of denosumab on bone mineral density and biochemical markers of bone turnover: 8-year results of a phase 2 clinical trial. Osteoporos Int. 2013;24(1):227–35.

86. *Bone HG, Chapurlat R, Brandi ML, Brown JP, Czerwinski E, Krieg MA, Mellström D, Radominski SC, Reginster JY, Resch H, Ivorra JA, Roux C, Vittinghoff E, Daizadeh NS, Wang A, Bradley MN, Franchimont N, Geller ML, Wagman RB, Cummings SR, Papapoulos S. The effect of three or six years of denosumab exposure in women with postmenopausal osteoporosis: results from the FREEDOM extension. J Clin Endocrinol Metab. 2013;98(11): 4483–92. *Long-term follow-up.

87. Khow KS, Yong TY. Atypical femoral fracture in a patient treated with denosumab. J Bone Miner Metab. 2015;33(3):355–8.

88. Ferrari-Lacraz S, Ferrari S. Do RANKL inhibitors (denosumab) affect inflammation and immunity? Osteoporos Int. 2011;22(2):435–46.

89. *Watts NB, Roux C, Modlin JF, Brown JP, Daniels A, Jackson S, Smith S, Zack DJ, Zhou L, Grauer A, Ferrari S. Infections in postmenopausal women with osteoporosis treated with denosumab or placebo: coincidence or causal association? Osteoporos Int. 2012;23(1):327–37. *Detailed description of adverse events related to infection with denosumab.

90. U.S. Food and Drug Administration. Prolia (Internet); 2014 (cited 2015 Jun 20). Available from: http://www.fda.gov/safety/medwatch/safetyinformation/safety-relateddruglabelingchanges/ucm307218.htm

91. Prolia (package insert). Thousand Oaks, CA: Amgen; 2015.

92. Shafqat H, Alquadan KF, Olszewski AJ. Severe hypocalcemia after denosumab in a patient with acquired Fanconi syndrome. Osteoporos Int. 2014;25(3):1187–90.

93. Sirvent AE, Enríquez R, Sánchez M, González C, Millán I, Amorós F. Extreme hypocalcaemia and hyperparathyroidism following denosumab. Is this drug safe in chronic kidney disease? Nefrologia. 2014;34(4):542–4.

94. Dave V, Chiang CY, Booth J, Mount PF. Hypocalcemia post denosumab in patients with chronic kidney disease stage 4–5. Am J Nephrol. 2015;41(2):129–37.

95. Okada N, Kawazoe K, Teraoka K, Kujime T, Abe M, Shinohara Y, Minakuchi K. Identification of the risk factors associated with hypocalcemia induced by denosumab. Biol Pharm Bull. 2013;36(10): 1622–6.

96. **Neer RM, Arnaud CD, Zanchetta JR, Prince R, Gaich GA, Reginster JY, Hodsman AB, Eriksen EF, Ish-Shalom S, Genant HK, Wang O, Mitlak BH. Effect of parathyroid hormone (1–34) on fractures and bone mineral density in postmenopausal women with osteoporosis. N Engl J Med. 2001;344(19):1434–41. **Pivotal trial.

97. Greenspan SL, Bone HG, Ettinger MP, Hanley DA, Lindsay R, Zanchetta JR, Blosch CM, Mathisen AL, Morris SA, Marriott TB, Treatment of Osteoporosis with Parathyroid Hormone Study Group. Effect of recombinant human parathyroid hormone (1–84) on vertebral fracture and bone mineral density in postmenopausal women with osteoporosis: a randomized trial. Ann Intern Med. 2007;146(5):326–39.

98. European Medicines Agency. Preotact (PTH (parathyroid hormone)). Withdrawal of the marketing authorisation in the European Union (Internet); 2011 (cited 2015 Jun 20). Available from: http://www.ema.europa.eu/docs/en_GB/document_library/Public_statement/2014/07/WC500169775.pdf

99. Saag KG, Zanchetta JR, Devogelaer JP, Adler RA, Eastell R, See K, Krege JH, Krohn K, Warner MR. Effects of teriparatide versus alendronate for treating glucocorticoid-induced osteoporosis: thirty-six-month results of a randomized, double-blind, controlled trial. Arthritis Rheum. 2009;60(11):3346–55.

100. Miller PD, Bilezikian JP, Diaz-Curiel M, Chen P, Marin F, Krege JH, Wong M, Marcus R. Occurrence of hypercalciuria in patients with osteoporosis treated with teriparatide. J Clin Endocrinol Metab. 2007;92:3535–41.

101. Forteo (package insert). Indianapolis, IN: Eli Lilly and Company; 2012.

102. Vahle JL, Long GG, Sandusky G, Westmore M, Ma YL, Sato M. Bone neoplasms in F344 rats given teriparatide [rhPTH(1–34)] are dependent on duration of treatment and dose. Toxicol Pathol. 2004;32(4):426–38.

103. Harper KD, Krege JH, Marcus R, Mitlak BH. Osteosarcoma and teriparatide? J Bone Miner Res. 2007;22(2):334.

104. Subbiah V, Madsen VS, Raymond AK, Benjamin RS, Ludwig JA. Of mice and men: divergent risks of teriparatide-induced osteosarcoma. Osteoporos Int. 2010;21(6):1041–5.

105. Cipriani C, Irani D, Bilezikian JP. Safety of osteoanabolic therapy: a decade of experience. J Bone Miner Res. 2012;27(12):2419–28.

106. Andrews EB, Gilsenan AW, Midkiff K, Sherrill B, Wu Y, Mann BH, Masica D. The US postmarketing surveillance study of adult osteosarcoma and teriparatide: study design and findings from the first 7 years. J Bone Miner Res. 2012;27(12):2429–37.

107. **Meunier PJ, Roux C, Seeman E, Ortolani S, Badurski JE, Spector TD, Cannata J, Balogh A, Lemmel EM, Pors-Nielsen S, Rizzoli R, Genant HK, Reginster JY. The effects of strontium ranelate on the risk of vertebral fracture in women with postmenopausal osteoporosis. N Engl J Med. 2004;350(5):459–68. **Pivotal trial.

108. **Reginster JY, Seeman E, De Vernejoul MC, Adami S, Compston J, Phenekos C, Devogelaer JP, Curiel MD, Sawicki A, Goemaere S, Sorensen OH, Felsenberg D, Meunier PJ. Strontium ranelate reduces the risk of nonvertebral fractures in postmenopausal women with osteoporosis: treatment of peripheral osteoporosis (TROPOS) study. J Clin Endocrinol Metab. 2005;90(5):2816–22. **Pivotal trial.

109. Blake GM, Fogelman I. Bone: strontium ranelate does not have an anabolic effect on bone. Nat Rev Endocrinol. 2013;9(12):696–7.

110. Recker RR, Marin F, Ish-Shalom S, Möricke R, Hawkins F, Kapetanos G, de la Peña MP, Kekow J, Farrerons J, Sanz B, Oertel H, Stepan J. Comparative effects of teriparatide and strontium ranelate on bone biopsies and biochemical markers of bone turnover in postmenopausal women with osteoporosis. J Bone Miner Res. 2009;24(8):1358–68.

111. Reginster JY, Felsenberg D, Boonen S, Diez-Perez A, Rizzoli R, Brandi ML, Spector TD, Brixen K, Goemaere S, Cormier C, Balogh A, Delmas PD, Meunier PJ. Effects of long-term strontium ranelate treatment on the risk of nonvertebral and vertebral fractures in postmenopausal osteoporosis: results of a five-year, randomized, placebo-controlled trial. Arthritis Rheum. 2008;58(6):1687–95.

112. European Medicines Agency. Strontium ranelate. Summary of product characteristics (Internet); 2009 (cited 2015 Jun 20). Available from: http://www.ema.europa.eu/docs/en_GB/document_library/EPAR-Product_Information/human/000560/WC500045525.pdf

113. Osborne V, Layton D, Perrio M, Wilton L, Shakir SA. Incidence of venous thromboembolism in users of strontium ranelate: an analysis of data from a prescription-event monitoring study in England. Drug Saf. 2010;33(7):579–91.

114. Breart G, Cooper C, Meyer O, Speirs C, Deltour N, Reginster JY. Osteoporosis and venous thromboembolism: a retrospective cohort study in the UK general practice research database. Osteoporos Int. 2010;21(7):1181–7.

115. Perrio M, Wilton L, Shakir S. Analysis of venous thromboembolism in the strontium ranelate prescription-event monitoring (PEM) cohort: interim results. Drug Saf. 2010;33(7):579–91.

116. Jonville-Béra AP, Crickx B, Aaron L, Hartingh I, Autret-Leca E. Strontium ranelate-induced DRESS syndrome: first two case reports. Allergy. 2009;64(4):658–9.

117. European Medicines Agency Assessment report – periodic safety update report (EPAR – Protelos-H-C-560-PSU31) www.ema.europa.eu/docs/en_GB/document_library/EPAR_-_Assessment_Report_-_Variation/human/000560/WC500147168.pdf. Accessed 3 Feb 2014.

118. Cooper C, Fox KM, Borer JS. Ischaemic cardiac events and use of strontium ranelate in postmenopausal osteoporosis: a nested case-control study in the CPRD. Osteoporos Int. 2014;25(2):737–45.

119. Reginster J-Y. Cardiac concerns associated with strontium ranelate. Expert Opin Drug Saf. 2014;13(9):1209–13.

120. European Medicines Agency. Recommendation to restrict the use of Protelos/Osseor (strontium ranelate) (Internet); 2013 (cited 2015 Jun 20). Available from: http://www.ema.europa.eu/docs/en_GB/document_library/Press_release/2013/04/WC500142507.pdf

121. European Medicines Agency. PRAC recommends suspending use of Protelos/Osseor (Internet); 2014 (cited 2015 Jun 20). Available from: http://www.ema.europa.eu/ema/index.jsp%3Fcurl=pages/news_and_events/news/2014/01/news_detail_002005.jsp%26mid=WC0b01ac058004d5c1

122. European Medicines Agency. European Medicines Agency recommends that Protelos/Osseor remain available but with further restrictions (Internet); 2014 (cited 2015 Jun 20). Available from: http://www.ema.europa.eu/ema/index.jsp?curl=pages/news_and_events/news/2014/02/news_detail_002031.jsp&mid=WC0b01ac58001d126

123. Rijks EB, Bongers BC, Vlemmix MJ, Boot AM, van Dijk AT, Sakkers RJ, van Brussel M. Efficacy and safety of bisphosphonate therapy in children with osteogenesis imperfecta: a systematic review. Horm Res Paediatr. 2015;84(1):26–42.

124. Green SB, Pappas AL. Effects of maternal bisphosphonate use on fetal and neonatal outcomes. Am J Health Syst Pharm. 2014;71(23):2029–36.

125. Evista (package insert). Indianapolis, IN: Eli Lilly and Company; 2011.

The Impact of Regulatory and Scientific Organizations' Recommendations on Clinical Decision-Making

Alexandra Papaioannou, Arnav Agarwal, and Sarah Karampatos

Summary

- Patients often experience a prodrome of dull aching pain weeks to months prior to atypical femur fracture.
- Although there is concern that long-term bisphosphonate use is associated with serious, rare adverse events, the benefits of using osteoporosis medication to prevent fracture outweigh the risks identified.
- Bisphosphonate drug holidays can be considered for patients who are a low-fracture risk after 3–5 years of therapy with bisphosphonates. For high-fracture risk patients with osteoporotic bone mineral density (BMD) and a history of fragility fracture, bisphosphonate therapy should be continued without drug holidays.
- Health professionals may report post-marketing adverse events to national and international bodies and highlight clinical recommendations.
- The development of an international registry to identify patients who have experienced these adverse events with bisphosphonates and denosumab is an important future direction.

A. Papaioannou, BScN, MD, MSc,
FRCP(C), FACP (✉)
Department of Medicine, McMaster University,
1280 Main St W, Hamilton, ON L8S 4L8, Canada

Geriatric Education and Research in the Aging
Sciences (GERAS) Centre, 88 Maplewood Avenue,
Hamilton, ON L8M 1W9, Canada

Department of Biostatistics and Epidemiology,
McMaster University, 1280 Main St W,
Hamilton, ON L8S 4L8, Canada
e-mail: papaioannou@hhsc.ca

A. Agarwal, BHSc
Faculty of Medicine, University of Toronto,
Toronto, ON, Canada
e-mail: arnav.agarwal@mail.utoronto.ca

Introduction

A growing prevalence of osteoporosis with an increasingly large geriatric population represents one of the modern healthcare system's prominent challenges [1]. Osteoporosis is characterized by

S. Karampatos, BASc, MSc(c)
Department of Medicine, McMaster University,
1280 Main St W, Hamilton, ON L8S 4L8, Canada

Geriatric Education and Research in the Aging
Sciences (GERAS) Centre, 88 Maplewood Avenue,
Hamilton, ON L8M 1W9, Canada

Department of Rehabilitation Sciences, McMaster
University, 1280 Main St W, Hamilton, ON
L8S 4L8, Canada
e-mail: karampatos@hhsc.ca

© Springer International Publishing Switzerland 2016
S.L. Silverman, B. Abrahamsen (eds.), *The Duration and Safety
of Osteoporosis Treatment*, DOI 10.1007/978-3-319-23639-1_21

low bone mass and microarchitectural deterioration of bone tissue that increases the risk of fracture [1]. Clinical complications of osteoporosis include increased risk of joint pain and fracture, particularly of the hip, vertebrae, and wrist [1]. A high prevalence of fractures among older adults has been noted in particular, and serious consequences of fractures in the geriatric population have been evidenced. One in four individuals suffering hip fractures dies within a 5-year period following their injury [2]. It is, therefore, important for physicians to not only diagnose patients with osteoporosis accurately and efficiently but also to appropriately prescribe appropriate medications targeted at improving bone density and reducing the risk of fracture.

The ultimate goal of clinical practice guidelines is to develop a more standardized approach and balance benefits, harms, and cost-effectiveness. Approaches to guideline development for osteoporosis have varied in terms of the use of systematic review methodology, of evidence-grading systems, and application of the Appraisal of Guidelines Research and Evaluation Framework (AGREE), resulting in different approaches and recommendations. Aside from the differences in methodology, the challenges in distilling the growing volume of guidelines is an issue for end users of these recommendations.

National and international regulatory organizations have developed and/or amended guidelines for assessment and treatment of osteoporosis in response to recent concerns regarding rare but serious adverse events associated with long-term utilization of widely prescribed osteoporosis pharmacotherapy. These adverse events include, but are not limited to, atypical fractures and osteonecrosis of the jaw (ONJ). The purpose of this chapter is to review recommendations of these scientific national and international bodies on the duration of safety of osteoporosis therapies of anabolic and antiresorptive medications. In particular, dosage recommendations, adverse events, drug holiday recommendations, and supporting research evidence considered by these national and international bodies in decision-making are explored.

Randomized Controlled Trials and the Evaluation of Efficacy and Harms

Randomized controlled trials are essential to establishing the efficacy of drugs. However, they may be underpowered to detect uncommon or rare but clinically significant adverse drug events, especially those that develop after prolonged exposure. A number of other study methodologies, including pragmatic trials, have been suggested to address this issue.

Randomized controlled trials on bisphosphonates for the prevention and treatment of osteoporosis represent one such case of the limitations of such studies to detect uncommon adverse drug events, even after prolonged exposure. Bisphosphonates were shown to reduce fracture risk in a number of randomized controlled trials involving 3000–7500 postmenopausal women over 3–5 year durations and subsequent meta-analysis [3–13]. With long-term bisphosphonate use, there were a number of post-marketing reports of atypical subtrochanteric fractures and ONJ. Black et al. (2012) reported that approximately 1 in 7 postmenopausal women in the United States was prescribed a bisphosphonate [13]. Ultimately, post-marketing reports resulted in a review by the Food and Drug Administration (FDA) to address the safety and efficacy of these medications beyond the 3–5-year periods of previously conducted clinical trials [14]. Internationally, a number of countries' health agencies addressing drug registration and approval subsequently revised their recommendations for this class of medications.

American Society for Bone and Mineral Research

The American Society for Bone and Mineral Research (ASBMR) is a medical society encompassing over 4000 researchers, physicians, and health professionals. Since the approval of bisphosphonates by the Food and Drug Administration (FDA), there have been a number of post-marketing studies reporting potential adverse effects of bisphosphonates. The ASBMR formed two task forces, one on ONJ in 2007 and a second on atypical fractures in 2010 [15–18]. The committees, which included international and multidisciplinary experts, reviewed both published (case reports, case series, and epidemiologic data) and unpublished data and interviewed pharmaceutical companies. The ASBMR provided testimony to the FDA Advisory Committee for Reproductive Health Drugs and the Drug Safety and Risk Management Committee with a focus on the two task forces on bisphosphonate use.

ASBMR Osteonecrosis of the Jaw

Bisphosphonates decrease fracture risk in patients with osteoporosis. However, they have been associated with potential risks, including ONJ and atypical femur fractures. Bisphosphate-related ONJ is defined by the ASBMR as being "associated with exposed bone in the maxillofacial region that did not heal within 8 weeks after identification by a health care provider, in a patient who was receiving or had been exposed to a bisphosphonate and had not had radiation therapy to the craniofacial region" [15]. The risk of ONJ is greatest in the oncology patient population (1–15 %), particularly with high doses or frequent doses. Overall, risk associated with oral bisphosphonate therapy for osteoporosis seems to be low, estimated between 1 in 10,000 and <1 in 100,000 patient-treatment years [19, 20]. However, the task force recognized that information on the incidence of ONJ is rapidly evolving and that the true incidence may be higher. Risk factors for ONJ include glucocorticoid use, maxillary or mandibular bone surgery, poor oral hygiene, chronic inflammation, diabetes mellitus, ill-fitting dentures, as well as antiangiogenic agents [16]. Prevention strategies for ONJ include elimination or stabilization of oral disease prior to initiation of antiresorptive agents and good oral hygiene [16]. Management of ONJ is based on the stage of the disease, size of lesions, comorbidity, and presence of

contributing drug therapy [16]. Ongoing reports and assessments of ONJ include independent international studies and post-marketing studies. In the future, improved diagnostic imaging modalities, such as MRI combined with contrast agents and the manipulation of image planes, may identify patients at preclinical or early stages of the disease.

The ASBMR has recently identified and reported an increased risk of ONJ with denosumab use.

ASMBR Atypical Femur Fracture

There has been considerable concern from clinicians and patients regarding atypical fractures involving the subtrochanteric and diaphyseal femur. ASBMR updated its original definition of atypical fractures of the femur in 2014 to include the following criteria: (1) associated with minimal or no trauma; (2) fracture line originating at the lateral cortex and running substantially transverse in its orientation, although it may become oblique as it progresses medially across the femur; (3) complete extension through both cortices and possible association with the medial spike; (4) non-comminuted or minimally comminuted fracture; and (5) localized periosteal or endosteal thickening of the cortex present at the fracture site [17]. Atypical fractures represent only 1 % of all hip and femur fractures and are thought to be stress fractures. These fractures seem to be more common in those exposed to bisphosphonates; however, they also occur in those without exposure. While there is evidence to suggest the occurrence of atypical subtrochanteric and diaphyseal femoral fractures, the magnitude of the effect is unknown, and events have primarily been noted with long-term bisphosphonate use, greater than 3 years with a median of 7 years [17, 18]. According to the ASBMR, the relative risk of atypical femur fractures is high in patients using bisphosphonates (3.1–128); however, the absolute risk remains low (3.2–50 cases per 100, 000). While a decrease in the risk for atypical fractures after bisphosphonates are discontinued has been considered, it is not well-evidenced [17]. The committee's recommendations for treatment of atypical fractures include discontinuation of bisphosphonates, dietary calcium and vitamin D assessment and supplementation, prophylactic reconstruction nail fixation for incomplete fractures accompanied by pain, limited weight bearing, and teriparatide (TPTD) therapy if conservative therapy does not result in healing. Randomized controlled trials are underway to determine if TPTD is beneficial in fracture healing [18, 21, 22].

Risk factors for atypical fractures include Asian ethnicity, lower limb geometry, and glucocorticoid use. Many patients experience a prodrome of dull aching pain weeks to months prior to fracture. ASBMR recommends that more information is needed to identify patients at high risk for atypical fractures and to inform decision-making on duration and adverse effects of bisphosphonates. Annual review on whether bisphosphonates are indicated, healthcare professional awareness of warning signs, and the development of an international registry to identify patients who have experienced these adverse events are pertinent [17, 18].

The ASBMR has recently identified and reported an increased risk of atypical fractures with denosumab use.

Food and Drug Administration

An agency within the US Department of Health and Human Services, the FDA strives to protect public health by promoting safety, effectiveness, quality, and security through regulation of medical products and tobacco, foods and veterinary medicine, global regulatory operations and policy, and operations. Post-marketing reports of atypical femur fractures, ONJ, and esophageal cancer resulted in the FDA completing a systematic review assessing bisphosphonates [14]. Other post-marketing reports of adverse events have included hypersensitivity reactions, musculoskeletal events (myalgias, bone joint muscle pain, and joint swelling), gastrointestinal events (esophagitis, esophageal ulcers, gastric or duode-

nal ulcers), skin rashes, pruritus, Stevens–Johnson syndrome, and toxic epidermal necrolysis, with rare reports of uveitis, scleritis, episcleritis, and hypocalcaemia.

The FDA also reviewed extension studies assessing bisphosphonates, including the Fosamax Fracture Intervention Trial Long-Term Extension (FLEX), the Reclast Health Outcomes and Reduced Incidence with Zoledronic Acid Once Yearly–Pivotal Fracture Trial (HORIZON-PFT), and the Actonel Vertebral Efficacy with Risedronate Therapy–Multinational Trial (VERT-MN) [14, 23–28]. These extension trials were primarily evaluated and were supplemented by long-term extension trials including 164–1233 participants and evaluated BMD as a surrogate outcome [23, 28]. These trials all demonstrated that 5 years of bisphosphonate treatment resulted in the stabilization of BMD at the femoral neck and continuing increases in lumbar spine BMD. In participants who were randomized to placebo thereafter, the BMD at the femoral neck decreased for the first 1–2 years and then remained stable, while lumbar spine BMD continued to increase.

The optimal duration of bisphosphonate treatment for osteoporosis is unknown based on FDA recommendations. Bisphosphonate medications approved for the prevention and/or treatment of osteoporosis have clinical trial data supporting fracture reduction efficacy through at least 3 years and, in some cases, through 5 years of treatment [29]. The regulatory body added a Limitations of Use statement in the indications and usage section of the labels for these drugs, based on its findings on atypical fractures and concerns regarding the duration of bisphosphonate use [30]. The FDA is continuing its evaluation of data examining the safety and effectiveness of long-term bisphosphonate use (greater than 3–5 years) for the treatment and prevention of osteoporosis.

The FDA has recently acknowledged that denosumab increases patients' risk of atypical fractures and ONJ and advised physicians to closely monitor patients prescribed with denosumab for these adverse events.

Agency for Healthcare Research and Quality

The Agency for Healthcare Research and Quality (AHRQ) is an agency that is part of the US Department of Health. The department supports healthcare research in order to disseminate information to healthcare professionals worldwide.

A clinical research summary was written in 2013 to update treatment and prevention recommendations for osteoporotic fractures. This update to the AHRQ's initial 2007 report included a systematic review of 567 clinical studies comparing safety and effectiveness of osteoporosis treatments [31]. The review notably found that (a) vertebral fractures were reduced by bisphosphonates (alendronate, risedronate, and zoledronic acid), denosumab, raloxifene, and TPTD; (b) non-vertebral fractures were reduced by bisphosphonates, denosumab, and TPTD; and (c) hip fractures were reduced by bisphosphonates and denosumab. The evidence for fracture reduction was greatest for those with BMD scores in the osteoporotic range (<-2.5) and those with preexisting vertebral fractures [31]. There was limited evidence for treatment beyond 5 years in reduction of vertebral fractures.

Although there is significant evidence that osteoporosis medications reduce fracture risk and increase BMD, there are also adverse events and side effects associated with the use of osteoporosis medications. Table 21.1 outlines adverse events associated with osteoporosis medications. Table 21.2 outlines possible side effects associated with osteoporosis medications. Dosage, duration, and frequency of medication can be associated with an increased risk of adverse events [31]. Post hoc analysis of major clinical trials included a review of all fractures below the lesser trochanter but above the distal metaphyseal flare [4, 8, 24, 32]. This included 284 cases of 14,195 women randomized to these trials. Twelve cases of atypical fractures were identified; however, results were not statistically significant, and the trials were underpowered to detect these adverse events [33].

National Osteoporosis Foundation

The National Osteoporosis Foundation (NOF) focuses on patient and professional education, advocacy, and research in the United States. Their recommendations target both healthcare providers and individuals with osteoporosis and are based on FDA recommendations to regularly monitor patients and individualize treatment plans. NOF's clinical guide to prevention and treatment of osteoporosis was updated in 2013 [34] and includes useful tools for clinicians on how to assess risk and when treatment should be indicated.

NOF Antiresorptive Therapy

Bisphosphonate medications have been known to involve adverse effects, most commonly gastrointestinal related. Unusually, there have been reports of bisphosphonate-related ONJ; however, ONJ risk in bisphosphonate-treated patients is unknown, and the risk appears to be low for at least up to 5 years of treatment [35]. The risk of ONJ also appears to increase in cancer patients receiving intravenous bisphosphonates. The NOF recommends that patients should speak to their doctors prior to discontinuing treatment. Atypical subtrochanteric and diaphyseal femoral fractures have been reported, although they are considered to be rare and associated with long-term use (>5 years). Symptoms of atypical subtrochanteric and diaphyseal femoral fractures include thigh and groin pain and should be reported immediately [35].

Alendronate has been approved by the FDA for the prevention and treatment of osteoporosis. It is recommended that patients receive 5 mg daily or 35 mg weekly for the prevention of osteoporosis and 10 mg daily (tablet) or 70 mg weekly (tablet) with 2800 IU or 5500 IU of vitamin D and 70 mg effervescent (tablet) for the treatment of osteoporosis. Alendronate has been shown to decrease the incidence of spine and hip fracture by 50 % and vertebral fracture by 48 % (without prior vertebral fracture) over 3 years [35].

Table 21.1 Adverse events with rated findings (AHRQ) [31]

Medication	Adverse event	Magnitude of association (from pooled analysis of clinical data)[a]
Bisphosphonates	Possible association with atypical subtrochanteric fractures of the femur	Not available—but the risk for this type of fracture is low Data is inconsistent, but the US Food and Drug Administration has issued a boxed warning about this possible adverse effect
Alendronate	Mild upper GI events[b]	OR = 1.08, 95 % CI: 1.01–1.15
	Hypocalcaemia	9/301 treatment vs. 0/207 placebo
Zoledronic acid	Hypocalcaemia	OR = 7.22, 95 % CI: 1.81–42.7
Intravenous forms of zoledronic acid and ibandronate	Osteonecrosis of the jaw (ONJ)	Less than one case per 100,000 person-years of exposure (nearly all cases of ONJ are reported in people being treated for cancer)
Raloxifene	Pulmonary embolism	OR = 5.27, 95 % CI: 1.29–46.4
	Thromboembolic events	OR = 1.63, 95 % CI: 1.36–1.98
	Myalgias, cramps, and limb pain	OR = 1.53, 95 % CI: 1.29–1.81
	Hot flashes	OR = 1.58, 95 % CI: 1.35–1.84
Menopausal hormone therapy: estrogen and estrogen–progestin combination	Cerebrovascular events[c]	Estrogen, OR = 1.34, 95 % CI: 1.07–1.68 Combination, OR = 2.27, 95 % CI: 1.05–1.57
	Thromboembolic events[c]	Estrogen, OR = 1.36, 95 % CI: 1.01–1.86 Combination, OR = 2.27, 95 % CI: 1.72–3.02
	Breast cancer	Estrogen: in the WHI [5], this hormone was associated with reduced incidence of breast cancer in women with hysterectomy when compared with placebo (HR = 0.77, 95 % CI: 0.62–0.95)[d], but subgroup analysis noted that risk reduction was concentrated in women without benign breast disease or family history of breast cancer. No risk reduction was seen in women at high risk for breast cancer Combination: in the WHI [15], estrogen–progestin was associated with more occurrences of invasive breast cancer than with placebo (HR = 1.25, 95 % CI: 1.07–1.46), tumors more likely to have lymph node metastases (HR = 1.96, 95 % CI: 1.00–4.04)[e]

Teriparatide	Hypercalcemia	OR = 12.9, 95 % CI: 10.49–16.0
	Headaches	OR = 1.44, 95 % CI: 1.24–1.67
Denosumab	Mild upper GI events[b]	OR = 2.13, 95 % CI: 1.11–4.4
	Rash	OR = 2.01, 95 % CI: 1.5–2.73
	Infection	OR = 1.28, 95 % CI: 1.02–1.60

[a]95 % CI = 95 % confidence interval; *HR* hazard ratio (in cancer research, a measure of how often a particular event happens in one group compared with how often it happens in another group over time); *OR* odds ratio (the odds of the condition developing in those taking the listed medications compared with the incidence in patients receiving placebo treatment; *WHI* Women's Health Initiative

[b]Mild upper GI events = conditions involving the upper gastrointestinal tract such as acid reflux, esophageal irritation, nauseam vomiting, and heart burn

[c]These finds are from the original 2007 report. *Note*: The WHI reported adverse effects associated with menopausal hormone therapy, including venous thromboembolic events, stroke, and a variable effect on breast cancer

[d]Anderson GI, Chlebowski RT, Aragaki AK et al. Conjugated equine oestrogen and breast cancer incidence and mortality in postmenopausal women with hysterectomy: extended follow-up of the Women's Health Initiative randomized placebo-controlled trial. Lancet Oncol 2012

[e]Chebowski RT, Anderson GL, Gass M et al.; WHI Investigators: Estrogen plus progestin and breast cancer incidence and mortality in postmenopausal women JAMA 2010

With permission from Treatment to Prevent Osteoporotic Fractures: An Update—Clinician Research Summary (AHRQ Publication No. 12-EHC023-3). Rockville, MD: Agency for Healthcare Research and Quality. May 2012. Available at http://effectivehealthcare.ahrq.gov/index.cfm/search-for-guides-reviews-and-reports/?productid=1048&pageaction=displayproduct#5272

Table 21.2 Additional possible side effects (AHRQ) [31]

Medications	Adverse effect(s)
Alendronate, risedronate, and ibandronate	Musculoskeletal pain Hypocalcemia Osteonecrosis of the jaw Severe irritation of upper gastrointestinal mucosa
Zoledronic acid	Severe musculoskeletal pain Renal toxicity and acute renal failure
Denosumab	Hypocalcemia Osteonecrosis of the jaw
Teriparatide	Increased risk of bone cancer

With permission from Treatment to Prevent Osteoporotic Fractures: An Update—Clinician Research Summary (AHRQ Publication No. 12-EHC023-3). Rockville, MD: Agency for Healthcare Research and Quality. May 2012. Available at http://effectivehealthcare.ahrq.gov/index.cfm/search-for-guides-reviews-and-reports/?productid=1048&pageaction=displayproduct#5272

Ibandronate has been approved by the FDA for the treatment of postmenopausal osteoporosis. The FDA recommends that patients receive a 150 mg monthly tablet and 3 mg every 3 months by intravenous injection. Ibandronate has shown to decrease the incidence of vertebral fractures by 50 % over 3 years; however, the reduction in risk of non-vertebral fracture has not been documented [36].

Risedronate is approved by the FDA for the prevention and treatment of osteoporosis in post-menopausal osteoporosis. It is recommended that patients receive 5 mg daily tablet, 35 mg weekly tablet, 35 mg weekly delayed release tablet, 35 mg weekly tablet packaged with six tablets of 500 mg calcium carbonate, 75 mg tablets on 2 consecutive days every month, or 150 mg monthly tablet. Risedronate has shown to reduce the incidence of vertebral fracture (41–49 %) and non-vertebral fracture (36 %) over 3 years [37].

Zoledronic acid has been approved for the treatment and prevention of osteoporosis in post-menopausal women, improved bone mass in men with osteoporosis, and for the prevention and treatment of osteoporosis for men and women expected to be on glucocorticoid therapy for at least 3 months. Zoledronic acid is administered intravenously for 15 min (5 mg) once a year for treatment and once every 2 years for prevention [38]. Zoledronic acid has been shown to reduce the incidence of vertebral fracture (70 %), hip fractures (41 %), and non-vertebral fractures (25 %) over 3 years [38]. Zoledronic acid can affect renal function and is contraindicated in patients with creatinine clearance less than 35 mL/min and with renal impairment [38]. Patients receiving zoledronic acid should be identified as at-risk and should have creatinine clearance monitored prior to each dose administered [38].

Estrogen (ET) and hormone therapy (HT) has been approved by the FDA for the prevention of osteoporosis. The Women's Health Initiative (WHI) found that ET/HT has been proven to reduce the risk of vertebral and hip fracture (34 %) and other osteoporotic fractures (23 %) over 5 years [39]. The FDA recommends that ET/HT be used only to treat moderately severe menopausal symptoms, for the shortest time necessary; ET and HT should only be used for the prevention of osteoporosis, and approved non-estrogen treatments should be considered first [39].

Denosumab has been approved by the FDA for the treatment of postmenopausal women at high risk of fracture. Denosumab is administered by a health professional twice a year at a dosage of 60 mg. Denosumab has been proven to reduce the risk of vertebral fracture (68 %), hip fracture (40 %), and non-vertebral fracture (20 %) over the course of 3 years. However, it has also been associated with ONJ and atypical femur fractures [40, 41].

NOF Anabolic Therapy

Parathyroid hormone TPTD has been approved by the FDA for the treatment of osteoporosis in postmenopausal women, men at high risk for fracture, and patients at high risk of fracture with osteoporosis associated with sustained systemic glucocorticoid therapy [34]. It is recommended that patients are administered a daily injection of 20 µg daily. TPTD has shown to decrease the incidence of vertebral fractures (65 %) and non-vertebral fractures (53 %) following 18 months of therapy. TPTD is not recommended for patients at risk for osteosarcoma (including those with Paget's disease, prior radiation of the skeleton, bone metastases, or hypocalcaemia) based on high osteosarcoma incidences identified in rat models. It is also recommended that patients do not receive TPTD treatment for more than 2 years and receive an antiresorptive agent such as a bisphosphonate to increase BMD [42].

Osteoporosis Canada

Osteoporosis Canada promotes osteoporosis risk reduction and treatment, providing medically accurate information to patients, healthcare professionals, and the public. The organization published guidelines in 2010, reviewing when osteoporosis pharmacotherapies including alendronate, risedronate, and zoledronic acid should be discontinued to prevent high-risk fracture in patients with osteoporosis [43]. According to Osteoporosis Canada, adverse events caused by bisphosphonates are considered to be rare, including ONJ and atypical fractures of the femur. The absolute risk of bisphosphonate-related ONJ is approximately 1 case per 100,000 person-years when bisphosphonates are administered for osteoporosis treatment [44]. The development of ONJ increases when individuals have poor oral hygiene and if oncology patients are receiving high-dose antiresorptive treatment. According to Osteoporosis Canada, little is known about features associated with atypical fractures of the femur. The absolute risk of bisphosphonate-associated atypical subtrochanteric diaphyseal femur fracture is between 2 and 78 cases per 100,000 persons [44]. However, while long-term clinical trial data has not shown an increase in atypical fracture of the femur risk, some studies have indicated that these trials are too small in nature to detect uncommon events [13, 44–46]. The most common bisphosphonate-associated with atypical femoral fractures is alendronate, likely due to its earlier availability relative to other currently used bisphosphonates.

Individuals at high risk for fracture are recommended to continue osteoporosis therapy without a drug holiday (Grade D evidence) as their anti-fracture benefits considerably outweigh potential for harm. This decision was based on rates of clinical vertebral fractures being reduced by 55 % for those who remained on alendronate therapy, compared to those who discontinued after 5 years in the FLEX trial [47]. High risk was identified as those over the age of 50 who had a prior fragility fracture of the hip or vertebrae, or those that suffered more than one fragility fracture, being offered a pharmacological therapy (Grade B evidence) or as greater than 20 % fracture probability, a major fracture probability over 10 years, using either FRAX or CAROC (Grade D evidence). Adverse effects were evidenced using Cochrane meta-analysis systematic reviews, as well as highlighting post-marketing surveillance [43].

A subsequent position statement on the duration of bisphosphonate use and drug holidays recommended that drug holidays should be considered for patients at low risk of fracture after 3–5 years of therapy with bisphosphonates [48]. For those at high risk of fracture with a history of fragility fracture or osteoporotic BMD, bisphosphonates should be continued without a drug holiday. A radiograph of the full length of the femur or a bone scan has been recommended for those with a history of thigh pain to assess for possible atypical subtrochanteric fractures [43]. Osteoporosis Canada findings and recommendations are in agreement with the ASBMR, FDA, and AHRQ.

Health Canada

Health Canada is the nation's federal regulator of therapeutic drugs and provides public information on human pharmaceutical and biological drugs, veterinary drugs, and disinfectant products approved for use in Canada. The organization is in agreement with Osteoporosis Canada and has encouraged practicing clinicians to recognize that while the risk of adverse events is higher with bisphosphonate use, it remains minor and osteoporosis-related fracture prevention benefits outweigh ONJ and atypical femoral fracture risks [43, 44].

European Medicines Agency

The European Medicines Agency (EMA) conducts scientific evaluations and European public assessment reports (EPARs) of pharmaceuticals developed for use. Authorization assessments are conducted based on scientific criteria related to quality, safety, efficacy, and risk–benefit standards, and EPARs establish the scientific criteria based on which a pharmaceutical was granted authorization, as well as a detailed summary of product characteristics, labeling/packaging, and assessment and authorization procedural steps [49].

An increased risk of atypical fracture of the femur with little or no trauma was noted by the CHMP's Pharmacovigilance Working Group in association with alendronic acid use in 2008, resulting in a warning addition to the product information of related medicines. The Working Group also decided to review this risk in other bisphosphonates (as a class effect) and identified published literature and post-marketing reports suggestive of atypical stress femoral fractures as a class effect by April 2010, leading to a further review by the CHMP to determine the need for regulatory action on bisphosphonate-containing medicines [50, 51].

The CHMP has examined all case reports, epidemiological studies, and other relevant data from published literature and industries relevant to bisphosphonate-related stress fractures. The optimal duration of bisphosphonate treatments has not been established by the EMA; the treatments have been recommended on a continual basis, with reevaluation of benefits and potential risks on an individual patient basis, particularly following 5 or more years of use [50, 51].

Authorized by the EU since April 15, 2005, zoledronic acid has been recommended as a single intravenous 5 mg infusion for osteoporosis in men at increased risk of fracture or with a recent low-trauma hip fracture, postmenopausal women, patients with long-term systemic glucocorticoid therapy, Paget's disease of the bone patients, and low-trauma hip fracture patients (initiated 2 or more weeks following fracture repair) [52]. Zoledronic acid has been contraindicated in patients with creatinine clearance of <35 ml/min (severe renal impairment), hypersensitivity to bisphosphonates or the drug's active substance, hypocalcaemia, and pregnant and breast-feeding women [52]. The HORIZON Pivotal Fracture Trial ($n=7736$ postmenopausal women with osteoporosis) identified one case of ONJ in both intervention and placebo-controlled groups. Compared to placebo, zoledronic acid was found to significantly reduce the days of limited activity ($p<0.01$) and the days of bed rest due to fractures ($p<0.01$) [26]. Overall, adverse reactions have been reported by 44.7 %, 16.7 %, and 10.2 % of patients following first, second, and third infusions, respectively. Fever (17.1 %), myalgia (7.8 %), flu-like symptoms (6.7 %), arthralgia (4.8 %), and headaches (5.1 %) were commonly reported mild or moderate adverse effects, particularly within the first three days following administration [26, 52, 53]. An increased incidence of serious atrial fibrillation adverse events was also reported (51/3862 vs. 22/3852 placebo patients). Other common adverse events associated with zoledronic acid use include ocular hyperemia, dizziness, nausea, vomiting, diarrhea, bone pain, back pain, extremity pain, chills, fatigue, asthenia, general pain, malaise, infusion site reactions, and C-reactive protein increases [26, 52, 53].

Alendronate sodium trihydrate was authorized by the EU on January 4, 2007, with a recommended dosage of one trihydrate tablet once weekly [54]. The pharmaceutical is contraindicated for patients with renal impairment, particularly for those with a glomerular filtration rate of less than 35 mL/min, as well as for those with hypersensitivity to the drug's active substances, an inability to stand or sit upright for a minimum of 30 min, and esophageal abnormalities or esophageal emptying delays [54]. The most commonly reported adverse reactions are upper gastrointestinal adverse reactions (>1 %), including abdominal pain dyspepsia, esophageal ulcer, dysphagia, abdominal distension, and acid regurgitation [54]. Headaches, dizziness, vertigo, alopecia, pruritus, bone/joint/muscle pain (sometimes severe), joint swelling, asthenia, and peripheral edema are other commonly reported adverse effects [54].

Denosumab was authorized by the EU on May 26, 2010 and is recommended as a single subcutaneous 60 mg injection into the thigh, abdomen, or upper arm once every 6 months; duration of treatment is unspecified [55]. Denosumab is not recommended for patients under the age of 18 years [55]. Hypocalcaemia and hypersensitivity to the drug's active substance are contraindicated, and adequate vitamin D and calcium intake are recommended as precautions [55]. Cellulitis and skin infections have also been identified as adverse events in postmenopausal osteoporosis patients (50/4041 placebo vs. 59/4050 denosumab), male osteoporotic patients (1/120 vs. 0/120), and breast or prostate cancer patients receiving hormone ablation (14/845 vs. 12/860). Clinical studies have reported ONJ as an occasional adverse effect in patients receiving 60 mg denosumab every 6 months, those with advanced cancer receiving a 120 mg dose monthly, and those simultaneously receiving hormone ablation [55]. Atypical femoral fractures have also been reported as well, particularly in patients with vitamin D deficiency, rheumatoid arthritis, hypophosphatemia, and bisphosphonate, glucocorticoid, or proton pump inhibitor use [55]. Other commonly associated adverse effects include urinary tract infection, upper respiratory tract infection, sciatica, cataracts, constipation, abdominal discomfort, rash, eczema, and pain in the extremities [55].

Authorized since June 10, 2003 by the EU, TPTD has been recommended at a dosage of 20 mg once daily for a maximum of 24 months without a second period of administration due to the risk of osteosarcoma [56]. Other bisphosphonate treatments and supplemental vitamin D and calcium have been recommended as necessary [56]. TPTD is not recommended for patients with severe renal impairment, is contraindicated for use during pregnancy and breast-feeding, and may be associated with reproductive toxicity and impaired fetal development based on animal studies [56]. Preexisting hypercalcemia, metabolic bone disease such as hyperparathyroidism and Paget's disease of the bone, unexplained alkaline phosphatase elevation, prior external beam or implant radiation therapy exposure, skeletal malignancies, and bone metastases are other reported contraindications [56]. Commonly reported adverse effects include nausea, limb pain, headaches, and dizziness [56]. Across several trials, 82.8 % of patients using TPTD reported at least one adverse event versus 84.5 % of patients administered a placebo. TPTD has also been associated with increased serum uric acid concentrations (2.8 vs. 0.7 % placebo patients) and cross-reacting antibodies, primarily in the first 12 months of therapy [56]. Other reportedly common adverse effects associated with TPTD include blood cholesterol level increases, depression, neuralgic leg pain, faintness, irregular heartbeats, breathlessness, increased sweating, muscle cramps, energy decreases, fatigue, chest pain, low blood pressure, heartburn, vomiting, esophageal hernia, and anemia [56].

Evaluating all available evidence on bisphosphonate use, the CHMP noted an increase in the number of reports of atypical fracture of the femur and a distinct X-ray pattern in users since its 2008 review, particularly with long-term use. This pattern might be related to bisphosphonate mode of action, which may cause in delayed repair of naturally occurring stress fractures [50].

Overall, the CHMP concluded that atypical fractures are likely a class effect of bisphosphonates, although they occur rarely and benefits outweigh risks involved with their use, based on currently available evidence. The European Commission put forward four recommendations as of July 13, 2011: (a) prescribing doctors should be aware that atypical fractures of the femur may occur rarely, particularly with long-term use, and should examine the other leg as well if an atypical fracture is suspected in one; (b) prescribing doctors should review continued treatment needs regularly, especially after 5 or more years of use; (c) patients receiving medicines should be aware of atypical fracture of the femur risks involved and should report any pain, weakness, or discomfort in the thigh or groin area to their doctor; and (d) patients should address questions with their doctor or pharmacist. Additionally, the CHMP recommended the amendment of product information to include warnings addressing this risk [50].

International Osteoporosis Foundation

International Osteoporosis Foundation (IOF) is a global alliance of patient societies, research organizations, and healthcare professionals working to promote bone, muscle, and joint health. The IOF initially published guidelines on the diagnosis and management of osteoporosis in 1997. The Scientific Advisory Board of the European Society for Clinical and Economic Aspects of Osteoporosis and Osteoarthritis (ESCEO) and the IOF have developed recent guidelines in 2013 to stimulate a cohesive approach to the management of osteoporosis in Europe. In 2011, the IOF and ESCEO came together to review evidence for a casual association between subtrochanteric fractures and long-term treatment of bisphosphonates and identified an association with atypical subtrochanteric femoral fractures, but recognized RCTs were insufficiently powered to identify meaningful associations. The risk–benefit ratio still remains in favor of use of bisphosphonates to prevent fractures [57]. Therefore, it is recommended that physicians continue assessing patients being treated with bisphosphonates for 5 or more years [57].

Conclusion

Ultimately guidelines and recommendations are intended to inform clinicians and their patients in decision-making on the benefits and harms of therapy. Although there is concern that long-term bisphosphonate use is associated with serious, rare adverse events, the benefits of using osteoporosis medication to prevent fracture outweigh the risks identified. Major medical societies and international bodies agree that it is important for patients at high risk of fracture to continue ongoing drug therapy. The dose and duration of osteoporosis medication should be determined on an individual patient basis. The ultimate goal of clinical practice guidelines is to develop a more standardized approach and balance benefits, harms, and cost-effectiveness.

References[1]

1. MacLean C, Newberry S, Maglione M, McMahon M, Ranganath V, Suttorp M, et al. Systematic review: comparative effectiveness of treatments to prevent fractures in men and women with low bone density or osteoporosis. Ann Intern Med. 2008;148(3):197–213.
2. Ioannidis G, Papaioannou A, Hopman WM, Akhtar-Danesh N, Anastassiades T, Pickard L, et al. Relation between fractures and mortality: results from the Canadian multicentre osteoporosis study. CMAJ. 2009;181(5):256–71.
3. Black DM, Cummings SR, Karpf DB, Cauley JA, Thompson DE, Nevitt MC, et al. Randomised trial of effect of alendronate on risk of fracture in women with existing vertebral fractures. Lancet. 1996; 348(9041):1535–41.
4. Cummings SR, Black DM, Thompson DE, Applegate WB, Barrett-Connor E, Musliner TA, et al. Effect of alendronate on risk of fracture in women with low bone density but without vertebral fractures: results from the fracture intervention trial. JAMA. 1998;280(24):2077–82.
5. Harris ST, Watts NB, Genant HK, McKeever CD, Hangartner T, Keller M, et al. Effects of risedronate treatment on vertebral and nonvertebral fractures in women with postmenopausal osteoporosis: a randomized controlled trial. JAMA. 1999;282(14):1344–52.
6. Reginster JY, Minne H, Sorensen O, Hooper M, Roux C, Brandi M, et al. Randomized trial of the effects of risedronate on vertebral fractures in women with established postmenopausal osteoporosis. Osteoporos Int. 2000;11(1):83–91.
7. McClung MR, Geusens P, Miller PD, Zippel H, Bensen WG, Roux C, et al. Effect of risedronate on the risk of hip fracture in elderly women. N Engl J Med. 2001;344(5):333–40.
8. Black DM, Delmas PD, Eastell R, Reid IR, Boonen S, Cauley JA, et al. Once-yearly zoledronic acid for treatment of postmenopausal osteoporosis. N Engl J Med. 2007;356(18):1809–22.
9. Lyles KW, Colón-Emeric CS, Magaziner JS, Adachi JD, Pieper CF, Mautalen C, et al. Zoledronic acid and clinical fractures and mortality after hip fracture. N Engl J Med. 2007;357(18):1799–809.
10. Chesnut CH, Skag A, Christiansen C, Recker R, Stakkestad JA, Hoiseth A, et al. Effects of oral ibandronate administered daily or intermittently on fracture risk in postmenopausal osteoporosis. J Bone Miner Res. 2004;19(8):1241–9.
11. Orwoll E, Ettinger M, Weiss S, Miller P, Kendler D, Graham J, et al. Alendronate for the treatment of osteoporosis in men. N Engl J Med. 2000;343(9): 604–10.

---

[1] *Important References

12. Wallach S, Cohen S, Reid D, Hughes R, Hosking D, Laan R, et al. Effects of risedronate treatment on bone density and vertebral fracture in patients on corticosteroid therapy. Calcif Tissue Int. 2000;67(4):277–85.

13. Black DM, Bauer DC, Schwartz AV, Cummings SR, Rosen CJ. Continuing bisphosphonate treatment for osteoporosis—for whom and for how long? N Engl J Med. 2012;366(22):2051–3.

14. Whitaker M, Guo J, Kehoe T, Benson G. Bisphosphonates for osteoporosis—where do we go from here? N Engl J Med. 2012;366(22):2048–51.

15. *Khosla S, Burr D, Cauley J, Dempster DW, Ebeling PR, Felsenberg D, et al. Bisphosphonate-associated osteonecrosis of the jaw: report of a task force of the American society for bone and mineral research. J Bone Miner Res. 2007;22(10):1479–91. *The report of the ASBMR task force on ONJ outlining definition and epidemiology.

16. Khan AA, Morrison A, Hanley DA, Felsenberg D, McCauley LK, O'Ryan F, et al. Diagnosis and management of osteonecrosis of the jaw: a systematic review and international consensus. J Bone Miner Res. 2015;30(1):3–23.

17. *Shane E, Burr D, Ebeling PR, Abrahamsen B, Adler RA, Brown TD, et al. Atypical subtrochanteric and diaphyseal femoral fractures: report of a task force of the American society for bone and mineral research. J Bone Miner Res. 2010;25(11):2267–94. *First of two reports of the ASBMR task force on atypical fractures. This report included incidence and definition of atypical femoral fracture.

18. Shane E, Burr D, Abrahamsen B, Adler RA, Brown TD, Cheung AM, Cosman F, et al. Atypical subtrochanteric and diaphyseal femoral fractures: second report of a task force of the American society for bone and mineral research. J Bone Miner Res. 2014;29(1):1–23. *Second of two reports of the ASBMR task force which updated epidemiology and definition of atypical femoral fracture.

19. Sambrook PN, Olver IN, Goss AN. Bisphosphonates and the osteonecrosis of the jaw. Aust Fam Physician. 2006;35(10):801–3.

20. Felsenberg D, Hoffmeister B, Amling M. Bisphosphonattherapie assoziierte. Kiefernekrosen Deutsches Arzteblatt. 2006;46:A3078–80.

21. Wernecke G, Namduri S, Dicarlo EF, Schneider R, Lane J. Case report of spontaneous, nonspinal fractures in a multiple myeloma patient on long-term pamidronate and zoledronic acid. Muskoloskelet J Hosp Spec Surg. 2008;4:123–7.

22. Visekruna M, Wilson D, McKiernan FE. Severely suppressed bone turnover and atypical skeletal fragility. J Clin Endocrinol Metab. 2008;93:2948–52.

23. Watts NB, Diab DL. Long-term use of bisphosphonates in osteoporosis. J Clin Endocrinol Metab. 2010;95(4):1555–65.

24. Black DM, Reid IR, Boonen S, Bucci-Rechtweg C, Cauley JA, Cosman F, et al. The effect of 3 versus 6 years of zoledronic acid treatment of osteoporosis: a randomized extension to the HORIZON-pivotal fracture trial (PFT). J Bone Miner Res. 2012;27(2):243–54.

25. Grbic JT, Landesberg R, Lin SQ, Mesenbrink P, Reid IR, Leung PC, et al. Incidence of osteonecrosis of the jaw in women with postmenopausal osteoporosis in the health outcomes and reduced incidence with zoledronic acid once yearly pivotal fracture trial. J Am Dent Assoc. 2008;139(1):32–40.

26. Black D, Boonen S, Cauley J, Delmas P, Eastell R, Reid I, et al. Effect of once-yearly infusion of zoledronic acid 5 mg on spine and hip fracture reduction in postmenopausal women with osteoporosis: the HORIZON pivotal fracture trial. J Bone Miner Res. 2006;21 suppl 1:S16.

27. Bilezikian JP. Efficacy of bisphosphonates in reducing fracture risk in postmenopausal osteoporosis. Am J Med. 2009;122(2):S14–21.

28. Kanis J, Barton I, Johnell O. Risedronate decreases fracture risk in patients selected solely on the basis of prior vertebral fracture. Osteoporos Int. 2005;16(5):475–82.

29. Abrahamsen B, Eiken P, Eastell R. Subtrochanteric and diaphyseal femur fractures in patients treated with alendronate: a register-based national cohort study. J Bone Miner Res. 2009;24(6):1095–102.

30. United States Food and Drug Administration. FDA drug safety communication: safety update for osteoporosis drugs, bisphosphonates, and atypical fractures. United States Department of Health and Human Services; 2010. Available from: http://www.fda.gov/Drugs/DrugSafety/ucm229009.htm

31. *Effective Health Care Program. Treatment to prevent osteoporotic fractures: an update. agency for healthcare research and quality; 2013. Available from: http://www.effectivehealthcare.ahrq.gov/ehc/products/160/1048/lbd_clin_fin_to_post.pdf. *A clinical research summary by ARHQ which updates treatment and prevention recommendations and includes adverse events and the magnitude of the association.

32. Schwartz AV, Bauer DC, Cummings SR, Cauley JA, Ensrud KE, Palermo L, et al. Efficacy of continued alendronate for fractures in women with and without prevalent vertebral fracture: the FLEX trial. J Bone Miner Res. 2010;25(5):976–82.

33. Effective Health Care Program. Treatment to prevent osteoporotic fractures: an update. Agency for Healthcare Research and Quality; 2012. Available from: http://effectivehealthcare.ahrq.gov/index.cfm/search-for-guides-reviews-and-reports/?productid=1048&pageaction=displayproduct

34. Cosman F, de Beur SJ, LeBoff MS, Lewiecki EM, Tanner B, Randall S, et al. Clinician's guide to prevention and treatment of osteoporosis. Osteoporos Int. 2014;25(10):2359–81.

35. Saag KG, Emkey R, Schnitzer TJ, Brown JP, Hawkins F, Goemaere S, et al. Alendronate for the prevention and treatment of glucocorticoid-induced osteoporosis. N Engl J Med. 1998;339(5):292–9.

36. United States Food and Drug Administration. Medication guide: Boniva (bon-EE-va) (ibandronate). United States Department of Health and Human Services; 2015. Available from: http://www.fda.gov/downloads/Drugs/DrugSafety/UCM241518.pdf

37. Eastell R, Devogelaer JP, Peel N, Chines A, Bax D, Sacco-Gibson N, et al. Prevention of bone loss with risedronate in glucocorticoid-treated rheumatoid arthritis patients. Osteoporos Int. 2000;11(4):331–7.

38. U.S. Food and Drug Administration. Reclast (zoledronic acid): drug safety communication – new contra-indication and updated warning on kidney impairment. United States Department of Health and Human Services; 2011. Available from: http://www.fda.gov/Safety/MedWatch/SafetyInformation/SafetyAlerts forHumanMedicalProducts/ucm270464.htm

39. Rossouw JE, Anderson GL, Prentice RL, LaCroix AZ, Kooperberg C, Stefanick M, et al. Risks and benefits of estrogen plus progestin in healthy postmenopausal women: principal results from the women's health initiative randomized controlled trial. JAMA. 2002;288(3):321–33.

40. Cummings SR, Martin JS, McClung MR, Siris ES, Eastell R, Reid IR, et al. Denosumab for prevention of fractures in postmenopausal women with osteoporosis. N Engl J Med. 2009;361(8):756–65.

41. McClung MR, Lewiecki EM, Cohen SB, Bolognese MA, Woodson GC, Moffett AH, et al. Denosumab in postmenopausal women with low bone mineral density. N Engl J Med. 2006;354(8):821–31.

42. Saag KG, Shane E, Boonen S, Marín F, Donley DW, Taylor KA, et al. Teriparatide or alendronate in glucocorticoid-induced osteoporosis. N Engl J Med. 2007;357(20):2028–39.

43. Papaioannou A, Morin S, Cheung AM, Atkinson S, Brown JP, Feldman S, et al. 2010 clinical practice guidelines for the diagnosis and management of osteoporosis in Canada: summary. Can Med Assoc J. 2010;182(17):1864–73.

44. Brown JP, Morin S, Leslie W, Papaioannou A, Cheung AM, Davison KS, et al. Bisphosphonates for treatment of osteoporosis expected benefits, potential harms, and drug holidays. Can Fam Physician. 2014;60(4):324–33.

45. Mellström D, Sörensen O, Goemaere S, Roux C, Johnson T, Chines A. Seven years of treatment with risedronate in women with postmenopausal osteoporosis. Calcif Tissue Int. 2004;75(6):462–8.

46. Bone HG, Hosking D, Devogelaer JP, Tucci JR, Emkey RD, Tonino RP, et al. Ten years' experience with alendronate for osteoporosis in postmenopausal women. N Engl J Med. 2004;350(12):1189–99.

47. Black DM, Schwartz AV, Ensrud KE, Cauley JA, Levis S, Quandt SA, et al. Effects of continuing or stopping alendronate after 5 years of treatment: the fracture intervention trial long-term extension (FLEX): a randomized trial. JAMA. 2006;296(24):2927–38.

48. Lentle B, Cheung AM, Hanley DA, Leslie WD, Lyons D, Papaioannou A, et al. Osteoporosis Canada 2010 guidelines for the assessment of fracture risk. Can Assoc Radiol J. 2011;62(4):243–50.

49. European Medicines Agency. What we do. European Union; 2015. Available from: http://www.ema.europa.eu/ema/index.jsp?curl=pages/about_us/general/general_content_000091.jsp&mid=WC0b01ac0580028a42

50. European Medicines Agency. Bisphosphonates. European Union; 2015. Available from: http://www.ema.europa.eu/ema/index.jsp?curl=pages/medicines/human/referrals/Bisphosphonates/human_referral_000266.jsp&mid=WC0b01ac05805c516f

51. European Medicines Agency. European medicines agency concludes class review of bisphosphonates and atypical fractures. European Union; 2011. Available from: http://www.ema.europa.eu/ema/index.jsp?curl=pages/news_and_events/news/2011/04/news_detail_001245.jsp&mid=WC0b01ac058004d5c1

52. European Medicines Agency Committee for Medicinal Products for Human Use. Aclasta-H-C-595-A20-0026: EPAR – assessment report – Article 20. European Union; 2011. Available from: http://www.ema.europa.eu/docs/en_GB/document_library/EPAR_-_Assessment_Report_-_Variation/human/000595/WC500111869.pdf

53. Lambrinoudaki I, Vlachou S, Galapi F, Papadimitriou D, Papadias K. Once-yearly zoledronic acid in the prevention of osteoporotic bone fractures in postmenopausal women. Clin Interv Aging. 2008;3(3):445.

54. European Medicines Agency Committee for Medicinal Products for Human Use. Adrovance: EPAR – procedural steps taken and scientific information after authorisation. European Union; 2013. Available from: http://www.ema.europa.eu/docs/en_GB/document_library/EPAR_-_Procedural_steps_taken_and_scientific_information_after_authorisation/human/000759/WC500022043.pdf

55. European Medicines Agency Committee for Medicinal Products for Human Use. Prolia: EPAR – procedural steps taken and scientific information after authorisation. European Union; 2015. Available from: http://www.ema.europa.eu/docs/en_GB/document_library/EPAR_-_Procedural_steps_taken_and_scientific_information_after_authorisation/human/001120/WC500107471.pdf

56. European Medicines Agency Committee for Medicinal Products for Human Use. Forsteo: EPAR – procedural steps taken and scientific information after authorisation. European Union; 2014. Available from: http://www.ema.europa.eu/ema/index.jsp?curl=pages/medicines/human/medicines/000425/human_med_000798.jsp&mid=WC0b01ac058001d124#documentation

57. Rizzoli R, Åkesson K, Bouxsein M, Kanis J, Napoli N, Papapoulos S, et al. Subtrochanteric fractures after long-term treatment with bisphosphonates: a European society on clinical and economic aspects of osteoporosis and osteoarthritis, and international osteoporosis foundation working group report. Osteoporos Int. 2011;22(2):373–90.

Integrated Clinical View on Long-Term Management of Patients with Osteoporosis

22

E. Michael Lewiecki

Summary

- Initiation of pharmacological therapy to reduce fracture risk should be a collaborative with the physician and patient considering available clinical information.
- Factors for selection of a therapeutic agent include the balance of expected benefits and potential risks, the likelihood of achieving an acceptable level of fracture risk, acceptability to the patient, and cost.
- Fracture liaison services (FLSs) provide a systematic method of identifying patients with fractures in order to initiate and manage care to reduce the risk of future fractures (secondary fracture prevention).
- Patients who are treated for osteoporosis should be periodically reevaluated to determine whether treatment should be continued or changed.
- For patients who have received long-term bisphosphonate therapy and are no longer at high risk for fracture, temporary withholding of bisphosphonate therapy (a "drug holiday") can be considered.

Introduction

The quality of interactions between healthcare professionals and patients is important in determining the success or failure of osteoporosis treatment. Patients at high risk for fracture can be identified by means of a directed medical history, limited physical exam, and the use of easily available clinical tools, such as bone mineral density (BMD) testing and FRAX, provided these resources are applied. Lifestyle modifications and pharmacological therapy can reduce fracture risk when patients are well informed on what to do (e.g., exercise, fall prevention, calcium and vitamin D intake), prescribed an effective medication, and then take the medication correctly (compliance) and long enough (persistence) to benefit. Patients are sometimes exposed to frightening media reports of possible adverse effects of osteoporosis treatment, often without consideration of the balance of expected benefits and potential risks. It is the role of the healthcare practitioner to see that patients are appropriately evaluated, educated on the disease state of osteoporosis and the consequences of fractures, and provided with

E.M. Lewiecki, MD (✉)
New Mexico Clinical Research and Osteoporosis Center, 300 Oak St. NE, Albuquerque, NM 87106, USA

Department of Medicine, University of New Mexico School of Medicine, Albuquerque, NM, USA
e-mail: mlewiecki@gmail.com

© Springer International Publishing Switzerland 2016
S.L. Silverman, B. Abrahamsen (eds.), *The Duration and Safety of Osteoporosis Treatment*, DOI 10.1007/978-3-319-23639-1_22

enough helpful information on the balance of benefits and risks to be active participants in making healthcare decisions. This chapter addresses the challenges faced by healthcare practitioners in the long-term management of osteoporosis and suggests strategies to improve clinical outcomes.

Challenges in the Management of Osteoporosis

Despite advances in methods to identify patients at high risk for fracture [1] and the availability of many pharmacological agents proven to reduce fracture risk of osteoporosis [2], osteoporosis is a disease that is underdiagnosed [3, 4] and undertreated [5]. In the United States, the osteoporosis testing/treatment rate in 2013 for women age 65 years and older after a fracture was 19.1–25.0 %, depending on the type of Medicare insurance coverage [6]. The difference between patients who could benefit from osteoporosis treatment and those who actually receive it has been called the treatment gap [7, 8]. There is also a gap in the quality of osteoporosis care due to misuse, overuse, and underuse of testing and treatment modalities [9]. There are numerous barriers to closing the treatment gap, including physician and patient attitudes toward osteoporosis care, competing healthcare priorities, cultural factors, insurance coverage, and cost. Clinical practice guidelines (CPGs) for osteoporosis care are sometimes confusing, variable, and fail to address important clinical issues [10]. Guidelines typically focus on BMD testing, evaluating secondary causes of osteoporosis, and initiating treatment but provide little if any help on selecting a specific medication, changing therapy, or stopping therapy. Measures to close the treatment gap must consider all potential barriers, with individualization of treatment decisions according to the circumstances of each patient.

Limited Time for Physician–Patient Encounters

In the 1980s, a study showed that physicians typically spent less than 1 min of a 20 min office visit discussing treatment plans [11]. In recent years,

with efforts to contain costs, maximize "productivity," and gather data for electronic medical records, the time allocated for primary care office visits is even less [12]. The time devoted to patient encounters is an important element of high-quality clinical care and is necessary for the development of trust between the physician and patient [13]. When complex and multiple problems, especially those that are symptomatic, must be addressed within a limited amount of time, chronic asymptomatic disorders such as osteoporosis may be neglected.

In the setting of limited office visit time, management of osteoporosis may be enhanced by designating a member of the office staff to be a "bone health advocate." This individual could be charged with screening for risk factors for fracture, ordering or suggesting a BMD test, educating patients on lifestyle changes and good nutrition, and responding to questions about osteoporosis. Posters, brochures, and other handouts with osteoporosis educational material can reinforce what is said in the office. The physician should be alerted when there has been a previous fracture, especially one that is recent, and when there is loss of height that might be due to a vertebral fracture. In offices with electronic medical records, reminders to order a BMD test or refill an osteoporosis medication can be generated.

Prioritizing Health Concerns

Osteoporosis is sometimes delegated to a low priority position compared with other health issues. The reasons for this may vary depending on perspective. Since osteoporosis causes no symptoms unless a fracture occurs, patients are more likely to focus on symptomatic disorders. If a fracture does occur, many patients attribute this to a level of trauma that might have caused any bone to break, rather than recognizing that they may have a bone disease that increases the risk of future fractures. Physicians often spend the majority of time during a patient encounter addressing matters that are symptomatic and of greatest concern to the patient. Perhaps the best time to consider evaluation and treatment of osteoporosis is soon after a fracture has occurred, when the pain and disability due to the fracture is receiving attention, or at the time of annual wellness visit, when preventive healthcare is major part of the healthcare agenda.

Assessing Fracture Risk

The assessment of fracture risk is an important feature for determining when treatment is likely to be beneficial and when consideration should be given to stopping treatment, at least temporarily (drug "holiday"—see Chap. 16). The clinical tools that are commonly used to assess fracture risk include BMD testing with dual-energy X-ray absorptiometry (DXA) and clinical risk factors (CRFs) for fracture, especially advanced age and previous fracture as an adult. Fracture risk algorithms, such as FRAX, can combine BMD and CRFs to provide a more robust estimate of fracture probability than BMD or CRFs alone. FRAX and other algorithms are incorporated into CPGs to aid physicians in identifying patients for starting treatment. The ordering of a BMD test and assessment of fracture risk can be facilitated by office staff, if delegated the responsibility to do so.

The evaluation of fracture risk in a treated patient may be helpful in guiding decisions to continue or stop treatment. FDA officials have recommended that decisions to continue treatment with a bisphosphonate be based on the balance of benefits and risk, with care to consider other factors, such as patient preference [14]. This concept has been operationalized by others, recognizing that data to support such clinical decisions are very limited. FRAX does not appear to be a good clinical tool for measuring reduction in fracture risk in treated patients [15]. Black et al. suggested that patients most likely to benefit from bisphosphonate treatment longer than 3–5 years are those with femoral neck T-score remaining below −2.5 and those with a somewhat higher T-score (−2.5 to −2.0) when there is a prevalent vertebral fracture [16]. When the femoral neck T-score is greater than −2.0, they suggest that discontinuation of treatment may be appropriate. It is reasonable to restart treatment with a bisphosphonate or other agent when fracture risk is again high. The optimal length of time for treating with a bisphosphonate is not known.

Teamwork

There is no single medical specialty with exclusive responsibility for the care of osteoporosis; almost all specialties, some more than others, encounter patients with osteoporosis or fractures, at least some of the time. When a patient has a fracture, low BMD, or CRFs for fracture, a healthcare professional should initiate appropriate care, with the long-term goal of preventing fractures. Most acute fractures are managed by an orthopedist, and for those that involve hospitalization and surgery, consultation with a hospitalist or other medical specialists is common. Other healthcare professionals, such as nurses, nutritionists, physical therapists, and physical medicine and rehabilitation specialists, play important roles in postfracture care. Teamwork is essential. The development of systems-based approaches has enhanced cooperation of all stakeholders involved in the care of patients with osteoporosis.

Systems-Based Management

Adults with a previous fracture are at increased risk of subsequent fractures [17], with a recent fracture being a more robust predictor of subsequent fractures than a remote fracture [18]. Fracture risk increases with the number [19] and severity of prevalent vertebral fractures [20]. Despite the availability of effective and safe treatments to reduce fracture risk, most patients with fractures, even those who are hospitalized in integrated healthcare systems with hip fractures, are not currently being selected for osteoporosis evaluation and treatment [21]. Because of this very great unmet need in the care of osteoporosis, the concept of a FLS has emerged [22–24]. This is a strategy for secondary fracture prevention whereby patients with fractures are systematically identified so that care can be delivered. The objectives of FLS are to assure that fracture patients are assessed for the risk of future fractures, evaluated for factors contributing to skeletal fragility, educated on skeletal health, started on treatment to reduce fracture risk when appropriate, and followed to assure that treatment is continued long enough for anti-fracture benefit to be achieved [22].

The central person associated with successful outcomes of FLS is a dedicated coordinator who is often a hospital-based nurse educator or discharge planner. The coordinator acts as a link among the patient, the orthopedic team, the osteoporosis and falls prevention services, and the primary care physician to assure the recommendations for care are fulfilled. Fall risk assessment may lead to a focus on weight-bearing exercise, core strengthening, and balance training which can be helpful [23]. Activities such as yoga [25] and Tai Chi [26] may improve balance and potentially reduce the risk of fall-related fractures. An experienced fitness trainer may be able to design a safe regimen of weight-bearing and muscle-strengthening physical activities. A nutritionist or nurse educator can be helpful in discussing lifestyle modifications that include adequate intake of calcium, vitamin D, and other skeletal nutrients. The coordinator is needed because the interventions for fracture prevention are typically incomplete or nonexistent, often with the expectation that it will be someone else who manages the osteoporosis. The use of FLS has the potential of enhancing the long-term care of patients with osteoporosis by providing a systematic method for evaluating and treating high-risk patients, including follow-up to facilitate long-term adherence to therapy.

Quality Matters

Throughout the spectrum of providers and services involved in the management of osteoporosis, quality is important. There is no better example than with bone density measurements. BMD testing by DXA is used to diagnose osteoporosis, assess fracture risk, and monitor the skeletal effects of therapy. The quality of the test determines its clinical utility [27]. An incorrect report may be harmful to patients due to needed therapy not being started, treatment being prescribed when it is not necessary, or unnecessary tests being ordered to evaluate conditions that are not present. The DXA technologist, working closely with an experienced clinician, must adhere to established quality standards for instrument calibration, acquisition of bone image, and analysis of the data [28]. Assessment of serial changes in BMD requires knowledge of the least significant change (LSC), the smallest change in value that is statistically significant, allowing clinicians to distinguish biologically meaningful changes from apparent changes that are within the range of error for the measurement. The LSC must be calculated following precision assessment, a standardized method for determining the reproducibility of BMD measurements [28].

Risk Communication

Consideration of risk in the care of patients with osteoporosis includes the risk (probability) of fracture, with or without treatment, and the risk (probability) of an undesirable medical occurrence, commonly called a "side effect," occurring as a result of treatment. Decisions to treat patients with osteoporosis are made after an assessment of the balance of benefits and risks [29, 30]. The primary benefit of treatment is reduction in fracture risk, recognizing that no treatment can ever totally eliminate the possibility of having a fracture. When the expected benefits of treatment outweigh the risks of side effects, then treatment is usually recommended.

Risk communication has been defined as "the study and practice of collectively and effectively understanding risks" [31]. It is a science-based discipline that is used by industry, government, and scientists in managing the fear and consequences of crises of all types, including natural disasters, bioterrorism, nuclear threats, and epidemics. Successful risk communication is reassuring when a hazard is not serious, yet the public is in a state of near-panic; when the risk is serious but the public is apathetic, it can generate a sense of urgency to take action. To be effective, risk communication must address a fundamental dilemma that is very familiar to healthcare professionals, i.e., the lack of correlation between the ranking of hazards according to statistics (the typical physician's perspective) and the ranking of the same hazards by how upsetting they are to patients [32].

The risk of an event that may cause serious harm or death (e.g., hip fracture) and the risk of rare possible adverse effect of an intervention (e.g., osteonecrosis of the jaw with long-term bisphosphonate therapy) to prevent that event may be perceived quite differently by physicians and their patients. These differences in perspective can lead to physician–patient misunderstandings and conflicts, with the end result being poor clinical outcomes; in the example used above, this could be a hip fracture that might not have occurred if a high-risk patient had been treated with a bisphosphonate. It is therefore an imperative for physician–patient interactions to include discussion and understanding of risk.

Risk communication for healthcare providers is a "one-to-one communication in which the intervention includes a stimulus to patients to weigh the risks and benefits of a treatment choice or behavioral (risk reducing) change" [33]. There are many obstacles to effective risk communication, including statistical illiteracy for both physicians and patients, complexity and uncertainty of the medical evidence, distrust of pharmaceutical companies, imbalanced reporting by news media, inaccurate information online, and numerous psychological and social factors that influence how we process information about risk [25]. The management of these obstacles begins with physicians understanding risk so that they can explain it to patients. As an example, a relative risk of fracture that is "ten times" that of an average women of the same age sounds very high but may actually represent a low probability of fracture when the average women of that age has a very low risk. It is for this reason that expressing fracture risk as absolute risk (fracture probability) offers greater clinical utility [34] and is the form that is used in current fracture risk algorithms, such as FRAX [35]. Since statistics of any sort may be difficult to understand, another strategy for communicating the level of an unfamiliar risk is to compare it with something that is more familiar. As an example, it might be helpful to explain that traveling in a passenger car or light truck, a daily non-frightening occurrence for many of us, is associated with accidents resulting in death in about 11 per 100,000 person-years [36] and then compare that to osteoporosis therapy. There is accumulating evidence that treatment of osteoporosis reduces mortality [37] and the risk of osteoporosis of the jaw, a nonfatal event associated with long-term bisphosphonate therapy that frightens many patients, is estimated to be between <1 and 10 per 100,000 patient-treatment years [38].

Uncertainty is a common companion of physicians attempting to make clinical decisions. The applicability of data from prospective randomized placebo-controlled trials to the care of individual patients is often in doubt, as many patients in need of treatment for osteoporosis would not qualify for participation in the registration studies that led to drug approval [39]. Healthcare journalists provide a valuable service by educating us all on important new developments in medicine, including new treatments and adverse effects of some treatments. However, news reports of terrifying "side effects" of medications sometimes fall short of achieving proper balance by failing to describe the rarity of an event, the possibility that the event may be unrelated to therapy, or the benefits of therapy in proportion to the risks. Patients who look for medical information on the Internet may find very helpful reliable information at some websites but risk being overloaded by too much information from highly biased websites that are ultimately attempting to sell a product or promote a point of view. It is important for physicians to stay current with news reports seen by their patients so that they are prepared to respond when asked questions about them (Table 22.1).

Decision Aids

Educational information to enhance physician–patient communication can take the form of graphs, brochures, videos, models, and other types of handouts, collectively called "decision aids." These can reinforce and expand on what was said during an office or hospital visit, potentially facilitating clinical decisions. Decision aids can be helpful with "close call" decisions, where the balance of treatment benefits and risks is uncertain or the clinical circumstances are complex.

Table 22.1 Clinical issues of interest with pharmacological therapy of osteoporosis

Medication	Short-term issues	Long-term issues	Comments
Estrogen[a]	Decreased hot flashes; breast tenderness	Venous thromboembolism; stroke	Benefit/risk most favorable in younger postmenopausal women; different estrogen preparations may have different clinical profiles
Estrogen+progesterone[b]	Decreased hot flashes; breast tenderness	Venous thromboembolism; breast cancer; stroke; coronary heart disease	Benefit/risk most favorable in younger postmenopausal women; different estrogen preparations may have different clinical profiles
Raloxifene	Increased hot flashes; no breast tenderness	Venous thromboembolism, decreased breast cancer	Not proven to reduce nonvertebral fractures or hip fractures
Conjugated estrogen+bazedoxifene[a]	Decreased hot flashes; no breast tenderness	Venous thromboembolism; no increase in breast cancer	Each agent individually proven to reduce fracture risk; combination increases BMD but not proven to reduce fractures
Oral bisphosphonates[c] (alendronate, risedronate, ibandronate)	GI upset	Associated with ONJ and AFF; long skeletal half-life	Ibandronate not proven to reduce nonvertebral fractures or hip fractures; dosing intervals daily, weekly, or monthly
Intravenous bisphosphonates[c] (zoledronic acid, ibandronate)	Acute phase reaction	Associated with ONJ and AFF; long skeletal half-life	Ibandronate not proven to reduce nonvertebral fractures or hip fractures; dosing interval every 3 months to every 2 years
Denosumab	Few short-term adverse effects	ONJ and AFF have been reported	Injection every 6 months; no limitations by renal function
Nasal calcitonin	Nasal irritation	Report of slightly increased cancer risk (controversial)	Not proven to reduce nonvertebral fractures or hip fractures
Teriparatide	Muscle cramps, hypercalcemia	Osteosarcoma in rats; decreased back pain in some patients	Only approved osteoanabolic agent; daily injectable dosing; limited to 24 months lifetime treatment; not proven to reduce hip fracture risk

These are examples, not an all-inclusive list, of skeletal and nonskeletal issues associated with osteoporosis medications, focusing on possible adverse effects of treatment that might alter the balance of benefits and risks. All available clinical information must be considered in individualizing treatment decisions. Each of these therapeutic agents is approved for prevention and/or treatment of osteoporosis. Two of them (zoledronic acid, denosumab) are used in higher doses for the treatment of cancer-related conditions, which are not considered here. Teriparatide is the only treatment with regulatory limitations on the duration of treatment. Data extracted from randomized placebo-controlled trials and post-marketing reports

[a]In women without a uterus

[b]In women with a uterus

[c]Persistence of antiresorptive effect after discontinuation of long-term bisphosphonate therapy allows for the possibility of a bisphosphonate holiday, where anti-fracture benefit may continue while risks may be diminished

ONJ osteonecrosis of the jaw

AFF atypical femur fracture

The effectiveness of decision aids were evaluated in a meta-analysis of 55 randomized controlled clinical trials [40]. Decision aids performed better than usual care in providing patients with a greater understanding of the treatment options. There were fewer decisional conflicts due to feeling uninformed, with more patients taking an active role in decision-making and fewer patients remaining undecided about treatment. Decision aids using risk probabilities resulted in a greater proportion of patients having accurate risk perceptions. The use of decision aids did not alter patient satisfaction with decision-making, anxiety, or health outcomes. The authors of the meta-analysis concluded that decision aids increased patient involvement in decision-making, leading to informed values-based decisions. Decision aids seemed to be most useful when more than one reasonable treatment option was available, with no clear advantage of one over the other, and each having potential benefits and harms.

In order for decision aids to be effective, the information provided must be accurate and unbiased. The quality of patient education material can be variable and is sometimes incorrect or biased. The quality of 165 printed consumer brochures about osteoporosis was evaluated according to criteria addressing evidenced-based content, risk communication, transparency of the development process, layout, and design [41]. The authors concluded that quality was "utterly inadequate," with failure to provide evidence-based data on diagnosis and treatment, regardless of the source of the brochure. In another study evaluating osteoporosis websites, a wide range of quality was observed [42]. Overall quality scores were significantly lower for websites with a uniform resource locator (URL) suffix of ".com" compared to those with ".gov," ".edu," and ".org."

Many decision aids present complex numerical information in a graphic format. The design features of graphs and the data scale may influence their effectiveness. A systematic review assessed the findings in 24 studies of graphs depicting probabilities, frequencies, or chances of occurrence of health-related events [43]. The best design for a graph depended on the purpose of the risk communication (e.g., understanding risk vs.

changing behavior) and the demographics of the recipients (e.g., educational level, literacy). For expressing probability data, "part-to-whole icon array graphs" appeared to be more useful than providing percentages or proportions. This type of graph displays icons (symbols or figures) to illustrate the population at risk and highlighted icons showing those experiencing an event of some kind. Bar graphs are often perceived as analytical and difficult to understand [44]. Other ways of depicting risk include risk tables, ladders, scales, and survival and mortality curves. Each of these may be effective in portraying risk, depending on the type of risk and the target population.

A multicenter randomized controlled trial in primary care practices evaluated the effectiveness of a decision aid to improve osteoporosis treatment decisions [45]. The intervention in this study was an icon array graph displaying each patient's FRAX 10-year probability of major osteoporotic fracture with and without bisphosphonate treatment, as well as listing possible side effects of treatment and out-of-pocket costs. Patients randomized to the control group received usual care and received an osteoporosis patient education brochure produced by the US National Osteoporosis Foundation. Cognitive, behavioral, and affective endpoints were assessed, with compliance and persistence measured at 6 months. It was concluded that the decision aid improved the quality of clinical decisions about bisphosphonate therapy by improving knowledge transfer and patient involvement. The decision aid did not alter medication start rates but may have improved adherence to therapy.

Shared Treatment Decision-Making

Methods for making treatment decisions have been classified in three forms [46, 47]. The first is "paternalism," where the physician has all the relevant information and is the sole decision-maker. The second is "independent choice," where the physician provides the patient with relevant information and the patient makes all decisions. The third is "shared treatment decision-making," where the physician and patient share information, discuss treatment options, and reach a collaborative decision. With shared treatment decision-making, it is appropriate and usually expected that the physician offers a recommendation. The patient is encouraged to respond to the recommendation. The physician should be receptive to verbal and nonverbal responses. A patient who expresses disagreement or discomfort with the recommendation is unlikely to be adherent to therapy, even if it is not rejected outright. The physician must be willing to offer an alternative recommendation if the first one is not acceptable and should be willing, as well, to consider the patient's proposal for a treatment plan. Shared treatment decision-making is often a negotiation between the physician and the patient, with the goal of developing a plan of action that is medically reasonable for the physician and acceptable for the patient.

Shared treatment decision-making has been shown to improve outcomes with some medical conditions [48, 49] and may be helpful in the care of osteoporosis [50]. A Cochrane review evaluated 43 randomized studies involving "patient-centered care" [51], which includes studies using models of shared decision-making. It was found that healthcare providers could be successfully trained to improve their ability to share control with patients about topics and decisions addressed during a consultation. The results were mixed on whether patients were more satisfied when providers applied these skills. Beneficial effects on health behavior and health status were seen with interventions that combined provider training with decision aids, although the conclusions were tentative due to the heterogeneity of outcomes in the studies.

Clinical Practice Guidelines

CPGs can be defined as "systematically developed statements to assist practitioner and patient decisions about appropriate healthcare for specific clinical circumstances" [52]. The purpose of CPGs is "to make explicit recommendations with a definite intent to influence what clinicians do" [53]. CPGs are commonly developed by a group of experts after evaluation of the best available medical evidence, often with consideration of healthcare policy and costs [54] using systematic approaches to achieve consensus [55]. Many professional societies and organizations have released CPGs for the treatment of osteoporosis, with updates subsequently needed to include new data, advances in diagnostic tools, and newly available treatments. These CPGs may improve health outcomes (i.e., fewer fractures in patients with osteoporosis) by advising physicians on when to measure BMD, how to assess fracture risk, what tests to order in evaluating for secondary causes of osteoporosis, when to start pharmacological therapy to reduce fracture risk, and sometimes what drug or drug class to consider for initiating therapy.

Despite the obvious benefits of CPGs, especially for practitioners who are unfamiliar with management of osteoporosis, there are limitations as well [56]. CPGs and the evidence from which they are derived are helpful for never sufficient for making clinical decisions with individual patients [57]. Data on efficacy and safety of osteoporosis treatments, for example, are applicable to groups of patients with specific demographics and allowable comorbidities, given the limitations of the study design and duration. Every patient seen in clinical practice is unique, each having his or her own cultural beliefs, biases, experiences, confounding health issues, concomitant medications, and concerns that must be considered alongside the CPGs and medical evidence.

Monitoring Therapy

Despite abundant evidence in clinical trials for efficacy and safety of medications approved for the prevention and treatment of osteoporosis, it remains uncertain whether each individual patient treated with one of these drugs in the clinical practice setting will achieve that same level of benefit and whether the balance of benefit and risk with long-term therapy is the same as reported for the relatively short duration of registration trials. For these reasons, patients treated for osteoporosis are monitored to provide some evidence that the treatment is effective and that adverse effects of therapy have not developed. Monitoring therapy and regular contact with a healthcare professional provide opportunities to assess the balance of benefit and risk, reassure the patient that taking the medication is worth the bother and the cost, and may improve adherence to therapy [58].

The most common measurements used to monitor therapy are BMD testing by DXA and bone turnover markers (BTMs). Stability or an increase in BMD, a decrease in BTMs with antiresorptive therapy, or an increase in BTMs with osteoanabolic therapy is generally considered to represent a favorable response to the therapy [59], with the caveat that the tests are conducted at facilities that follow quality standards and that the LSC is known.

Adherence to Therapy

Pharmacological therapy for osteoporosis must be taken correctly and for a sufficient length of time for patients to achieve the expected reduction in fracture risk. There are many studies showing that adherence and persistence with osteoporosis is suboptimal, with many or most patients discontinuing treatment within 1 year after a prescription is written [60] and poor adherence being associated with poor clinical outcomes [61]. A recent systematic review evaluated 20 studies of interventions intended to improve adherence and persistence in adult users of osteoporosis medications [62]. It was concluded that simplification of dosing regimens, electronic prescriptions, decision aids, and patient education may improve adherence and persistence, noting many limitations of the studies. There was wide variation in the quality of the studies, with differences in study design, inconsistent definitions for measurement of adherence and persistence, limited reporting of relevant information reported, lack of data on clinical outcomes, and short duration of follow-up. More vigorous investigation of likely interventions in large randomized controlled trials was recommended.

Until more definitive data are available, it is prudent for healthcare practitioners to customize approaches to improving adherence and persistence with consideration and understanding of issues of greatest importance to each individual patient. Potentially useful clinical strategies include patient education, effective risk communication, shared decision-making, monitoring therapy, and periodic reevaluation of the balance of benefit and risk with treatment.

Treat-to-Target

A good response to therapy (stability or an increase in BMD or an appropriate change in BTMs) does not necessarily represent achievement of an acceptable level of fracture risk. For example, in a patient with a very high pretreatment fracture risk, the expected fracture risk reduction with the medication chosen for initial therapy may still leave the patient with a higher than desirable risk. Recognition of this concept has led to consideration of developing a treat-to-target strategy for osteoporosis [63, 64], as has been effectively used for other chronic asymptomatic disorders, such as hypertension and diabetes mellitus. An osteoporosis treatment target (e.g., a T-score or BTM value) might help physicians in the selection of an initial agent that is most likely to reach that target. If the treatment target is reached with bisphosphonate therapy, then a drug holiday may be considered. If there is a failure to reach the treatment target with initial therapy, a change in treatment might be indicated. At this time, treat-to-target for osteoporosis is being investigated, with no consensus and no guidelines on the use of treatment targets in clinical practice.

Duration of Osteoporosis Therapy

Few medical issues in the field of skeletal health have generated as much controversy, discussion, and confusion as the duration of treatment of osteoporosis. The question of "how long to treat?" is not often raised in association with other chronic asymptomatic disorders, such as hypertension and hypercholesterolemia. However, with osteoporosis, rare but disturbing bone-related occurrences (e.g., osteonecrosis of the jaw, atypical femur fractures) associated with long-term therapy have received a great deal of attention in scientific journals and news media, resulting in some patients stopping medication of their own accord and some being told to stop by their physicians. The concept of bisphosphonate holidays has emerged because this class of drugs has a long skeletal half-life, with discontinuation after years of therapy followed by persistence of antiresorptive effect for an undetermined period of time. The anti-fracture benefit may also persist, at least in low-risk patients, for a period of time, while the risk of some adverse events associated with long-term therapy, such as AFF, may rapidly diminish.

The management of drug holidays is addressed in detail in another chapter. It is important for clinicians to recognize that the levels of evidence for beginning and ending a bisphosphonate holiday are low. Decisions regarding drug holidays should be individualized according to the balance of expected benefits and potential risks of therapy (Table 22.1), with consideration of all available clinical information.

Conclusion

The long-term management of osteoporosis is most likely to be successful when a compassionate knowledgeable physician and a well-informed motivated patient collaborate to develop a treatment plan that is medically sound and acceptable to the patient. The evaluation of osteoporosis includes assessment of fracture risk and investigation for secondary causes of osteoporosis. Nonpharmacological management includes attention to maintaining a healthy lifestyle, good nutrition, preventing falls, and avoiding drugs that have harmful skeletal effects. Selection of the initial drug for osteoporosis therapy, the duration of therapy, and changes in therapy should be individualized with consideration of the balance of benefits and risks for the patient. A drug holiday should be considered for patients who have

received long-term bisphosphonate therapy and are no longer at high risk for fracture. Long-term adherence to therapy may be enhanced through regular contact with a healthcare professional.

References[1]

1. Lewiecki EM. Bone density measurement and assessment of fracture risk. Clin Obstet Gynecol. 2013; 56(4):667–76.
2. Warriner AH, Saag KG. Osteoporosis diagnosis and medical treatment. Orthop Clin North Am. 2013;44(2):125–35.
3. Delmas PD, van de Langerijt L, Watts NB, Eastell R, Genant H, Grauer A, et al. Under diagnosis of vertebral fractures is a worldwide problem: the IMPACT study. J Bone Miner Res. 2005;20(4):557–63.
4. Kamel HK, Hussain MS, Tariq S, Perry III HM, Morley JE. Failure to diagnose and treat osteoporosis in elderly patients hospitalized with hip fracture. Am J Med. 2000;109(4):326–8.
5. Curtis JR, McClure LA, Delzell E, Howard VJ, Orwoll E, Saag KG, et al. Population-based fracture risk assessment and osteoporosis treatment disparities by race and gender. J Gen Intern Med. 2009;24(8): 956–62.
6. National Committee for Quality Assurance. Improving quality and patient experience-the state of health care quality; 2013. http://www.ncqa.org/Portals/0/Newsroom/SOHC/2013/SOHC-web%20version%20report.pdf. Accessed 21 Dec 2013.
7. US Department of Health and Human Services. Bone health and osteoporosis: a report of the surgeon general. Rockville, MD: US Department of Health and Human Services, Office of the Surgeon General; 2004.
8. Strom O, Borgstrom F, Kanis JA, Compston J, Cooper C, McCloskey EV, et al. Osteoporosis: burden, health care provision and opportunities in the EU: a report prepared in collaboration with the international osteoporosis foundation (IOF) and the European federation of pharmaceutical industry associations (EFPIA). Arch Osteoporos. 2011;6(1–2):59–155.
9. Curtis JR, Adachi JD, Saag KG. Bridging the osteoporosis quality chasm. J Bone Miner Res. 2009; 24(1):3–7.
10. Lewiecki EM. Review of guidelines for bone mineral density testing and treatment of osteoporosis. Curr Osteoporos Rep. 2005;3(3):75–83.
11. Waitzkin H. Doctor-patient communication. Clinical implications of social scientific research. JAMA. 1984;252(17):2441–6.

---

[1] *Important References
**Very important References

12. Tai-Seale M, McGuire TG, Zhang W. Time allocation in primary care office visits. Health Serv Res. 2007;42(5):1871–94.

13. Braddock 3rd CH, Snyder L. The doctor will see you shortly. The ethical significance of time for the patient-physician relationship. J Gen Intern Med. 2005;20(11):1057–62.

14. Whitaker M, Guo J, Kehoe T, Benson G. Bisphosphonates for osteoporosis – where do we go from here? N Engl J Med. 2012;366(22):2048–51.

15. Leslie L, Lix L, Morin S, Majumdar S, Johansson H, McCloskey E, et al. Can changes in FRAX probability be used to "treat-to-target"? A clinical feasibility study. J Bone Miner Res. 2013;28 Suppl 1:S157.

16. Black DM, Bauer DC, Schwartz AV, Cummings SR, Rosen CJ. Continuing bisphosphonate treatment for osteoporosis – for whom and for how long? N Engl J Med. 2012;366(22):2051–3.

17. Gehlbach S, Saag KG, Adachi JD, Hooven FH, Flahive J, Boonen S, et al. Previous fractures at multiple sites increase the risk for subsequent fractures: the global longitudinal study of osteoporosis in women. J Bone Miner Res. 2012;27(3):645–53.

18. van Geel TA, Huntjens KM, van den Bergh JP, Dinant GJ, Geusens PP. Timing of subsequent fractures after an initial fracture. Curr Osteoporos Rep. 2010;8(3):118–22.

19. Gallagher JC, Genant HK, Crans GG, Vargas SJ, Krege JH. Teriparatide reduces the fracture risk associated with increasing number and severity of osteoporotic fractures. J Clin Endocrinol Metab. 2005;90(3):1583–7.

20. Black DM, Arden NK, Palermo L, Pearson J, Cummings SR. Prevalent vertebral deformities predict hip fractures and new vertebral fractures but not wrist fractures. J Bone Miner Res. 1999;14:821–8.

21. Shibli-Rahhal A, Vaughan-Sarrazin MS, Richardson K, Cram P. Testing and treatment for osteoporosis following hip fracture in an integrated U.S. healthcare delivery system. Osteoporos Int. 2011;22(12): 2973–80.

22. **Akesson K, Marsh D, Mitchell PJ, McLellan AR, Stenmark J, Pierroz DD, et al. Capture the fracture: a best practice framework and global campaign to break the fragility fracture cycle. Osteoporos Int. 2013;24(8):2135–52. **This is an excellent presentation of the concept of a fracture liaison service with advice on how to initiate and maintain it.

23. Lee DB, Lowden MR, Patmintra V, Stevenson K. National bone health alliance: an innovative public-private partnership improving America's bone health. Curr Osteoporos Rep. 2013;11(4):348–53.

24. Tosi LL, Gliklich R, Kannan K, Koval KJ. The American orthopaedic association's "own the bone" initiative to prevent secondary fractures. J Bone Joint Surg Am. 2008;90(1):163–73.

25. Galantino ML, Green L, Decesari JA, Mackain NA, Rinaldi SM, Stevens ME, et al. Safety and feasibility of modified chair-yoga on functional outcome among elderly at risk for falls. Int J Yoga. 2012;5(2):146–50.

26. Lee MS, Ernst E. Systematic reviews of t'ai chi: an overview. Br J Sports Med. 2012;46(10):713–8.

27. Lewiecki EM, Binkley N, Petak SM. DXA quality matters. J Clin Densitom. 2006;9(4):388–92.

28. **Schousboe JT, Shepherd JA, Bilezikian JP, Baim S. Executive summary of the 2013 international society for clinical densitometry position development conference on bone densitometry. J Clin Densitom. 2013;16(4):455–66. **The ISCD Official Positions provide standards for quality control, acquisition, analysis, and interpretation of bone density tests.

29. *Lewiecki EM, Miller PD, Harris ST, Bauer DC, Davison KS, Dian L, et al. Understanding and communicating the benefits and risks of denosumab, raloxifene, and teriparatide for the treatment of osteoporosis. J Clin Densitom. 2014;17(4):490–5. *This is a review of the balance of benefits and risks of non-bisphosphonate therapies for osteoporosis.

30. *McClung M, Harris ST, Miller PD, Bauer DC, Davison KS, Dian L, et al. Bisphosphonate therapy for osteoporosis: benefits, risks, and drug holiday. Am J Med. 2013;126(1):13–20. *This is a review of the balance of benefits and risks of bisphosphonate therapies for osteoporosis.

31. Radonich M. Communicating radiation risk to the public. In: Community environmental monitoring program 25th anniversary annual workshop (Internet); 2006. http://www.cemp.dri.edu/cemp/workshop2006/presentations/Radonich-Communicating_Radiation_Risk_to_the_Public-Part_1.pdf. Accessed 2 Jan 2014.

32. Covello VT, Sandman PM. Risk communication: evolution and revolution. The Peter Sandman Risk Communication Website (Internet); 2001. http://www.psandman.com/articles/covello.htm. Accessed 10 Jan 2014.

33. Edwards A, Elwyn G. How should effectiveness of risk communication to aid patients' decisions be judged? A review of the literature. Med Decis Making. 1999;19(4):428–34.

34. Kanis JA, Hans D, Cooper C, Baim S, Bilezikian JP, Binkley N, et al. Interpretation and use of FRAX in clinical practice. Osteoporos Int. 2011;22(9):2395–411.

35. World Health Organization. FRAX WHO fracture risk assessment tool. World Health Organization (Internet); 2012. http://www.shef.ac.uk/FRAX/. Accessed 17 Sept 2012.

36. Cohen JT, Neumann PJ. What's more dangerous, your aspirin or your car? Thinking rationally about drug risks (and benefits). Health Aff (Millwood). 2007; 26(3):636–46.

37. Grey A, Bolland MJ. The effect of treatments for osteoporosis on mortality. Osteoporos Int. 2013;24(1):1–6.

38. Khosla S, Burr D, Cauley J, Dempster DW, Ebeling PR, Felsenberg D, et al. Bisphosphonate-associated osteonecrosis of the jaw: report of a task force of the American society for bone and mineral research. J Bone Miner Res. 2007;22(10):1479–89.

39. Dowd R, Recker RR, Heaney RP. Study subjects and ordinary patients. Osteoporos Int. 2014;17(4):490–5.

40. O'Connor AM, Bennett CL, Stacey D, Barry M, Col NF, Eden KB, et al. Decision aids for people facing health treatment or screening decisions. Cochrane Database Syst Rev. 2009;3:CD001431.

41. Meyer G, Steckelberg A, Muhlhauser I. Analysis of consumer information brochures on osteoporosis prevention and treatment. Ger Med Sci. 2007;5:1–9.

42. Lewiecki EM, Rudolph LA, Kiebzak GM, Chavez JR, Thorpe BM. Assessment of osteoporosis-website quality. Osteoporos Int. 2006;17(5):741–52.

43. Ancker JS, Senathirajah Y, Kukafka R, Starren JB. Design features of graphs in health risk communication: a systematic review. J Am Med Inform Assoc. 2006;13(6):608–18.

44. Schapira MM, Nattinger AB, McHorney CA. Frequency or probability? A qualitative study of risk communication formats used in health care. Med Decis Making. 2001;21(6):459–67.

45. Montori VM, Shah ND, Pencille LJ, Branda ME, Van Houten HK, Swiglo BA, et al. Use of a decision aid to improve treatment decisions in osteoporosis: the osteoporosis choice randomized trial. Am J Med. 2011;124(6):549–56.

46. Charles C, Gafni A, Whelan T. Decision-making in the physician-patient encounter: revisiting the shared treatment decision-making model. Soc Sci Med. 1999;49(5):651–61.

47. Charles C, Gafni A, Whelan T. Shared decision-making in the medical encounter: what does it mean? (or it takes at least two to tango). Soc Sci Med. 1997;44(5):681–92.

48. Wilson SR, Strub P, Buist AS, Knowles SB, Lavori PW, Lapidus J, et al. Shared treatment decision making improves adherence and outcomes in poorly controlled asthma. Am J Respir Crit Care Med. 2010;181(6):566–77.

49. Loh A, Leonhart R, Wills CE, Simon D, Harter M. The impact of patient participation on adherence and clinical outcome in primary care of depression. Patient Educ Couns. 2007;65(1):69–78.

50. *Lewiecki EM. Risk communication and shared decision making in the care of patients with osteoporosis. J Clin Densitom. 2010;13(4):335–45. *Strategies for applying effective risk communication and shared decision making in the care of osteoporosis are reviewed here.

51. Dwamena F, Holmes-Rovner M, Gaulden CM, Jorgenson S, Sadigh G, Sikorskii A, et al. Interventions for providers to promote a patient-centred approach in clinical consultations. Cochrane Database Syst Rev. 2012;12:CD003267.

52. National Research Council. Clinical practice guidelines: directions for a new program. In: Field J, Lohr K, editors. Committee to advise the public health service on clinical practice. Washington, DC: The National Academies Press; 1990.

53. Hayward RS, Wilson MC, Tunis SR, Bass EB, Guyatt G. Users' guides to the medical literature. VIII. How to use clinical practice guidelines. A. Are the recommendations valid? The evidence-based medicine working group. JAMA. 1995;274(7):570–4.

54. O'Brien Jr JA, Jacobs LM, Pierce D. Clinical practice guidelines and the cost of care. A growing alliance. Int J Technol Assess Health Care. 2000;16(4):1077–91.

55. Nair R, Aggarwal R, Khanna D. Methods of formal consensus in classification/diagnostic criteria and guideline development. Semin Arthritis Rheum. 2011;41(2):95–105.

56. *Lewiecki EM, Binkley N. Evidence-based medicine, clinical practice guidelines, and common sense in the management of osteoporosis. Endocr Pract. 2009;24(10):1643–6. *This describes the benefits and limitations of evidence-based medicine and clinical practice guidelines in the care of individual patients with osteoporosis.

57. Swiglo BA, Murad MH, Schunemann HJ, Kunz R, Vigersky RA, Guyatt GH, et al. A case for clarity, consistency, and helpfulness: state-of-the-art clinical practice guidelines in endocrinology using the grading of recommendations, assessment, development, and evaluation system. J Clin Endocrinol Metab. 2008;93(3):666–73.

58. Clowes JA, Peel NF, Eastell R. The impact of monitoring on adherence and persistence with antiresorptive treatment for postmenopausal osteoporosis: a randomized controlled trial. J Clin Endocrinol Metab. 2004;89(3):1117–23.

59. Lewiecki EM, Watts NB. Assessing response to osteoporosis therapy. Osteoporos Int. 2008;19(10):1363–8.

60. Imaz I, Zegarra P, Gonzalez-Enriquez J, Rubio B, Alcazar R, Amate JM. Poor bisphosphonate adherence for treatment of osteoporosis increases fracture risk: systematic review and meta-analysis. Osteoporos Int. 2010;21(11):1943–51.

61. Siris ES, Selby PL, Saag KG, Borgstrom F, Herings RM, Silverman SL. Impact of osteoporosis treatment adherence on fracture rates in North America and Europe. Am J Med. 2009;122 Suppl 2:S3–13.

62. Hiligsmann M, Salas M, Hughes DA, Manias E, Gwadry-Sridhar FH, Linck P, et al. Interventions to improve osteoporosis medication adherence and persistence: a systematic review and literature appraisal by the ISPOR medication adherence & persistence special interest group. Osteoporos Int. 2013;24(12):2907–18.

63. Lewiecki EM, Cummings SR, Cosman F. Treat-to-target for osteoporosis: is now the time? J Clin Endocrinol Metab. 2013;98(3):946–53.

64. Cummings SR, Cosman F, Eastell R, Reid IR, Mehta M, Lewiecki EM. Goal-directed treatment of osteoporosis. J Bone Miner Res. 2013;28(3):433–8.

Conclusions

Stuart L. Silverman and Bo Abrahamsen

This is an exciting time in the world of osteoporosis treatment with an increasing opportunity to individualize osteoporosis therapies for our patients based on efficacy, safety, and convenience and potential for adherence. However, there are also new challenges within long-term efficacy and safety as we are moving toward the possibility of "treat-to-target" algorithms. Firstly, the algorithms are not yet agreed upon [1, 2]. Can the task be simplified so that clinicians can simply look for certain target BMD? This could perhaps be a BMD threshold where patients would have been too healthy to be candidates for the clinical trials that were proof of efficacy or one that was shown in trials to separate at least partly between those who would benefit from an extension of the treatment period and those who likely would not as in the alendronate FLEX study [3] or zoledronic acid HORIZON extension [4]. This could also be a ten-year fracture risk threshold such as FRAX [5] with the fracture risk threshold being derived from a given health care system's willingness to treat.

Our first step is to "target-to-treat" patients. Our first target is patients with fragility fracture who are at high risk for further fracture of which only a minority are being treated [6–8]. The development of system-wide interventions such as fracture liaison services is slowly helping us to better identify patients at need of intervention due to increased fracture risk.

A patient with a fragility fracture has had a sentinel event which tells us that patient is at increased risk. But we also identify patients based on BMD and other clinical risk factors such as falls, medications, or conditions associated with osteoporosis.

We now recognize that bone strength is related to both bone quantity and bone quality. Newer measurement techniques such as trabecular bone score [9] or microindentation [10] as well as bone turnover markers may provide some insight into bone quality. Bone turnover markers may also provide insight into rate of predicted BMD loss and do in themselves add to BMD and clinical risk factors in predicting the risk of fractures [11].

There is increased recognition that osteoporosis is not perhaps best defined by DXA T score alone. We now recognize that osteoporosis is not only characterized by low bone density but also by microarchitectural deterioration of bone leading to decreased bone strength (NIH consensus conference [12]). Unfortunately payors

S.L. Silverman, MD, FACP, FACR (✉)
Division of Rheumatology, Cedars-Sinai Medical Center, UCLA School of Medicine and the OMC Clinical Research Center, 8641 Wilshire Blvd, suite 301, Beverly Hills, CA 90211, USA
e-mail: stuarts@bhillsra.com

B. Abrahamsen, MD, PhD (✉)
Institute of Clinical Research, OPEN, University of Southern Denmark,
JB Winslowsvej 9,3, Odense DK-5000, Denmark
e-mail: b.abrahamsen@physician.dk

© Springer International Publishing Switzerland 2016
S.L. Silverman, B. Abrahamsen (eds.), *The Duration and Safety of Osteoporosis Treatment*, DOI 10.1007/978-3-319-23639-1_23

sometimes determine eligibility for an osteoporosis medication based only on decreased BMD. A recent US working group paper by Siris has redefined osteoporosis not only based on BMD but on FRAX and/or prevalent fragility fracture [12].

We want to prevent further fracture in our patients, recognizing the costs and loss of quality of life. However, fracture prevention is not simply choosing the right medication. Some aspects of fracture prevention are not related to the skeleton at all, but focus on maintaining muscle strength and body balance, hence reducing the risk of fall-related fractures. Thus despite populations' aging, the age-adjusted risk of hip fracture—the archetypal fall-related fracture—is decreasing in large parts of the world, probably less due to pharmaceutical intervention than to improvement in functional status, nutrition, and general health [13–15].

The recent few years have brought about new anabolic and antiresorptive drugs (see Chaps. 3 and 4), some of which are in widespread clinical use at the time of writing while others are in phase II and phase II trials. In Chap. 10, Bouxsein discusses how antiresorptive therapies work by reducing bone turnover and by mineralizing old bone. In contrast, in the simplest terms, anabolics (please see Chap. 3) work by a different mechanism by stimulating the formation of new, young bone, while antiresorptive agents (Chap. 2) improve the strength of bone by keeping older bone tissue in service for longer, hence increasing the mean age of bone [16] where anabolics do the opposite. This has practical implications in terms of concern over the ultimate toughness of older bone tissue and monitoring issues because older bone is more highly mineralized than young bone, producing a slight negative bias against anabolics when monitoring by methods where mineral alone is the unit of currency, such as DXA. Antiresorptive agents differ in their residence time in bone and reversibility (see Russell Chap. 2).

Osteoporosis medications have both short- and long-term adverse events (AEs) [17]. Long-term adverse events usually have a low incidence and increase with duration of use of therapy. There may be an inflection point for rare long-term AEs such as atypical femoral fracture (AFF) and osteonecrosis of the jaw (ONJ). Also, ONJ may be preventable in some cases with use of antibiotics and primary closure (see Sedghizadeh Chap. 12).

In patients at high risk of fractures due to osteoporosis, intervention with osteoporosis medications generally produces benefits that far outweigh what can be achieved by non-pharmaceutical means. On a group basis, these benefits strongly offset any known risks of side effects, though they can be devastating in the rare instances that they occur and it is hard for the patient and health provider to compare a real occurrence of ONJ or AFF with the less tangible benefit of having avoided major osteoporotic fractures. This is particularly challenging as all patients will not be at equal risk of these events, with the risk of ONJ, for example, far larger in patients with poor dental status or ill-fitting dentures who have an invasive dental procedure such as dental extraction and the risk of AFF being influenced by baseline characteristics such as race and femur geometry.

Although side effects such as ONJ and AFF are rare, they are of great concern to our patients based on the bias of media coverage to publicize new findings about risk more than established benefit. Our patients do a risk benefit analysis where they may often weigh risks higher than benefits, making it harder to convince patients to start osteoporosis therapies and to continue them. Concerns over certain salient side effects such as ONJ and AFF have led some patients to believe that all osteoporosis medications are unsafe and should be avoided, resulting in both primary and secondary nonadherence (see Chap. 17), an example of categorical bias.

Clearly the best we can strive for is for drugs to provide high efficacy and a solid margin of safety. Hence, properties of the ideal osteoporosis drug would include not only efficacy but understanding of mode of action, excellent short- and long-term safety, simple monitoring, excellent tolerance, low cost, and small environmental footprint.

The major thrust of this book has been to help clinicians understand the safety and duration of use of osteoporosis therapies. We tried to provide in-depth current understanding of both general safety concerns (see McClung Chap. 20) as well as medication and disease-specific adverse events seen with antiresorptives such as ONJ (see Chaps. 12–14) and AFFs (see Chaps. 6–11) by discussing epidemiology, pathophysiology, and treatment. Although, newer anabolic agents may avoid some of the long-term AEs such as AFF and ONJ, they may present with newer AE concerns such as osteosarcoma. But there are also clear concerns with long-term use of anabolics that follow directly from their mechanism of effect. Will patients be at risk of excessive bone growth, expanding bone size, foraminal closing, nerve entrapment, and even neoplasms, skeletal or nonskeletal? These issues also need to be resolved before we can arrive at a strong, coherent long-term management strategy for osteoporosis treatment.

We hope that this book will become a step toward better understanding of safety issues allowing patients to make better informed decisions about osteoporosis therapies with their health-care providers. This book was written to give the perspective not only of the clinician but that of regulatory agencies who oversee safety (see Papaioannou Chap. 21). There is no suggestion of increased mortality with osteoporosis medications (see Chap. 19)—indeed observational studies and one intervention study have found a reduction in mortality in patients who are treated with bisphosphonates.

Osteoporosis treatment is different than many medical conditions because everyone can be treated using the same dose despite the differences in the size of the skeleton and the body between individuals. In other therapeutic fields, doses of medications are often reduced for Asian populations. Have we been oversimplifying dosage requirements because we learned from bisphosphonates that the main concern is making sure the dose is large enough for a large person, as the skeleton is capable then of auto-dosing with the kidneys quickly clearing any bisphosphonate that is in excess of what can be stored in the skeleton?

Some medications such as denosumab or estrogen are reversible, so we need to continue them indefinitely until we begin a maintenance therapy. Bisphosphonates are associated with certain AES such as AFFs which although rare may have an inflection point in their incidence after 5 years [18]. This combined with known long-term residence in bone has led us to the concept of a bisphosphonate holiday (see Chap. 16) with alendronate and risedronate after 5 years. However, though based on relatively short-term data, the risk of rare events such as AFF has been reported to disappear within three years of cessation, suggesting that we could then perhaps consider restarting bisphosphonate therapy. However, in some individuals at high risk such as low BMD or fracture while on therapy, a holiday may not be the best choice (see Chap. 16).

We do not know as yet how best to monitor a holiday. There is a lack of clinical evidence, but from the point of the clinician, however, bone loss and incident fracture should be reasons to at least reevaluate the holiday and do a reappraisal of the likelihood that restarting osteoporosis treatment would confer an overall benefit to the patient.

How do we judge the response to therapy? A change in BMD is an imperfect measure of the reduction in risk, and the BMD attained after treatment may translate to a different (probably lower) risk than estimated with FRAX and other tools, especially for drugs that have a long transit time in bone and have residual effect after pausing. As discussed in Chap. 4, while FRAX can be useful even when used in patients on some forms of osteoporosis treatment, a reduction in FRAX score itself is generally not an appropriate target for goal-directed therapy. Hence, we need tools that can extrapolate from change in readily available clinical parameters such as BMD or bone turnover on a given drug to the reduction in the risk of fractures before goal-directed treatments would be realistically available to patients. A target algorithm has challenges as antiresorptive drugs are not simply BMD modifiers but drugs that act by reducing bone remodeling. The filling of the remodeling space results in a BMD change that can be measured, but which varies between anatomic sites, and a reduction in the number of stress risers on the bone surfaces, which is difficult to measure in vivo even with advanced radiology techniques and which we may have to approximate using (global) biochemical markers. There is a need for better communication to patients (and better tools for doctors) about risks with medication as we move toward shared decision-making and as our patients rely more heavily on the Internet for information.

It is beyond dispute that some patients fail to respond adequately [19–21] to an osteoporosis drug even if they adhere fully to treatment or more appropriately that some drugs fail to achieve the level of protection against fracture that could reasonably be expected based on clinical experience and clinical trials. Diez Perez, in Chap. 5, discusses proposed IOF nonresponder criteria. Treatment failure criteria need to be refined further and be based on evidence rather than expert opinion and clinical experience alone. After all, patients who sustain many fractures despite being treated with what is generally a good and effective osteoporosis drug may have been at an exceptionally high base risk of fracture due to comorbid conditions, perhaps recurrent falls, and have responded with a large risk reduction, yet still remain at high immediate fracture risk compared with most other patients. But it is difficult for clinicians to determine if the patient simply failed to respond—so maintained their base risk—or if they reduced a base risk that was simply very high indeed. Goal-directed therapy encompasses this issue and also recognizes that severe disease may need therapies that are more potent than milder cases.

Does the use of osteoporosis medications affect fracture healing? When should we start osteoporosis medication in a patient with fragility fracture? Bukata and colleague discuss the impact of osteoporosis medication on fracture healing in Chap. 18. In general, the use of osteoporosis medications does not delay fracture healing; although there is some concern that when we give an antiresorptive therapy within the first 2 weeks after fracture, particularly an IV therapy such as zoledronic acid which is only given yearly, all the medication goes to the fracture site, and little goes to other skeletal sites. There is the potential that our anabolic medications may be helpful in patients with delayed fracture healing.

We conclude that the first 25 years of widespread clinical use of specific osteoporosis drugs have left us with the challenge to develop a coherent evidence-based strategy not for deciding whether to treat or not but for deciding when to stop, change, or reinitiate osteoporosis treatment and how to monitor the response to such changes in the individual patient. The area is challenging. There is a lack of strong clinical evidence supporting drug holidays, but there is almost as little evidence supporting long-term treatment, hence such decisions are currently based more on personal experiences, preferences, hope, and fears than on rigorous science. With the coming of new potent anabolic and antiresorptive drugs, we are of course facing additional possibilities but also additional challenges in knowing when to change treatment to the new drugs and how they will perform in a long-term scenario.

References

1. Boonen S, Ferrari S, Miller PD, Eriksen EF, Sambrook PN, Compston J, et al. Postmenopausal osteoporosis treatment with antiresorptives: effects of discontinuation or long-term continuation on bone turnover and fracture risk-a perspective. J Bone Miner Res. 2012;27(5):963–74.
2. Cummings SR, Cosman F, Eastell R, Reid IR, Mehta M, Lewiecki EM. Goal-directed treatment of osteoporosis. J Bone Miner Res. 2013;28(3):433–8.
3. Black DM, Schwartz AV, Ensrud KE, Cauley JA, Levis S, Quandt SA, et al. Effects of continuing or stopping alendronate after 5 years of treatment: the fracture intervention trial long-term extension (FLEX): a randomized trial. JAMA. 2006;296:2927–38.
4. Cosman F, Cauley JA, Eastell R, Boonen S, Palermo L, Reid IR, et al. Reassessment of fracture risk in women after 3 years of treatment with zoledronic acid: when is it reasonable to discontinue treatment? J Clin Endocrinol Metab. 2014;99(12):4546–54. doi:10.1210/jc.2014-1971.
5. Lewiecki EM, Compston JE, Miller PD, Adachi JD, Adams JE, Leslie WD, et al. Official positions for FRAX® bone mineral density and FRAX® simplification from joint official positions development conference of the international society for clinical den-

sitometry and international osteoporosis foundation on FRAX®. J Clin Densitom. 2011;14(3):226–36.

6. Roerholt C, Eiken P, Abrahamsen B. Initiation of anti-osteoporotic therapy in patients with recent fractures: a nationwide analysis of prescription rates and persistence. Osteoporos Int. 2009;20:299–307.

7. Wilk A, Sajjan S, Modi A, Fan C-PS, Mavros P. Post-fracture pharmacotherapy for women with osteoporotic fracture: analysis of a managed care population in the USA. Osteoporos Int. 2014;25(12):2777–86.

8. Akesson K, Marsh D, Mitchell PJ, McLellan AR, Stenmark J, Pierroz DD, et al. Capture the fracture: a best practice framework and global campaign to break the fragility fracture cycle. Osteoporos Int. 2013;24(8):2135–52.

9. Silva BC, Leslie WD, Resch H, Lamy O, Lesnyak O, Binkley N, et al. Trabecular bone score: a noninvasive analytical method based upon the DXA image. J Bone Miner Res. 2014;29(3):518–30.

10. Güerri-Fernández RC, Nogués X, Quesada Gómez JM, Torres Del Pliego E, Puig L, García-Giralt N, et al. Microindentation for in vivo measurement of bone tissue material properties in atypical femoral fracture patients and controls. J Bone Miner Res. 2013;28(1):162–8.

11. Naylor K, Eastell R. Bone turnover markers: use in osteoporosis. Nat Rev Rheumatol. 2012;8(7):379–89.

12. Siris ES, Adler R, Bilezikian J, Bolognese M, Dawson-Hughes B, Favus MJ, et al. The clinical diagnosis of osteoporosis: a position statement from the national bone health alliance working group. Osteoporos Int. 2014;25(5):1439–43.

13. Cooper C, Cole ZA, Holroyd CR, Earl SC, Harvey NC, Dennison EM, et al. Secular trends in the incidence of hip and other osteoporotic fractures. Osteoporos Int. 2011;22(5):1277–88.

14. Abrahamsen B, Vestergaard P. Declining incidence of hip fractures and the extent of use of anti-osteoporotic therapy in Denmark 1997–2006. Osteoporos Int. 2009;21:373–80.

15. Rosengren BE, Ahlborg HG, Mellström D, Nilsson J-Å, Björk J, Karlsson MK. Secular trends in Swedish hip fractures 1987–2002. Epidemiology. 2012;23(4):1.

16. Boskey AL, Spevak L, Weinstein RS. Spectroscopic markers of bone quality in alendronate-treated postmenopausal women. Osteoporos Int. 2009;20(5):793–800.

17. Hermann AP, Abrahamsen B. The bisphosphonates: risks and benefits of long term use. Curr Opin Pharmacol. 2013;21.

18. Shane E, Ebeling PR, Abrahamsen B, Adler RA, Brown TD, Cheung AM, et al. Atypical subtrochanteric and diaphyseal femoral fractures: second report of a task force of the American society for bone and mineral research. Osteoporos Intl 2012;23:2709–14.

19. Diez-Perez A, Adachi JD, Agnusdei D, Bilezikian JP, Compston JE, Cummings SR, et al. Treatment failure in osteoporosis. JBMR 2014;29:1–23.

20. Díez-Pérez A, Adachi JD, Adami S, Anderson FA, Boonen S, Chapurlat R, et al. Risk factors for treatment failure with antiosteoporosis medication: the global longitudinal study of osteoporosis in women (GLOW). J Bone Miner Res. 2014;29(1):260–7.

21. Abrahamsen B, Rubin KH, Eiken PA, Eastell R. Characteristics of patients who suffer major osteoporotic fractures despite adhering to alendronate treatment: a national prescription registry study. Osteoporos Int. 2013;24(1):321–8.

Index

© Springer International Publishing Switzerland 2016

S.L. Silverman, B. Abrahamsen (eds.), *The Duration and Safety
of Osteoporosis Treatment*, DOI 10.1007/978-3-319-23639-1